S0-ARM-499

SECOND EDITION

Rehabilitative Audiology: Children and Adults

SECOND EDITION

Rehabilitative Audiology: Children and Adults

....

EDITORS

JEROME G. ALPINER, Ph.D.

Coordinator of Audiology
Veterans Administration Medical Center
Denver, Colorado

PATRICIA A. McCARTHY, Ph.D.

Associate Professor
Department of Communication Disorders and Sciences
College of Health Sciences
Rush-Presbyterian-St. Luke's Medical Center
Rush University
Chicago, Illinois

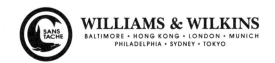

WILLIAMS & WILKINS
BALTIMORE · HONG KONG · LONDON · MUNICH
PHILADELPHIA · SYDNEY · TOKYO

Editor: John P. Butler
Managing Editor: Linda S. Napora
Copy Editor: Melissa Andrews
Designer: Norman W. Och
Illustration Planner: Wayne Hubbel
Production Coordinator: Anne Stewart Seitz
Cover Designer: Norman W. Och

Copyright (c) 1993
Williams & Wilkins
428 East Preston Street
Baltimore, Maryland 21202, USA

All rights reserved. This book is protected by copyright. No part of this book may
be reproduced in any form or by any means, including photocopying, or utilized
by any information storage and retrieval system without written permission from
the copyright owner.

Accurate indications, adverse reactions, and dosage schedules for drugs are
provided in this book, but it is possible that they may change. The reader is urged
to review the package information data of the manufacturers of the medications
mentioned.

Printed in the United States of America

First Edition 1987

Library of Congress Cataloging in Publication Data

Rehabilitative audiology : children and adults / editors, Jerome G. Alpiner,
Patricia A. McCarthy. — 2nd ed.
p. cm.
Includes index
ISBN 0–683–00078–0
1. Hearing impaired—Rehabilitation. 2. Deaf—Rehabilitation. 3. Audiology.
I. Alpiner, Jerome G., 1932–   . II. McCarthy, Patricia A.
[DNLM: 1. Hearing Disorders—rehabilitation. WV 270 R3452]
RF297.R44   1993
617.8′9—dc20
DNLM/DLC   92–49408
                                                           CIP

97 96 95 94
2 3 4 5 6 7 8 9 10

To my wife, Victoria, and our family: David, Sharon, Susan, Steven, Carol, Dan, Bill, and Boomer who have supported me with their love. Victoria has shared the moments that mean so much for all of our family. This book is also dedicated to my students, colleagues, and other family members who have meant much to me and have provided continuing inspiration for the things I do from day to day.

J. G. A.

To my husband and son, Richard and Kevin Peach, and my parents, Joanne and Daniel McCarthy, who provide unconditional support and love.

P. A. M.

Preface

In the six years that have elapsed since the first edition of *Rehabilitative Audiology,* there have been numerous changes in the field of audiology. Emphasis has shifted even further from the early traditional aspects of speechreading and auditory training. Indeed, one of our authors points out that this second edition has no dedicated chapters about these two topics.

Rehabilitative audiology has seen expanded and sophisticated advances for both children and adults. A review of early texts on this subject could be perused quickly and without intensive concentration. Today, a greater number of professional audiologists have become involved in rehabilitation. Some new topic areas have emerged; there are more options for clients in need of professional help. Chapter 19 on research needs makes us aware of our progress as well as clarifying the need to study new areas as we approach a new century. Students of past generations would be amazed at the "content" which has become part of an "aural rehab" course. Rehabilitative audiology has come of age in our profession.

This book is organized in five sections: Philosophy and Service Provision; Rehabilitative Audiology: Children; Rehabilitative Audiology: Adults; Technology in Rehabilitative Audiology; and Future Directions. Chapter 5 on amplification for children makes its debut. Chapter 9 on the counseling process for children and parents is also new to this edition. Current information covers rehabilitative audiology in private practice, cochlear implants, assistive technology, computers in hearing rehabilitation, needs of the geriatric population, and research needs in rehabilitative audiology.

The contributors to this edition represent a variety of audiology work environments: universities, hospitals (public, private, and government), schools, hearing aid dispensing practices, private practice, and industry. These authors bring many years of experience and hands-on treatment with clients and provide a comprehensive view of rehabilitative audiology in the United States. We are fortunate to have so many authorities represented as well as comprehensive references to other experts in the profession.

For our readers, we hope that rehabilitative audiology becomes a typical part of day-to-day work life. Come and experience *Rehabilitative Audiology* with us. The real benefactors of our efforts will be those children and adults with loss of hearing.

J.G.A.
P.A.M.

Contributors

....

Jerome G. Alpiner, Ph.D., Coordinator of Audiology, Veterans Administration Medical Center, Denver, Colorado

Anne L. Beiter, M.S., Clinical Services Manager, Cochlear Corporation, Englewood, Colorado

Ruth A. Bentler, Ph.D., Assistant Professor, Department of Speech Pathology and Audiology, University of Iowa, Iowa City, Iowa

Judith A. Brimacombe, M.A., Director of Clinical and Regulatory Affairs, Cochlear Corporation, Englewood, Colorado

Arlene Earley Carney, Ph.D., Director, Center for Childhood Deafness, Boys Town National Research Hospital, Omaha, Nebraska

Cynthia L. Compton, M.S., Director, Assistive Devices Center, Department of Audiology and Speech Language Pathology, Gallaudet University, Washington, D.C.

Sue Ann Erdman, M.A., Research Associate, Department of Psychology, University of Maryland, Baltimore County, Baltimore, Maryland

Carol Flexer, Ph.D., Associate Professor of Audiology, Department of Communicative Disorders, The University of Akron, Akron, Ohio

Dean C. Garstecki, Ph.D., Professor and Head, Audiology Program, Director, The Hugh Knowles Center, Northwestern University, Evanston, Illinois

Kenneth W. Grant, Ph.D., Research Audiologist, Army Audiology and Speech Center, Walter Reed Army Medical Center, Washington, D.C.

Alison M. Grimes, M.A., Private Practice, Clinical Audiologist, Nova Care, Inc., Poudre Valley Hearing Center, Fort Collins, Colorado

Perry C. Hanavan, M.A., Audiology and Speech Pathology Service, Veterans Administration Medical Center, Sioux Falls, South Dakota

Suzanne Hasenstab, Ph.D., Associate Professor, Audiology and Speech Pathology, Medical College of Virginia, Richmond, Virginia

Kristen J. Kaufman, M.S. Audiology and Speech Pathology Service, Veterans Administration Medical Center, Sioux Falls, South Dakota

O.T. Kenworthy, Ph.D., Executive Director, Providence Speech and Hearing Center, Orange, California

Patricia B. Kricos, Ph.D., Professor of Audiology, Department of Communication Processes and Disorders, University of Florida, Gainesville, Florida

Joan Laughton, Ph.D., Associate Professor, Department of Communication Sciences and Disorders, University of Georgia, Athens, Georgia

Patricia A. McCarthy, Ph.D., Associate Professor, Department of Communication Disorders and Sciences, College of Health Sciences, Rush University, Rush-Presbyterian-St. Luke's Medical Center, Chicago, Illinois

Mary Pat Moeller, M.S., Coordinator, Center for Childhood Deafness, Boys Town National Research Hospital, Omaha, Nebraska

Allen A. Montgomery, Ph.D., Research Professor, Department of Communication Disorders, University of South Carolina, Columbia, South Carolina

H. Gustav Mueller, Ph.D., Research Associate, University of Northern Colorado, Clinical Faculty, University of Colorado Health Sciences Center, Denver, Colorado, Adjunct Associate Professor, Vanderbilt University, Nashville, Tennessee, Senior Audiology Consultant, Siemens Hearing-Instruments.

Julie Vesper Sapp, M.S., Department of Communication Sciences and Disorders, University of Georgia, Athens, Georgia

Ronald L. Schow, Ph.D., Professor, Department of Speech Pathology and Audiology, Idaho State University, Pocatello, Idaho.

H. Christopher Schweitzer, Ph.D., Senior Audiologist, Family Hearing Center, Karistech, Inc., Boulder, Colorado

Joseph A. Smaldino, Ph.D., Professor and Head, Department of Communicative Disorders, University of Northern Iowa, Cedar Falls, Iowa

Sharon E. Smaldino, Ph.D., Associate Professor, Department of Curriculum and Instruction, University of Northern Iowa, Cedar Falls, Iowa

Brian E. Walden, Ph.D., Director of Research, Army Audiology and Speech Center, Walter Reed Army Medical Center, Washington, D.C.

Barbara E. Weinstein, Ph.D., Associate Professor of Audiology, Department of Speech and Theatre, Lehman College, CUNY, Bronx, New York

Contents

Preface... vii
Contributors ix

SECTION 1
PHILOSOPHY AND SERVICE PROVISION

1. Overview of Rehabilitative Audiology............. 3
   JEROME G. ALPINER, Ph.D., KRISTEN J. KAUFMAN, M.S.,
   and PERRY C. HANAVAN, M.A.

   Appendix 1.1   Definition of and Competencies for Aural
                   Rehabilitation (Position Statement)............... 16

2. Rehabilitative Audiologists and the Hearing-
   Impaired Population: Continuing and New
   Relationships.................................... 17
   DEAN C. GARSTECKI, Ph.D.

3. Rehabilitative Audiology in the Private Practice
   Dispensing Office 35
   H. CHRISTOPHER SCHWEITZER, Ph.D.

   Appendix 3.1   Sample Diary for Use After Purchase of a New
                   Hearing Aid................................... 46

SECTION 2
REHABILITATIVE AUDIOLOGY: CHILDREN

4. Early Identification: Principles and Practice 53
   O.T. KENWORTHY, Ph.D.

5. Amplification for the Hearing-Impaired Child 72
RUTH A. BENTLER, Ph.D.

    Appendix 5.1   DSL Selection Approach for Children (Version 3.0)...   102
    Appendix 5.2   Testing with Five Tasks   104

6. Assessment and Intervention with Preschool
Hearing-Impaired Children 106
MARY PAT MOELLER, M.S., and ARLENE EARLEY CARNEY, Ph.D.

7. Assessment and Intervention with School-Age
Hearing-Impaired Children 136
JOAN LAUGHTON, Ph.D., and M. SUZANNE HASENSTAB, Ph.D.

    Appendix 7.1   Language Tests   168

8. Management of Hearing in an Educational
Setting..176
CAROL FLEXER, Ph.D.

    Appendix 8.1   History of Ear and Hearing Problems.............   207
    Appendix 8.2   Speech Information Available at 250 Hz, 500 Hz,
                1000 Hz, 2000 Hz, 4000 Hz   208
    Appendix 8.3   Evaluation of Children with Suspected Listening
                Difficulties....................................   209

9. The Counseling Process: Children and Parents..211
PATRICIA B. KRICOS, Ph.D.

SECTION 3

REHABILITATIVE AUDIOLOGY: ADULTS

10. Rehabilitative Evaluation of Hearing-Impaired
Adults...237
JEROME G. ALPINER, Ph.D., and RONALD L. SCHOW, Ph.D.

    Appendix 10.1   Self-Assessment of Communication (SAC)   260
    Appendix 10.2   Significant Other Assessment of Communication
                (SOAC)   261
    Appendix 10.3   Denver Scale of Communication Function   262
    Appendix 10.4   Quantified Denver Scale   266
    Appendix 10.5   McCarthy-Alpiner Scale of Hearing Handicap
                (M-A Scale).................................   268
    Appendix 10.6   Hearing Handicap Inventory for Adults (HHIA)   271
    Appendix 10.7   California Consonant Test.....................   273
    Appendix 10.8   Central Institute for the Deaf (CID) Everyday Speech
                Sentences..................................   275
    Appendix 10.9   University of Iowa Tinnitus Questionnaire   278

Appendix 10.10a Alpiner-Meline Aural Rehabilitation (AMAR)
               Screening Scale Instructions.................... 281
Appendix 10.10b Alpiner-Meline Aural Rehabilitation (AMAR)
               Screening Scale.............................. 282

11. Hearing Aid Selection and Assessment.........284

H. GUSTAV MUELLER, Ph.D., and ALISON M. GRIMES, M.A.

12. Management of the Hearing-Impaired Adult......311

ALLEN A. MONTGOMERY, Ph.D..

Appendix 12.1   Adult Aural Rehabilitation Group Outline 328
Appendix 12.2   Specific Goals and Purposes for the Class........ 329
Appendix 12.3   Ways to Maximize Your Chances of Lipreading in
                Combination with Your Hearing Aid 329
Appendix 12.4   Goals and Methods in Adult Aural Rehabilitation 330

13. Rehabilitative Considerations with the Geriatric Population 331

PATRICIA A. McCARTHY, Ph.D., and JULIE VESPER SAPP, M.S.

Appendix 13.1   The Denver Scale of Communication Function for
                Senior Citizens Living in Retirement Centers 358
Appendix 13.2   The Denver Scale of Communication Function—
                Modified 362
Appendix 13.3   Nursing Home Hearing Handicap Index (NHHI):
                Self Version for Resident...................... 366
Appendix 13.4   Communications Assessment Procedure for Seniors
                (CAPS).. 368
Appendix 13.5   The Hearing Handicap Inventory for the Elderly 371
Appendix 13.6   Hearing Handicap Inventory for the Elderly—
                Screening Version (HHIE-S).................... 373

14. Counseling Hearing-Impaired Adults 374

SUE ANN ERDMAN, M.A.

SECTION 4

TECHNOLOGY IN REHABILITATIVE AUDIOLOGY

15. Cochlear Implants.................................417

ANNE L. BEITER, M.S., and JUDITH A. BRIMACOMBE, M.A.

Appendix 15.1   Sample Expectations Questionnaire for an Adult
                Candidate 438
Appendix 15.2   Sample Expectations Questionnaire for the Family
                Member of an Adult Candidate.................. 438
Appendix 15.3   Sample Expectations Questionnaire for a Pediatric
                Candidate 439
Appendix 15.4   Sample Expectations Questionnaire for the Family
                Member of a Pediatric Candidate................ 440

16. Assistive Technology for Deaf and
    Hard-of-Hearing People 441
    CYNTHIA L. COMPTON, M.S.

        Appendix 16.1   Resources..................................... 469

17. Computers in Hearing Rehabilitation 470
    JOSEPH A. SMALDINO, Ph.D., and SHARON E. SMALDINO, Ph.D.

SECTION 5

FUTURE DIRECTIONS

18. Needs of the Geriatric Population................489
    BARBARA E. WEINSTEIN, Ph.D.

19. Research Needs in Rehabilitative Audiology 500
    BRIAN E. WALDEN, Ph.D., and KENNETH W. GRANT, Ph.D.

    Author Index 529
    Subject Index... 541

1

PHILOSOPHY AND SERVICE PROVISION

1

Overview of Rehabilitative Audiology

JEROME G. ALPINER, Ph.D., KRISTEN J. KAUFMAN, M.S.,
PERRY C. HANAVAN, M.A.

There are millions of persons in this country who have varying degrees of hearing loss, which may affect their performance in everyday living situations. These persons include both children and adults, many of whom have acquired hearing loss due to one of many etiologies, while others were born with hearing loss. Hearing impairment is one of the most handicapping conditions in this country, yet it often goes unnoticed if a hearing aid is not seen on the individual or if one does not hear the speech production of a congenitally deaf youngster. Among those with significant hearing loss, for example, may be the school child failing a class in English, the husband whose wife always yells at him for turning up the TV volume, a congregant who stops going to church because of an inability to understand the minister, or the office worker who cannot hear the supervisor's instructions very well.

The National Center for Health Statistics in 1987 (Smith, 1991) estimated that approximately 21 million persons have hearing loss. Other estimates indicate that up to 24 million people in the United States have hearing loss that affects the ability to understand speech. Of those, about 1 million are children under the age of 18 years.

The most common causes of hearing loss for adults are presbycusis and noise exposure. Middle ear problems represent the main etiology of child hearing loss. It is anticipated that the incidence of hearing loss in children, especially teenagers, will increase as a result of the "boom box" era of loud noise.

Figure 1.1 indicates the percentage of people with hearing loss by age range. Presbycusic trends are demonstrated with 14% of the 45- to 64-year-old group having hearing loss, increasing to 30% in those older than 65 and to 35% in those over 75 years. Only 3.5 million of the 21 million persons with hearing loss wear hearing aids. The need for aural rehabilitation appears to be great, but people may not seek out rehabilitation services for a number of reasons:

1. They may be unaware that hearing loss exists.
2. Hearing aids cost too much money.
3. Hearing aids are a sign of old age.
4. Hearing aids will not help.
5. A stigma of mental ability emerges.
6. They may not be emotionally ready for hearing aids.

Definitions

A variety of definitions have been used to describe the remediation process for persons with hearing loss. In a position statement by the American Speech-Language-Hearing Association (1984), a definition of aural rehabilitation is offered:

Aural rehabilitation refers to services and procedures for facilitating adequate receptive and

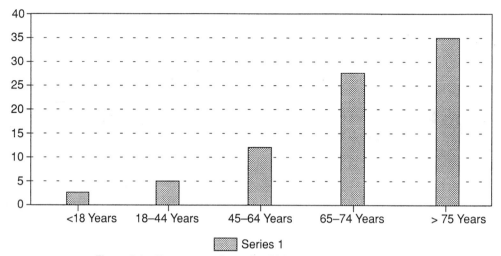

Figure 1.1. Percentage of people with hearing loss by age range
(National Center for Health Statistics, 1987).

expressive communication in individuals with hearing impairment. These services and procedures are intended for those persons who demonstrate a loss of hearing sensitivity or function in communicative situations as if they possess a loss of hearing sensitivity.

Excerpts of procedures and services are found in Appendix 1.1. For the purposes of this text, we use *rehabilitative audiology*, *habilitative audiology*, and *aural rehabilitation* interchangeably. The term *rehabilitative audiology* is preferred. It has been favored by some because it suggests a more comprehensive terminology in working with the "whole person" (Alpiner & McCarthy, 1987).

Rehabilitative Audiology and the Audiologist's Role

We know that many persons with hearing loss need assistance such as amplification, speechreading, communication training, counseling, or other professional services when the problem results in a handicap. Through the years, many terms have been used that attempt to describe what rehabilitative audiologists do. Wood and Miettinen (1988) discuss the role of the hearing therapist in the United Kingdom as it relates to the needs of persons with hearing loss. They outline services that may be provided:

1. An assessment of the rehabilitative needs of the hearing-impaired person that includes:
   a. Assessment of residual hearing and the further use that can be made of it;
   b. Assessment of lipreading ability;
   c. Assessment of "communication lifestyle" (for example, the communication needs of a young executive will differ from those of a housebound retiree).
2. The formulation of a program designed to maximize the patient's ability to communicate. The patient and his or her family will be instructed in communication skills, including the use of hearing aids, environmental aids, lipreading, auditory training, and hearing treatment strategies.
3. The provision of information and help concerning aural rehabilitation to the general public, contact with professional and nonprofessional groups, and counseling for the patient and the family.
4. Employment as a member of a multidisciplinary team that will include clinical and social work staff, as well as work in hospital, community, and domiciliary situations.

According to Wood and Miettinen (1988), good rehabilitative audiology provided at the right time can prevent a hearing impairment from becoming a major handicap. It can prevent withdrawal of the hearing-impaired person from his or her social, domestic, and occupational roles, and all that this withdrawal would imply. Further, financial and domestic pressures, premature retirement, stress-related problems, and emotional withdrawal also may be minimized. It is clear that rehabilitative audiology is a broad-based area that is an extension of the diagnostic process. The diagnostic process defines the numerical audiology problem. Rehabilitative audiology then defines social and emotional "people" problems and the procedures that can be used to help minimize these problems. The audiologist who engages in rehabilitation assumes major responsibility for identifying "people" needs and strategies that should be implemented.

The primary responsibility for audiologic rehabilitation of children and adults rests with the audiologist. Other specialists are involved in the rehabilitation process, but their responsibilities are defined in a more narrow sense. For example, the physician is concerned with medical and surgical treatment for the hearing loss. The psychologist may be concerned with problems manifested by the hearing loss that require counseling. Social workers may be involved to the extent that appropriate services are provided for the person and the family. Overall management, however, rests with the audiologist, who makes sure that appropriate referrals are made for ancillary services as well as ensuring that clients in need receive diagnostic services, hearing aids, and aural rehabilitation. Further, the needs of the consumer must be met. The major consumer interest group in the United States is the Self-Help for Hard of Hearing People, Inc. (SHHH). Thousands of consumers belong to SHHH. Community SHHH chapters throughout the United States are dedicated to ensuring that appropriate services are provided. Their interests include hearing aid costs, provision of assistive devices for theaters and churches, tinnitus, hearing aid banks, and stress management.

A Communication Model

Many authorities recognize that there is a direct relationship between effective communication and quality of life. Effective communication is a dynamic process of exchanging ideas with both expressive and receptive characteristics. Audiologists are concerned primarily with the receptive aspects of communication behavior. Alpiner and Meline (1989) have developed a communication model (see Fig. 1.2) that emphasizes the receptive process. This model attempts to illustrate factors that are pertinent to the quality of life of persons with hearing loss by exemplifying the multifaceted issues that an audiologist must address in clinical service delivery.

There are four levels of concern in this model. Level 1 is *message expression*. A communication event is transmitted through sound, touch, and movement. It must transcend environmental barriers to reach the receiver. These barriers to reception may include telephone lines that have static or a room with a high level of background noise.

Level 2 deals with *message encoding*. The individual must have the ability to receive the communication. The integrity of the receiver's auditory, tactile, and visual systems must be intact to receive whatever message is being sent.

Level 3 involves *message decoding*. Once the message has reached the receiver, it must be interpreted. These interpretations are often determined by internal cognitive factors and by the social, vocational, and emotional needs of the individual.

Level 4 is *message perception*. The receiver of the communication internalizes the message, may ask for clarification, may observe the speaker's feedback, and may repair the perceived meaning of the message prior to formulating a response.

In essence, this model demonstrates that the message is sent to a person who is a listener; is encoded by the visual and tactile systems; is related to the environment of the individual as a social, vocational, or emotional need; and, finally, is perceived by the receiver.

Historical Aspects

The Academy of Rehabilitative Audiology observed its 25th anniversary in 1991. In reviewing the archives of the Academy,

Communication Block Diagram
Emphasis: Receptive Process

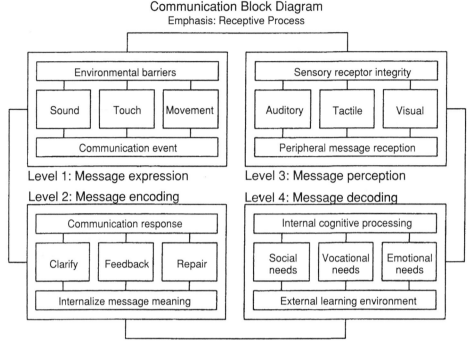

Environmental barriers			Sensory receptor integrity		
Sound	Touch	Movement	Auditory	Tactile	Visual
Communication event			Peripheral message reception		

Level 1: Message expression   Level 3: Message perception
Level 2: Message encoding   Level 4: Message decoding

Communication response			Internal cognitive processing		
Clarify	Feedback	Repair	Social needs	Vocational needs	Emotional needs
Internalize message meaning			External learning environment		

Figure 1.2. Communication model.

it is interesting to view the transitions that have occurred in rehabilitative audiology. During the first 30 years of this century, there was extensive emphasis on the visual modality, including speechreading, and on manual communication because of the lack of sophisticated amplification systems. A transition to more widespread use of amplification occurred in the 1940s and 1950s with the development of the transistor.

In the 1960s and 1970s, audiologists viewed lipreading and auditory training as aural rehabilitation processes that were largely independent of amplification. With improving technology and evolving philosophies, many audiologists began to regard hearing aids as a definite part of the aural rehabilitation process. A major event that occurred in the late 1970s is probably responsible for hearing aids becoming an integral part of rehabilitative audiology. The American Speech-Language-Hearing Association (ASHA) approved a resolution that allowed audiologists to dispense hearing aids. Prior to that time, ASHA-certified audiologists could not dispense hearing aids; the responsibility was solely that of the commercial hearing aid dealer.

That single event appeared to change the profession of audiology. Previously, audiologists performed hearing aid evaluations and then referred clients to hearing aid dealers. Usually there was little rehabilitation follow-up. Only in the last 15 years has the ASHA audiologist been able to assume the entire aural rehabilitation process from evaluation through hearing aid dispensing.

The role of the rehabilitative audiologist in the present era centers on amplification. Curran (1990) indicates that hearing aid dispensing is now the most viable aspect of audiology, and it is the one activity that almost all new graduates find themselves doing immediately on graduation. In a recent survey, Curran states that audiologists now account for the distribution of approximately 60 to 65% of the aids dispensed (Kochkin, 1990). Additionally, more than 45% of the active dispensers today (approaching 5000) are audiologists (Cranmer, 1990). Even considering these trends, it should be noted that only about 18% of all persons who need hearing aids obtain them (English, 1991). With all of the developments in aural rehabilitation, we must be cognizant that there are many persons who need our help and are not receiving it. We continue into the 1990s and approach the year 2000 with new missions. It would seem that we still need to continue our outreach to the public, just as we did 50 years ago.

The Present Status of Rehabilitative Audiology

In the 1990s, hearing loss is being viewed as a high-profile health care issue (Kirkwood, 1991). In the early 1960s, patients would be told that there was nothing that could be done about their nerve deafness. The situation is certainly much different 30 years later with the technological advances that have occurred with regard to amplification.

It should be emphasized, however, that many obstacles still need to be overcome to raise public consciousness about hearing loss, which affects more than 21 million Americans. Kirkwood has cited several reasons why awareness has been delayed. First, quoting Geraldine Dietz Fox, whose lobbying helped create the National Institute on Deafness and Other Communication Disorders (NIDCD), "When you don't die from something, people aren't so anxious to provide funds for it." Second, hearing loss is invisible, and some people prefer to keep their disability hidden. Third, the confusion of hearing loss with senescence causes many persons to avoid being labeled mentally inferior. Fourth, quoting from John House, M.D., "Part of the problem is that unless people experience hearing loss, they don't know how devastating it can be. Even blindness you can relate to more. You can see how it affects people, or you can close your eyes and have an idea of what it's like to be blind. You can't do that very well with deafness."

Considerable progress, however, has been made. Rizzo (1991), executive director of the Better Hearing Institute (BHI), states that more progress has been made in the past decade than in the previous 50 years in terms of public awareness of hearing loss. Rizzo indicates that one of the responsible factors is that famous people have volunteered their efforts by going public with their hearing loss. Some of these individuals have been Nanette Fabray, Johnny Ray, Bob Hope, Phyllis Diller, football star Mike Singletary, actor Richard Thomas, race car driver Al Unser, and Mark Herndon of the country music band Alabama. The federal government also has been involved in increasing public awareness with passage of the Americans with Disabilities Act.

The impact of amplification in the rehabilitative audiology process continues to expand with both conventional and digital hearing aid technology. The implantable hearing aid is a promising new development in hearing amplification. The cochlear implant is another significant step in the understanding and treatment of sensorineural hearing loss. In addition to conventional hearing aids, the number of assistive devices has increased dramatically in the past decade. Each of these developments has helped shape the present status of rehabilitative audiology.

Rehabilitative audiology can be seen as a broad-based process in which all of these developments can be incorporated. Alpiner and Meline (1989) present major points to be considered for an aural rehabilitation program:

1. Review the anatomy and physiology of the hearing mechanism as it applies specifically to group members.
2. Provide prognostic information regarding hearing loss relevant to group members.
3. Discuss the importance of interpersonal relationships and individual group members' responsibility in management of associated problems.
4. Assess the impact of hearing loss on group members and significant others' life-style in areas of attitude, communication breakdown, and hearing handicap.
5. Determine goals of aural rehabilitation group therapy designed to meet group members' specific needs.
6. Conduct pre- and postassessment of group members' awareness levels and communication skills as they relate to their specific problems in areas of listening, environmental considerations, lipreading activities, and personal assertiveness.

7. Provide listening training. Emphasize effects of distance, noise, and poor visibility of the speaker's face and the optimum management of these problems present in specific communication environments and situations.
8. Provide lipreading training. Emphasize the benefits of using visual cues available in the communication environment such as facial, gestural, contextual, and situational cues to optimize communication events.
9. Provide assertiveness training. Emphasize the communication strategies and techniques needed in specific situations to facilitate successful communication.
10. Reinforce individual group members' progress and the importance of establishing a stress-free communication pattern complemented by personal confidence in effective communication skills.

Service Delivery in the 1990s

The actual delivery of services often depends on the location and type of clinic. Rehabilitative audiologic services are provided in hospital clinics, university hearing and speech centers, physician offices (usually Ear, Nose, and Throat), Veterans Administration (VA) Medical Center clinics, military clinics, hearing aid dispensers, school programs, and private practitioners' offices.

We live in a cost-conscious society: Medical expenses have soared, health insurance programs have limited services, and premiums have increased. Medicare and Medicaid have faced restrictions in what health problems can be covered and to what extent. And although diagnostic audiology fees usually are covered, rehabilitative services generally have not been covered for reimbursement. Private sector clinics, therefore, emphasize diagnostics and minimize rehabilitative audiology. The issue is not the value of the service; it is cost-effectiveness. Hearing aid programs, an integral process of rehabilitative audiology, are in large part cost-effective because of the sale of products.

Unfortunately, a total rehabilitation program as part of hearing aid dispensing tends to be the exception rather than the rule. However, the Aural Rehabilitation Program at the Veterans Administration Outpatient Clinic in Los Angeles typifies a model comprehensive program (Daguio & Steckler, 1987) that can be developed around hearing aid dispensing. Daguio and Steckler have described the goal of aural rehabilitation, which is to provide hard-of-hearing individuals with a greater understanding of hearing problems. Other goals are to improve communication skills and to provide a realistic estimate of progress in overcoming the problem. Their aural rehabilitation program also includes a lecture on the medical aspects of hearing problems: how the ear works, what can go wrong with it, and what can be done to correct hearing problems. Most important is the establishment of a hearing conservation program to prevent further hearing loss.

The Los Angeles VA program provides lectures on hearing aids and discussion of client capabilities and limitations, followed by descriptions of other devices for hearing with some instruction and practice in their use. Considerable emphasis is placed on describing the speechreading process by outlining general principles rather than conducting intensive drills. In auditory training sessions, listening habits are discussed and tests are administered to identify specific types of errors that are made. In speech conversation, clients are taught to evaluate each other's speech in terms of clarity and understandability. Counseling on individual problems related to occupation or environment is emphasized. An analysis of the problem is conducted for each client, and possible solutions are outlined for each problem.

This VA program consists of 30 hours of instruction over several days following hearing aid dispensing. Because of clients' work schedules, transportation needs, and so forth, there are problems. The primary focus, however, is to be cognizant of the value of rehabilitative audiology. It is not a one- or two-time event as typically seen with an audiologic evaluation followed by a hearing aid evaluation. It is an ongoing process focusing on education, counseling, and management of the hearing loss.

For the past several years, we have presented a service delivery model that may

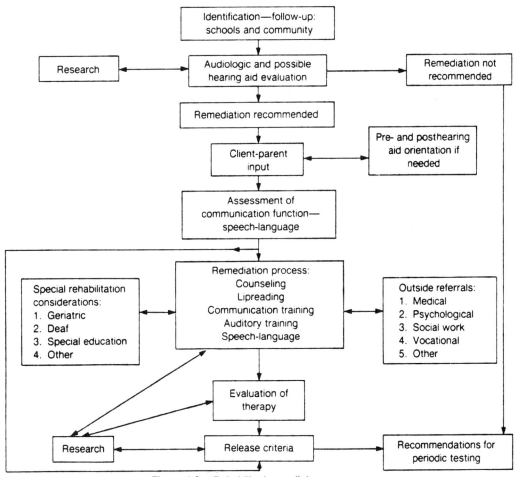

Figure 1.3. Rehabilitative audiology process.

help in the establishment of an effective program. The complexities of the rehabilitation process can be narrowed by use of this model, which permits us to develop and use the philosophies with which we are most comfortable. Figure 1.3 presents this model.

The first phase in the model is the identification of the child or the adult. Children in school programs usually are screened on a periodic basis and identified in this manner. Infants may be identified in hospitals with newborn testing procedures. Adults with hearing loss have less chance of being identified, since there are no mandatory adult testing programs. Adults usually have to take the initiative to have their hearing tested. Many adults, however, are not terribly interested in knowing about their hearing, probably because hearing loss for

most is gradual and not obvious to them. Many general practitioners do not screen hearing as part of physical examinations.

Whatever the identification program, the audiologist needs to make some clinical judgments when hearing loss exists:

1. Is remediation necessary after completion of the audiologic evaluation?
2. Should a hearing aid evaluation be administered to determine if the hearing impairment can be minimized by amplification? Should assistive devices be recommended?
3. Is rehabilitation indicated after completion of the hearing aid evaluation? Here and in item 1, remediation is not recommended if, on the basis of the audiologist's information and judgment, the client is able to communicate

effectively without assistance. Conversely, on the same basis, remediation is recommended when the client needs assistance to improve communication ability or to minimize any concomitant problems resulting from hearing loss.

4. What are the client's communication needs? In the initial stages of rehabilitation, client input and parent input help to provide significant information regarding communication status. Pre- and postorientation may be necessary if amplification is considered.

5. Should the client be released? An assessment of communication function, including speech-language development for the child, is considered in the process to determine the need for continued rehabilitation. At this point, on the basis of established criteria of the measuring instruments, the client is released from rehabilitation. When treatment is terminated, recommendations are made for periodic hearing and educational rechecks. We recommend that this occur once a year or sooner if a change is noticed in the ability to communicate.

6. Which rehabilitative procedures should be recommended? The implementation of remediation may include counseling, language stimulation groups, auditory training, speech-language treatment, and hearing aid orientation.

7. Should referrals be made? The child's or adult's situation may require referral to other professional persons such as psychologists, family counselors, pediatricians, vocational counselors, and so forth. Generally, professionals in other disciplines will refer directly back to the audiologist or work with the client concurrently.

8. Are special treatment considerations necessary? Additional procedures may be indicated when dealing with profoundly deaf children, geriatric clients in extended care facilities, multihandicapped persons, and clients with additional problems due to stroke and other disorders. It is desirable to include family members in aural rehabilitation for both children and adults.

9. Has therapy been successful? During the course of therapy, periodic assessment measures need to be made with regard to both success and termination from rehabilitation. Release from therapy can be made on the basis of the criteria established in items 4 and 6.

10. How can research serve this process? Research in the total rehabilitative program is suggested for more meaningful and valid approaches. Research applications are more easily made in the university setting, since most research efforts are done in this setting. It is important to devise ways to relate developments to those in other settings, such as private clinics and private practitioner offices, where a majority of time is spent in service delivery.

General Effects of Hearing Loss

Now that we have some information about rehabilitative audiology, let us consider the effects of hearing loss. Yantis (1985) discusses the matter of describing hearing impairment and/or handicap. An *impairment* refers to a structural or functional abnormality. A *handicap* occurs when one's personal efficiency in daily living activities is affected by an impairment (AAO-ACO, 1979). These activities relate to social, emotional, intellectual, and occupational situations. Numerical classification systems have been used for medical-legal purposes. The numerical system generally is based on averages for pure tone air conduction audiometry. A practical application, for example, might be the amount of compensation paid to a veteran for service-connected hearing loss, or to a construction worker under workman's compensation who incurs hearing loss due to industrial noise exposure.

We need to consider the effects of the hearing loss on everyday living activities. Numerical hearing measures do not provide us with this information. Self-Assessment Scales of Hearing Handicap have increased in popularity. They can determine how a loss interferes in an individual's daily

Table 1.1
Classes of Hearing Handicap[a]

Hearing Threshold Level	Class	Degree of Handicap	Average Hearing Threshold Level for 500, 1000, and 2000 Hz in the Better Ear[b]		Ability to Understand Speech
			More Than	Not More Than	
dB			dB	dB	
ISO					
25	A	Not significant		25	No significant difficulty with faint speech
40	B	Slight handicap	25	40	Difficulty only with faint speech
55	C	Mild handicap	40	55	Frequent difficulty with normal speech
70	D	Marked handicap	55	70	Frequent difficulty with loud speech
90	E	Severe handicap	70	90	Can understand only shouted or amplified speech
	F	Extreme handicap	90		Usually cannot understand even amplified speech

[a] Reprinted by permission from Davis, H., and Silverman, S. R., *Hearing and Deafness*. 4th Ed. New York: Holt, Rinehart and Winston (1978).
[b] Whenever the average for the poorer ear is 25 dB or more than that for the better ear in this frequency range, 5 dB is added to the average for the better ear. This adjusted average determines the degree and class of handicap. For example, if a person's average hearing threshold level for 500, 1000, and 2000 Hz is 37 dB in one ear and 62 dB or more in the other, his adjusted average hearing threshold level is 42 dB and his handicap is Class C instead of Class B.

activities. Assessment scales are discussed in Chapter 10.

One example of a numerical classification is a modification proposed by Goodman (1965) and modified by Clark (1981). It is based on an average threshold level re ANSI (1986) for 500, 1000, and 2000 Hz. The categories range from normal hearing (−10 to 15 dB) to profound hearing loss (91 dB plus). It should be noted that the numerical designation describes how a person hears auditory messages; for example, "I can hear but it is not very loud" to "I can't hear anything." Table 1.1 (Davis & Silverman, 1978) presents classifications describing the ability to understand speech. The Veterans Administration (1990), with regard to Compensation and Pension Examinations, presents a numerical classification that takes into account higher frequencies, previously neglected in other classifications. For example, 500 Hz is dropped, and 3000 and 4000 Hz are added. A four frequency average is then computed using 1000, 2000, 3000, and 4000 Hz. There

are varying philosophies regarding numerical classifications. It is appropriate to use a numerical classification with numerical descriptors and assessment scales of hearing handicap that describe more fully a client's everyday communication problems.

It also is necessary to more specifically define hearing loss in children. Northern and Downs (1984) ask the question "What then is the beginning of a handicapping hearing loss for a child?" Is it 10 dB, 15 dB, 20 dB? Reference was made to the American Academy of Otolaryngology (AAO, 1979), which defined a permanent handicap as "the disadvantage imposed by an impairment sufficient to affect a person's efficiency in the activities of daily living." The committee thought that a loss greater than 25 dB represented an impairment in everyday living.

Northern and Downs (1984) state that a handicapping hearing loss in a child is any degree of hearing loss that reduces the intelligibility of a speech message to a degree inadequate for accurate interpretation or learning. Of importance is the situation in which a 10-dB loss may be handicapping to one child, whereas a 25-dB loss may not be handicapping to another child.

Regardless of classifications and assessment scales, the main point to be emphasized is that each person, child or adult, needs to be evaluated individually, not necessarily in comparison to others. Aural rehabilitation goals then may be established for each individual in terms of the aural rehabilitation model presented previously.

Areas of Rehabilitative Audiology

We consider five major areas of study in this text: *(1)* philosophy and service provision, *(2)* rehabilitative audiology for children, *(3)* rehabilitative audiology for adults, *(4)* technology in rehabilitative audiology, and *(5)* future directions.

In the philosophy and service provision section, trends in rehabilitative audiology since its inception are presented. It is interesting to compare the first chapter of the author's text *Handbook of Adult Rehabilitative Audiology* (Alpiner, 1978) with this text. In that edition there were no chapters dealing with consumer and professional relationships, reimbursement issues, cochlear implants, assistive devices, and computers in rehabilitative audiology. We have come a long way since the early days when speechreading and auditory training dominated aural rehabilitation. Hearing-impaired clients are the ones who will benefit from these advances.

Audiologists still have the task of convincing hearing-impaired persons that hearing aids will help and that additional procedures such as counseling and auditory training will provide additional benefit. We continue our efforts to show clients that there is help beyond hearing loss.

Garstecki (1991) focuses on the relationship between rehabilitative audiologists and hearing-impaired individuals. This is done in terms of habits and attitudes of adults toward professional services. Ideal relationships between clients and audiologists are considered. We need to know that

clients do not always welcome us with open arms. Audiologists need to take into account client feelings toward the rehabilitation process. Clients do not always agree, as we do, with the worth of our service.

Audiologists often encounter clients who are interested in our services but quickly reject rehabilitation when they learn that insurance does not cover the service. Diagnostic audiology procedures usually are reimbursed, but rehabilitation services are not. At the conference of the Academy of Rehabilitative Audiology, a discussion ensued regarding aural rehabilitation services in private practice. An audiologist was professing the advantages of rehabilitation. When asked if these services were a part of his practice, the response was negative. The reason cited was lack of reimbursement. We need to be aware of this issue so that we can involve ourselves in legislative issues that ultimately will enable our clients to receive needed rehabilitative audiology services.

A section focusing on hearing-impaired children discusses the identification, evaluation, and impact of hearing loss in children; amplification for the hearing-impaired child; assessment and intervention with preschool and school-age hearing-impaired children; and the counseling process for both children and parents.

Although hearing-impaired students are commonly perceived to be a low-incidence handicapped population, this population may be one of the largest of all handicapping conditions found in school-age children (Hull & Dilka, 1984; Ross, Brackett, & Maxon, 1982). Allard and Golden (1991) define audiology services according to the following categories:

1. Comprehensive screening programs designed to identify students in need of evaluation
2. Comprehensive assessment programs designed to evaluate and diagnose auditory disorders and provide program planning information
3. Comprehensive habilitation programs designed to provide auditory intervention, management, and skill development.

It is possible that the numbers of children with hearing impairment may increase. Reports of elevated high-frequency hearing thresholds in children have appeared in the literature repeatedly (Chermak & Peters-McCarthy, 1991). Roche et al. (1978) attributed elevated auditory thresholds observed among children age 4 to 18 years to noise exposure associated with farm machinery and amplified musical instruments. Although the presence of high-frequency hearing loss in school-age children has been known for a long time, little has been done to remedy the problem (Chermak & Peters-McCarthy, 1991). It appears that considerable numbers of children from infancy through the teenage years may benefit from the services of the audiologist.

Rehabilitative Audiology: Adults

One of the goals of rehabilitation for adults is to provide support therapy. For a number of years, audiologists have used two approaches to rehabilitative audiology. These approaches supplement the use of hearing aids:

1. The traditional approach, which primarily involves auditory training and speechreading
2. The progressive approach (Alpiner, 1982), which is primarily a counseling-oriented methodology.

While we address different approaches to rehabilitation, we must also address other issues that relate to the treatment process for adults. Assessing the impact of deafness on the individual is a good starting point. Assessment scales allow us to determine how hearing loss affects the emotional, social, and vocational aspects of everyday living. This type of assessment, discussed in Chapter 10, provides a baseline for treatment and a measure by which we may determine how effective rehabilitative audiology has been.

Hearing aids are a crucial part of the rehabilitation process. Many audiologists think that the hearing aid is the major aspect of our service. This may be true to a certain degree, particularly in view of the fact that hearing aid technology has provided a much better product than in previous years. Yet we need to remember that hearing aids still are not the same as new ears and that ancillary rehabilitation services may be necessary to provide optimum assistance for clients. Our goal should be to provide all resources for maximum benefit.

Resources other than the hearing aid may include speechreading instruction, auditory training, counseling, speech conservation, and other procedures. These are discussed in detail in Chapter 12. Some audiologists believe that a knowledge of audiology, coupled with a skill for interpersonal relationships, is a requisite for success for those professionals who emphasize aural rehabilitation. Special considerations may be indicated for the geriatric client who no longer has complete independence for everyday living. For all persons with hearing loss, the need arises occasionally for counseling because of problems that may arise in family situations at home, because of work difficulties due to hearing loss, or because of frustrations in dealing with social situations.

A variety of individuals may be involved in the rehabilitative audiology of adults. The audiologist assumes a major role in the areas of evaluation, hearing aid selection, therapy, communication training, and hearing aid follow-up. If the need exists for vocational rehabilitation counselors, social workers, and others to be involved, then a case manager needs to assume coordination responsibility. Not having a coordinator for services results in conflicts that ultimately affect the client. It is a little like the old saying, "There can only be one cook in the kitchen," even though there may be other helpers. All of these areas of adult rehabilitative audiology will be of interest in this section.

There are three areas in rehabilitative audiology that have not been covered in previous editions. Cochlear implants have been of significant help to both children and adults. Only a few years ago, there was little, if anything, that could be done for the profoundly deaf individual short of some amplification and sign language. How exciting it must be for a profoundly deaf person who can now communicate in varying degrees with the hearing world. Think also of those persons who may be able to carry on limited telephone conversations. The positive impact of the cochlear implant cannot be denied. Audiologists and speech-language pathologists are challenged to assimilate the vast amounts of information being made available in the implant field today.

Assistive devices for the hearing impaired are really of recent vintage when we think of the number of audiologists who are aware of them. It was not very long ago that these devices existed but not many persons knew much about them. The increased interest is positive, since our clients may benefit further by participating in everyday communication activities. Such devices include special alarm clocks, light indicators, TV/radio amplifiers, telephone typewriters for the hearing impaired, telephone amplifiers, closed-caption television, FM systems, and so forth. There is a responsibility to educate the public about these devices now that audiologists are more familiar with them and learning more as time passes.

We are all aware of the impact computers have made on all aspects of society. It is no different in audiology. We can observe computerization of audiology tests, real ear measurements to evaluate the effectiveness of hearing aids, and treatment programs for clients to help them improve communication. The computer has been feared by some who were never exposed to it during school and college. Yet the future belongs, in part, to those who are willing to learn about and use hardware and software so that clients will be better communicators. For this reason, we explore the world of computers in this text. It will be exciting for us to partake of new knowledge in this area.

The final section of this text covers future directions in rehabilitative audiology. As we approach the year 2000, we need to consider the needs of the geriatric population. People are living longer, and we need to address the issue of quality of life. The population will continue to increase and the incidence of hearing loss will continue to be a national health problem because of major factors like the aging process and noise exposure. We can all have an opportunity to participate in this important area.

All of our treatment and evaluation procedures are based on research endeavors to find meaningful and better ways to do things. Chapter 19 on research needs in audiology will consider this aspect of audiology, not always the favorite of clinicians but a necessity for future success for all persons with hearing loss. We think that you will find this chapter both interesting and stimulating.

Educational Directions for Rehabilitative Audiology

We would be remiss if we did not consider significant events that have occurred in recent years concerning the "new" audiologist, the making of the "Doctor of Audiology (Au.D.)." A major proponent of the Au.D. (Goldstein, 1989) states that current audiology programs do not allow students to earn a professional degree. The Master of Science or the Master of Arts degrees are academic degrees, not professional degrees. The issue may be clarified by indicating that the degree does not represent a clinical or service delivery degree. There are differences between academic and professional degrees. Goldstein (1989) emphasizes that not being able to be an Au.D. is not consistent for those who are providing a doctoring service. Reference is made to other professions. Physicians (M.D.s) are doctors of medicine, dentists are doctors of dentistry (D.D.S), and optometrists earn an O.D. degree. Audiologists also are health care professionals who wish to be able to earn a professional degree with its associated obligations and opportunities. Various training models have been presented for the Au.D. degree.

At this time, there has been considerable emphasis on the implementation of the Au.D. program. It appears that this new program will soon begin in some universities in the country. Those persons presently possessing a Master's degree will have options that will enable them to become Doctors of Audiology. Cunningham and Windmill (1991) state that the Au.D. proposal purports to educate a completely new level of audiologic practitioner. These audiology doctors will be required, for example, to complete some 2000 or more clock hours of clinical training before graduation. It is hoped that much of this practicum will be devoted to rehabilitative audiology. It is appropriate to indicate that advances in audiology are accompanied by new developments in the training of audiologists who will serve persons with hearing impairment.

As a final note to this overview, we make mention of the various contributors to this book on rehabilitative audiology. The information is presented in a format that allows them to use their individual styles. We think that this will give us a greater appreciation and understanding of rehabilitative audiology.

References

Allard, J.B., and Golden, D.C., Educational audiology: a comparison of service delivery systems utilized by Missouri schools. *Lang. Speech Hear. Serv. Schools*, 22, 5–11 (1991).

Alpiner, J.G., *Handbook of Adult Rehabilitative Audiology*, Baltimore, MD: Williams & Wilkins (1978).

Alpiner, J.G., and McCarthy, P.A., *Handbook of Rehabilitative Audiology: Children and Adults*. Baltimore, MD: Williams & Wilkins (1987).

Alpiner, J.G., and Meline, N.C., A self-assessment scale of hearing handicap (AMAR Scale). Paper presented to annual convention of Alabama Speech and Hearing Association. Birmingham, Alabama (1989).

American Academy of Otolaryngology (AAO) Committee on Hearing and Equilibrium and the American Council of Otolaryngology (ACO) Committee on the Medical Aspects of Noise, Guide for the evaluation of hearing handicap. *JAMA*, 251, 2055–2059 (1979).

American Speech-Language-Hearing Association. Position statement on the definition and competencies for aural rehabilitation. *Asha*, 26, 37–41 (1984).

Chermak, G.D., and Peters-McCarthy, E.P., The effectiveness of an educational hearing conservation program for elementary school children. *Lang. Speech Hear. Serv. Schools*, 22, 308–312 (1991).

Clark, J.G., Use and abuses of hearing loss classification. *Asha*, 23, 493–500 (1981).

Cranmer, K.S., Hearing instrument marketing analysis. *Hear. Instru.*, 41, 6–10 (1990).

Cunningham, D.R., and Windmill, I., The AuD degree: clinical instructors wanted. *Audiol. Today*, 3, 18–20 (1991).

Curran, J.P., Editorial. *Audiol. Today*, 2, 6–11 (1990).

Daguio, M., and Steckler, J., *Veterans Administration Outpatient Clinic Aural Rehabilitation Desk Guide*. Los Angeles: Veterans Administration (1987).

Davis, J., and Silverman, S.R., *Hearing and Deafness*. New York: Holt, Rinehart and Winston (1978).

Department of Veterans Affairs, Standard procedures for audiology compensation and pension examinations. Circulat. 10–89–103. Washington, DC (September 25, 1989).

English, B., Personal communication (December 1991).

Garstecki, D.C., Rehabilitative audiologists and hearing-impaired persons; continuing new relationships. In J. Alpiner and P. McCarthy, *Rehabilitative Audiology: Children and Adults*. Baltimore, MD: Williams & Wilkins (1993).

Goldstein, D., The doctoring degree in audiology. *Asha*, 31, 33–35 (1989).

Goodman, A., Reference zero levels for pure-tone audiometers. *Asha*, 7, 262–263 (1965).

Hull, R., and Dilka, K., *The Hearing Impaired Child in School*, Vol. 4. New York: Grune & Stratton (1984).

Kirkwood, D.H., Hearing loss emerges as a high-profile health care issue. *Hear. J.*, 44(17), 9–11, 14–17 (1991).

Kochkin, S., Introducing marketrak: consumer tracking survey of the hearing instrument model. *Hear. J.*, 43(5), 17–27 (1990).

Northern, J.L., and Downs, M.P., *Hearing in Children*. Baltimore, MD: Williams & Wilkins (1984).

Rizzo, J., cited in Kirkwook, D.H., Hearing loss emerges as a high-profile health care issue. *Hear. J.*, 44(7), 10–11 (1991).

Roche, A.F., Siervogel, R.M., Himes, J.H., and Johnson, D.L., Longitudinal study of hearing in children; baseline data concerning auditory thresholds, noise exposure, and biological factors. *J. Acoust. Soc. Am.*, 64, 1593–1601 (1978).

Ross, M., Bruckett, D., and Maxon, A., *Hard of Hearing Children in Regular Schools*. Englewood Cliffs, NJ: Prentice-Hall (1982).

Smith, R.D., *About Hearing Aids and Hearing Loss*. Denver, CO: Ramie Publishing Corporation (1991).

Wood, C., and Miettinen, I., Why you should have a hearing therapist. *J. Laryngol. Otol.*, 102, 142–143 (1988).

Yantis, P.A., Pure tone air-conduction testing. In J. Katz (au.), *Handbook of Clinical Audiology*. Baltimore, MD: Williams & Wilkins (1985).

APPENDIX

1.1 Definition of and Competencies for Aural Rehabilitation (Position Statement)*

I. Identification and Evaluation of Sensory Capabilities
  A. Identification and evaluation of the extent of the impairment, including assessment, periodic monitoring, and re-evaluation of auditory abilities.
  B. Monitoring of other sensory capabilities as they relate to receptive and expressive communication.
  C. Evaluation, fitting, and monitoring of auditory aids and monitoring of other sensory aids.
  D. Evaluation and monitoring of the acoustic characteristics of the communicative environments confronted by the hearing-impaired person.
II. Interpretation of Results, Counseling, and Referral
  A. Interpretation of audiologic findings to the client, family, employer, teachers, and significant others involved in communication with the hearing-impaired person.
  B. Guidance and counseling for the client, family, employer, caregiver, teachers, and significant others concerning the educational, psychosocial, and communicative effects of hearing impairment.
  C. Guidance and counseling for the parent/caregiver regarding:
    1. educational options available;
    2. selection of educational programs; and
    3. facilitation of communicative and cognitive development.
  D. Individual and/or family counseling regarding:
    1. acceptance and understanding of hearing impairment;
    2. functioning within difficult listening situations;
    3. facilitation of effective strategies and attitudes toward communication;
    4. modification of communicative behavior in keeping with those strategies and attitudes; and
    5. promotion of independent management of communication-related problems.
  E. Referral for additional services.
III. Intervention for Communicative Difficulties
  A. Development and provision of an intervention program to facilitate expressive and receptive communication.
  B. Provision of hearing and speech conservation programming.
  C. Service as a liaison between the client, family, and other agencies concerned with the management of communicative disorders related to hearing impairment.
IV. Re-evaluation of the Client's Status
 V. Evaluation and Modification of the Intervention Program

---

*Excerpts from: Position Statement, Definition of and competencies for aural rehabilitation. *Asha*, 26, 37–41 (1984).

2

Rehabilitative Audiologists and the Hearing-Impaired Population: Continuing and New Relationships

DEAN C. GARSTECKI, Ph.D.

Relationships between clinicians and clients are influenced by many factors. Some factors are easy to control, like appointment schedules, fees, and where services are provided. Other factors are not controllable, like personal conviction and mutual respect. This chapter focuses on the relationship between rehabilitative audiologists and hearing-impaired individuals. First, prevailing habits and attitudes of hearing-impaired adults toward professional services are considered. Next, recent federal legislation mandating nondiscrimination of individuals with disabilities, including the hearing disabled, is examined. The result describes where the rehabilitative audiologist/hearing-impaired person relationship is now, what the relationship ought to be, and how we might begin to close the gap.

Habits and Attitudes of Hearing-Impaired Persons

HEARING AID USE

It is estimated that only 10 to 18% of the hearing-impaired population uses hearing aids (Gallup, 1980; Ries, 1982; Wilder, 1975). Hearing aid industry estimates suggest that under 5 million hearing-impaired children and adults use hearing aids (Goldstein, 1984). When low, mid, and high hearing loss prevalence rates are applied to estimated hearing aid use rates, the unmet need (i.e., the number of hearing-impaired individuals who do not use hearing aids) ranges from 93.8% to 92.0% to 85.7%, respectively. Also, since 80% of all hearing-impaired children use hearing aids (Karchmer & Kirwin, 1977), the unmet need is considered to be almost entirely among the adult hearing-impaired population (Goldstein, 1984). Currently, the number of hearing-impaired nonusers of hearing aids is estimated at 18.4 million people (Kochkin, 1991).

Why do so few people who might benefit from amplification choose to use hearing aids? Goldstein (1984) reviewed factors generally considered to affect hearing aid consumption. These included (1) the stigma associated with hearing loss, (2) the cost of obtaining and using a hearing aid, (3) hearing aid delivery systems, (4) the "medical funnel," and (5) the behavior of hearing care professionals.

In regard to the stigma, age at onset of hearing loss must be considered. If hearing loss occurs in midlife, there is a strong likelihood that it will negatively affect occupational goals and social prowess, and, therefore, hearing loss occurring at this time is likely to be denied. If hearing loss occurs in later life, there is a strong chance that it will be regarded as inevitable and unremediable (Humphrey, Herbst, & Faurqui, 1981). Rehabilitative audiologists must be aware of these differences, as they affect counseling strategy. However, regardless of age at onset, when hearing loss occurs, the embarrassment created by related problems and by the need to wear hearing aids is the most frequently cited difficulty in the acceptance and use by adults (Barcham & Stephens, 1980; Bevan, 1981). Tyler, Baker, and Armstrong-Bednall (1983) reported that hearing aids communicate weakness to others. They draw attention to hearing loss (Franks & Beckmann, 1985), and for some they serve as a sign of advancing age (Maurer, 1982). Studies by Blood, Blood, and Danhauer (1978) and Lass (1989) demonstrate a "hearing aid effect" in that those who use hearing aids are perceived by others to be less intelligent, lower achieving, less attractive, and more likely to demonstrate negative personality traits.

Obviously, the stigma of hearing loss and the desirability of hearing aid use do not affect all hearing-impaired individuals in the same way. Morgan (1990) reported that in the population of older adults considered to be most highly motivated toward hearing care, a group labeled as the "pro-actives," 23% of those age 50 to 64 years wore hearing aids, as did 46% of those over age 65 years. Among the next least motivated group, the "faithful patient" segment of the older population, 13% of those between 50 and 64 years and 21% of those over 65 years wore hearing aids. Only 6% of the "optimist" group between ages 50 and 64 and only 10% of those age 65 years and older wore hearing aids. Finally, among those least likely to take advantage of health aids and services, the "disillusioned" group, 1% or less wore hearing aids.

Although not a concern to the pro-actives in the Morgan report, cost is often cited as one of the more common reasons why relatively few individuals use hearing aids. However, Goldstein (1984) described a loose relationship between hearing aid cost and take-up rate. Citing increasing hearing aid sales during times of severe recession, coupled with a 25% decrease in third-party reimbursement for hearing aid purchases since 1980, he stated that economic stress should not be considered to be a critical factor in explaining low hearing aid consumption. In fact, only 5% of the hearing-impaired individuals interviewed in the 1980 Gallup Poll complained of hearing aid cost. Cost may be a factor some need to consider in deciding on a hearing aid purchase, but apparently it is not the major factor accounting for the gap between the potential and actual number of hearing aid users.

Despite the increasing number of clinical audiologists and growing acceptance of hearing aid dispensing in the clinical practice of audiology, some audiologists continue to harbor mixed feelings about their role in the sale of hearing aids (Goldstein, 1984). These feelings may range from skepticism to negativism regarding the legitimate cost of an aid as compared with the level of assistance the aid provides. For example, they may ask, "Can I honestly say that my clients' best interests will be served by my selling a product having greater mark-up value than a comparable product having a lower mark-up value?" Goldstein reports that audiology textbooks and examples from clinic files suggest a highly conservative attitude toward hearing aid dispensing on the part of the audiology profession at large.

The hearing aid delivery system may be another factor contributing to the gap between the comparatively low level of hearing aid consumption and the high number of hearing-impaired individuals. Not long ago, procuring a hearing aid within the "system," that is, not through newspaper ads, flea markets, or another's discard, required one or more visits to a referring general physician, an ear specialist or otologist, an audiologist, and/or a hearing aid salesperson. In the past 15 to 20 years, this process has been streamlined and currently may involve only one or two visits. So, while all hearing aid delivery systems are not the same, the current system is not as likely to be at fault in accounting for low consumption of hearing aids as had been the case years ago. In contemporary clinical practice, it is common for hearing aid users to strive to develop a working relationship with a dispensing audiologist to ensure quick access to hearing aid replacement and repair services as the need occurs. Further testimony to this shift toward a symbiotic relationship is evidence in the failure of shopping mall "one-stop" hearing aid dispensing offices. Although this was an attempt to increase the convenience of hearing care to the general population, few of these offices have demonstrated long-term staying power (Jaquett, 1988).

Another factor cited by Goldstein (1984) is the "medical funnel" (Haggard, 1982). The purchaser of a hearing aid in the United States must first receive a medical examination from a physician (FDA, 1977). While certain conditions apply to a waiver of this examination, this occurs only after expressed admonition from the dispenser. This service delivery procedure may create a bottleneck in the flow of services to potential hearing aid users. According to Goldstein, the problem is in linking the hearing aid to medicine and illness when, in fact, fewer than 10% of all hearing problems are medically or surgically treatable (Laux, 1983), and that number may be nearer to 5% (Magielski, 1982). Again, although this is not likely to account entirely for the gap in hearing aid candidacy versus consumption, it may factor into the equation and should be acknowledged in counseling and consumer information provided to those interested in hearing loss management.

Finally, hearing aid sales practices will influence the relationship between hearing-impaired hearing aid consumers and audiologists. The hearing aid industry's response to low sales typically has been to persuade the potential consumer to purchase the aid through promises of improved products (e.g., noise reduction systems, "invisible" hearing aids), free hearing exams, and discounted prices rather than by attempting to understand the underlying motivational differences between users and nonusers. Smirga (1990) advised hearing aid dispensers to regard hearing loss as a medical problem and assume the affect of a health professional.

PARTICIPATION IN REHABILITATIVE SERVICES

Rehabilitative services may include lipreading or speechreading classes, self-help group activities, hearing aid orientation and counseling services, and more traditional clinical programs emphasizing delivery of comprehensive, long-term rehabilitative services. Although it would be difficult to estimate how many hearing-impaired individuals take advantage of one or more rehabilitative service options, the following observations apply.

Lipreading/speechreading classes are commonly offered in community senior activity centers, providing an opportunity for improved communication and adjustment to hearing loss. They are offered in an "adult education" environment that enables individuals experiencing similar communication difficulty to socialize. Enrollment typically is low, and there may be little change in group composition over long periods of time. Alternately, in a clinical setting, speech-language pathologists and audiologists incorporate speechreading training in programs concentrating on communication skill building. Participants in a clinic-based program may be more interested in optimizing their communication potential than in peer socialization. Small group sessions may be held, but it is as likely that such training will be provided on an individual basis.

Support groups centering on physical, mental, or emotional conditions and on social status have demonstrated steady growth since World War II (Levy, 1982). Such groups are known to help increase feelings of self-esteem (Yahne and Long, 1988) and social support. For the hearing-impaired person, support groups provide an opportunity to deal with consumer issues, including access to public meeting places, legislation regulating access to telephone communication, availability and use of assistive listening devices, and access to closed-captioned films and television programs. Self-help groups also provide an opportunity for peer socialization. In large cities, they may be organized as chapters of a national network or as one of a program of special services offered by a community hearing center. Perhaps the most successful, nationally based self-help group for hearing-impaired individuals is SHHH (Self-Help for the Hard of Hearing). This organization has over 225 chapters in 44 states (Anon., 1988), 19,000 dues-paying members, and a journal with a 1986 circulation of just under 50,000 (Bebout, 1986). Self-help groups provide a mechanism for transition from clinical management of hearing loss to self-management.

Hearing aid orientation, counseling services, and traditional rehabilitative service programs offered in a clinical setting (e.g., university, Veterans Administration hospital, or hearing society) typically are provided on a one-to-one basis. Participants represent a disproportionately small number of hearing clinic patrons (Marrer and Garstecki, 1985). Although the demand for these programs is constant, the overall volume of interest is low. Binnie (1977) surveyed a group of adult aural rehabilitation program participants in regard to their reaction to speechreading lessons and found that although no significant improvement was noted in performance, respondents reacted positively to information on hearing loss. They reported increased confidence in communication situations and welcomed the support they received from each other. Smaldino and Smaldino (1988) studied the effects of an aural rehabilitation program on reducing feelings of hearing handicap by first-time hearing aid users and found greater reduction in self-perception of hearing handicap by those who participated in the rehabilitation experience over those who did not participate in such a program.

Stephens and Goldstein (1983) postulated that attitude toward hearing care determines who participates in a rehabilitation program. They developed a patient rating scale that is used to classify categories of patient attitude toward rehabilitative service. The first category describes the majority of hearing-impaired adults and represents the "straightforward" case. These are individuals who are positively motivated to obtain help, may have previously had successful rehabilitative care, and probably have relatively uncomplicated hearing losses. The second category includes individuals who are positively motivated but who may have had a poor previous experience with rehabilitation, have a relatively mild hearing loss, or have found it difficult to benefit from hearing aid use. The third category consists of those who have a negative predisposition toward the rehabilitative process and use of a hearing aid. These individuals may demonstrate a shred of motivation and may move toward consid-

eration of a hearing aid by first concentrating on communication strategies and environmental aids. The final category consists of individuals with strong negative attitudes toward rehabilitation who participate solely as a result of pressure from a spouse, other family members, or associates. Many do not return for a second session. If they are fitted with a hearing aid, they are not likely to wear it. Clearly, an audiologist who is concerned with rehabilitative care must be cognizant of the fact that each individual brings a different level of motivation and interest in self-improvement to the task. When approaches to rehabilitation acknowledge different attitudes toward the process, more of those in need of such services will be likely to take advantage of them. Finally, while rehabilitative service programs are available in a variety of settings and formats, almost nothing is reported in the professional literature about the benefits of such services (ASHA Committee on Rehabilitative Audiology, 1990).

RELATED FACTORS

Age is another factor contributing to habits in hearing care. According to a Communications Omnibus survey (Anon., 1984), 77% of all respondents rated themselves as good or excellent in taking care of their health, yet 64% had not had a hearing test within the previous year. Of those over age 65 years, 67% had not had their hearing tested. Income level also is associated with attention to health care. Survey results revealed that of the respondents earning more than $40,000 annually, 33% rated themselves in excellent health compared to 15% of those earning less than $10,000. Similarly, the higher an individual's formal education, the greater the likelihood of excellent health (33% of the respondents with college degrees were reported to be in good health versus 18% of those with less than a high school diploma). While 62% reported having received one general physical and eye examination, and 69% had at least one dental checkup in the previous year, only 34% reported at least one ear or hearing exam during that time period. The 64% who had not had a recent hearing test were asked when they last had their hearing checked.

Among the responses, 10% said more than 1 but less than 2 years ago; 15% responded between 2 and 3 years ago; 58% said more than 3 years ago; and 17% said they did not recall when their hearing was last tested.

General neglect of hearing care was common in every demographic segment studied. Men and women differed only slightly in their attention to hearing tests and ear examinations. In contrast, 27% of the male respondents and 40% of the female respondents understood the potential threat to hearing posed by loud noise.

Among those age 65 and over who had not been tested in the previous year, 48% reported that their last hearing test occurred more than 3 years ago, and 29% did not recall when they were last tested. Of those age 50 to 64, 64% reported no recent hearing examination, while 35% said they had had at least one exam in the last 12 months. Of those not examined, however, 48% had not been tested for more than 3 years, and 28% did not recall when their hearing was last tested.

Respondents in the highest income group reported a significantly higher degree of attention to hearing care: 38% of those earning $30,000 to $40,000 annually were examined at least once in the previous year, and 43% of those earning more than $40,000 annually reported the same. However, only 30% of those respondents earning less than $10,000 annually reported having undergone a recent hearing exam, and 28% of those who earned $20,000 to $30,000 annually had been examined in the previous year. In contrast, 35% of those in the $10,000 to $15,000 annual income bracket had been examined, as had 39% of those who earned $15,000 to $20,000 annually. Respondents who earned less than $10,000 annually expressed the least concern about potential dangers of loud noise: 47% did not consider noise to be a serious concern, while 40% considered noise to be a potential hearing hazard.

Unlike annual income, level of education had little to do with how conscientious one was about hearing checks. Only 32% of the college graduates surveyed reported that their hearing had been examined within the previous year, compared with 38% of those with some college education and 35% of those who were high school graduates. The lowest scoring group consisted of those who had completed an eighth grade education or less, 68% of whom had no recent ear exam. Among college graduates, 30% reported they had had a hearing test within the previous 3 years. Those with the least education, eighth grade or lower, recorded the highest "don't know" percentage (33%) when asked when they last had a hearing test.

The least educated respondents also were the least concerned about potential hazards of loud noise: 49% indicated that loud noise and street noise did not present a serious threat to their hearing; 44% seriously considered the potential danger; and 7% did not have an opinion. At all other education levels, the majority of respondents indicated that noise presented a potentially serious danger to their hearing—from 57% of those with high school education to 70% of those with college degrees.

Marrer and Garstecki (1985) examined the hearing care preferences of a group of 200 older adults living in the Chicago area northern suburbs. Of this group, 65% failed a community hearing screening. Of those who failed the hearing screening, only 52% participated in follow-up lectures on self-management of problems related to hearing loss; only 40% participated in further audiologic assessment; and a mere 8% participated in hearing aid evaluations. Of the 65% who failed the hearing screening, only 25% participated in an adult aural rehabilitation program. Each of these services was made available at no cost to each participant. Overall, the result of this investigation highlighted the need to increase older adults' awareness of the need for and potential benefit from participation in hearing service programs provided in both community and clinic settings.

PERCEIVED PSYCHOLOGICAL CONTROL

It is agreed that the number of hearing-impaired individuals who use hearing aids is comparatively small and stable. The reason for this behavior can only partially be explained by the stigma associated with hearing loss, hearing aid purchase and maintenance costs, behaviors and practices of hearing care professionals, the hearing aid delivery system, and the medical funnel. None of these reasons fully accounts for the substantive discrepancy between the number of users and nonusers, and there is an astounding unmet need. Similarly, the number of individuals who participate in speechreading classes, support group activities, hearing aid orientation and counseling programs, and traditional audiologic treatment programs is unspecified but is observed to be small and stable. Also, it has been demonstrated that some hearing-impaired older adults lack information regarding hearing assessment, hearing loss prevention, personal impact of hearing loss, and treatment of problems related to hearing loss. The older the individual, the more likely this condition will apply. Hearing care is generally neglected among older adults of average income, yet is not as likely to be neglected by those with higher income. Level of education does not correlate closely with hearing care. Finally, there is evidence of diminishing interest in hearing service as an individual progresses along the chain of audiologic service options.

The term "psychological control" refers to how individuals experience and regulate their behavior in terms of reasons and causes for action and consequences of action. Rotter (1966) applied social learning theory to the study of perception in developing the concept of locus of control. Locus of control refers to whether or not one perceives a causal relationship between a given behavior and a reward. When a person perceives an event to be contingent on personal behavior or relatively permanent personal characteristics, locus of control is internal. When an event is considered to be the result of luck, chance, fate, under the control of others, or unpredictable, locus of control is external. Any personal event can be perceived as primarily externally or internally controlled. A clear and positive relationship between a tendency toward internal locus of control and life satisfaction (Kuypers, 1972; Mancini, 1980; Palmore & Luikart, 1972; Schulz, 1976), physical health (Mancini, 1980; Rodin & Langer, 1977), and happiness (Schulz, 1976) has been reported in psychology literature.

Perception of control is demonstrated by the physically ill. Janis and Rodin (1979) reported that the sensations and experiences encountered by ill individuals may be unfamiliar and frightening. Their ability to regulate physiological processes may be threatened (Brody, 1980). In addition, these individuals may be threatened by their relationship with their physician. They may be made to feel that they do not have the competency to deal with their condition alone. Patients may feel they are in a "one-down" position in relation to the medical practitioner.

Locus of control has received limited attention in literature on communication disorders. Dowaliby, Burke, and McKnee (1983) modified the Rotter (1966) scale for use with college freshmen and found that deaf students were substantially more external in their locus of control than hearing freshmen. Similar findings were reported in an earlier study of deaf and normal hearing college students (Bodner & Johns, 1977). Locus of control has been examined in stutterers (Craig, Franklin, & Andrews, 1985; Madison, Budd, & Itzkowitz, 1986). Those who moved toward internality of control were judged more likely to maintain improvement in their fluency over time. Shrilberg et al. (1977) examined locus of control in communication disorders majors and found that students who were more internal in their locus of control were rated as better clinicians. Learning-disabled populations have been reported to have more external locus of control (Hallahan et al., 1978), and blind individuals have been found to have more external orientation than sighted individuals (Land & Vineberg, 1965). Luterman (1991) stated that the finding of external locus of control in disabled populations is not surprising when one sees how professionals tend to interact with the disabled. It is not uncommon to see professionals who are routinely rescuing their clients. In doing so, the clinician makes the client feel even more externally controlled.

Aging individuals would appear to be particularly vulnerable to the processes described above. First, as a function of age, older adults are exposed to various social and personal conditions that are a challenge to their sense of personal control (e.g., retirement, bereavement, separation from family, relocation, decreased mobility, greater dependence on others, loss of spouse, reduced physical strength and vigor, possible institutionalization). Second, older individuals undergo physiological changes as a function of aging that make them more vulnerable to the effects of general loss of control (e.g., immune system depression, decline in metabolism of adrenocortical hormones, increase in chronic illness, and increase in memory loss). Aging individuals with hearing loss would appear to be at even greater risk for loss of control than others in that their condition does not enable them to communicate efficiently with others in attempting to deal with life changes and manage problems relating to overall physiological deterioration. Hearing loss may exacerbate the problems related to personal control and physiological change.

Four studies are particularly noteworthy for having considered the relationship between locus of control and hearing loss. Hunter et al. (1980) found that an individual's self-perceived ability to hear discriminated significantly between internally and externally oriented groups. Subjects with poorer self-perceived hearing ability were more likely to be external in their perceived locus of control. A second study reported by McDavis (1983–1984) hypothesized that the amount of control individuals feel they have over their life, health, and hearing loss would affect their denial levels. McDavis predicted that internally controlled individuals would be more likely to deny their hearing loss than externally controlled individuals. However, only the results on one of the items in the control measure were significantly correlated with amount of denial. In a third study, Kuller (1976) found no significant relation between locus of control and self-perceived hearing handicap in institutionalized aging individuals. There is some indication that institutionalized aging adults, as a group, demonstrate more external locus of control than their noninstitutionalized counterparts. Kuller made the point that there may have been a different relationship between hearing handicap and locus of control if the subjects had been noninstitutionalized. In the fourth study, Garstecki et al. (1989) found that responses to selected items from the Communication Profile for the Hearing Impaired (Demorest & Erdman, 1987) can be used to predict a hearing-impaired adult's locus of control. Two groups of subjects, one containing 19 adults age 29 to 85 years demonstrating moderate to profound hearing loss and another consisting of 20 adults ranging in age from 65 to 79 years with normal hearing, were examined. The hearing-impaired group members perceived themselves to be moderately handicapped by problems relating to hearing loss and in control over factors in their environment at a level of only half of what was desired. The group with age-appropriate hearing did not experience communication difficulty relating to hearing, nor did they consider themselves to be hearing impaired. Members of this group regarded themselves to be more in control of environmental influence on their lives than the hearing-impaired group but in less than optimal control. The results of this study suggested that hearing handicap, as currently understood, may be explained, at least in part, by an individual's global locus of control.

Indeed, for hearing-impaired aging adults, there appear to be multiple advantages in developing a sense of control over their everyday world. The implications for rehabilitative audiologists are clear. Concerted effort needs to be directed toward educating society at large and hearing-impaired older adults in particular, in understanding hearing and hearing loss, in preventing hearing loss, and in compensating for hearing loss through hearing aids, assistive devices, and rehabilitative services. Understanding hearing loss paves the way for self-management of problems associated with hearing loss and potentially helps restore control in communication and life events by those with hearing disability.

Americans with Disabilities Act of 1990

BACKGROUND AND LEGISLATIVE HISTORY

Physical and mental disabilities affect not only those so afflicted and their families but also all of society. For example, consider the fact that disabled individuals participate in the work force at a rate *half* that of nondisabled individuals, according to the President's Committee on Employment of People with Disabilities (Goozner, 1990).

In 1987, the Social Security system paid $28.2 billion to 5.7 million unemployed disabled individuals (Goozner, 1990). And, a 1986 Harris Poll (Bebout, 1990) revealed that approximately two-thirds of the disabled population is *not* employed when two-thirds of that group *wants* to be employed. The chief reason for nonemployment was employer bias. Clearly, the need to address and eliminate discrimination against individuals with disabilities is not only a matter of civil responsibility and timeliness but also a matter of increasing fiscal concern.

To address this matter, former President Ronald Reagan's National Council on Disability drafted the bill that was to become the Americans with Disabilities Act (ADA). The ADA was to provide a national mandate for the elimination of discrimination against individuals with disabilities. In this law, an "individual with a disability" was defined as someone who *(1)* has a physical or mental impairment that substantially limits one or more major life activities, *(2)* has a record of such an impairment, or *(3)* is regarded as having such an impairment (Rovner, 1990). The ADA, in effect, was expected to serve as an enforceable standard for addressing discrimination. It was to ensure the central role of the federal government in its enforcement, and it would invoke congressional authority in addressing major areas of discrimination. The ADA was to guarantee equal opportunity for individuals with disabilities in employment, public accommodations, transportation, state and local government services, and telecommunications (Brotmon 1991).

COMPONENTS OF THE AMERICANS WITH DISABILITIES ACT

To understand how hearing-disabled individuals may potentially benefit from this law and how rehabilitative audiologists might assist in its implementation, each of the five components (Titles) of the ADA is described below.

Title I: Employment

The intent of Title I is to protect qualified individuals with disabilities from discrimination in all aspects of employment from the point of job application through hiring, job orientation, advancement, and dismissal (Rovner, 1990). An individual is deemed to be qualified for any job in which the essential job functions can be performed, with or without special accommodation. Job functions are those duties and responsibilities specified by a potential employer prior to initiating job advertisement and applicant interviews.

Under provisions of Title I, employers may ask about a job applicant's ability to perform job tasks, but employers cannot rightfully inquire if an applicant has a disability or attempt to screen out individuals with disabilities in the employee selection process. For example, employers may not ask if an applicant has a hearing impairment, but they may ask if an applicant can efficiently manage interpersonal or telephone communication. Employers are expected to provide "reasonable accommodation" to individuals with disabilities. This may involve making existing facilities and/or equipment accessible and usable. A hearing-disabled individual may require a telephone amplifier, interpreter, or visual alerting signals, for example. Reasonable accommodation also applies to job restructuring and work schedule modification. Employers do not need to provide accommodations that impose an "undue hardship" or significant difficulty or expense on their business operation.

Regulations governing compliance with Title I were prepared by the Equal Employment Opportunity Commission (EEOC) and published in the *Federal Register* on July 26, 1991. In these regulations, hearing loss is listed as a potentially disabling physical impairment. An individual with hearing loss is regarded as having a physical impairment, regardless of mitigating measures such as use of hearing aids or assistive listening devices. However, a hearing-impaired individual is not regarded as *disabled* until it is determined that hearing loss substantially limits one or more major life activities. For example, if hearing loss precludes efficient telephone communication, it limits a major life activity and must be regarded as disabling. If telephone communication can occur efficiently and accurately with use of hearing aids and telephone amplifiers or decoders, hearing loss does not limit a major life activity and is not regarded as disabling.

Determining whether an individual with a hearing disability qualifies for special consideration under the law is a two-step process. First, a judgment is made in regard to the individual's qualifications for meeting job requirements. The first step is an employer–job applicant concern. The second step is to determine whether the individual can perform the essential functions of a job with or without special accommodation. The second step may require consultation between the owner or operator of a public entity and an audiologist or noise specialist in resolving problems created by noise conditions in a work area. Besides addressing noise damping and attenuation concerns, consideration may need to be given to modification of work schedules, use of interpreters, selection and use of assistive devices (including personal and group amplifiers), selection and use of visual alerting and warning systems, and selection and use of amplified telephones or telephone message decoding systems. The audiologist may also need to be involved in demonstrating to a potential employer how a hearing-impaired job candidate is able to perform essential job functions with or without any of the above assistive devices and services.

Complaints against those failing to comply with Title I regulations of the ADA may be filed with the EEOC and by private lawsuit. In response, employers may be ordered to hire or promote qualified individuals, accommodate these individuals on the job, and pay back wages and attorney's fees. These are the same remedies as are available under Title VII of the Civil Rights Act of 1964 (Equal Employment Opportunity Commission, 1991).

Title II: Public Services

Under Title II, new buildings and alterations to existing buildings must allow for accessibility by individuals with disabilities, effective January 26, 1992 (Department of Justice, 1991a). The Attorney General's office issued relevant regulations on July 26, 1991. Individuals who believe that their rights have been withheld, ignored, or violated may file complaints with federal agencies designated by the Attorney General and/or file a private lawsuit to enforce this regulation. The court may order that facilities be made accessible, provide auxiliary aids or services, modify policies and pay attorney's fees. These remedies are the same as those available under Section 505 of the Rehabilitation Act of 1973 (Department of Justice, 1991a).

In addition, under Title II, new public transit buses and rail cars ordered after August 26, 1990 must be accessible by individuals with disabilities. Existing rail systems must have one accessible car per train by July 26, 1995. Key stations in rapid, light, and commuter rail systems must be made accessible by July 23, 1993. Commuter rail systems may receive an extension of up to 20 years to comply with this regulation, and rapid and light rail systems may receive up to a 30-year extension. Special transportation services must be provided to those who cannot used fixed route bus services, unless an undue burden would result. Finally, all existing Amtrak stations must be accessible by July 26, 2010 (Department of Justice, 1991a).

The Department of Justice published regulations for implementing Title II in the July 26, 1991 issue of the *Federal Register*. However, since Title II applies to state and local governments and most programs and activities of state and local governments are assisted by federal funding agencies, discrimination on the basis of physical or mental handicap is already prohibited by Section 504 of the Rehabilitation Act of 1973 (Department of Justice, 1991a).

Title II guarantees that auxiliary aids and services will be made available to ensure communication access. These include videotext displays that provide a means of accessing auditory information through public address systems, transcription services to relay aurally delivered material in written form, and closed and open captioning for relay of televised messages. Other aids and services include interpreters, notetakers, written materials, telephone handset amplifiers, assistive listening devices, hearing aid compatible telephones, and telephone devices for deaf persons (TDDs). The rehabilitative audiologist has a vital role to play in selection, fitting, and orienting others in the use of devices to accommodate individuals with hearing disability.

In public hearings held during the drafting of Title II regulations, requests were made to include a guarantee of currency of auxiliary aids and services, a statement to ensure that new and emerging services and technological advances would be made available to qualified individuals. The Department of Justice declined to incorporate this request in its definition of auxiliary aids and services, indicating that public entities are not obliged to provide "state of the art" devices or services, only devices and services that afford effective communication—that is, devices and services that would make aurally and visually delivered information available to persons with hearing, speech, and vision impairments (Department of Justice, 1991a).

Although provision of auxiliary aids and services is required under Title II, it is not required that aids and services be provided to qualified disabled individuals for private or personal use. That is, the law does not require provision of prescription sunglasses or hearing aids, for example, which are considered to be personal aids. However, this does not preclude loan of personal receivers that may be part of an assistive listening system, for example. It also is the case that individuals with disabilities must be allowed to request auxiliary aids and services of their choice. By allowing freedom of choice, the disabled individual may determine which of the range of available devices would work best in a given communication circumstance. For example, in some lecture hall situations an amplifying device will be of benefit to some hearing-impaired individuals, whereas others may require use of a sign language interpreter. Under Title II, consideration is given to provision of interpreting services and, accordingly, a qualified interpreter is defined as someone who is able to interpret effectively, accurately, and impartially both receptively and expressively, using any necessary specialized vocabulary. Rehabilitative audiologists will have responsibility for educating hearing-impaired individuals in the selection and use of alternative devices and possibly advising in the selection of qualified interpreters. The reader is referred to Chapter 16 for a thorough discussion of assistive devices.

Despite requests to replace the term "telecommunication device for deaf persons (TDD)," with the term "text telephone (TT)," the Department of Justice declined to do so on the basis that it would be inconsistent with the Federal Communications Commission's (FCC) use of the term "TDD" in final regulations for implementing Title IV of the ADA (Department of Justice, 1991a). The FCC, however, decided to use the term "text telephone (TT)" in place of TDD, so there is a slight discrepancy in terminology between Title II and Title IV in reference to this system (Federal Communications Commission, 1991). The term "text telephone (TT)" will be used in place of TDD in the remainder of this chapter to refer to graphic telephone communication systems.

When a public entity communicates with individuals by telephone, TTs or equally effective telecommunication systems must be available for hearing- or speech-disabled individuals. A problem occurs when one party in a telephone communication does not have a TT. Title IV addresses this concern through use of a relay operator (termed "communication assistant [CA]" in the final regulation), who would use both a standard telephone and a TT to type voice messages to the TT user and read TT messages to the standard telephone user. The Department of Justice received many comments regarding the inefficiencies of such a relay system. In addition, they received complaints concerning the inability of a TT user to access automated systems that require a caller to respond by pushing buttons on a touch tone phone. Also, CAs cannot act fast enough to convey messages on answering machines, and they are not permitted to leave recorded messages. Finally, communication through a relay system may not be appropriate in crisis situations, such as in instances of reporting violent crime or health emergencies. Where the intent of Title II is to ensure access to telephone emergency service (i.e., 911 calls), which may be accomplished using a relay system, the final rule mandates direct caller access. Access through a third party or through a relay service does not satisfy this requirement. (It is interesting to note that the Department of Justice encourages use of speech amplification devices for use in the event that a hearing-disabled individual does not have a telephone amplifier, suggesting a basic lack of understanding of the nature of hearing loss and how best to compensate for hearing loss in telephone communication.) These problems were referred to the FCC to be addressed under Title IV (Department of Justice, 1991a). However, as part of a comprehensive program of hearing care, rehabilitative audiologists will want to educate hearing-impaired individuals in optimizing their use of available relay services and telephone technology.

Individuals may file complaints concerning Title II with the Attorney General, by private lawsuit, or with any of the following federal agencies: Department of Agriculture for complaints regarding programs, services, and regulatory activities relating to farming; Department of Education for concerns relating to elementary and secondary education, institutions of higher education and vocational education, and libraries; Department of Health and Human Services for concerns relating to health care and social services, including schools of medicine, dentistry, nursing, and other health-related schools; Department of Housing and Urban Development for concerns relating to state and local public housing; Department of Interior for concerns relating to lands and natural resources, including historic buildings; Department of Justice for concerns relating to law enforcement, public safety, commerce and industry, planning and development, state and local government support services, and all government functions not assigned to other designated agencies; Department of Labor for concerns relating to labor and the work force; Department of Transportation for concerns relating to transportation. The remedies for complaints levied against those in noncompliance with Title II are the same as those available under Section 505 of the Rehabilitation Act of 1973 (Department of Justice, 1991a).

Title III: Public Accommodations

This section of the ADA ensures nondiscrimination toward individuals with disabilities in the full and equal enjoyment of goods, services, facilities, privileges, advantages, and accommodations of any public entity as of January 26, 1992 (Department of Justice, 1991b). Auxiliary aids and services must be provided to individuals with vision or hearing impairments and other individuals with disabilities, unless undue burden would result. In determining level of burden, the nature and cost of required action, overall financial resources of the facility, overall size of the business, and number, type, and location of facilities are considered.

The Department of Justice published Title III regulations in the *Federal Register* on July 26, 1991. Rehabilitative audiologists involved in implementing Title III regulations will need to consider the types of assistive devices and audiologic services that would guarantee access to the following types of facilities listed under the rubric of Title III (Department of Justice, 1991b):

1. Places of lodging (e.g., inn, motel, hotel)
2. Establishments serving food or drink (e.g., restaurant, bar)
3. Places of exhibition or entertainment (e.g., motion picture house, theater, concert hall, stadium)
4. Places of public gathering (e.g., auditorium, convention center, lecture hall)
5. Sales or rental establishments (e.g., bakery, grocery store, clothing store, hardware store, shopping center)
6. Service establishments (e.g., laundromat, dry-cleaner, bank, barber shop, beauty shop, travel service, shoe repair service, funeral parlor, gas station, office of an accountant or lawyer, pharmacy, insurance office, professional office of a health care provider, hospital)
7. Stations used for specified public transportation (e.g., terminal, depot)
8. Places of public display or collection (e.g., museum, library, gallery)
9. Places of recreation (e.g., park, zoo, amusement park)
10. Places of education (e.g., nursery, elementary, secondary, undergraduate, or postgraduate private school)
11. Social service center establishments (e.g., day care center, senior citizen

center, homeless shelter, food bank, adoption agency)
12. Places of exercise or recreation (e.g., gymnasium, health spa, bowling alley, golf course)

In public accommodations equipped with audible emergency alarms, the alarm signal must exceed the prevailing sound in an area by 15 dBA, or it must exceed the maximum sound typically occurring in an area by 5 dBA with a duration of 60 seconds. Audible alarms having a periodic element to their signal such as single-stroke bells (clang-pause-clang-pause), high-low (up-down-up-down), or fast whoop (on-off-on-off) are easiest for a hearing-impaired person to detect. Continuous and reverberant alarm signals should be avoided (United States Architectural & Transportation Barriers Compliance Board, 1991).

Public accommodations are required to modify policies, practices, and procedures to allow the use of "service animals." A service animal is any guide dog or other animal trained to provide assistance to an individual with a disability. A hearing ear dog is an example of a service animal that will need to be accommodated in public entities visited by hearing-disabled individuals. Other examples include animals used to guide individuals with impaired vision, provide protection or conduct rescue work, pull a wheelchair, or fetch dropped items. If a restaurant tenant of a building refuses to accommodate a disabled person with a service animal, the restaurant can be held responsible. If a restaurant tenant refuses to modify its landlord's "no pets" policy, then both the tenant and the landlord are liable for violation of Title III of the ADA. Finally, it is the disabled individual's responsibility to supervise or care for any service animal (Department of Justice, 1991b).

Under Title III, telephones must be hearing aid compatible. Telephone amplifier volume controls must allow for a minimum signal intensity increase of 12 dBA and a maximum increase of 18 dBA. If an automatic volume control reset feature is provided, the 18-dBA limit may be exceeded. Telephones must have push-button controls where such service is available. Tele-

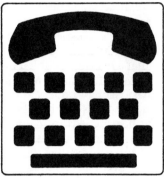

Figure 2.1. International TDD symbol. (U.S. Architectural & Transportation Barriers Compliance Board. Americans with Disabilities Act [ADA]: accessibility guidelines for buildings and facilities. *Federal Register*, 56, 144, July 26, 35512 [1991].)

phones equipped with amplifiers must be identified by a sign containing a depiction of a telephone handset with radiating sound waves. Text telephones (TTs) used along with pay telephones must be permanently affixed to the telephone enclosure. TTs are required to be identified by the international TDD symbol (see Fig. 2.1). In addition, signage indicating the location of a public TT must be placed adjacent to banks of telephones that do not contain a TT (United States Architectural & Transportation Barriers Compliance Board, 1991).

Places of lodging and hospitals providing televisions in five or more guest rooms are required to provide a television program decoding device for hearing-disabled individuals. Hotels should also provide a TT at the front desk to take calls from guests who use TTs in their room. Hotels providing 1 to 25 sleeping rooms must equip a minimum of one room with devices for hearing-disabled individuals (i.e., visual alarms, notification devices, amplified or text telephones); with 26 to 50 sleeping rooms, two rooms must be accessible; with 101 to 150 rooms, five rooms must be accessible; and, with 501 to 1000, 2% of the total must be accessible. Visual alarms should be located and oriented so that they spread signals and reflections throughout a space or raise overall light level sharply. Visual alarms are not the best means to alert sleepers. A flashing light seven times brighter than required to alert awake individuals in normal daylight is required to wake a sleeper. For sleepers, a sound-activated mattress/box spring vi-

Figure 2.2. International symbol of access for hearing loss. (U.S. Architectural & Transportation Barriers Compliance Board. Americans with Disabilities Act [ADA]: accessibility guidelines for buildings and facilities. *Federal Register*, 56, 144, July 26, 35512 [1991].)

brator is more effective than a visual system. Sound-activated devices respond to alarm clocks, clock radios, wake-up calls and smoke detectors. Remote light control systems also provide an effective means of transmitting warning signals through an existing electrical power line (United States Architectural & Transportation Barriers Compliance Board, 1991).

Title III also ensures that no individual with a disability is discriminated against because of absence of auxiliary aids and services unless it can be demonstrated that taking such steps would alter the nature of the accommodations being offered or result in undue hardship. The type of aid that would be appropriate for a particular application depends on the characteristics of the setting. For example, if a listening system is to serve individuals in fixed seating, seats must be located within a 50-foot viewing distance of a target area. In areas where permanently installed assistive listening systems are required, the availability of such systems must be identified with signage that includes the international symbol of access for hearing loss (see Fig. 2.2). Appropriate messages may include (United States Architectural & Transportation Barriers Compliance Board, 1991):

INFRARED ASSISTIVE LISTENING
  SYSTEM AVAILABLE—PLEASE ASK;
AUDIO LOOP IN USE, TURN T-SWITCH
  FOR BETTER HEARING—OR ASK
  FOR HELP;

FM ASSISTIVE LISTENING SYSTEM
  AVAILABLE—PLEASE ASK.

Assistive listening devices should be permanently installed at all sales and service counters, teller windows, box offices, and information kiosks where a physical barrier separates service personnel and customers. Some advantages, disadvantages, and applications of alternative assistive listening systems include the following:

Induction loop system.
  Advantages
    Cost-effective; low maintenance; ease of use; unobtrusive; may integrate into existing public address system; some hearing aids function as receivers.
  Disadvantages
    Signal spillover from adjacent rooms; electrical interference; limited portability; inconsistent signal strength; lack of standards for induction coil performance.
  Applications
    Meeting areas; theaters; religious meeting halls; conference rooms; classrooms; television viewing areas.

FM system.
  Advantages
    Highly portable; multiple channels for multiple group usage in single room; high user mobility; accommodates wide range of hearing loss.
  Disadvantages
    High cost of receivers; lack of equipment durability; obtrusive; high maintenance (incidence and cost); custom fitting may be required.
  Applications
    Classrooms; tour groups; meeting areas; outdoor events; one-on-one communication.

Infrared system
  Advantages
    Ease of use; ensures privacy; moderate cost; can be integrated into existing public address system.
  Disadvantages
    Line of sight required between emitter and receiver; ineffective outdoors; limited portability; requires installation.
  Applications
    Theaters; religious meeting halls; auditoriums; meetings requiring confidentiality; television viewing.

Complaints concerning Title III ensurances may be filed with the Attorney General and by private lawsuit. Remedies are the same as available under Title II of the Civil Rights Act of 1964. In remedying concerns under Title III, the court may order that facilities be made accessible, auxiliary aids or services be provided, policies be modified, and attorney's fees be paid (Department of Justice, 1991b).

Title IV: Telecommunications Relays

Title IV of the ADA amends Title II of the Communications Act of 1934 by making available to all individuals in the United States a rapid, efficient communication service. Under Title IV, the Federal Communications Commission (FCC) ensures that inter- and intrastate telecommunications relay services (TRS) are available. Telecommunications relay services are transmission services that enable a speech- or hearing-impaired individual to communicate by wire or radio with a hearing individual in a manner functionally equivalent to that of someone without a speech or hearing impairment.

Title IV requires that the FCC's regulations become effective by July 26, 1993. These regulations, published on August 1, 1991 in the *Federal Register*, address operational standards that may be summarized as follows:

1. Telecommunications relay system providers are responsible for supplying communications assistants (CAs) who are trained to meet the specialized needs of individuals with speech or hearing disability. The CA must demonstrate skill in typing, English grammar usage, spelling, interpretation of typewritten American Sign Language (ASL), and familiarity with the culture, language, and etiquette of speech- and hearing-disabled individuals.
2. CAs are prohibited from disclosing the content of any relayed conversation and from keeping records of the conversation beyond the duration of a telephone call. They may not intentionally alter a message and must relay all messages verbatim, unless the relay user requests a summarized message.

3. CAs are prohibited from refusing single or sequential calls or limiting the length of calls using a relay service. The relay system must be capable of handling any type of call normally provided by common carriers. If credit authorization is denied, CAs are permitted not to complete a call. Emergency calls must be handled in the same manner as other calls.

Finally, the FCC developed a set of functional standards, which are summarized below:

1. The FCC will resolve any complaint alleging a violation within 180 days of it being filed.
2. TRS carriers will publicize the availability of their services.
3. TRS users will pay rates no greater than rates paid for functionally equivalent voice communication services.
4. Costs caused by interstate TRS will be recovered from subscriber fees. Costs caused by intrastate TRS providers will be recovered from the intrastate jurisdiction.
5. Complaints will be handled by the state in which the problem occurred and/or by the FCC.

Under Title IV, the FCC is required to issue regulations governing jurisdictional separation of costs of such services and to resolve complaints alleging violations within 180 days of when the complaint is filed (Federal Communications Commission, 1991).

Title V: Miscellaneous

This section ensures that the rights and protections provided by the ADA, the Civil Rights Act of 1964, the Age Discrimination in Employment Act of 1967, and the Rehabilitation Act of 1973 will apply to members of the Senate, House of Representatives, and all offices of Congress. It provides whistleblower protection in regard to reporting discriminatory practices. It requires the Architectural and Transportation Barriers Compliance Board to issue guidelines to further ensure accessibility by individuals with disabilities. Title V addresses issues relating to alteration of historic buildings, payment of attorneys' fees, provision of technical assistance from various other agencies, wilderness land management practices, illegal drug usage, and alternative means of dispute resolution (Rovner, 1990).

Summary

The relationship between rehabilitative audiologists and hearing-impaired persons can be summarized by answering three interrelated questions.

First, what is the current relationship? At present, rehabilitative audiologists provide a range of clinical services focusing on the selection, fitting, and use of hearing aids. In clinical practice, it is apparent that successful hearing aid use obviates the need for other types of rehabilitative services. However, on the average, fewer than one out of five hearing-impaired persons who might benefit from hearing aid use wear hearing aids. Reasons for this low take-up rate have been suggested, but none is conclusive in and of itself. Similarly, a variety of rehabilitative services are available to hearing-impaired individuals, yet relatively few individuals seek these services of their own volition. While client testimony supports rehabilitative service, true benefits in terms of measured improvement in communication efficiency, for example, remain to be documented in the professional literature. The relationship between rehabilitative audiologists and hearing-impaired persons is a long way from reaching its maximum potential, both in terms of volume and in terms of scope of professional practice.

Second, what ought to be the relationship? Hearing-impaired persons ought to consider rehabilitative audiologists as important resources for all information regarding management of hearing loss. They ought to avail themselves of the audiologist's professional knowledge and skill. Hearing-impaired persons should use the resources of the audiologist to learn how to compensate for hearing loss and overcome any of its related problems. Audiologists ought to be regarded as champions of the hearing-impaired person's cause.

In turn, audiologists need to take an eclectic view toward their professional relationship with hearing-impaired individu-

als. They must broaden their scope of practice and individualize their approach in addressing a potentially wide range of rehabilitative needs. Finally, audiologists must tailor their treatment approach to fit the life-style interests and needs of those they purport to serve.

How can the gap between what the current relationship is and what it ought to be be closed? In part, the gap will close as involved parties realize the benefits of a symbiotic relationship. For some, federal legislation will foster new relationships. In all, the following must be considered:

1. The number of hearing aid users must increase to be more in parity with the estimated number of hearing-impaired individuals. Efforts will need to be directed toward more effective public education of potential hearing aid consumers in regard to the benefits of hearing aid use. Audiologists must be aware of the differential impact of acquired hearing loss on an individual by age at onset, tendency toward health care management, and personal reaction to wearing a hearing aid. Audiologists must consider how to make hearing aids more acceptable to hearing-impaired persons. They also need to consider how to make the acquisition of a hearing aid affordable to those on fixed or low incomes. They must examine their own attitude toward comprehensive hearing care and be cognizant of the image they present to those seeking audiologic service. Audiologists must work to widen the medical funnel and educate others in understanding the difference between hearing loss as a medical problem and hearing loss as an irreversible human condition.
2. The number of hearing-impaired individuals who take advantage of available rehabilitative service programs must increase. Efforts will need to be directed toward determining treatment efficacy of various service options, educating potential consumers in the advantages and disadvantages of service options, and effectively marketing rehabilitative services. Rehabilitation programs must be affordable yet cost-effective.
3. The general public should have improved understanding of hearing and

hearing loss, prevention of hearing loss, the impact of hearing loss on communication, and the various treatments available for hearing loss, including hearing aids. Efforts will need to be directed toward educating older adults and their families in regard to the above. The benefits of routine hearing examinations and noise abatement need to be publicized among individuals in all age, education, and income brackets.

4. Better understanding of the psychological factors influencing behavior in self-management of hearing loss is needed. Why is it that some people take advantage of opportunities to overcome hearing problems and others (the large majority) choose to ignore available aids and services? Consideration should be given to study of perceived psychological control as a basis for behavioral difference in self-management of hearing loss.

5. Implementation of the ADA will extend the scope of audiologic practice well outside the confines of hearing clinics and well beyond compensation for hearing loss through use of hearing aids. It will become increasingly more common for audiologists to carry their practice to the community at large, interacting with engineers, architects, transit authority officials, potential employers of hearing-disabled individuals, assistive device manufacturers and distributors, telecommunication service representatives, proprietors of businesses serving individuals with hearing disability, and attorneys. It also is likely that with implementation of the ADA, audiologists will assume the responsibility of "case worker" in championing the rights of hearing-disabled individuals in the workplace.

In conclusion, rich and exciting challenges and opportunities lay ahead for the relationship between rehabilitative audiologists and hearing-impaired persons in co-management of hearing loss. The remainder of this text provides information that will help make these challenges and opportunities a reality.

References

Anon., American hearing health habits & attitudes. *Hearing J.*, December, 13–19 (1984).

Anon., SHHH and hearing access 2000. *Hearing Instruments*, **39**, 34 (1988).

ASHA Committee on Rehabilitative Audiology, Aural rehabilitation: Thoughts and challenges. *J. Speech-Language-Hearing Assoc.*, **32**, 49 (1990).

Barcham, L.J., and Stephens, S.D.G., The use of an open-ended problem questionnaire in auditory rehabilitation. *Br. J. Audiol.*, **14**, 49–54 (1980).

Bebout, J.M., Hearing health consumerism: Advocacy groups in the 80s. *Hearing J.*, April, 7–11 (1986).

Bebout, J.M., The Americans with Disabilities Act: American dream achieved for the hearing impaired? *Hearing J.*, **43**, 11–19 (1990).

Bevan, M.A., The effects of hearing aids on interpersonal perceptions: credibility, employability, and interpersonal attraction. Ph.D. dissertation, University of Connecticut (1981).

Binnie, C.A., Attitude changes following speechreading training. *Scandinavian Audiol.*, **6**, 13–19 (1977).

Blood, G.W., Blood, I.M., and Danhauer, J.L., Listeners' impressions of normal-hearing and hearing-impaired children. *J. Communication Disorders*, **11**, 513–518 (1978).

Bodner, B., and Johns, J., Personality and hearing impairment: a study in locus of control. *Volta Rev.*, **79**, 362–368 (1977).

Brody, D.S., Psychological distress and hypertension control. *J. Human Stress*, **6**, 2–6 (1980).

Brotman, S.N., *Extending Telecommunications Service to Americans with Disabilities: A Report on Telecommunications Services Mandated Under the Americans with Disabilities Act of 1990*. Washington: The Annenberg Washington Program in Communications Policy Studies of Northwestern University (1991).

Craig, A., Franklin, J.G., and Andrews, J., The prediction and prevention of relapse in stuttering. *J. Behav. Modification*, **9**, 422–442 (1985).

Demorest, M.E., and Erdman, S.A., Development of the Communication Profile for the Hearing Impaired. *J. Speech Hear. Dis.*, **52**, 129–143 (1987).

Department of Justice (DOJ), 28 CFR Part 35, Nondiscrimination on the basis of disability in state and local government services; final rule. *Federal Register*, **56**, 144, July 26, 35694–35723 (1991a).

Department of Justice (DOJ), 28 CFR Part 36, Nondiscrimination on the basis of disability by public accommodations and in commercial facilities; final rule. *Federal Register*, **56**, 144, July 26, 35544–35604 (1991b).

Dowaliby, F., Burke, N., and McKee, B., A comparison of hearing impaired and normally hearing students on locus of control, people orientation and study habits and attitudes. *Am. Ann. Deaf*, **128**, 53–59 (1983).

Equal Employment Opportunity Commission (EEOC), 29 CFR Part 1630, Equal employment opportunity for individuals with disabilities; final rule. *Federal Register*, **56**, 144, July 26, 35726–35755 (1991).

Federal Communications Commission (FCC), 47 CFR Parts 0 and 64, Telecommunications services for hearing and speech disabled; final rule. *Federal Register*, **56**, 148, August 1, 36729–36733 (1991).

Food and Drug Administration (FDA), Hearing aid devices—professional and patient labeling and conditions for sale. *Federal Register*, **42**, February 15, 9286–9296 (1977).

Franks, J.R., and Beckmann, N.J., Rejection of hearing aids: attitudes of a geriatric sample. *Ear Hear.*, **6**, 161–166 (1985).

Gallup, F., *A Survey Concerning Hearing Problems and Hearing Aids in the United States*. Washington: Hearing Industries Association (1980).

Garstecki, D., Kobrin, M., Erler, S., and Palmer, C., Predicting locus of control using selected items from the Communication Profile for the Hearing Impaired. Academy of Rehabilitative Audiology Summer Institute, Austin, TX (1989).

Goldstein, D.P., Hearing impairment, hearing aids, and audiology. *J. Am. Speech-Language-Hearing Assoc.*, **9**, 24–35, 38 (1984).

Goozner, M., Workplace doors opening to disabled. *Chicago Tribune Business Section*, July 22 edition, 1–2 (1990).

Haggard, M.P., What should be done about hearing impairment? *J. Royal Soc. Med.*, **75**, 211–212 (1982).

Hallahan, P., Gasar, A., Cohen, S., and Tarver, S., Selective attention and locus of control in learning disabled and normal children. *J. Learn. Dis.*, **11**, 47–57 (1978).

Humphrey, C., Herbst, K.G., and Faurqui, S., Some characteristics of the hearing impaired elderly who do not present themselves for rehabilitation. *Br. J. Audiol.*, **15**, 25–30 (1981).

Hunter, K., Linn, M., Harris, R., and Pratt, T., Discriminators of internal and external locus of control orientation in the elderly. *Res. Aging*, **2**, 49–60 (1980).

Janis, I.L., and Rodin, J., Attribution control and decision making: social psychology and health care. In G.C. Stone, F. Cohen, and N.E. Adler (Eds.), *Health Psychology*. San Francisco: Jossey-Bass (1979).

Jaquett, Z., The graying of America: a new dimension in hearing impairment. *Hear. Instruments*, **39**, 24–25 (1988).

Karchmer, M., and Kirwin, L., *The Use of Hearing Aids by Hearing-Impaired Children in the United States*, **5**, 2. Washington: Gallaudet College Office of Demographic Studies (1977).

Kochkin, S., MarkeTrak II: more MDs give hearing tests, yet hearing aid sales remain flat. *Hearing J.*, **44**, 24–35 (1991).

Kuller, J., The relationships among self-assessment of hearing handicap, locus of control, and audiologic measures of hearing impairment in presbycusic individuals. Ph.D. dissertation, New York University (1976).

Kuypers, J.A., Internal-external locus of control, ego functioning, and personality characteristics in old age. *Gerontologist*, **1**, 168–173 (1972).

Land, S.L., and Vineberg, S.E., Locus of control in blind children. *Exceptional Child*, **31**, 257–263 (1965).

Lass, N.J., Speech-language pathologists' knowledge of, exposure to, and attitudes toward hearing aids and hearing aid wearers. *Lang. Speech Hear. Serv. Schools*, **20**, 115–132 (1989).

Laux, D.M., What's in a name? *Hearing J.*, **36**, 4 (1983).

Levy, L., Mutual support groups in Great Britain: a survey. *Social Sci. Med. (Oxford)*, **16**, 1265–1275 (1982).

Luterman, D.M., *Counseling the Communicatively Disordered and Their Families* (second ed.). Austin: Pro-Ed (1991).

Madison, L., Budd, L., and Itzkowitz, J., Changes in stuttering in relation to children's locus of control. *J. Genetic Psychol.*, **147**, 233–240 (1986).

Magielski, J., Positive communication game rules. Part 1: Auditory reach. *Hear. Instruments*, **33**, 34 & 64 (1982).

Mancini, J., Effects of health and income on control orientation and life-satisfaction among aged public housing residents. *Internat. J. Aging Hum. Develop.*, **12**, 215–220 (1980).

Marrer, J.L., and Garstecki, D.C., Community/clinic management of hearing-impaired aging adults. Illinois Speech-Language-Hearing Association Convention, Chicago (1985).

Maurer, J.F., The psychosocial aspects of presbycusis. In R.H. Hull (Ed.), *Rehabilitative Audiology*. New York: Grune & Stratton (1982).

McDavis, K.C., The effects of severity of hearing impairment and locus of control on the denial of hearing impairment in the aged. *Internal. J. Aging Hum. Develop.*, **1**(1), 47–60 (1983–1984).

Morgan, C.M., The over 50 population and their attitude toward health care. *Hear. Instruments*, **41**, 8–9 (1990).

Palmore, E., and Luikart, C., Health and social factors related to life satisfaction. *J. Health Soc. Behav.*, **13**, 68–79 (1972).

Ries, P.W., Hearing ability of persons by sociodemographic and health characteristics: United States (Vital and Health Statistics, Series 10, No. 140, DHHS Publication No. [PHS] 82–1568). Washington: U.S. Government Printing Office (1982).

Rodin, J., and Langer, E., Long-term effect of a control-relevant intervention. *J. Personality Soc. Psychol.*, **35**, 897–902 (1977).

Rotter, J.B., Generalized expectancies for internal versus external control of reinforcement. *Psychological Monographs*, **80** (1966).

Rovner, J., Americans with Disabilities Act. *Congressional Quarterly: For the Record*, July 28 edition, 2437–2444 (1990).

Schulz, R., Effects of control and predictability on the physical and psychological well-being of the institutionalized aged. *J. Personality Soc. Psychol.*, **33**, 563–573 (1976).

Shriberg, L., Diabless, D., Carlson, K., Filley, F., Kwiatkowski, J., and Smith, M., Personality characteristics, academic performance and clinical competence in communication disorders majors. *J. Am. Speech-Language-Hearing Assoc.*, **19**, 311–315 (1977).

Smaldino, S.E., and Smaldino, J.J., *Amplified Hearing-Impaired Adults*. Association for Educational Communications and Technology, Annual Meeting. New Orleans (1988).

Smirga, D.J., The psychology of the hearing instrument "non-buyer." *Hear. Instruments*, **41**, 6–7 (1990).

Stephens, S.D.G., and Goldstein, D.P., Auditory rehabilitation for the elderly. In R. Hinchcliffe (Ed.), *Hearing and Balance in the Elderly.* London: Churchill Livingstone, pp. 201–226 (1983).

Tyler R.S., Baker, L.J., and Armstrong-Bednall, G., Difficulties experienced by hearing aid candidates and hearing aid users. *Br. J. Audiol.,* **17,** 191–201 (1983).

United States Architectural & Transportation Barriers Compliance Board, Americans with Disabilities Act (ADA): accessibility guidelines for buildings and facilities. *Federal Register,* **56,** 144, July 26, 35455–35542 (1991).

Wilder, C.S., Prevalence of selected impairments: U.S.-1971. *Vital and Health Statistics,* **10,** 99, DHWE Publication No. HRA 75–1526 (1975).

Yahne, C.E., and Long, V.O., The use of support groups to raise self-esteem for women clients. *J. Am. College Health (Washington),* **37,** 79–84 (1988).

3

Rehabilitative Audiology in the Private Practice Dispensing Office

H. CHRISTOPHER SCHWEITZER, Ph.D.

The audiology private practice that specializes in hearing aid dispensing is necessarily steeped in rehabilitation on a full-time basis. The entire premise and mission of such a business is to improve the probabilities that consumers will understand spoken messages. In such a practice, auditory diagnostics play a considerably less important role, in terms of revenue flow, than in a more medically oriented setting. Rehabilitation, through the provision of appropriate wearable instrumentation and counseling, is unfailingly foremost as an everyday objective.

In another regard, a small private practice is a microcosmic convergence of market enterprise and the profession of audiology. A dispensing practice must compete in the free market to provide services and products. The extent that it is successful as a business entity establishes the boundaries of its capabilities to render professional services. In other words, competent audiologists may have a very limited opportunity to exercise their expertise if they are incapable of managing cash flow to pay the rent and utilities.

Perhaps because there is a closeness of economic interchanges in a private practice, as compared to an institutional setting where salaries seem to flow independent of the moment-to-moment care for patients,

a philosophical foundation appears essential for success. After all, unless the client is asked to trade negotiable currency for improved hearing, there is no salary in such a business. Schweitzer (1986) developed the concept of EVE, equivalent value exchange, in the process of articulating a particular practice's philosophical reasons for existence. Such a concept injects an underlying tenet of "fairness" into the daily demands of collecting money to stay in business. It may be a common misconception that business and philosophy don't routinely intermingle. Experience suggests that nothing could be further from the truth. Blending ethics and well-examined human values with solid business principles is a synergistic formula for success (Blanchard & Peale, 1988), for both consumers and providers.

Apart from the business-oriented issues (see Curran, 1986; Teter & Schweitzer, 1991), such as resource allocation and legal considerations, there are three major practical and interconnected focal points of consideration in the private practice dispensing office (Fig. 3.1). These are *product*, *service*, and *counseling*. The audiologist must strive to achieve excellence in each of these areas.

The remainder of this chapter will attempt to elucidate activities and delineate

35

attributes regarding those three contributors to success that compose the "success triangle."

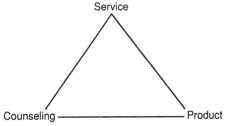

Figure 3.1. Success in a dispensing-oriented private practice will likely require a balanced dedication to achieving excellence in each of these interrelated areas.

Service

Much has been said in the recent business literature about the need to concentrate on service-oriented (Hawken, 1987) customer-driven activities. The postindustrial age has driven many thousands of professionals into the "service sector" of the economy (*Business Week*, August 19, 1991), and simultaneously attention to service has rocketed as a provisionary issue. A progressive, service-oriented business has a willfully enlarged perception of customer relationships. In a hearing aid focused practice, the term "dispense" must be expanded from the limited connotative meaning (i.e., to distribute, vend) to an affirmative, educational proposition fitting for the "Information Age" economy of the late 20th century.

The issuing of a hearing aid is rarely, if ever, a single transaction event as in the vending of other consumer goods, such as clothing. Furthermore, the provision of hearing aids is the formation of a contractual relationship that often lasts many years. In the militaristic jargon of the business educator, the mission is to "capture and control" market segments. In the lighter view of progressive entrepreneurs (Hawken, 1987), the "mission" is to gain the permission of the marketplace to practice the profession of rehabilitative audiology.

ACCESSIBILITY

Traditional hearing aid offices, operated by business people without graduate degrees in audiology, have a notable attribute that consumers appreciate—accessibility. Accessibility is identified as a key component in the delivery of goods and services to the aging American population (Dychtwald, 1990). Accessibility for the present purpose suggests that clients have the comforting assurance that minor problems and questions can be handled on short notice and that barriers to such service are minimized.

Some barriers are psychological and may appear less obvious to those not closely attuned to the senior consumer market. One example of a barrier is the simple requirement of advanced appointments for minor service. Other examples include gated parking lots at high-rise professional buildings that have imposing security stations in the lobby and protective receptionists who insulate the audiologists from time-demanding "intrusions."

Dychtwald (1990) argues persuasively that accessibility may be "as important as the product or service itself" for the senior segment of the American consumer market.

CLARITY OF PURPOSE

Regrettably at this time in the developing profession of audiology, "XYZ Audiology Center" is almost certainly less comprehensible on an immediate basis than "XYZ Hearing Center" for a large segment of consumers of audiologic products and services. In a time when consumers are virtually bombarded with daily messages, clarity of purpose is particularly important and there is little opportunity for unclear messages to penetrate. Mackay (1990) describes an example of some well-intentioned physicians who opened an "Ambulatory Care Clinic" in a laudably "accessible" shopping center location. After several months of virtually no patient activity it was determined that most prospective clinic users believed "ambulatory care" meant that patients were expected to arrive in an ambulance.

Clarity of purpose means discarding technical jargon to communicate with the public. "Aural rehabilitation" may be just such a term that could conceivably confuse the public to a greater extent than the more recognizable terms "hearing" or "auditory." Obviously, professionally unique terms used within the domain of education and peer exchange are unlikely to create problems and are quite useful for purposes of precision and succinctness. But transferring such terms to the consumer public should be undertaken with careful appreciation of the need for uncomplicated messages. Physicians and pharmacists have persisted for centuries with the use of "secretive" prescriptions that mostly serve to keep a guarded mystique separating consumers from professionals. The "Information Age" tendency is for consumers to migrate to those providers who provide the most comprehensible, and therefore valuable, information. The entrepreneurial audiologist can be viewed then as an interpreter of an obscure (to the public) knowledge base to the lay consumer.

Clarity is a form of service, and greater service is good business, which in turn generates more opportunities for service. Great service, one of the cornerstones of the success triangle, means adopting a consumer perspective. Imagine for a moment that you are a hearing aid client and that you have come to depend on your aids as your virtual link to interpersonal communication and acoustical stimulation. Now imagine that one of your hearing aids stops working this morning. You would probably not want to be told that you can see the audiologist next Thursday at 4:00 p.m. and further that the hearing aid will most likely have to be sent away to a laboratory for 2 to 3 weeks. The typical consumer, particularly an individual over the age of 55, is more likely to develop loyalty to the audiologist who welcomes "walk-in" service problems and is sufficiently flexible to conduct some on-site service (see Fig. 3.2).

Product

Providing the best possible product is the second attribute of the successful audiologist in private practice. Because the audiologist is typically not in a position of actually manufacturing the hearing product, the alternative is to become vigorously insistent on superior products from the suppliers. A paternal attitude must be devel-

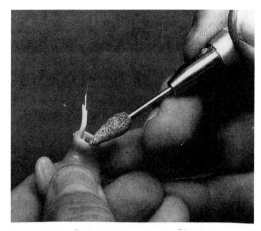

Figure 3.2. The ability to accomplish a number of minor repairs on hearing aids is an important indication of a "service-oriented" dispensing practice. (Photo courtesy of Electone, Inc.)

oped on behalf of the clients. Their auditory well-being is at stake, and a fierce, uncompromising sense of urgency is fully appropriate and certainly appreciated.

Developing close relationships with manufacturers is an essential (and seldom taught) behavior of the modern dispensing audiologist. Such relationships with customer service personnel and with engineering and technical staff at selected suppliers leaves the dispenser less at the mercy of a manufacturer's lottery. The audiologist must choose suppliers that are not only dependable but also solicitous and appreciative of suggestions to improve their products. The primary source of information on the quality and effectiveness of a manufacturer's products is undeniably the audiologist who consummates the fittings and observes the results. Consumers rarely enter into dialogue directly with the manufacturer, so the audiologist is the critical liaison and transmitter of crucial information in both directions.

Product performance measures, particularly the acoustical characteristics obtained by use of probe microphone instruments, are vital to a dispensing practice in the "Information Age" (see Fig. 3.3). There are many sources of error in estimating hearing aid outputs on a particular client's ear from a standardized coupler measure. These will not be detailed at this time, but it must be stressed that far too much guess-

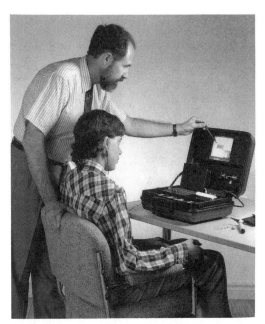

Figure 3.3. In the "Information Age," an essential item of information is the acoustical transformer at the tympanic membrane that results from the application of a hearing aid. (Photo courtesy of the Audioscan Company.)

ing, often incorrectly, about a hearing aid's in situ performance must be done in the absence of such measures. The reader is referred to Chapters 5 and 11 for further discussions of this issue.

Another important contribution of a probe microphone measurement system is the monitoring of modifications done by the audiologist to improve an unsatisfactory fit. Many times the resultant changes are exactly the *reverse* of expectations because of the complex and difficult to predict individual acoustical characteristics of the user. One good example is the effect of venting. Often intended to reduce low frequency gain, venting may, in fact, create a Helmholtz resonance that actually increases gain where it was meant to be attenuated.

The incessant advance of technological progress has recently resulted in the development of programmable hearing devices (see Fig. 3.4). These systems allow the clinician in the office to make highly diverse adjustments to the electroacoustics of the aid. That capacity, of course, moves greater responsibility to the fitter. Moreover, fitting expertise is enlarged and sharpened by the

very rapid feedback that is given by the client as various output schemes are tried.

Dedication to superior products for the client is essentially a guarantee that the audiologist will continue to learn and expand his or her technical understanding. In the recent past, far too many fittings have been designed and built on specifications generated at the factory, based on minimal audiologic information provided by dispensers of various backgrounds. Programmable systems clearly necessitate greater technical understanding of hearing aid electroacoustics. Such a development is most certainly advantageous for the profession of audiology.

Counseling

Other chapters in this text deal with counseling both in general and for specific populations. There are, however, some unique counseling issues that must be addressed in the dispensing-oriented private practice. These comments will pertain primarily to the active adult population hearing aid consumers.

It cannot be overstressed that the provision of hearing aids is a multistage process, and the economics of the exchange must account for the need for frequent follow-up counseling and minor adjustments.

THE AUDIOLOGIST AS FACILITATOR AND COACH

One popular dictionary defines the word "counsel" as follows: "noun: a mutual exchange of ideas." Too often, it seems, clinicians approach the counseling (verb form) process as something that must be *done* to, or on behalf of, the client. It is argued here that it is the *process* of interaction in mutual exchange that is the "doing" and that the appropriate verb is "facilitate."

To further this concept it is proposed that a metaphor of "coaching" is quite appropriate. Whereas it is all too obvious that audiologists do not actually "fix" their clients' ears, it would seem that what they often do accomplish is a guided improvement in hearing function and the provision of the right equipment. This behavior and

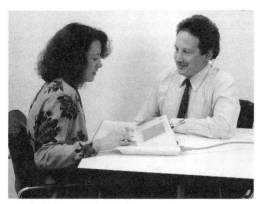

Figure 3.4. The dispensing audiologist will likely assume greater responsibility in client satisfaction through the increasing use of programmable hearing aids. (Photo courtesy of Siemens Hearing Instruments.)

responsibility has many similarities to coaching. In this case, the audiologist as coach attempts to facilitate the process whereby the client, player, or pupil improves the probability of communicating effectively.

ALIGNMENT OF COACH/PUPIL GOALS

A coach and a pupil must have a shared alignment of goals. The following are suggested in this context:

To strive (to hear) competitively
To reach for maximum potential
To strive for excellence

A great coach must expect nothing less from him(her)self or from the pupil. Of course, the metaphor can only be extended to a reasonable extent, but the author has found it quite useful. If a client with uncertainties about the wisdom of investing considerable money in hearing aids approaches a coach-oriented audiologist, it is easy to develop a dialogue such as the following:

Mr. Anderson, you've come to me about your hearing problem, and I do have expertise in providing assistance for that type of problem. But then you tell me that you're not sure if you want to buy a hearing aid for both ears, and you may want an inexpensive one for just one ear. Mr. Anderson, I take great pride in my work, and you're asking me to lower my standards of success. It's as if I were an ice-skating coach and you wanted me to teach you

how to skate. But you wanted to buy only one skate and a used one at that! Obviously, neither of us is going to look very good, and I can't afford to have such poorly performing students representing my coaching abilities. Now, if you are genuinely interested in hearing with greater confidence and ending each day with less accumulated stress from difficult listening, then you and I can challenge the apparent "mumblers" and the competing noises . . . and win.

ATTRIBUTES OF A GOOD COACH

A number of attributes of a good coach can be identified. Five of these are discussed in the following sections.

A Coach Knows the Assets and Limitations of the Pupil

Clearly, diagnostic audiometric information is important, but a good coach has an appreciation for the physical and psychological characteristics of the client. With regard to the latter, threshold values describe the shoreline between hearing and not hearing, but the most comfortable level (MCL) for speech may yield the greatest descriptors for amplification designs. A reliably obtained MCL for speech essentially describes the gain target for a hearing aid. For example, if the MCL is 80 dB hearing level (HL), given the 20 dB calibration pad, the client is indicating that speech levels around 100 dB sound pressure level (SPL) are desirable. Further, given the typical spoken average level at the listener's ear of about 65 dB SPL, a quick estimate of gain is 35 dB (to reach the 100 dB SPL comfort level).

The rehabilitative process would be far less complicated if clients heard with their ears, but regrettably most actual hearing is done with the brain. Therefore, there is a vast range of responses to the same acoustic pattern for persons with nearly identical audiometric thresholds. Hence, a good coach develops some intuitive wisdom about the personality features that may contribute to greater success with a client. For example, a particular style of aid might be appropriate for one person who is especially concerned with cosmetics. A hearing aid with a greater gain range might be recommended for the client who is insecure about missing the slightest bit of information. At another extreme are those individuals devoted to deep contemplation who may prefer the acoustic insulation of hearing loss to the "demands" of a more fully interactive life (see Edison anecdote later in this chapter).

A Coach Has Appropriate Experience

Far too often hearing aids are fitted by individuals who never have actually worn an aid or experienced diminished hearing. Both are essential experiences that every good coach/audiologist should conscientiously arrange. A week with a pair of well-fitted ear plugs is a critical experience for the developing audiologist. Moreover, hearing aids should be routinely worn in a variety of circumstances to develop the experiential base necessary for good counseling. (Appropriate precautions should be taken to avoid acoustic trauma during the experiment.) Occasional listening to a hearing aid through a stethoscopic device with a long length of tubing is a quite different experience than actually having hearing aids in the ear while driving a car. Complaints about sound quality in hearing aids are often based on undeniable realities that must be genuinely appreciated by the clinician at more than academic levels.

A Coach Has a Good Sense of Timing

It does little good to describe many of the technical details of otopathology and/or amplification if a client is still struggling with the acceptance/denial components in the rehabilitative construct. Providing information as the client is ready to receive it is the issue here. A competent gymnastics coach would never push a novice student into dangerous high bar routines. Similarly, the hearing coach cannot suggest or expect a first-time hearing aid user either to prosper in difficult noise conditions or to fully comprehend all aspects of the fitting.

A Coach Exhibits "Tough Love"

A masterful balance of empathy and encouragement is greatly desired in counseling adults with hearing aids. Empathy taken to an extreme becomes unproductive sympathy. An excess of empathy results in the audiologist morosely agreeing with every complaint of new and "unnatural" sounds when actually some cognitive accommodation quite routinely is needed.

Conversely, a surplus of encouragement might be construed as a lack of sensitivity. A good counselor often has to "pull" a client to higher levels of performance, encouraging participation in challenging listening situations, but "pushing" may be unproductive. Hard-driving drill sergeants are not good role models. A "tough love" coach is.

Every practicing audiologist fully appreciates the enormous diversity of human reaction to similar experiences. The good coach learns to distinguish between unjustified "whining" and genuine anxiety or confusion. Some clients are overly stoic about problems with their fittings and need to be scrutinized by the hearing coach for abrasions or pressure sores. Others wince and whimper at even the most cursory examination of the ear. Again, it is extremely valuable for audiologists occasionally to undergo an otoscopic examination, have probe tubes inserted, and have impression material injected into their auditory canals. This will help audiologists develop a full sensitivity to the experiences they are responsible for producing in their clients.

A Coach Experiments with New Methods

No doubt, successful coaches often may be tempted to continue to use tactics that have yielded good results in the past. But truly great coaches are always seeking to push to higher levels of performance. A private "practice" is just that—an eternal practicing to become increasingly masterful. There is an instinctive burning desire among successful dispensing audiologists to strive continuously for better results. What more can be learned about hearing aid fittings? What new ways can be implemented to modify an instrument for better results? What other information about my clients' hearing can be obtained? What new technology should be studied and mastered to better care for my clients? These are the kinds of questions that are constantly pursued by the audiologist/coach destined for greatness and success. Failure to strive to examine new methods often reduces counseling to what this author calls the ancient YGUTI method of counseling, which is simply, "You'll Get Used To It!" Although there is an undeniable need for psychological accommodation, a client may never adjust to a hearing aid with a horribly peaky frequency response.

CLOSING THE EXPECTATIONS-TO-REALITY GAP

A crucial role assumed in the counseling process is to shrink undesirable gaps between the true performance benefits that might be delivered with the use of hearing aids and the client's often unrealistic expectations. This, again, cannot be accomplished by an audiologist conducting a one-sided monologue. Recall that history cites both Epictetus and Zeno with having said, "People have two ears and only one tongue so that they might listen twice as much as they speak."

The counseling clinician needs to solicit from prospective purchasers a portrait of their expectations. The interactive discussion then often can lead, in the "mutual exchange of ideas," to a more appropriate and realistic set of expectations.

"Under-Promise and Over-Deliver"

Continuing the theme of closing the expectation/reality gap, the above quotation from a business text is of great value. It can be expressed alternatively as, "Always give more than is expected." In this regard, the successful clinician must greatly downgrade the likely benefits from amplification. The deliverable auditory enhancements are then enjoyed more.

A useful means to bridge the gap of expectations to reality is the user diary. Appendix 3.1 presents an example of one developed by this author and is available from a hearing aid manufacturer. This tool encourages purchasers of new hearing aids to participate in the adjustment process by recording significant new sounds noticed with their instruments. It further alerts them to the expectation that the hearing aids are not an instant-fix device and that accommodation and flexibility are essential aspects of putting them to good use.

Five Essential Concepts

A great educator was once quoted as saying, "In teaching it is the drawing out that counts, not the pumping in." There are several essential concepts that a good coach/audiologist can guide the hearing aided adult to understand. This author has observed that when these concepts are understood, the hearing aid user's flexibility, tolerance, and skill with the instruments are greatly augmented.

THE WORLD IS A VERY NOISY PLACE

Thomas Edison (1948) indicated that he believed his hearing impairment actually increased his productivity and creativity because it provided a buffer from the distractions and noises around him. Some of his diary notes of 1930 include the following:

From the start I found that deafness was an advantage. . . . I could not hear . . . distracting sounds. It may be said that I was shut off from that particular kind of social intercourse, which is small talk. I am glad of it. I couldn't hear, for instance, the conversations at the dinner tables of the boarding-houses and hotels where, after I became a telegrapher, I took my meals. Freedom from such talk gave me an opportunity to think out my problems. I have no doubt that my nerves are stronger and better today than they would have been if I had heard all the foolish conversation and other meaningless sounds that normal people hear.

Edison's belief, of course, can be neither proved nor disputed, but the undeniable fact is that the technological and high-density dwelling world is, indeed, a very noisy place. Furthermore, it is quite true that even a mild threshold loss removes a large proportion of everyday sounds from a person's experience. A prominent hearing aid engineer (Goldberg, 1988) once estimated that as much as 90% of common everyday sounds, such as clothes rubbing, quiet fans running, and distant dogs barking, are less than 50 dB SPL. That would imply clearly that a clinically mild loss would remove a great proportion of auditory experiences from one's daily listening. It is no wonder, then, that so many first-time users are quick to take notice of the vast number of common sounds that do not arouse the attention of normal hearing persons.

It is vital that the user be prepared for the onslaught of new sounds. Further, an extension of this first concept is that most of the world's noises are not communicative priorities. In other words, a client invests a substantial amount of money to hear the vocal messages of significance and he or she may discover that most of the newly audible sounds are of little interest and may be a great distraction. This naturally leads to the ill-conceived marketing tactics that feature "automatic noise canceling" circuits. This is a somewhat preposterous proposition, since "noise" is almost always a moment-to-moment decision on the part of the listener.

Signal processing specialists talk about "target to jammer ratios" (TJR) in the scientific journals. These TJR experiments may use highly contrived signals, or targets, and evaluate their audibility in the presence of certain noises, or jammers. Imagine, though, a male client who at one moment is interested in his wife's speech. Minutes later she may be conversing with someone else, and he now wants to hear the football score on the TV. Should the hearing aid be optimized electroacoustically for the wife's speech acoustics or for the sportscaster on the TV? Although it may be true that a circuit adaptively adjusts the bass or treble according to the level detected at some stage in the processor, it hardly can be claimed that it "focuses on what you want to listen to," since that is usually a dynamic and varying target within some potentially wide limits. It is somewhat frightening to imagine a world with an artificially imposed deletion of many nonspeech sounds that inform us, for example, of the velocity of the wind, the nearness of a shout, the integrity of a machine, or the completion of a microwave's cook cycle.

THE BRAIN HEARS, AND THE EARS CONVEY

How is it that anyone, with normal or impaired ears, can extract a meaningful signal out of the noise in a common, high-level, uncorrelated noise? The answer relates to the capacity of the "incredible listening brain." By use of its phased array bilateral difference detectors (Schweitzer, 1989), the brain is able to "deverberate," inhibit, squelch, and modify the middle and inner ears to alter differentially the flow of noises as opposed to those judged

to be message units. This physiological reality, that hearing is ultimately a central nervous system process modulated by conscious mental processing, contributes to the fact that many clinically "good" fittings are often rejected as sounding so "unnatural." To some extent, those cases represent the mental adaptation that accompanies threshold losses. As a result of having high frequencies filtered from cognitive awareness for some period of time, the filtered experience has become "normal," and partial recovery of them then seems "unnatural." In such cases, of course, the rehabilitative process requires a guided reintroduction to recently unfamiliar sounds.

But there may be more to the situation than simple refamiliarization with normal acoustical experience. One of the consequences of many hearing aid fittings is to shift the image of the auditory process to the peripheral area of the ears. This is particularly true of monaural fittings but also with binaural fittings, where the phase of one hearing aid may be 180° in reverse of the other. The simple shifting of the image of sounds is likely to occur concomitantly with other alterations in the ability of the brain to manage complex signals when the interaural relations have been altered in the aided condition. Certainly, this is an area of clinical speculation that merits rigorous study (Smith & Schweitzer, 1991).

Another example of how the brain hears and the ears convey is the following: A young mother is napping on a warm afternoon. The window is open, and at her tympanic membranes are the minuscule acoustic motions caused by dogs barking, children playing, and cars starting. For a conscious person with good hearing, motions of less than the diameter of a hydrogen molecule in the audible frequency region can be heard. But the young mother continues to sleep. Until, at less than the sound pressure levels of the ongoing sounds, the baby whimpers. Instantly, the woman arouses and speeds into the nursery. Is it the reticular formation that serves as the alerting device, as some neuroscientists suggest (Curtis, Jacobsen, & Marcus, 1972)? Perhaps, but the relevance to the rehabilitative audiologist is that it is not only the levels of sounds at the eardrum that determine reactions but also the *significance* attached by the mid- and higher processing centers (the reticular formation being the central core of the medulla, pons, and midbrain tegmentum). The mother's brain "knows" that the baseline "familiar" noises are unimportant, so sleep was permitted to continue. But the specific acoustics of the baby's voice are obviously deemed significant enough for inner alarms to go off.

Similarly, initial reactions to many unfamiliar sounds may demand that the hearing aid user pay attention to them. But after the familiarization process, they may be heard without requiring attention. The alerting function probably relates to biologic survival functions of the auditory system. Without it, few humans might have evolved from their sleeping, cave-dwelling ancestors if soft-footed predators approached them without detection. The audiologist should encourage the new hearing aid user to "make friends" with the various audible intrusions that, on identification, often fade into the background where they often belong . . . except when survival is at stake.

HEARING AIDS SHRINK THE AUDITORY DISTANCES

Improving someone's hearing threshold invariably also means expanding his or her auditory distance. To the extent that the inverse square law holds true, which is greatly influenced by reflective surfaces, every 6 dB of increased sensitivity might double the distance at which something can be heard. Compression circuits that maximize the gain for soft sounds may even compound the experience. To the new hearing aid user, this is both good news and bad. The hum of the refrigerator, which might have previously been heard only when standing right next to it, now can be heard in the living room. The neighborhood dogs suddenly may seem to multiply.

The coach/clinician often needs to celebrate the expanded auditory distance with the client to accelerate the adjustment process. Growth is commonly affiliated with pain and fear. The first time a figure-skating pupil makes a difficult leaping spin, the great coach rushes in to celebrate, discussing both the fear and the accomplishment

even if the pupil has fallen. The very word *encourage* is related to the French, *coer*, heart. To encourage is to assist the progress of the heart's desire to excel. It is a concept that should not be overlooked in the counseling process. Furthermore, it is an extension of other counseling-inspired adjustments, such as adjustments to noise, that might come under the heading, "Make friends of your enemies."

THE AIDED INJURED EARS ARE STILL INJURED

Besides the obvious fact that hearing aids do not stimulate the regrowth of hair cells and that audiologists do not "fix" injured ears, there is an important functional consideration regarding hearing aided performance. It may not be evident immediately to new audiology students that most hearing aid fittings leave the user with a mild threshold impairment. This probably results from a combination of many of the adjustment problems mentioned above and the considerable nonlinearity that is not fully mapped in the injured ear. In other words, it may be possible to bring a client's thresholds down to normal levels, but it would be rare for the user actually to adjust the gain to such a level for typical use. The preferred gain for suprathreshold sounds often is much less than a gain setting that enables normal threshold ability. Routine functional gain and real ear insertion responses taken at "use volume control" positions generally confirm the truth that "aided injured ears are still injured," at least for linear amplifiers. Often, users indicate very satisfactory benefit when sound field functional gain measures show only a 10- or 15-dB threshold improvement for hearing losses of 55 and 65 dB.

However, where gain is inverse to input, nonlinear amplification schemes often can be shown to allow the user to have thresholds near normal while still tolerating a typical dynamic range. Methods that map the suprathreshold performance of hearing aid candidates seem especially useful in that regard. The Resound Company has an important tool for that purpose. An example of the Loudness Growth for Octave Bands centered at four frequencies is shown in Figure 3.5. The data provide a useful coun-

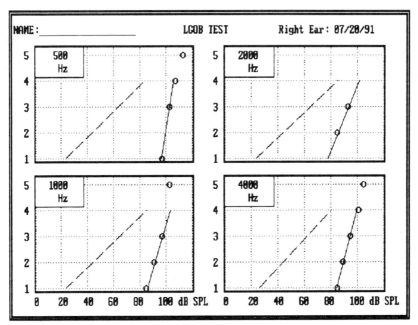

Figure 3.5. An example of loudness mapping for four octave bands using the Resound Digital Hearing System. The vertical numbers correspond to the client's loudness impressions for one ear (1 = Very Soft; 5 = Very Loud). Sound pressure levels are shown on the horizontal scale at the bottom. The dashed diagonal line represents an expected normal ear response.

seling tool for any hearing-impaired client. The rehabilitative audiologist is vigorously encouraged to move beyond the basic audiogram, which was developed originally for medical diagnostic purposes not for hearing aid fitting, and to incorporate progressive tools that are more fundamentally oriented toward hearing aid fitting.

BALANCE IS VITAL

Counseling the adult hearing aid user should include developing methods by which the user can quickly ascertain whether the sound levels to the two ears are reasonably balanced. With asymmetrical hearing losses that is often difficult but nevertheless important. Harris (1980) points out that the animal kingdom has great diversity in the number of legs, eyes, and other organs, but auditory detectors always come in twos, with definite interconnections in the nervous system. Engineers are hard pressed to exceed nature when it comes to the signal detection capabilities of the uninjured human hearing system. But there is a host of evidence that such a capacity requires a fairly close interaural balance to accomplish the neat trick of ex-

tracting a single voice from a diffusion of many.

Remember, the premise of the Stenger test for pseudohypocusis is that an ear will perceive a diotic signal only in the ear in which it is the loudest. If one hearing aid is haphazardly turned to a moderately higher gain than the other, it presumably disrupts the binaural signal processing ability of the listening brain. It further shifts the image of what is heard to an unnatural lateral location.

The use of highly directional sound field speakers is an excellent way to establish balance at several frequencies. In the absence of such equipment as the Dyna-Aura Sound Field Audiometer, which easily maps balance for tones and speech-shaped noise, other simpler measures can and should be made. For example, a repeated click from a single speaker can be used to test whether the client can locate the sound correctly, proving some ability to localize that is naturally confounded by unbalanced aids. The striking of a spoon on a ceramic coffee cup provides a similar stimulus. The client should be asked to close his or her eyes while the audiologist moves the cup and strikes the spoon to determine whether the client can point to the sound source.

Once away from the office, the user should be encouraged to check for balance by choosing a particular localized sound source such as a ticking clock, small radio, or tapping of a utensil on a glass. After some experience, most users develop a fairly well-established internal criterion for proper, balanced gain levels.

Conclusion

Balance is one of nature's greatest virtues and lessons. Besides the need for auditory balance there are other levels of balance needed in the dispensing audiologist's office to ensure success. Professional skill must be balanced with business skill. Empathy must be balanced with an education in market economics (also known as "trade skill" by some; see Hawken, 1987; Teter & Schweitzer, 1991). Tenderness must be balanced with toughness, and the ledgers must be balanced.

Rehabilitation in the private practice hearing aid office offers the enjoyment of routinely engaging the "problem solution" side of audiology versus the "problem description" aspect that is characteristic of the diagnostic-type setting. But the price of entry includes a well-developed ability to work independently and a notable amount of courage. High-level empathy is accompanied by substantial agonizing over the shortcomings of current technology but great elation when progress is observed. Cicero said that "the ears are the doorway to the mind." A profession that stands with the keys to the mind when ears are injured should take great pride in its mission.

References

Blanchard, K., and Peale, N.V., *The Power of Ethical Management.* New York: Fawcett Crest (1988).

Business Week, cover article "Young Americans," August 19, 1991.

Curran, J., The ten commandments of hearing aid dispensing. In J. Curran (Guest Ed) J. Northern and W. Perkins (Eds.-in-Chief), *Seminars in Hearing,* 7, No. 2. New York: Thieme, Inc., pp. 219–228 (1986).

Curtis, B., Jacobson, S., and Marcus, E., *An Introduction to the Neurosciences.* Philadelphia: W. B. Saunders (1972).

Dychtwald, K., *Age Wave.* New York: Bantam Books (1990).

Edison, T., *Thomas Edison, the Diary and Observations.* D.D. Runes (Ed.). New York: The Philosophical Library, Inc. (1948).

Goldberg, H., Dyna-Aura Engineering, San Diego, personal communication (1988).

Harris, J.D., Psycho-acoustics and neurophysiology of binaural hearing. In E. Robert Libby (Ed.), *Binaural Hearing and Amplification,* Vol. 1. Chicago: Zenetron (1980).

Hawken, P., *Growing a Business.* New York: Simon & Schuster (1987).

Mackay, H., *Beware the Naked Man Who Offers You His Shirt.* New York: Ivy Books (1990).

Schweitzer, H.C., Reflections on the significance of private practice dispensing. In J. Curran (Guest Ed.), J. Northern and W. Perkins (Eds.-in-Chief), *Seminars in Hearing,* 7, No. 2. New York: Thieme, Inc., pp. 205–212 (1986).

Schweitzer, H.C., The incredible listening brain. Presentation at the national Self-Help for the Hard of Hearing convention, Washington, DC (1989).

Smith, D.A., and Schweitzer, H.C., An electronic solution to the "occlusion effect" and a clinician adjustable phase circuit. Paper presented at the International Hearing Conference, University of Iowa (1991).

Teter, D.L., and Schweitzer, H.C., Private practice hearing aid dispensing. *Audiol. Today,* 3, No. 5 (1991).

Returning to the World of Sound.

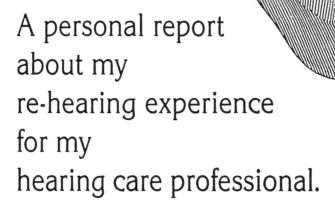

A personal report
about my
re-hearing experience
for my
hearing care professional.

_____   _____
CLIENT NAME   DATE

PLEASE FILL IN QUESTIONNAIRE ON INSIDE PAGES.

Dear _____:

Now that you have been fitted with your new hearing instruments, you have completed the first step in your hearing rehabilitation program and are ready for more. You will notice that you may have to make some re-adjustments in your life style, but that is perfectly natural, as you become more closely coupled to our wonderful world of sound. You can help in this period if you will take a few minutes to fill out this report of your daily hearing experiences and return it to our office at your convenience.

| DAY 1 | How long did you wear your aids today (hours)? _____ |

What new or different sounds did you hear today? _____

_____

Where did you put your hearing aids when you took them off? _____

| DAY 2 | How long did you wear your aids today (hours)? _____ |

Did you have trouble putting on or taking off your aids?_____

Did you check your aids for ear wax?_____

| DAY 3 | How long did you wear your aids today (hours)? _____ |

How did you get along in social groups today?

_____

Do you enjoy TV/radio now? _____

DAY 4

Are you hearing your spouse and your relatives more clearly now? _____

Can you understand them from a greater distance? About how far away? _____

Are their voices more distinct? _____

DAY 5

Can you distinguish these sounds?

Refrigerator? ____ Furnace? ____

Running water? ____ Motorcycle? ____

Doorbell? ____ Keys jingling? ____

Are there sounds you can't identify? Please specify. _____

_____

DAY 6

When riding in a car, do traffic sounds bother you? _____

Do you wipe your hearing aids when you retire at night? ____ Remove the battery? ____

How long did you wear your instruments today (hours)? _____

DAY 7

How does your own voice sound to you?

_____

What do you like most about using your new hearing aids? _____

_____

What help do you need? _____

_____

_____

Thank you for completing this repòrt. It is an important part of your Auditory Awareness Re-education. We have re-engineered the sounds available to the brain, improving your hearing function considerably, even though the unaided sensitivity deficit remains. Now, because hearing is a mental process as well as a physiological one, your conscious effort and attention are required. It is your attitude toward returning to the world of sound which will become the most significant factor in your successful hearing rehabilitation. We are very appreciative of your efforts.

_____

Dispensing Professional

Please deliver this report on
your next scheduled visit to your
Authorized UHS Hearing care Professional:

UHS Form 1024 · 9/91 Printed in U S A.

United Hearing Systems, Inc. • Plainfield, Connecticut 06374

2

REHABILITATIVE AUDIOLOGY: CHILDREN

Early Identification: Principles and Practices

O.T. KENWORTHY, Ph.D.

According to Piagetian theory, classification is a process that is fundamental to logico-mathematical development (Gruber & Voneche, 1977). Perhaps contrary to one's first instincts, sorting and counting are the very basis of higher level mathematics such as calculus and statistics. Customarily, though, we tend to think of classification in what Piaget refers to as its simple, *additive* form, that is, the binary operation of sorting one class from another along a single attribute. For example, one might differentiate two groups of objects based on color (e.g., red versus not red). The process becomes much more complex, however, when considered in its *multiplicative* form whereby classification is done relative to multiple attributes. An example of this might be sorting objects by both shape and color (red/not red, triangle/not triangle). Of course, one can break down the underlying attributes into more discrete sets (e.g., red/blue/green, triangle/circle/square) with the result being a multiplying of the potential outcomes, or sorting bins. From this, it is easy to see that the seemingly simple process of sorting can result in very different outcomes depending on one's approach.

Definition of Terms for Classification of Hearing Status

It is not surprising then that the classification of hearing status may be accomplished from two quite different perspectives. On the one hand, the *medical/epidemiologic* perspective tends to apply an additive approach. The testing is referred to as screening, and the outcomes tend to be binary, or a two-alternative, forced choice. The objective is to precisely select those individuals affected by a certain disease when the symptoms of that disease are not readily observable (Rogers, 1986). The focus is generally on disease rather than on disability and on medical rather than rehabilitative treatment. The precision of the applicable test method is evaluated through analysis of a tetrachoric (2×2) table, as discussed later under "Psychometric Considerations."

The strength of this method is in its systematic approach to measurement. When the object of interest is a disease for which a medical treatment regimen is well specified, then this approach is applicable. For example, early detection and treatment of hypertension in high-risk populations can lead to significant reductions in cardiac disease. In general, an epidemiologic approach works most effectively when:

1. the methods of identification and treatment are well recognized and standardized;
2. the disease being screened for exists primarily in isolation; and
3. the affected individual's response to treatment is predicated on well-understood biomedical principles.

These conditions are less frequently observed in the case of developmental disabilities such as communicative disorders. Accordingly, an *educational* perspective on identification offers a multiplicative approach to testing for disabilities (Tjossem, 1976). In an educational model, the focus is programmatic and is aimed at establishing a continuum of services rather than a single test/treatment protocol. The process is generally referred to as identification and incorporates such elements as case finding (screening), tracking, referral, follow-up, and advocacy, particularly public education. The primary goal is to ensure a smooth transition between the identification, assessment, and intervention components of the program based more on the affected individual's functional needs than on symptomatology. To that end, monitoring and verification of referral outcomes are crucial aspects of the identification process and ensure continuity between identification, assessment, and intervention. The identification process remains nondiagnostic but often results in more than binary outcomes, depending on the individual's complex of needs and on the assessment and intervention resources (i.e., referral options) available. For instance, a child presenting with abnormal hearing may be simultaneously referred for an audiologic evaluation, a speech/language screening or evaluation, a developmental evaluation, and/or medical follow-up depending on the needs detected through case-finding (screening) methods.

As defined above, the educational approach to identification is consistent with a rehabilitative posture and offers certain advantages to the clinician providing aural rehabilitation. In particular, it leads to more efficient and effective routing of patients and, hence, to earlier intervention. This, in turn, incorporates the rehabilitative specialists more effectively into case management and facilitates coordinated and functional intervention rather than fragmented treatment. The result is improved treatment efficacy and accountability.

This kind of comprehensive and coordinated care is especially crucial within the context of current public policy. Recently, several public-policy forces have converged in ways that suggest movement beyond the debate of whether early identification is justified. The U.S. Public Health Service has adopted Health Objectives for the Year 2000 that include early identification and management of hearing loss. Federal legislation has been adopted (Public Law 99–457) that requires interagency coordination of services and provides funding incentives for comprehensive identification. Congress is currently considering legislation that would mandate hearing testing for all newborns. The American Speech-Language-Hearing Association (ASHA) has also adopted Guidelines for the Audiologic Screening of Newborn Infants Who Are at Risk for Hearing Impairment (ASHA, 1989a) and Guidelines for the Audiologic Assessment of Children from Birth Through 36 Months of Age (ASHA, 1991a). In addition, the Joint Committee on Infant Hearing has revised the high-risk register (HRR) to reflect more current thinking on what criteria constitute high risk of hearing impairment (ASHA, 1991b). Together, these items represent an unprecedented level of policy-making activity in the area of early identification and intervention. One would hope that these activities indicate that state and federal mandates for early identification are imminent.

Statement of Purpose

It would seem prudent to assume that any mandate for early identification will be accompanied by increased demands for accountability. Hence, if we are to effect early identification and intervention, there is a need to incorporate both the programmatic orientation of the educational perspective and the measurement precision of the epidemiologic approach. Therefore, the intent of this chapter is to draw from each of these perspectives in addressing the *psychometric, epidemiologic, programmatic,* and *procedural considerations* necessary to the implementation of a comprehensive early identification program.

The topic of this chapter is early identification of hearing impairment, but methods for screening speech/language delay will also be addressed. This stems from the author's underlying belief that the problem confronting the hearing-impaired child is not just hearing impairment. Our professional commitment to hearing-impaired children not only must address their sensory deficit but must facilitate their speech/language acquisition as well. To screen for and treat only the hearing loss without addressing the concomitant delay in communicative development is analogous to treating the symptoms and not the disease. Therefore, in keeping with the broad perspective on early identification discussed above, our focus will be on the complex of hearing impairment and speech/language delay.

Public school audiometry plays an important role in the process of identification. The procedures suited to such a program have been well documented elsewhere, however (ASHA, 1979, 1985, 1989b; Bluestone, Berry, & Paradise, 1973; Brooks, 1978, 1982; FitZaland & Zink, 1984; Lous, 1983; Lucker, 1980; Melnick, Eagles, & Levine, 1964; Roeser & Northern, 1981; Roush & Tait, 1985; Wilson & Walton, 1974, 1978). Therefore, this chapter will focus on the importance of screening in the preschool period of life and on the issues related to accomplishing that task.

Psychometric Considerations

Table 4.1 presents a general-case 2 × 2 (tetrachoric) table of the type used to evaluate screening procedures. Several measures of interest may be derived from such a table. The measures most pertinent to this discussion fall into two categories: *measures of association* and *measures of test operating characteristics*.

Measures of association indicate the degree to which two or more measurement sources agree. These indices may be used to express interobserver agreement and such measures of intertest association as concurrent validity, co-positivity, co-negativity, and test-retest reliability.

Measures of test operating characteristics quantify the efficacy and precision of a given screening test. In slight contrast to measures of agreement between tests, measures of test operating characteristics are predicated on the assumption that the confirmative test (criterion measure or "gold standard") is error free. In general, this condition can be met when measuring hearing

sensitivity. The lack of a true diagnostic standard presents a problem when other aspects of hearing or speech/language are screened. In particular, we will return to this issue when discussing screening for middle ear disease. (See "Procedural Considerations" for further discussion.)

Among the measures of association that can be calculated from a 2 × 2 table are percentage of overall agreement, Cohen's kappa coefficient of agreement (K), the chi-square statistic (χ^2), and the phi coefficient (θ), or its more familiar parametric counterpart, the Pearson product-moment correlation (r). Percent of overall agreement is probably the most frequently used index of association and is the easiest to compute. The formula for determining overall agreement (OA) is provided in Table 4.1. Each of these measures has specific properties and limitations that should be taken into consideration when selecting an appropriate measure of agreement. Marascuilo (1971), Marascuilo and McSweeney (1977), and Nie et al. (1975) provide understandable reviews of the statistical reasoning behind several of these measures. Hollenbeck (1978) also presents a cogent review of their properties, computation, and respective limitations.

Several specific indices of test operating characteristics also may be computed from the general-case decision matrix shown in Table 4.1. The most familiar of these measures are the measures of test precision: *sensitivity* and *specificity*. Sensitivity indicates how well the test detects affected persons. By contrast, specificity reflects the ability of the test to distinguish those persons who are not affected by the disease. Mathematically, sensitivity and specificity are the complement of the false-negative and false-positive rates, respectively. Thus, if one subtracted the percent of false-positive cases from 100, it would yield the specificity of the test. Conversely, if one subtracted the percent of false-negative cases from 100, it would result in the sensitivity of the test.

It is also important to recognize that the false-positive and false-negative rates are *not* equivalent to the over- and underreferral rates for the test. Rather, the over- and underreferral rates are expressed as a percentage of the marginal value shared by the true positive and true negative values (cells

Table 4.1

A General-Case Decision Matrix and Accompanying Terminology Associated with Test Operating Characteristics[a]

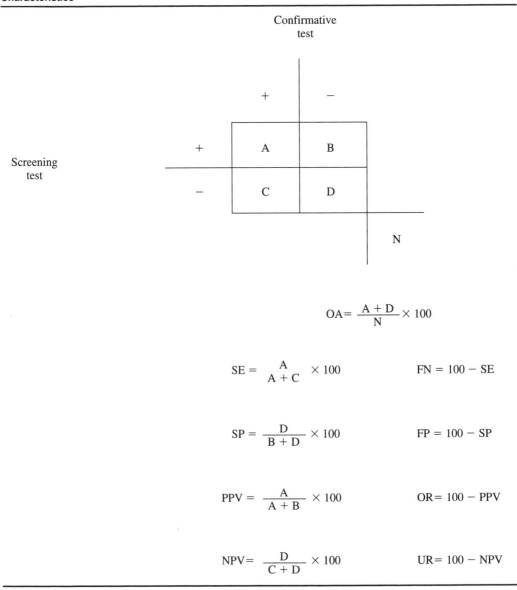

$$OA = \frac{A + D}{N} \times 100$$

$$SE = \frac{A}{A + C} \times 100 \qquad\qquad FN = 100 - SE$$

$$SP = \frac{D}{B + D} \times 100 \qquad\qquad FP = 100 - SP$$

$$PPV = \frac{A}{A + B} \times 100 \qquad\qquad OR = 100 - PPV$$

$$NPV = \frac{D}{C + D} \times 100 \qquad\qquad UR = 100 - NPV$$

[a] Test operating characteristics: overall agreement (OA), sensitivity (SE), specificity (SP), positive predictive value (PPV), negative predictive value (NPV), false-negative rate (FN), false-positive rate (FP), overreferral rate (OR), and underreferral rate (UR).

A and D) and their respective false counterparts (cells B and C). These various measures and their mathematical formulae are summarized in Table 4.1.

It should be clear from studying Table 4.1 that these measures share certain trade-off relationships (Frankenburg, 1974; Northern & Downs, 1984). Consequently, it is not possible to design a perfect screen-ing test that has 100% sensitivity and 100% specificity. Acceptable values for these various test operating characteristics are largely determined by the consequences of the disease. For example, a screening test for AIDS (acquired immune deficiency syn-drome) might require a higher sensitivity (lower false-negative rate) and a lower spec-ificity than a screening test for hearing or

Table 4.2
Summary of Test Operating Characteristics for Auditory Brainstem Response (ABR) Screening in a Sample of Randomly Selected Infants for Whom the Prevalence of Sensorineural Hearing Loss (SNHL) Is Assumed to Be 0.4% (1:250)

		Diagnostic result		
		+	−	
Screening result	+	2	50	52
	−	0	448	448
		2	498	500

Overall agreement = 90%

Sensitivity = 90%[a]	False-negative rate = 10%
Specificity = 90%	False-positive rate = 10%
Positive predictive value = 4%	Underreferral rate < 1%
Negative predictive value > 99%	Overreferral rate = 96%

[a] The sensitivity and specificity of the test are assumed to remain constant at 90% for both Table 4.2 and 4.3 and are noted accordingly. Because of sample size and prevalence rate, however, the observed sensitivity and the false-negative rate for Table 4.2 are actually 100% and 0%, respectively.

speech/language delay, since the ultimate consequence of AIDS is death. There are, to this author's knowledge, no hard data or established standards for appropriate test operating characteristics. Usually, screening tests for behavioral or developmental impairments are considered most appropriate when they demonstrate very high specificity (>0.95) to minimize overreferral. Hence, the criteria for sensitivity (>0.80) and underreferral are more relaxed. This impression comes only from this author's clinical experience, informal discussions with colleagues from the medical profession, and review of several articles on this topic.

To alter the sensitivity and specificity of the test requires redesigning the content of the test or resetting the cutoff criterion. For example, Brooks (1978) discusses how resetting the cutoff criterion for pure tone screening from 25 dB HL to 15 dB HL improves the sensitivity of the test for locating children with otitis media. The accompanying result is to inflate the false-positive rate substantially. Assuming that the prev-

alence of hearing loss remains stable during such an adjustment, there is also a resultant decrease in the specificity of the test.

There are circumstances whereby the prevalence rate of the disease can be altered. The impact on test operating characteristics is not as one might expect though. An example of the results is provided in Tables 4.2 and 4.3. Table 4.2 estimates the results from application of an auditory brainstem response (ABR) screening test to a sample of 500 children for whom the prevalence of hearing impairment is assumed to be 1:250 (after Robins, 1990). Sensitivity and specificity were taken from the literature summarized in Table 4.8. The resulting underreferral rate was less than 1%, and the overreferral rate was 96%. Table 4.3 indicates the estimated outcome if the same test were applied in a high-risk population for whom the prevalence rate is 1:50 (after Gerkin, 1984). As may be expected, a slight increase in the underreferral rate (less than 1%) and a significant

Table 4.3

Summary of Test Operating Characteristics for Auditory Brainstem Response (ABR) Screening in a Sample of Randomly Selected Infants for Whom the Prevalence of Sensorineural Hearing Loss (SNHL) Is Assumed to Be 2% (1:50)

		Diagnostic result		
		+	−	
Screening result	+	9	49	58
	−	1	441	442
		10	490	500

Overall agreement = 90%

Sensitivity = 90%	False-negative rate = 10%
Specificity = 90%	False-positive rate = 10%
Positive predictive value = 16%	Underreferral rate < 1%
Negative predictive value > 99%	Overreferral rate = 84%

decrease in the overreferral rate (84%) occur. Note, however, that there is no change in the sensitivity and specificity of the test.

The simple explanation for this effect is that when the prevalence rate of the disease is altered, the marginal values in the table are simultaneously shifted such that the sensitivity and specificity values remain unchanged. The point of raising this issue is that the specificity and sensitivity of a screening test may operate independently of the under- and overreferral rates. In other words, test precision and test efficacy may function as independent measures under certain conditions. Hence, a test with excellent sensitivity and specificity may still overrefer a high percentage of cases because of a low prevalence rate for the disease. Under these circumstances, it would be unrealistic to expect that changing the test content would substantially affect the problem of overreferral. On the other hand, if the prevalence rate can be altered somehow, then further examination of test efficiency (e.g., positive and negative predictive value) should be carried out to determine the need for and effect of altering the test design.

What this further suggests is the importance of clinicians understanding clearly the various relationships between test operating characteristics and the characteristics of the disease being identified. We will return to this issue later in the discussion when we consider program content (see Programmatic Considerations). Further review of these relationships is also offered by Fria (1985) in his discussion of screening using the auditory brainstem response (ABR).

Epidemiologic Considerations

SENSORINEURAL HEARING LOSS (SNHL)

It has been commonly reported that the incidence of sensorineural hearing loss (SNHL) approximates 1:1000 live births (Northern & Downs, 1984; Simmons 1980a, 1980b). By comparison, infants presenting with high-risk prenatal or perinatal history present with an incidence of hearing impairment around 1:50 (Gerkin, 1984; Northern & Downs, 1984; Ruth, Dey-Sigman, & Mills, 1985). Robins (1990) further observes that the combined incidence approaches 1:300 live births for all neonates irrespective of risk category.

It remains uncertain to what degree increases in survival rate of high-risk infants (Seaborg, 1985; Shenai, 1992) have altered the incidence and prevalence of SNHL. Contrary to what one might predict, the overall prevalence of SNHL appears to have remained stable, based on reports on the numbers of hearing-impaired children served under the auspices of Public Law 94-142 (U.S. Department of Education, 1979–1989). It should be recognized, however, that other factors, such as funding patterns, may account for the stability of the rate of children served; in that respect, it may not accurately reflect the actual prevalence of SNHL. It is interesting to note though that a large-scale study of hearing aid prescription data in Australia also noted a stable prevalence rate for SNHL in the decade from 1975 to 1985 while the survival rate for high-risk infants was increasing (Upfold, 1986). An interesting concomitant finding of the Upfold study was that actual decreases in the prevalence of severe to profound losses attributable to teratogenic agents, such as maternal rubella, were offset by equally large increases for SNHL in the mild to moderate categories. Certainly, this kind of shift in the demographics of hearing loss has significant implications relative to the kind of procedures applied (see Procedural Considerations).

When one extends the focus of inquiry to measures of prevalence and increases the age interval to include school-age children, it is interesting to note that the rate of SNHL increases to the 1 to 2% range (Healey et al., 1981; Hull et al., 1976). Given the incidence rate reported for neonates, it is interesting to speculate to what degree this increase in rate of occurrence might represent latent or progressive onset of SNHL. At the very least it seems prudent to account for latent and/or progressive onset by incorporating periodic monitoring, rather than single-point measurement, into our program design.

In general, the follow-up interval applied should vary depending on the suspected etiology of the hearing loss. Grundfast (1983), Northern and Downs (1984), and Jones (1988) review several dimorphisms and syndromes that are known to be associated with differing types of hearing loss. Similarly, certain risk factors, such as persistent fetal circulation (PFC) or persistent pulmonary hypertension in the newborn (PPHN), are believed to be associated with progressive or latent onset (ASHA, 1989a; Gerkin, 1984). In these cases, more frequent monitoring, say on a 6-month basis, seems warranted until one feels comfortable that progressive or latent onset has been ruled out. For example, in our own early identification program we have followed children believed at risk of progressive loss on a 6-month interval until the second birthday and then on an annual basis thereafter, unless other developmental concerns arise. These children are followed until school age, when care is transferred to the public schools.

Some caution should be exercised in the application of high-risk factors in an early identification program. In particular, several studies have observed that up to 46% of infants identified as hearing impaired presented no evidence of a high-risk history (Jacobson & Morehouse, 1984; Stein, Clark, & Kraus, 1983; Tell, Levi, & Feinmesser, 1977). It remains to be seen whether recent changes in the risk criteria will alter this finding (ASHA, 1991b). Even if this drawback were resolved, concerns about the test operating characteristics of the HRR would remain (Kenworthy, 1990). Taken as a whole, these observations suggest that although risk factors may be used to improve the yield from a screening procedure such as ABR, the use of risk factors alone is not sufficient to accomplish comprehensive early identification. Furthermore, recent work by Turner and Cone-Wesson (1992) has raised some interesting questions about the cost-effectiveness of high-risk factors.

MIDDLE EAR EFFUSION (MEE)

Middle ear effusion (MEE) is unquestionably one of the most prevalent diseases in early childhood. Studies have reported that between 60 and 80% of children may evidence a single bout of the disease prior to their third birthday. The prevalence rate drops sharply if only recurring cases are considered. Nonetheless, approximately one-third (35%) of the population has been estimated to experience more than three bouts of MEE prior to their third birthday (Klein, 1983; Teele, Klein, & Rosner, 1980). Moreover, the incidence of MEE has been found to peak between 6 and 8 months of age (Marchant et al., 1985). Data from several studies have suggested that between 30 and 40% of all neonates present with MEE (Jacobson & Morehouse, 1984; Keith, 1973, 1975; Zarnoch & Balkany, 1978).

This presents a challenge to early identification for several reasons. First, it has been suggested that up to 60% of children with MEE have associated hearing loss in excess of 20 dB HL (Bess, 1984; Fria, Cantekin, & Eichler, 1985). Yet many of the children who contract MEE will resolve spontaneously without the benefit of medical intervention (Bavosi & Rupp, 1984; Cantekin et al., 1983). From the standpoint of test operating characteristics, this means that the overreferral rate for any given protocol is apt to be high unless children with MEE are selected out of the sample and subjected to different referral, tracking, and monitoring procedures (Fria, 1985; Jacobson & Morehouse, 1984). In addition, the cutoff criterion applied and the timing of testing may need to be altered to account for MEE throughout infancy and the preschool period (Brooks, 1978, 1982; Jacobson, Jacobson, & Spahr, 1990). Whether one includes some measure of middle ear function and/or adjusts cutoff criterion to rule out or rule in MEE cases will be determined by the resulting test operating characteristics as well as the identified goals and objectives of the identification program (see Procedural Considerations and Programmatic Considerations).

The inclusion of measures of middle ear function in the screening protocol will also be influenced by one's perceptions of the risk of leaving the disease untreated. Previous mention has been made of the tendency for MEE to resolve spontaneously. This should not be taken to mean that the disease is without consequence. The medical consequences of untreated, recurrent MEE are well understood and include cholesteotoma, mastoiditis, meningitis, and ossicular necrosis to mention just a few (Bluestone et al., 1983; Harford et al., 1978). In addition, recent evidence has suggested that

other developmental sequelae such as cognitive (Ruben, 1984) and speech/language delays (Finitzo, Friel-Patti, & Lindgren, 1991; Shriberg & Smith, 1983; Teele, Klein, & Rosner, 1980) may be linked to recurrent middle ear disease. Whether these sequelae are causally linked to MEE and prevalent enough to warrant mass screening remains a matter of controversy (Bluestone, Fria, & Arjona, 1986; Ventry, 1980, 1983).

Programmatic Considerations
CALCULATING COSTS

The rationale for establishing comprehensive early identification programs is well recognized (Kenworthy, 1987), and public policy has turned favorably toward the goal of early identification. Nevertheless, we still face some formidable budgetary obstacles within the current fiscal context. We cannot hope to surmount these obstacles without a clear understanding of both the required budgetary allocations and the unit (per case) costs of our services. Cooper et al. (1975) offer the following formula as a method of computing unit costs:

$$\text{Unit Cost} = (S/R) + (C + (M \times L)/(N \times L))$$

where S = salary for the person(s) conducting the screening, in dollars per hour; R = rate, or number of children screened per hour; C = cost of the equipment and supplies, in total dollars expended; M = annual maintenance costs, in dollars; L = lifetime of the equipment, in years; and N = number of children screened (or accurately referred), per year.

Two unit costs might be derived from this formula, depending on the value assigned to N. We can determine the unit cost per child screened by setting the value of N equal to the total population. Or, we can establish the costs per child identified by setting N equal to the number of children accurately referred. By using the latter value, we account for variance in test operating characteristics between screening measures and provide a clearer picture of how test precision and yield affect program effectiveness. Tables 4.4 to 4.7 offer examples of how this formula might be used to

Table 4.4
A Sample Cost Analysis of ABR Screening for All Live Births Versus Only High-Risk Births

Assumptions

1. Incidence of SNHL for high-risk infants = 1:50

2. Incidence of SNHL for all live births = 1:250

3. Test operating characteristics and all other cost parameters are constant across the two approaches

   Sensitivity (SE) = 98%
   Specificity (SP) = 90%
   S/R = 0   M = $200/yr
   C = $10,000   L = 5 yr

Unit Costs for Screening High-Risk Births

N1 (Children screened) = 500/yr
N2 (Children referred) = 10

UC1 (Unit cost/child screened) = $ 4.40
UC2 (Unit cost/child referred) = $220.00

Unit Costs for Screening All Live Births
N1 = 500/yr   UC1 = $ 4.40
N2 =   2/yr   UC2 = $1100.00

evaluate program strategies, outcomes, and equipment.

Table 4.4 provides a sample cost comparison of screening by ABR all live births versus only infants considered at high risk of hearing loss. This analysis provides some insight into the impact of prevalence not only on yield but also on program costs. The resulting reduction in unit cost when screening only high-risk infants is striking, providing one compares the cost per child referred. As might be expected, the cost decreases by the same factor of five as the prevalence rate increase.

Table 4.5 displays estimates of the cost differential for screening by ABR versus the HRR. Note that the cost differential for unit cost based on children screened is in favor of the HRR by a factor of four. When one takes into account test operating characteristics and computes the costs per child referred, the costs are more comparable. This particular analysis also points up an interesting characteristic of the formula proposed by Cooper et al. (1975). Because this method accounts only for children accurately referred, it is influenced by the results

of the main diagonal (cells A and D) and not by the off-diagonal results.

The off-diagonal results are important to consider when comparing two methods with different test operating characteristics, as in this case. Based on the test operating characteristics reported in Table 4.8 and assuming that the same sample of 500 infants with a prevalence rate of 1:50 was screened by each method independently, one would derive a false-positive (cell B) value of 39 cases for the ABR but 122 cases for the HRR. If the cost of providing diagnostic follow-up were $100 per referral, then the total costs for the two programs would differ by $9400 in favor of ABR screening. This does not take into consideration both the tangible and intangible costs related to the failure of the HRR to identify four children with SNHL. Certainly, these costs should be included in the decision-making process.

Table 4.6 details a sample costs analysis of two different acoustic immittance meters. This example points out the importance of considering all aspects of the cost formula. Although ZA1 is the more costly machine by nearly a factor of two, its unit cost is actually lower. This is attributable to slight differences in annual maintenance costs, an increased life expectancy, and improved yield (N1).

Finally, Table 4.7 shows what potential impact the use of paraprofessionals might have on program costs. The hourly cost differential of nearly $5.00 per hour offers no significant impact on the unit costs for the test, once a slight difference in rate (10 seconds per child) is factored in. It is interesting to further consider that this example does not take into consideration the training and supervision costs that might accrue if paraprofessionals were employed.

POPULATION SELECTION

The overriding goal of any identification program is to ensure that all individuals exposed to the disease are screened and accurately referred. Universal access is, however, an ideal that is compromised by psychometric limitations and by logistical factors that limit enrollment and follow-up. Accordingly, our implementation of an identification program represents a series of

Table 4.5
A Sample Cost Comparison of Screening by Means of the Auditory Brainstem Response (ABR) and by Applying a Computerized High-Risk Register (HRR)

Assumptions

1. Salary and rate of screening are equal across the two programs and are set equal to zero (0).

2. Test operating characteristics and cost parameters are as follows:

Parameter	ABR	HRR
Cost (C)	$10,000	$ 4,000
Maintenance (M)	200/yr	200/yr
Life (L)	5 yr	5 yr
Sensitivity (SE)	98%	65%
Specificity (SP)	90%	75%
N1 (Screened)	500/yr	5000/yr
N2 (Referred)[a]	10/yr	5/yr

Associated Unit Costs

	ABR	HRR
UC1	$ 4.40	1.00
UC2	$ 220.00	166.00

[a] The N2 value for the high-risk register is further predicated on the assumption that application of the risk criteria to a sample of 5000 infants will result in a screening sample of 425 infants, or 8.5%, to which the applicable test operating characteristics are applied to obtain the true positive yield. (See Kenworthy, 1990, for further discussion.)

Table 4.6
A Sample Cost Analysis for Two Acoustic Immittance Meters (ZA1 and ZA2) for Screening Middle Ear Function

Assumptions

1. Salary and rate of screening are constant across the two machines and are set equal to zero.

2. Test operating characteristics are slightly different across the two machines because of a manual (ZA1) versus automated (ZA2) cutoff criterion, thus resulting in a slight difference in yield (N1).

3. Pertinent cost parameters are as follows:

Parameter	ZA1	ZA2
Cost (C)	$ 4500	2500
Maintenance (M)	$ 100/yr	200/yr
Life (L)	5 yr	3 yr
N1 (Referred)	500/yr	450/yr

Associated Unit Costs per Machine

	ZA1	ZA2
UC1	$2.00	2.30

compromises that seeks to maximize yield and minimize obstacles. In the case of early identification of hearing loss, we must choose between mass screening of all infants and selective screening of subsamples of children. From the foregoing examples and the discussion of psychometric principles, the advantage of increasing the prevalence rate of the population screened should be evident. What should be similarly evident, however, is that the test operating characteristics of the preselection method are equally as important as the actual screening method (Turner, 1990). Consider, for example, our earlier observation that nearly 50% of the children with SNHL present without high-risk histories. While recent revisions to the HRR may alter this finding, it seems prudent to account for it until research can document the impact of those revisions. Therefore, use of the HRR as a preselection device may need to be augmented by other procedures that accurately select those children who evidence an increased likelihood of SNHL but are not considered otherwise "at risk" by traditional criteria. (For further discussion, see Mencher, 1977; Turner, Frazer, & Shephard, 1984; and Turner, 1990.)

In that regard, we might consider routine speech/language screening as an appropriate supplement. There are several good reasons for implementing this strategy. First, we know that speech/language delay is closely associated with the presence of hearing loss. Second, this association appears to operate independently of the severity of the hearing loss (Davis et al., 1986) or the etiology of the hearing loss (Finitzo, Friel-Patti, & Lindgren, 1991). Third, parental concern over the child's speech/language development has been found to be associated with referral of children for audiologic evaluation (Kenworthy, 1987). Fourth, there are methods of screening available that are efficient, easy to administer, and of proven reliability (Coplan, 1983; Ireton & Thwing, 1974; Matkin, 1984). Accordingly, these measures allow implementation in numerous settings by professionals of varied background (e.g., physicians and other allied-health professionals). This, in turn, increases accessibility and may minimize obstacles to follow-up (Kenworthy, 1987, 1990).

Table 4.7
A Sample Cost Analysis of Two Staffing
Strategies: Use of an Audiologist (MA) Versus
an Audiometrist (AU)

Assumptions

1. Test operating characteristics are assumed to be equal across examiners. Differences in N1 are attributable only to rate differences over the time allotted.

2. Total time allotted is set arbitrarily to one full work week (40 hours) of direct patient contact.

3. Rates (R) are predicated on per-patient rates of 30 seconds for MA and 40 seconds for AU.

4. Pertinent cost parameters are as follows:

Parameter	MA	AU
Hourly salary (S)	$ 15.60	11.00
Hourly test rate (R)	120	90
Cost (C)	$ 4500	4500
Maintenance (M)	$100/yr	100/yr
Life (L)	5/yr	5/yr
N1 (Screened)	4000	3600

Associated Unit Costs

	MA	AU
UC1	$ 0.34	0.40

A slight variation on this theme arises when screening for MEE. In this case, the prevalence of the disease is less at issue. As noted previously, over two-thirds of all children will experience MEE prior to their third birthday, and, more to the point, over 60% of those children with MEE will present with abnormal hearing. What presents as a concern in this case is the clinical course of the disease. Specifically, two-thirds of those children who present with MEE will recover subsequent to medical treatment and will not be further affected by the disease (Klein, 1983). In addition, many of those children who contract the disease, even on a recurrent basis, will spontaneously recover without the benefit of medical intervention (Bavosi & Rupp, 1984; Cantekin et al., 1983). Accordingly, it seems prudent to develop criteria for those children considered at risk of recurrence of the disease and its developmental sequelae. (For further discussion, see Brooks, 1982; Lous, 1983; and Kenworthy, 1990).

PROGRAM FOCUS AND EFFECTIVENESS

It should be clear from the foregoing discussion that there are numerous decisions related to implementation of a comprehensive early identification program that require technical consideration and professional input. Further examples of these technical issues are also advanced below in our discussion of procedural considerations. It goes without saying though that even the most technically sophisticated program can become the victim of the infamous budget cut if the program's rationale and aims are not clearly articulated (Bess & McConnell, 1981; Wilson & Walton, 1978). The viability of any service may be predicated as much on its adherence to its stated goals (and budgetary allocations) as its level of technical excellence. It is crucial to establish a clear action plan and to develop a consensus of support for the program's objectives **prior** to implementation. Using such a plan and administrative mandate as one's guide will, in fact, assist in technical decision making. For example, if the aim of a particular program is to identify **all** children with abnormal hearing, then screening for middle ear disease would be appropriate for inclusion, *and* screening all live births might be suitable. On the other hand, if the program's aim were to identify all children with significant SNHL, then the inclusion of middle ear screening might seem more questionable or would at least require formulation of a different rationale than in the first case. To proceed with such decisions without a clearly formed action plan and administrative mandate would seem to be a classic example of missing the forest for the trees and may generate unnecessary obstacles to success.

PROGRAM SCOPE

In addition to developing an appropriate focus to our program, we must also recognize its accompanying scope. If our goal is to provide services to all affected cases, then we need to be sensitive to limitations on full access. In particular, we need to recognize the etiology and natural history of the disease and develop procedures that account for these variables. In addition, we must recognize and account for barriers to

Table 4.8
A Summary of Selected Screening Measures and Their Respective Test Operating Characteristics

Method	Source	Age Range (mo.)	Test Operating Characteristics		Cutoff Criterion
			Sens.	Spec.	
High-risk register	Mahoney & Eichwald (1979)	Birth	65	75	Positive on one or more factors
Behavioral: arousal	Downs & Sterritt (1967)	0–4	63	29	50 dB HL
Behavioral: VRA	Kenworthy et al. (1986)	>6	80	86	30 dB HL
Auditory brainstem response	Fria (1985)	Birth–Adult	98	95	60 and 30 dB nHL
Individual pure-tone	Wilson & Walton (1978)	>36	63	97	20 dB HL
	Melnick et al. (1964)		85	98	20 dB HL
ELM scale	Coplan (1983)	0–36[a]	90	93	Failure on any item at 90% point of emergence

[a] The reader should be aware that Walker and her co-workers (1989) have suggested that test operating characteristics of the ELM scale may be age dependent. Accordingly, there may be an optimal age range for application of the scale (18 months and above) that does not correspond with the full age range of the published scale.

appropriate follow-up. In the case of SNHL, this necessitates procedures that account for latent and progressive onset and that ensure parental compliance with screening recommendations. To accomplish these two ends may go beyond the scope of any single program and require interagency coordination. That is, identification and screening will be required across numerous disciplines and settings such as hospitals, clinics, physicians' offices, and the schools (Kenworthy, 1990). Along with this system-wide effort, centralized lines of communication and authority will be needed.

Procedural Considerations

TEST SELECTION

Once our goals, objectives, and supporting rationale are clearly formulated, then the selection of appropriate procedures is simplified greatly. In essence, we must simply match the test operating characteristics, developmental level, and other measure-

ment constructs of each available instrument with the demographics, etiology, natural history, and developmental sequelae of the disease. To assist in this effort, Table 4.8 offers a summary of test operating characteristics of some well-recognized screening methods that might be appropriate to a comprehensive early identification program, as discussed above. The discussion that follows also provides some procedural hints that may assist in fine-tuning the screening protocol.

PROTOCOL CONSIDERATIONS.

Behavioral Methods

In developing a screening protocol for early identification of hearing loss, it is important to recognize that the demographics of SNHL may be shifting toward an increase in the prevalence of milder losses (Upfold, 1986) and sloping, high-frequency losses. To respond appropriately to this trend, our screening protocols must incorporate more frequency-specific procedures and lower cutoff criteria (e.g., 30 dB HL) than may have been previously acceptable. This, in turn, places some limitations on the use of behavioral methods, both behavioral observation audiometry (BOA) and visual reinforcement audiometry (VRA), as screening procedures (ASHA, 1989a, 1991a).

For infants under 5 months of age, it should be recognized that their responses to external stimuli are prone to be reflexive in nature and correspondingly variable. Consequently, it has been generally observed that elicitation of clearly evident behavioral responses from these infants necessitates the use of signals that exceed 50 dB HL (Eisenberg, 1976; Northern & Downs, 1984). This principle has applied whether the testing has been conducted in vivo (e.g., Downs & Sterritt, 1967) or has been automated (Bennett, 1979; Simmons, 1980a, 1980b). Olsho and her colleagues (1988) have provided recent data relative to behaviorally derived hearing thresholds in neonates and young infants that contradict this finding. It would appear, however, that the time and instrumentation required to acquire these results would preclude application of Olsho's methodology to the screening process. Until such an adaptation might be accomplished and proved, available methods of behavioral testing in this age range would not appear consistent with the cutoff criterion required to capture milder losses.

The use of noisemakers and other broadband stimuli is also a questionable practice when identification of mild to moderate losses or sloping, high-frequency losses is a concern. Coleman and Pelson (1977) observed that noisemakers calibrated for hearing screening emitted signal transients that departed significantly from the expected frequency and intensity characteristics. This raises the question of whether the use of even calibrated noisemakers might best be restricted to selecting cases with flat, moderate-to-severe losses.

Application of a 30-dB HL criterion, to allow for identification of milder losses, also raises concerns about ambient noise levels when applying behavioral methods, including VRA. Customarily, the ambient noise levels in most screening environments comply only with standards for the "ears covered" condition. This assumes that the attenuation characteristics of the earphone cushion enter into play. It seems less likely that these same screening environments will comply with the standards for an "ears uncovered" (sound-field) measurement. This concern has been raised specifically with regard to neonatal intensive care units (Fria, 1985). To address this concern, a properly sound-treated environment may be required. If this proves necessary, it raises the overall costs of screening, and, in the case of NICU patients, it necessitates additional personnel to ensure safe and appropriate transport and monitoring.

Finally, as the cutoff criterion is lowered, more children with MEE are identified as screening failures (Brooks, 1978). Because MEE tends to resolve spontaneously, the tracking and referral of infants with MEE will need to vary from those infants who fail screening but are clear of MEE (Harford et al., 1978; Lucker, 1980; Roeser & Northern, 1981). Specifically, to maintain acceptable under- and overreferral rates may require some measure of middle ear function (Jacobson, Jacobson, & Spahr, 1990). Most often, acoustic immittance measures have been proposed to fulfill this function.

Acoustic Immittance

Although the data are not universal in support of acoustic immittance, it has been generally accepted as a valid and reliable measure of middle ear function for preschool and school-age children (see Kenworthy, 1987, 1990 for further discussion). If one is screening infants under 7 months of age, the limitations of tympanometry should be well understood (Paradise, Smith, & Bluestone, 1976; Sprague, Wiley, & Goldstein, 1985). In particular, the use of 220-Hz probe tone may result in an inordinately high number of false-negatives due to the flaccidity of the young infant's ear canal and the sensitivity of lower frequency probe tones to stiffness. The use of higher frequency probe tones (e.g., 660 or 678 Hz) has provided some encouraging results, but these are preliminary in nature and do not represent full test operating characteristics (Sprague, Wiley, & Goldstein, 1985). Similarly, acoustic reflexes (Schwartz & Schwartz, 1978), reflectometry (Teele & Teele, 1984), and otoscopy have all been suggested as potential alternatives, but the data relative to their test operating characteristics are either inadequate or discouraging (Kenworthy, 1990).

Another difficulty in evaluating middle ear screening methods is that there is a lack of a clear "gold standard" on which to base test operating characteristics. Traditionally, pneumatic otoscopy has been accepted as the criterion measure, providing that the examiner's observations have been validated against the findings of typanocentesis or myringotomy (e.g., Orchik, Morff, & Dunn, 1985). Although not ideal, this approach has been well accepted in the research literature as a reasonable compromise of the various ethical and practical considerations involved. Because of logistical and fiscal limitations, this method has not been applied in other than experimental settings. This would be of no concern except that comparisons of tympanometry with validated otoscopy have yielded quite different results than comparisons between tympanometry and routine clinical judgments.

For example, when Cooper et al. (1975) compared tympanometry with the findings of a validated otoscopist who classified ears as normal/abnormal, they found sensitivity of 94% and specificity of 61%. By contrast Schow et al. (1984) compared tympanometry with routine clinical otoscopy whereby ears were classified as treat/no treat. Under these conditions, the resulting sensitivity and specificity were 82% and 85%, respectively. The discrepancy in findings between these studies may be attributed to the differing classification systems used interacting with *(1)* the poor reliability reported previously for routine otoscopy (Paradise, 1976; Reichert et al., 1978; Roeser et al., 1977) and *(2)* a tendency for physicians to avoid overtreatment. In the study by Cooper et al., the validated otoscopist needed only to classify ears as normal/abnormal without regard to treatment. By contrast, the physicians in the study by Schow et al. had to make a determination about whether to treat any noted deviations from normal. Consequently, when faced with uncertainty or with resolving MEE, physicians in the study by Schow et al. might classify an ear as not requiring treatment, whereas the validated otoscopist in the study by Cooper et al. might classify a similar ear as abnormal. The classification scheme applied in each case is defensible, but the outcomes relative to test operating characteristics would be quite different. Hence, until more efficient and effective means of validating test performance are made available, our evaluations of programs that screen for MEE should remain mindful of the discrepancies between clinical and research findings in this area and the limitations of using clinical otoscopy as our criterion measure (Paradise & Smith, 1978).

Auditory Brainstem Response (ABR)

For screening infants under 5 months of age, the ABR has emerged as the clear method of choice (ASHA, 1989a, 1991a; Fria, 1985; Jacobson, Jacobson, & Spahr, 1990; Ruth, Dey-Sigman, & Mills, 1985). In fact, ASHA Guidelines for Audiologic Screening for Newborn Infants Who Are at Risk for Hearing Impairment (ASHA, 1989a) spell out quite clearly a protocol that includes the following recommendations:

- *Application of high-risk criteria.* All children identified at risk of hearing impairment, based on criteria at the Joint Infant Hearing Committee, are preselected for audiologic screening.
- *Parent/caregiver education.* All parents are to be alerted to risk factors and provided with information that will facilitate appropriate referral.
- *Audiologic screening.* All newborns identified as at risk are to be screened by ABR prior to discharge from the hospital. Pass criterion is a "response from both ears at intensity levels 40 dB nHL or less" (p. 91).
- *Immediate referral, evaluation, management, and follow-up.* Infants who fail the ABR screening are to receive immediate referral for evaluation and follow-up. All infants who fail on follow-up evaluation are to be referred for comprehensive medical evaluation. Electrophysiologic findings are to be confirmed by means of behavioral testing. Intervention services are to be initiated by 6 months of age, when indicated.
- *Continued monitoring for progressive loss.* Infants who pass the initial ABR but are considered at risk of latent-onset or progressive hearing loss "should receive au-

diologic monitoring on a periodic basis and probably through the preschool years" (p. 91).

In addition to these recommendations, our own efforts in this area have led us to adopt some additional procedural precautions. First, we screen all NICU infants by ABR without applying the HRR. Consistent with arguments raised by Turner (1990), we view application of the HRR to NICU populations as adding costs without appreciable benefit. Second, we have come to recognize that the "objectivity" of the ABR is compromised in cases where wave morphology is not well developed. In our experience, such is the case in a substantial number of our neonates. Accordingly, we employ a second, independent reading of all ABRs for which wave morphology is questionable. In addition, our quality review procedures require us to provide second, independent readings on a random sample of all ABRs done in the NICU. Third, we always monitor the input rather than wave acquisition. It has been our observation, especially in certain subsamples, such as drug-exposed infants, that the ABR input may reflect a high level of spurious activity, or noise, that does not register as artifact or overload. This may occur even in fully sedated babies. The result of this noise can be waveforms that resemble the classic waveform template, even though no stimulus is presented. Finally, we observe the added precaution of including no-stimulus, or control, trials in our protocol. We do this to counteract the effects of spurious activity that may or may not be visible on the ABR input screen. In cases where we can get interobserver agreement, low noise level on the input, and no identifiable "responses" during control trials, we feel confident our results will reflect the precision and "objectivity" that has been reported in the literature on ABR screening.

In spite of well-developed protocols and the high acceptance of the ABR as a screening procedure, unit costs for this procedure limit its application to other than high-risk populations. With an average test time of 40 to 60 minutes the resulting unit costs easily exceed $200 per child referred (see Table 4.4). The need for occasional sedation even in neonates and infants presents an additional concern. Recently, the measurement of otoacoustic emissions has emerged as a cost-effective alternative that may allow expansion of neonatal screening into well-child nurseries.

Otoacoustic Emissions (OAE)

In 1978, Kemp first reported his observation of signals emitted *from* the inner ear into the external auditory meatus in response to auditory stimulation with clicks. Since that time, numerous investigators have confirmed Kemp's original observations in both adults and children. (See Cope and Lutman, 1988, for a review.)

Two general classes of OAE have been observed: *spontaneous* and *evoked*. Spontaneous emissions (SOAE), as the name implies, occur without any external stimuli. Although quite common, they appear in only about 40% of subjects with normal hearing (e.g., Probst et al., 1986; Strickland, Burns, & Tubis, 1985). Accordingly, SOAEs appear useful in further explicating cochlear mechanics but impractical as a screening response. By contrast, evoked otoacoustic emissions (EOAEs) have been nearly universally observed in ears with normal hearing (e.g., Johnsen et al., 1988) and have not been observed in the presence of peripheral hearing loss greater than 30 to 40 dB HL (Collet et al., 1989; Kemp, Ryan, & Bray, 1990). Unlike SOAEs, the presence of EOAEs is directly linked to the intensity of an external eliciting signal. As such, EOAEs have direct application to the screening process.

Until recently, the clinical application of OAE has been most widespread in the United Kingdom and Europe. Kemp and his colleagues (e.g., Bray & Kemp, 1987) have developed instrumentation for measuring delayed EOAEs that is now commercially available in the United States. This instrumentation uses a probe system similar to acoustic immittance meters and transient stimulation and signal-averaging techniques similar to the ABR. Like acoustic immittance, the time required for acquiring results is quite brief, around 1 to 3 minutes per ear (Bonfils, Uziel, & Pujol, 1988; Bray & Kemp, 1987).

Test operating characteristics of the test when applied to infants have also been quite encouraging. Two studies are of par-

Table 4.9
A Summary of Combined Results from Two Studies Comparing the ABR and Evoked Otoacoustic Emissions

		Diagnostic result (ABR)		
		+	−	
Screening result (OAE)	+	41	16	57
	−	8	196	204
		49	212	261

Overall agreement = 91%

Sensitivity = 84%	False-negative rate = 24%
Specificity = 92%	False-positive rate = 8%
Positive predictive value = 72%	Underreferral rate = 4%
Negative predictive value = 96%	Overreferral rate = 28%

ticular relevance to this discussion. Bonfils and co-workers (1988) studied a sample of 46 ears from 30 normally hearing infants and 16 infants with SNHL, as measured by ABR. Using a cutoff criterion of 30 dB nHL for both tests, these authors noted overall agreement between ABR and EOAE of 98% with sensitivity of 100% and specificity of 97%. Similarly, Stevens and colleagues (1987) performed EOAE and ABR measures on 215 ears of 112 infants admitted to a special care nursery and found overall agreement of 89%, sensitivity of 76%, and specificity of 92%, using cutoff criteria of 31 dB nHL for OAE and 43 dB nHL for ABR.

Table 4.9 summarizes the combined results of the two studies. The resulting overall agreement was 91%, with sensitivity of 84% and specificity of 92%. With an estimated prevalence of 19%, the underreferral rate was 4%, and the overreferral rate was 28%. Based on an estimated hourly compensation (salary plus benefits) of $25 per hour, a screening rate of 10 infants per hour, equipment costs of $11,000, maintenance and supply costs of $300 per year, an equipment life of 5 years, and 6 solid hours of testing per day, the resulting unit costs for

this test would be $2.67 and would not vary significantly whether based on number of children tested or number of children referred.

There are some limitations to these findings that should be taken into account in future studies. In particular, neither study employed a blind design, both applied the ABR as the confirmative test, and both samples evidenced a prevalence rate that exceeds that reported for the general population (Frankenburg, Chen, & Thornton, 1988). Nevertheless, these results offer some encouraging prospects for the future of early identification.

Acknowledgments. The author gratefully acknowledges the assistance of Tom Campbell, Ph.D., Allan Diefendorf, Ph.D., and Vicki Jax, Ph.D., in critiquing ideas presented in this manuscript. Heartfelt gratitude is also due to Christine Carpenter and Donna Stockbridge for their help in preparing this manuscript.

References

American Speech-Language-Hearing Association (ASHA), Committee on Audiometric Evaluation,

Guidelines for Acoustic Immittance Screening of Middle-Ear Function. *Asha*, **21**, 283–291 (1979).

American Speech-Language-Hearing Association (ASHA), Committee on Audiologic Evaluation, Guidelines for Identification Audiometry. *Asha*, **27**, 49–52+ (1985).

American Speech-Language-Hearing Association (ASHA), Committee on Infant Hearing, Guidelines for Audiologic Screening of Newborn Infants Who Are at Risk for Hearing Impairment. *Asha*, **31**, 89–92 (1989a).

American Speech-Language-Hearing Association (ASHA), Committee on Audiologic Evaluation and Working Group on Acoustic Immittance Measurements, Guidelines for Screening for Hearing Impairment and Middle Ear Disorders. *Asha*, **31**, 71–92 (1989b).

American Speech-Language-Hearing Association (ASHA), Committee on Infant Hearing, Guidelines for the Audiologic Assessment of Children from Birth Through Thirty-Six Months of Age. *Asha* (Suppl. 5), 37–43 (March 1991a).

American Speech-Language-Hearing Association (ASHA), Joint Committee on Infant Hearing, 1990 Position Statement. *Asha*, (Suppl. 5), 3–6 (March 1991b).

Bavosi, R., and Rupp, R., Otitis media in children: further findings on spontaneous resolution. *Hear. J.*, **37**(2), 18 (1984).

Bennett, M., Trials with the auditory response cradle: 7. Neonatal response to auditory stimuli. *Br. J. Audiol.*, **13**, 125–134 (1979).

Bess, F., Hearing loss associated with middle ear effusion. *Pediatrics*, **75**, 206–216 (1984).

Bess, F., and McConnell, F., *Audiology, Education and Hearing Impaired*. St. Louis, MO: C.V. Mosby (1981).

Bluestone, C., Berry, Q., and Paradise, J., Audiometry and tympanometry in relation to middle ear effusions in children. *Laryngoscope*, **83**, 594–604 (1973).

Bluestone, C., Fria, T., Arjona, S., et al., Controversies in screening for middle ear disease and hearing loss in children. *Pediatrics*, **77**, 57–77 (1986).

Bluestone, C., Klein, J., Paradise, J., et al., Workshop on effects of otitis media on the child. *Pediatrics*, **71**, 639–652 (1983).

Bonfils, P., Uziel, A., and Pujol, R., Screening for auditory dysfunction in infants by evoked oto-acoustic emissions. *Arch. Otolaryngol. Head Neck Surg.*, **114**, 887–890 (1988).

Bray, P., and Kemp, D., An advanced cochlear echo technique suitable for infant screening. *Br. J. Audiol.*, **21**, 191–204 (1987).

Brooks, D., Acoustic impedance testing for screening auditory function in school children: part II. *Maico Audiological Library Series*, **15**, Report 9 (1978).

Brooks, D., Acoustic impedance studies on otitis media with effusion. *Int. J. Pediatr. Otorhinolaryngol.*, **4**, 89–94 (1982).

Cantekin, E., Mandel, E., Bluestone, C., et al., Lack of efficacy of a decongestant-antihistamine combination for otitis media with effusion ("secretory" otitis media) in children. *N. Engl. J. Med.*, **308**, 297–301 (1983).

Coleman, R., and Pelson, R., Marked high frequency hearing loss in children: a problem for early identification. *J. Speech Hear. Dis.*, **42**, 335–339 (1977).

Collet, L., Gartner, M., Moulin, A., et al., Evoked otoacoustic emissions and sensorineural hearing loss. *Arch. Otolaryngol. Head Neck Surg.*, **115**, 1060–1062 (1989).

Cooper, J.C., Jr., Gates, G., Owen, J., and Dickson, H., An abbreviated impedance bridge screening technique for school screening. *J. Speech Hear. Dis.*, **40**, 260–369 (1975).

Cope, Y., and Lutman, M., Oto-acoustic emissions. In B. McCormick (Ed.), *Paediatric Audiology 0–5 Years*. London: Taylor & Francis (1988).

Coplan, J., *The Early Language Milestone (ELM) Scale*. Tulsa, OK: Modern Education Corporation (1983).

Davis, J., Elfenbein, J., Schum, R., and Bentler, R., Effects of mild and moderate hearing impairments on language, educational and psychosocial behavior of children. *J. Speech Hear. Dis.*, **51**, 53–62 (1986).

Downs, M., and Sterritt, G., Identification audiometry for neonates. *Arch. Otolaryngol.*, **85**, 15–22 (1967).

Eisenberg, R., *Auditory Competence in Early Life: The Roots of Communicative Behavior*. Baltimore, MD: University Park Press (1976).

Finitzo, T., Friel-Patti, S., and Lindgren, B., Early tympanostomy tube intervention in OME: protection for future language development? Paper presented at the International Symposium on Screening Children for Auditory Function, Vanderbilt University, Nashville, TN (July 1991).

FitZaland, R., and Zink, G.D., A comparative study of hearing screening procedures. *Ear Hear.*, **5**, 205–210 (1984).

Frankenburg, W., Selection of diseases and tests in pediatric screening. *Pediatrics*, **54**, 612–616 (1974).

Frankenburg, W., Chen, J., and Thornton, S., Common pitfalls in the evaluation of developmental screening tests. *J. Pediatrics*, **113**, 1110–1113 (1988).

Fria, T., Identification of congenital hearing loss with the auditory brainstem response. In J. Morehouse (Ed.), *The Auditory Brainstem Response*. San Diego, CA: College-Hill Press, pp. 317–334 (1985).

Fria, T., Cantekin, E., and Eichler, J., Hearing acuity of children with otitis media with effusion. *Arch. Otolaryngol.*, **111**, 10–16 (1985).

Gerkin, K., The high risk register for deafness. *Asha*, **26**, 17–23 (1984).

Gruber, H.E., and Voneche, J.J., *The Essential Piaget*. New York: Basic Books, Inc. (1977).

Grundfast, K., The role of the audiologist and otologist in the identification of the dysmorphic child. *Ear Hear.*, **4**, 24–30 (1983).

Harford, E., Bess, F., Bluestone, C., and Klein, J., *Impedance Screening for Middle Ear Disease in Children*. New York: Grune & Stratton (1978).

Healey, W., Ackerman, B., Chappell, C., Perrin, K., and Stormer, J., *The Prevalence of Communicative Disorders: A Review of the Literature*. Rockville, MD: American Speech-Language-Hearing Association (1981).

Hollenbeck, A., Problems of reliability in observational research. In G. Sackett (Ed.), *Observing Behavior, Vol. II, Data Collection and Analysis Methods*. Baltimore, MD: University Park Press, pp. 79–98 (1978).

Hull, J., National speech and hearing survey: final report. Colorado State University, Project No. 50978, Grant No. OE-32-15-0050-5010 (607), U.S. Department of Health, Education and Welfare, Bureau of Education for the Handicapped (1969).

Ireton, H., and Thwing, E., *Manual for the Minnesota Child Development Inventory*. Minneapolis, MN: Behavior Sciences System (1974).

Jacobson, J., and Morehouse, C., A comparison of auditory adapted screening in high risk and normal newborn infants. *Ear Hear.*, **5**, 247–253 (1984).

Jacobson, J., Jacobson, C., and Spahr, R., Automated and conventional ABR screening techniques in high-risk infants. *J. Am. Acad. Audiol.*, **1**, 187–195 (1990).

Johnsen, N., Bagi, P., Parbo, J., and Eberling, C., Evoked acoustic emissions from the human ear. *Scand. Audiol.*, **17**, 27–34 (1988).

Jones, K.L., *Smith's Recognizable Patterns of Human Malformation* (4th ed.). Philadelphia: W.B. Saunders (1988).

Keith, R., Impedance audiometry in neonates. *Arch. Otolaryngol.*, **97**, 465–467 (1973).

Keith, R., Middle ear function in neonates. *Arch. Otolaryngol.*, **101**, 376–379 (1975).

Kemp, D., Stimulated acoustic emission from within the human auditory system. *J. Acoust. Soc. Am.*, **64**, 1388–1391 (1978).

Kemp, D., Ryan, S., and Bray, P., A guide to the effective use of otoacoustic emissions. *Ear Hear.*, **11**, 93–105 (1990).

Kenworthy, O.T., Identification of hearing loss in infancy and early childhood. In J. Alpiner and P. McCarthy (Eds.), *Rehabilitative Audiology: Children and Adults*. Baltimore: Williams & Wilkins (1987).

Kenworthy, O.T., Screening for hearing impairment in infants and young children. *Semin. Hear.*, **11**, 315–332 (1990).

Kenworthy, O.T., Bess, F., Schaffer, M., and Fainberg, J., Screening for speech, language and hearing impairment in early childhood: an analysis of established and emerging techniques. Presentation to the Annual Meeting of the Robert Wood Johnson Foundation National Collaborative Project on Identification and Management of Communication Disorders in Children. Keystone, CO (May 14–16, 1986).

Klein, J., Epidemiology and natural history of otitis media. *Pediatrics*, **71**, 639–640 (1983).

Lous, J., Three impedance screening programs on a cohort of seven-year-old children: can serial impedance screening reveal chronic middle ear disease? *Scand. Audiol.*, **17**, 60–64 (1983).

Lucker, J., Application of pass-fail criteria to middle ear screening results. *Asha*, **22**, 839–840 (1980).

Mahoney, T., and Eichwald, J., Newborn high-risk hearing screening by maternal questionnaire. *J. Am. Aud. Soc.*, **5**, 41–45 (1979).

Marascuilo, L.A., *Statistical Methods for Behavioral Science Research*. New York: McGraw-Hill (1971).

Marascuilo, L., and McSweeney, B., *Non-parametric and Distribution Free Statistics for the Behavioral Sciences*. Berkeley, CA: Brooks Cole (1977).

Marchant, C., Shurin, P., Turczyk, V., et al., Course and outcome of otitis media in early infancy: a prospective study. *J. Pediatr.*, **104**, 826–831 (1985).

Matkin, N., Early recognition and referral of hearing-impaired child. *Pediatr. Rev.*, **6**(5), 151–156 (1984).

Melnick, W., Eagles, E., and Levine, H., Evaluation of a recommended program of identification audiome-

try with school-age children. *J. Speech Hear. Dis.*, **29**, 3–13 (1964).

Mencher, G., Screening the newborn infant for hearing loss: a complete identification program. In F. Bess (Ed.), *Childhood Deafness: Causation, Assessment and Management*. New York: Grune & Stratton (1977).

Nie., N., Hull, C., Jenkins, J., et al., *Statistical Package for the Social Sciences*. New York: McGraw-Hill (1975).

Northern, J., and Downs, M., *Hearing in Children*. Baltimore, MD: Williams & Wilkins (1984).

Olsho, L.W., Koch, E.G., Carter, E.A., Halpern, C.F., and Spetner, N.B., Pure-tone sensitivity of human infants. *J. Acoust. Soc. Am.*, **84**(4), 1316–1324 (1988).

Orchik, D., Morff, R., and Dunn, J., Middle ear status at myringotomy and its relationship to middle ear immittance measurements. *Ear Hear.*, **6**, 324–328 (1985).

Paradise, J., Pediatricians' view of middle-ear effusions. More questions than answers. *Ann. Otol.*, (Suppl. 25), 20–24 (1976).

Paradise, J., and Smith, C.G., Impedance screening for preschool children—state of the art. In E. Harford et al. (Eds.), *Impedance Screening for Middle Ear Disease in Children*. New York: Grune & Stratton, pp. 113–124 (1978).

Paradise, J., Smith, C.G., and Bluestone, C., Tympanometric detection of middle ear effusion in infants and young children. *Pediatrics*, **58**, 198–209 (1976).

Probst, R., Coats, A., Martin, G., and Lounsbury, Martin, B., Spontaneous, click- and toneburst-evoked otoacoustic emissions from normal ears. *Hear. Res.*, **21**, 261–275 (1986).

Reichert, T., Cantekin, E., Riding, K., Chon, B., and Bluestone, C., Diagnosis of middle ear effusions in young infants by otoscopy and tympanometry. In E. Harford et al. (Eds.), *Impedance Screening for Middle Ear Disease in Children*. New York: Grune & Stratton, pp. 81–90 (1978).

Robins, D.S., A case for infant hearing screening. *Neonatal Intensive Care*, 24–29+ (November/December 1990).

Roeser, R., Dunckel, D., Soh, J., et al., Comparison of tympanometry and otoscopy in establishing pass/fail referral criteria. *J. Am. Audiol. Soc.*, **3**, 20–25 (1977).

Roeser, R., and Northern, J., Screening for hearing loss and middle ear disorders. In R. Roeser and M. Downs (Eds.), *Auditory Disorders in School Children*. New York: Thieme-Stratton, pp. 120–150 (1981).

Rogers, K., Screening for middle ear disease. *Pediatrics*, **77**, 57–70 (1986).

Roush, J., and Tait, C., Pure-tone and acoustic immittance screening of preschool-aged children: an examination of referral criteria. *Ear Hear.*, **6**, 245–249 (1985).

Ruben, R., An inquiry into the minimal amount of auditory deprivation which results in a cognitive effect in man. *Acta Otolaryngologica* (Stockholm), **414** (Suppl.), 157–164 (1984).

Ruth, R., Dey-Sigman, S., and Mills, J., Neonatal ABR screening. *Hear. J.*, **38**, 39–45 (1985).

Schow, R., Pederson, J., Nerbonne, M., and Boe, R., Comparison of ASHA's acoustic immittance guidelines and standard medical diagnosis. *Ear Hear.*, **2**, 251–255 (1984).

Schwartz, D., and Schwartz, R., A comparison of tympanometry and acoustic reflex measurements for detecting middle ear effusion in infants below seven months of age. In E. Harford et al. (Eds.), *Impedance Screening for Middle Ear Disease in Children.* New York: Grune & Stratton, pp. 91–96 (1978).

Seaborg, J., Tennessee perinatal care system status report. State of Tennessee, Department of Health and Environment, Bureau of Health Services, Division of Maternal and Child Health, Nashville, TN (1985).

Shenai, J., Changing demographics of infants in the neonatal intensive care unit: impact on auditory function, In F. Bess and J. Hull (Eds.), *Screening Children for Auditory Function.* Nashville: Bill Wilkerson Press (1992).

Shriberg., L., and Smith, A., Phonological correlates of middle-ear involvement in speech-delayed children: a methodological note. *J. Speech Hear. Res.*, **26**, 293–297 (1983).

Simmons, F., Patterns of deafness in newborns: part I. *Laryngoscope*, **90**, 448–453 (1980a).

Simmons, F., Diagnosis and rehabilitation of deaf newborns: part II. *Asha*, **22**, 475–479 (1980b).

Sprague, B., Wiley, T., and Goldstein, R., Tympanometric and acoustic-reflex studies in neonates. *J. Speech Hear. Res.*, **28**, 265–272 (1985).

Stein, L., Clark, S., and Kraus, N., The hearing-impaired infant: patterns of identification and habilitation. *Ear Hear.*, **4**, 232–236 (1983).

Stevens, J., Webb, H., Smith, M., et al., A comparison of oto-acoustic emissions and brain stem electric response audiometry in the normal newborn and babies admitted to a special care baby unit. *Clin. Physics Physiol. Meas.*, **8**, 95–104 (1987).

Strickland, E., Burns, E., and Tubis, A., Incidence of spontaneous otoacoustic emissions in children and infants. *J. Acoust. Soc. Am.*, **78**, 931–935 (1985).

Teele, D., Klein, J., and Rosner, B., Epidemiology of otitis media in children. *Ann. Otol. Rhinol. Laryngol.*, **89** (Suppl. 68) (1980).

Teele, D., Klein, J., Rosner, B., et al., Otitis media with effusion during the first three years of life and development of speech and language. *Pediatrics*, **74**, 282–287 (1984).

Teele, D.W., and Teele, J., Detection of middle ear effusion by reflectometry. *J. Pediatr.*, **104**, 832–838 (1984).

Tell, L., Levi, C., and Feinmesser, M., Screening infants for deafness in baby clinics. In F. Bess (Ed.), *Childhood Deafness: Causation, Assessment, and Management.* New York: Grune & Stratton, pp. 117–126 (1977).

Tjossem, T.D. (Ed.), *Intervention Strategies for High Risk Infants and Children.* Baltimore, MD: University Park Press (1976).

Turner, R., Recommended guidelines for infant hearing screening: analysis. *Asha*, **32**, 63–67 (1990).

Turner, R., and Cone-Wesson, B., Prevalence rates and cost effectiveness of risk factors. In F. Bess and J. Hall (Eds.), *Screening Children for Auditory Function.* Nashville: Bill Wilkerson Press (1992).

Turner, R., Frazer, G., and Shephard, N., Formulating and evaluating audiological test protocols. *Ear Hear.*, **5**, 321–330 (1984).

Upfold, L.J., Children with hearing aids in Australia: prevalence, hearing characteristics, age at fitting, and etiologies. Unpublished Master's thesis. MacQuarie University, North Ride, New South Wales, Australia (1986).

U.S. Department of Education, Progress toward a free and appropriate education. Report to Congress on the implementation of Public Law 94–142. Washington, DC: U.S. Government Printing Office (1979–1989).

Ventry, I., Effects of conductive hearing loss: fact or fiction? *J. Speech Hear. Dis.*, **45**, 143–156 (1980).

Ventry, I., Research design issues in studies of effects of middle ear effusion. *Pediatrics*, **71**, 644 (1983).

Walker, D.W., Gugenheim, S., Down, M.P., Northern, J.L., Early language milestone scale and language screening of young children. *Pediatrics*, **83**, 284–288 (1989).

Wilson, W.R., and Walton, W., Identification audiometry accuracy: evaluation of a recommended program. *Language, Speech Hear. Services Schools*, **5**, 132–142 (1974).

Wilson, W.R., and Walton, W., Public school audiometry. In F. Martin (Ed.), *Pediatric Audiology.* Englewood Cliffs, NJ: Prentice-Hall, pp. 389–455 (1978).

Zarnoch, J., and Balkany, T., Tympanometric screening of normal and intensive care unit newborns: validity and reliability. In E. Harford, F. Bess, C. Bluestone, and J. Klein (Eds.), *Impedance Screening for Middle Ear Disease in Children.* New York: Grune & Stratton (1978).

5

Amplification for the Hearing-Impaired Child

RUTH A. BENTLER, Ph.D.

···

We *need* to question ourselves, because a child cannot go back and make up years two through six of his or her life.*

According to the Office of Demographic Studies approximately 1 in 1000 children is born with severe or profound bilateral sensorineural hearing impairment; relative to mild or moderate hearing loss "estimates range from 6 children per 1000 to 16 per 1000, depending upon who you include" (Matkin in Mahon, 1987). With these statistics and current Public Law 99-457 at hand, the audiologist needs to become cognizant of the issues surrounding amplification decisions for the hearing-impaired child, whatever the age or degree of impairment. It is the intent of this chapter to examine some of those issues. Although we cannot take back earlier decisions made, neither can we be faulted for continually striving to understand the process.

Limited Data to Define Hearing Loss

It is often the attentive parent who gets the first clue that a newborn or young child is not responding appropriately to environmental stimuli. Yet, Elssmann, Matkin, and Sabo (1987) have reported that across all socioeconomic levels and degrees of hearing loss the average age of *formal* identifi-

cation is 19 months, with a 6-month average delay before amplification. Other investigators have reported similar findings (Bergstrom, 1976; Shah, Chandler, & Dale, 1978; Simmons, 1980). Diagnostic evaluation of the very young child must be viewed as an ongoing process whereby the audiologist uses a battery of test procedures appropriate to the age and abilities of the client, including conditioned play audiometry, tangible reinforcement audiometry, and visual reinforcement audiometry. Refer to Chapter 4 for an overview of diagnostic procedures. If, in fact, the child is too young or manifests any of a number of mental or physical limitations, a more objective approach may be needed to ascertain hearing levels.

Urgency

Northern and Downs (1991) and Ross and Seewald (1988) provide reviews of studies of sensory deprivation in animals. Findings of incomplete maturation of brainstem auditory neurons (Webster & Webster, 1977, 1979), pathological changes in the brainstem (Evans, Webster, & Cullen, 1983), inability to resolve differences in sound patterns (Tees, 1967), and an increase in the latency of the auditory neural response and abnormal binaural interaction (Clopton & Silverman, 1977; Silverman & Clopton, 1977) provide convincing evidence of the urgency of early intervention. While there are few human studies

---

*Quote is from Julia Davis in Mahon, W., Hearing care for infants and children. *Hear. J.*, 40, 7–10 (September 1987).

corroborating these findings (e.g., Dobie & Berlin, 1979), recent investigations of the impact of temporary auditory deprivation, such as can occur with prolonged otitis media in infants and young children, suggest the strong possibility of central detriment (Eisen, 1962).

Besides sensory deprivation and its physiological consequences, the effect on language acquisition during this "critical period" is of great concern. Northern and Downs (1991, p. 117) define the "critical period" as "certain period(s) in development when the organism is programmed to receive and utilize particular types of stimuli and that subsequently the stimuli will have diminishing potency in effecting the organism's development in the function represented." Although some controversy exists as to the exact timing of the period (Benedict, 1979; Dennis, 1973; Greenstein et al., 1976), most investigators pinpoint the time prior to age 2 as being essential to development of auditory functioning and speech/language development.

Matkin (1986, p. 172) poses another potential deprivation possibility: "Does the lack of auditory input during early developmental periods have detrimental effects with respect to the hearing impaired child's psychosocial development?" The evidence is overwhelming in that, regardless of the degree of impairment, the earlier invervention is initiated, the greater the likelihood of success. To deny an infant some amplification system because of limited audiologic information rather than approaching the entire diagnostic/rehabilitative process as an ongoing process is without merit. As Ross and Lerman (1967, p. 60) so aptly stated, "Denying a child a hearing aid during the critical language years may only be saving his or her hearing for no good purpose."

Candidacy

Any child with a *significant* hearing loss is a candidate for amplification. While a number of authors have attempted to describe candidacy in terms of the degree or configuration of hearing loss, the rules are not easily defined. Hearing-impaired children are a heterogeneous group, and the ef-

fects of hearing impairment on intellectual status, academic achievement, and social skills vary from child to child (Davis et al., 1986). Davis et al. have indicated that "even minimal hearing loss places children at risk for language and learning problems" (p. 53). Further, they found that hearing-impaired children of all degrees and ages were concerned about being accepted by their peers (50% of a hearing-impaired group compared to 15.5% of normal hearing children). Any hearing loss that places a child at a disadvantage in an academic, social, or, in the case of the older child, occupational setting warrants amplification consideration. Candidacy cannot be dictated a priori on the basis of thresholds.

Candidacy for the profoundly hearing-impaired child may become an issue as well. With the advent of cochlear implantation of children and vibrotactile units of multichannel design, the candidacy for a variety of amplification systems must be considered (refer to Chapter 15 for further discussion of cochlear implantation and vibrotactile stimulation).

One cannot discuss candidacy issues without considering the plight of the unilaterally hearing-impaired child. Prevalence data suggest that 3 children in 1000 exhibit unilateral losses in excess of 45 dB HL, and 13 children in 1000 exhibit losses from 26 to 45 db HL (Bergman, 1957). Whether the unilateral loss is conductive or sensorineural in nature, evidence is growing as to the potential for academic failure, lower language performance, and behavioral disorders (refer to entire monograph, *Ear and Hearing*, 7(1), 1986). Auditorily, the problems are obvious (Bess, 1985; Mueller & Hawkins, 1990).

1. *Binaural summation.* With two equally sensitive ears, threshold is 3 dB better than with either ear alone; relative to loudness judgments, a stimulus presented simultaneously to both ears at 40 dB SL will require a 46 dB SL presentation level for equal loudness when presented to either ear alone. As pointed out by Bess and Tharpe (1986), this "advantage becomes rather substantial when one considers the effect on speech recognition." Eighteen to 30% improvement in speech recognition can be ex-

Table 5.1a
Formula for Calculating Required Real-Ear Gain (Insertion Gain or Functional Gain), for Volume Control Setting 15 dB Below Maximum

1. Calculate $X = 0.05 (H_{500} + H_{1k} + H_{2k})^a$

2. $G_{250} = X + 0.31 H_{250} - 17b$
$G_{500} = X + 0.31 H_{500} - 8$
$G_{750} = X + 0.31 H_{750} - 3$
$G_{1k} = X + 0.31 H_{1k} + 1$
$G_{1.5k} = X + 0.31 H_{1.5k} + 1$
$G_{2k} = X + 0.31 H_{2k} - 1$
$G_{3k} = X + 0.31 H_{3k} - 2$
$G_{4k} = X + 0.31 H_{4k} - 2$
$G_{6k} = X + 0.31 H_{6k} - 2$

pected from binaural listening over monaural listening, depending on the stimulus used (Konkle & Schwartz, 1981).

2. *Head shadow effects.* Head shadow refers to the reduction in signal intensity that occurs as the signal moves from one side of the head to the other; this effect is more substantial in the high frequencies. For the unilaterally hearing-impaired child, any signal presented on the side of the impaired ear may be attenuated 10 to 16 dB above 1000 Hz by the time it reaches the functional ear (Festen & Plomp, 1986). Obviously this magnitude of attenuation can have significant impact on speech intelligibility (Mueller & Hawkins, 1990), since that area of the speech spectrum may account for 60% of speech intelligibility (Bess & Tharpe, 1986).

3. *Localization.* The importance of localization, or directionality, is generally considered to be a binaural phenomenon, the result of interaural time and intensity differences. For low-frequency stimuli, the primary cue for localization is the interaural time difference, while for high frequencies (above 1500 Hz) the primary cue is the interaural intensity difference.

The typical clinical management approach over the past 20 years has been relatively nonaggressive; that is, children with unilateral hearing loss have been provided preferential seating with an occasional referral for a Contralateral Routing of Signal (CROS)-type hearing aid (Bess & Tharpe,

1986). It was generally assumed that because one ear was normal, normal cognitive, academic, and social development would prevail. Recently, a more aggressive approach has been taken toward management of the unilaterally hearing-impaired child. Preferential seating and/or use of amplification will not restore these auditory deficits, but closer monitoring of potential areas of weakness may preclude more serious ramifications.

Gain/Output/Frequency Response Considerations

Children under the age of 10 or 12 cannot be expected to provide extensive input into the hearing aid fitting process (refer to Chapter 11 for adult hearing aid selection procedures). As a result, a formula approach toward determining and setting frequency response characteristics may be necessitated. With the advent of probe microphone technology, a clearer understanding of the results of our efforts is possible.

A number of gain-targeting approaches have been forwarded over the years, including the *Berger* (Berger, Hagberg, & Rane, 1977), *POGO* (Prescription of Gain and Output) (McCandless & Lyregaard, 1983), and *NAL* (National Acoustics Laboratory) (Byrne & Dillon, 1986) procedures, to name only a few. Each formula purports to provide the electroacoustic characteristics necessary for maximizing speech intelligibility, yet different response characteristics are typically derived from each formula for the same audiogram. The clinician is often in the situation of determining which formula most favorably suits which client. For the pediatric population, the theoretical considerations of the NAL approach deserve consideration. The National Acoustic Laboratory's (NAL) formula derived by Byrne and Tonnison (1976) was originally developed for use with young children (Byrne & Fifield, 1974). More recently, a revision of that prescriptive approach has been provided by Byrne and Dillon (1986). The premise of the approach is to amplify the long-term speech spectrum so that it is most com-

Table 5.1b
Formulas for Calculating Required 2-cc Coupler and Ear Simulator Gain

	2-cc Coupler[b]			Ear Simulator		
	BTE	ITE	Body	BTE	ITE	Body
1. Calculate $X = 0.05 (H_{500} + H_{1k} + H_{2k})^a$						
2. $G_{250} = X + 0.31 H_{250} +$	1	−1	0	5	2	0
$G_{500} = X + 0.31 H_{500} +$	9	9	2	13	12	6
$G_{750} = X + 0.31 H_{750} +$	12	13	8	17	16	12
$G_{1k} = X + 0.31 H_{1k} +$	16	16	13	22	21	19
$G_{1.5k} = X + 0.31 H_{1.5k} +$	13	14	22	19	21	28
$G_{2k} = X + 0.31 H_{2k} +$	15	14	25	24	23	35
$G_{3k} = X + 0.31 H_{3k} +$	22	15	26	29	25	33
$G_{4k} = X + 0.31 H_{4k} +$	18	13	17	24	25	23
$G_{6k} = X + 0.31 H_{6k} +$	12	4		21	19	

[a] H, HTL (ISO standard).
[b] G, insertion gain.
Reprinted with permission from Byrne, D., and Dillon, H., The National Acoustic Laboratories (NAL) new procedure for selecting the gain and frequency response of a hearing aid. *Ear Hear.,* 7, 257–265 (1986).

Table 5.2
Modifications to NAL Hearing Aid Selection Procedure (Byrne & Dillon, 1986) for Application to Severe/Profound Hearing Losses

1. $X = 0.05 \times$ HTL $(0.5 + 1 + 2k)$ up to 180 dB (i.e., 3FA = 60 dB)
   $+ 0.116 \times$ combined HTL in excess of 180 dB.

2. Where the 2000 Hz HTL is 95 dB or greater, add the following:

2 kHz HTL	250	500	750	1k	1.5k	2k	3k	4k	6k
95	4	3	1	0	−1	−2	−2	−2	−2
100	6	4	2	0	−2	−3	−3	−3	−3
105	8	5	2	0	−3	−5	−5	−5	−5
110	11	7	3	0	−3	−6	−6	−6	−6
115	13	8	4	0	−4	−8	−8	−8	−8
120	15	9	4	0	−5	−9	−9	−9	−9

Reprinted with permission from Byrne, D., Parkinson A., and Newall, P., Modified hearing aid selection procedure for severe/profound hearing loss. In G. Studebaker, F. Bess, and L. Beck (Eds.), *The Vanderbilt Hearing Aid Report II.* Parkton, MD: York Press, Inc. (1991).

fortably loud and equally loud across frequency. That is, the speech spectrum is shaped so that each frequency band contributes equally to its loudness; this, presumably, will lead to maximum intelligibility. As shown in Table 5.1, insertion gain targets (or functional gain targets, if a probe microphone system is not accessible) are derived based on the degree of hearing loss at each frequency. The same table provides a formula for converting these gain values to 2-cc coupler values, if necessary, to select hearing aids from manufacturer's specifications. While the required insertion gain will be the same regardless of aid style—body, behind-the-ear (BTE), or in-the-ear (ITE)—the coupler gain required to give that insertion gain will vary, as a result of different microphone locations on the different styles. Recent investigations (Byrne & Cotton, 1988; Byrne, Parkinson, & Newall, 1990, 1991; Pascoe, 1988; Schwartz, Lyregaard, & Lundh, 1988) have suggested that for severely impaired listeners (adults as well as children), more gain may be required than is prescribed by this formula. In Table 5.2 a modification of the NAL prescriptive formula is shown for losses in excess of 60 dB HL. Preferred gain was typically found to be about 10 dB greater than

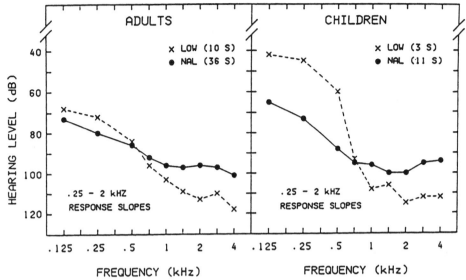

Figure 5.1. Average audiograms of subjects who preferred the NAL response and those who required more low-frequency amplification. [Reprinted with permission from Byrne, D., Parkinson, A., and Newall, P., Modified hearing aid selection procedures for severe/profound hearing loss. In G. Studebaker, F. Bess, and L. Beck (Eds.), *The Vanderbilt Hearing Aid Report II*. Parkton, MD: York Press, Inc. (1991).]

the NAL prescribed gain for hearing losses greater than 60 dB HL (Byrne et al., 1991). In addition, approximately half of their subjects who exhibited steeply sloping hearing losses as shown in Figure 5.1 preferred more low-frequency gain than prescribed by the formula, based on judgments of intelligibility, home trials, and speech recognition testing.

Of more utility in the fitting of young children may be a strategy based on the philosophy of making as much of the speech spectrum audible as possible without exceeding discomfort. The difference in these approaches is subtle: While the NAL prescription places the speech spectrum at approximately half the hearing loss for mild to moderate hearing losses (0.46 HTL) and at equal loudness across the frequency range, the following approaches attempt to make as much of the speech spectrum audible as possible—presumably at a preferred listening level—without exceeding discomfort. The underlying difference here is that the audiologist is working with measured sensation levels of amplified speech spectra, rather than the targeting of some gain values derived from threshold estimates. Thresholds of hearing do not change with the use of amplification; therefore, it may

be more practical to begin to look at how the amplified speech range fits into the child's usable hearing range. Three such methods have repeatedly been suggested for use with young children:

1. Version 3.1 MSU Hearing Instrument Prescription Formula
2. CID method: Phase IV
3. Desired Sensation Level (DSL) approach

The original version of the Memphis State University (MSU) prescriptive method (Cox, 1983) required measurements of thresholds as well as suprathreshold measures of the *upper level of comfortable loudness (ULCL)* or *highest comfortable loudness level (HCL)*.* The basis of the MSU procedure is to place the amplified speech spectrum in the middle of the listener's long-term listening range (LTLR), defined as the halfway point between threshold and HCL. The speech spectrum used by the MSU procedure and shown in Figure 5.2 has an overall level of

---

*In more recent publications (e.g., Cox & Alexander, 1990), ULCL has been replaced with highest comfortable loudness level (HCL), to avoid confusion with uncomfortable loudness (UCL).

Table 5.3
Comparison of One-Third Octave Levels of Speech (in dB SPL) for Following Hearing Aid Prescription
Formulas: National Acoustics Laboratories (NAL), Memphis State University (MSU Version 3.1), Desired
Sensation Level (DSL Version 3.1), Central Institute of the Deaf (Phase IV)

Freq (Hz)	NAL	MSU	DSL	CID
100.0	0.0	0.0	39.1	
125.0	0.0	0.0	39.9	
160.0	0.0	0.0	46.3	
200.0	63.0	0.0	59.6	
250.0	62.0	60.0	62.8	62.0
315.0	60.0	57.0	60.1	
400.0	62.0	61.0	61.6	
500.0	61.0	62.0	64.3	66.0
630.0	58.0	59.0	63.1	
800.0	55.0	56.5	60.1	
1000.0	50.0	55.0	56.4	56.0
1250.0	51.0	54.5	53.7	
1600.0	51.0	52.0	52.1	
2000.0	49.0	49.0	51.0	50.0
2500.0	48.0	48.0	48.8	
3150.0	47.0	46.5	45.0	
4000.0	48.0	46.0	42.3	49.0
5000.0	45.0	44.0	41.5	
6300.0	46.0	45.5	42.1	
8000.0	0.0	0.0	40.9	
10000.0	0.0	0.0	38.0	
Overall	70.0	70.0	70.9	70

70 dB SPL. Cox found that 16 adults with moderate, moderately severe, and severe hearing impairments preferred to listen to amplified speech at this midpoint. For frequencies above 1600 Hz where the long-term listening range tends to be narrow, she noted a preference for a gain setting at a level lower than the midpoint of the LTLR. As a result, the target was modified so that "the target level for amplified speech is reduced from the midpoint of the long-term listening range at frequencies where this range is narrower than 30 dB" (Cox, 1988, p. 6). Target values for setting SSPL90 are generated by adding the value for speech peaks (derived from Dunn & White, 1940) to HCL − 12 at each frequency. Correction factors for the 6-cc-to-eardrum and eardrum-to-2-cc transformations are included in the SSPL90 equation in order to compare resultant prescribed gain and output value to coupler specifications. One obvious advantage of the MSU prescription formula is that it is available on a computer disk. Based on as few as two thresholds, entered in dB SPL, the program will predict HCL,

display target 2-cc "use" gain, 2-cc SSPL90 values, aided soundfield thresholds (in dB SPL), and target insertion gain values for those entered thresholds. Because the insertion gain target values are calculated by subtracting the aided soundfield threshold goal from the unaided soundfield threshold, the values can be used for functional gain targeting when a probe system is not available. Use of a functional gain approach to measuring hearing aid advantage, however, may be subject to a number of inherent disadvantages when used with young children, including limited frequency specificity and its time-consuming nature (Haskell, 1987).

Another selection method gaining increased attention is the Desired Sensation Level (DSL) approach, originally proposed by Seewald, Ross, and Spiro (1985). Based on the premise that "suprathreshold measures of auditory perception" in young children lack reliability and validity, these authors attempt to place the amplified long-term speech spectrum between the child's threshold and the predicted loudness dis-

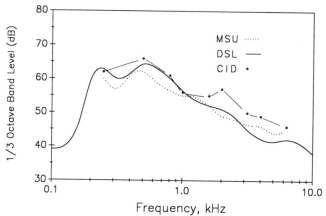

Figure 5.2. Speech spectra (1/3 octave band levels) used by MSU (Version 3.1), DSL (Version 3.0), and CID (Phase IV) hearing aid fitting strategies. Refer to text for further explanation. Values for CID (Phase IV) given only for octave and midoctave frequencies used in audiometric testing.

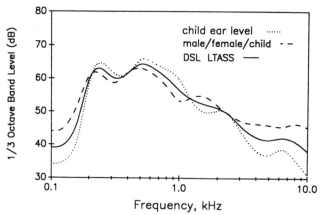

Figure 5.3. Long-term average speech spectrum (LTASS) used by Seewald et al. (1991a, 1991b) in the DSL (Version 3.0) hearing aid fitting strategy composed of the average of male/female/child recordings obtained directly in front of the talker (30 cm) and recordings taken at ear level of a child.

comfort level (LDL) across the frequency range. In generating a long-term average speech spectrum (LTASS) specifically related to children, Seewald et al. (1991a) considered two issues: first, the relationship between the hearing aid microphone and the source of the speech, and second, the self-monitoring that children do of their own vocalizations. Typically, the spectral characteristics of speech used in the calculation of amplification characteristics are obtained from recordings taken directly in front of a talker rather than at the ear level of the hearing-impaired listener (Byrne & Dillon, 1986; Cox & Moore, 1988). As Cornelisse, Gagne, and Seewald (1991) point out, the hearing-impaired child must monitor his or her own voice as well, and any

algorithm based on the former LTASS may result in inappropriate gain characteristics for self-monitoring of speech. In fact, these investigators found that ear-level measures of LTASS taken for three groups of subjects (adult males, adult females, and children) consisted of more low-frequency energy (below 1000 Hz) and less high-frequency energy (above 2500 Hz) than previous estimates obtained directly in front of the talker. As a result of the findings, the DSL approach now incorporates a speech spectrum that is composed of the average of male/female/child recordings of speech obtained directly in front (30 cm) of the talker and recordings taken at the ear level of the child. This speech spectrum has an overall level of 70.9 dB SPL and is shown in Figures 5.2 and 5.3. The relative weightings of the prescribed sensation levels for this spectrum are similar to Pascoe's (1978) "perceived speech spectrum" with two exceptions: reduced low frequency emphasis and slightly increased midfrequency emphasis (1500 to 3000 Hz). The latter is intended to restore natural amplification that is associated with external ear resonance in that range but that is eliminated with an occluding mold.

The DSL computerized procedure involves several stages: In the first stage, the thresholds obtained using insert earphones, circumaural earphones, or soundfield presentation are entered. The program will make calculations on entered thresholds only; no interpolation at other frequencies is done. If the client's real-ear unaided response (REUR*) and RECD values are known, those values are entered as well. If no REUR and RECD measures are available, the program will use default age-appropriate values for children (Feigin et al., 1989; Kruger, 1987) or adult values (Hawkins et al., 1990; Shaw, 1974; Shaw & Vaillancourt, 1985). Loudness discomfort values, if available, are also entered; default values for adults (Skinner, 1988) are used for the calculation of a prescribed saturation sound pressure level with a 90-dB input (SSPL90) and real-ear saturation response (RESR). On the basis of these entered/default values, the program determines the amount of gain required to place the idealized speech spectrum at the desired sensation levels for each of nine frequency regions. The prescribed real-ear saturation response (RESR) at each frequency is selected on the basis of the prescribed level of amplified speech. As with the MSU method, these maximum output values are related to threshold levels and fall below the mean LDL values for differing degrees of loss as reported by Pascoe (1988) and Skinner (1988). Since the program provides for

---

*Although probe microphone technology is not covered in this chapter, a number of the standard terms are used, for example, *real-ear unaided response*, or REUR, referring to the open ear resonance; real-ear to coupler difference, or RECD, referring to the difference in output measured in a coupler and in the ear of the hearing aid user; *real-ear insertion response*, or REIR, referring to the gain of the hearing aid measured in the ear canal; and, *real-ear saturation response*, or RESR, referring to the maximum output of the hearing aid measured in the ear, a real-ear correlate of SSPL90.

recommended electroacoustic specifications of gain and output as well as preferred sensation levels and real-ear output levels, all prescribed values are corrected for their 2-cc equivalent (Feigin et al., 1989; Hawkins, Cooper, & Thompson, 1990). As shown in Figure 5.4, the amplified long-term speech spectrum target and prescribed output at 1000 Hz are derived from threshold values. Target sensation levels, output, in situ gain, and functional gain can be found in the tables in Appendix 5.1.

If a probe microphone system is used, the derived "in situ" gain necessary for preferred sensation levels across frequency can be plotted as real ear targets, and adjustments can be made to the hearing aid to match the desired target with minimal cooperation from the child. Output measures can also be verified quickly using the probe system. The DSL program will be optimally useful when interfaced with a probe microphone system. In that way, thresholds and individual transformation values entered into the hearing aid software program will result in target values for probe mic measures without having to manually enter these target values.

A final method often suggested for use with children is the Central Institute for the Deaf (CID) Phase IV procedure. This computerized fitting program does not prescribe hearing aid characteristics but rather provides articulation index (AI) values for any hearing aid whose gain/output is entered for a particular hearing-impaired client. The "articulation index" is a theoretical construct that attempts to quantify the contribution of different frequency bands to the overall intelligibility of the speech signal (refer to Pavlovic, 1989). There are several different proposed methods for calculating the AI (French & Steinberg, 1947; Kryter, 1962a, 1962b; Pavlovic, 1988, 1991), each proposing slightly different bands and weighting. The Phase IV procedure uses the standardized method (ANSI, 1969), with a long-term average speech spectrum as shown in Figure 5.2. The overall level is assumed to be approximately 70 dB SPL. Using this program, AI calculations for an unaided audiogram can be compared to those obtained for any number of hearing aids. The strategy used is based on the following premises: First, conversational

DSL 3.0: 1000 Hz

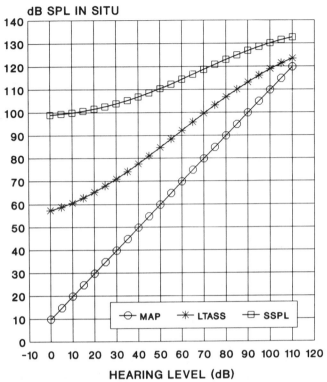

Figure 5.4. Threshold (0 – 0), the amplified long-term average speech spectrum target levels (* – *) and the desired maximum real-ear sound pressure levels (–) in dB SPL at the eardrum as a function of decibels Hearing Level for the 1000-Hz frequency region, as prescribed by Desired Sensation Level (DSL). [Reprinted with permission from Seewald, R.C., Zelisko, D.L.C., Ramji, K., and Jamieson, D.G., *Computer Assisted Implementation of the DSL Approach: Version 3.0.* Poster presented at the International Hearing Aid Conference, Iowa City, Iowa (1991).]

speech falls within the frequency region of 200 to 6000 Hz with approximately 30 dB amplitude variation; second, this speech spectrum should be amplified so that as much as possible is above the individual's threshold; and third, the hearing aid should be so limited that incoming stimuli are not amplified above thresholds of discomfort. The computerized protocol involves entering thresholds obtained under earphones (TDH 39 or 49) and in the sound field in hearing level (HL) (ANSI, 1989). Functional and/or insertion gain measures are taken with a chosen hearing aid coupled to the individual's own earmold and are likewise entered. This procedure provides a graphic display of the amplified speech spectrum in HL with either a soundfield or earphone reference based on the gain values

entered. Unlike the DSL method and its SPL-at-the-eardrum graphic representation, this procedure provides for transformation of the speech spectrum and its resultant gain onto an audiogram-type form. And unlike the MSU program, which requires that all threshold information be entered in dB SPL, audiometric data can be entered without first correcting for SPL. The AI is computed and displayed in the upper right-hand corner of the screen. The gain obtained from any combination of hearing aids, earmolds, and volume control wheel (VCW) settings can be entered and the resultant AI obtained. As the authors point out, this fitting method "only quantifies speech audibility." It is not intended as an accurate prediction of the individual's speech recognition performance (Popelka,

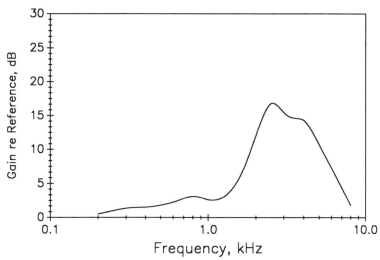

Figure 5.5. Average sound pressure transformation for free field to eardrum, frontal incidence (0° azi- muth). Data obtained from 12 studies covering 100 adult subjects (Shaw, 1974).

1983, 1988; Popelka & Engebretson, 1983). Investigations of that relationship continue to support a monotonic one rather than a direct one (Fabry & Van Tasell, 1990; Humes et al., 1986; Pavlovic, Studebaker, & Sherbecoe, 1986).

Of current interest in hearing aid fitting procedures is the involvement of individual ear acoustics in the attempt to match some prescriptive formula. Of particular interest is the external ear resonance measure. Shaw (1974) compiled data from 12 contemporary investigations to show the average sound pressure transformation from a free field. His data for frontal incidence (0° azimuth), shown in Figure 5.5, indicate that the primary resonance of the adult ear is around 2600 Hz with an average pressure gain of 17 dB. Probe microphone measures of hearing aid performance (in particular, gain or REIR) require some initial measure of this transformation.

Kruger (1987) noted that the external ear resonant frequency is higher at birth (note in Figure 5.6 that the resonant peak is at approximately 6000 Hz) and decreases with age to adult values by the second year. Other investigators (Bentler, 1989; Dempster & MacKenzie, 1990) have studied the change in resonant frequency and peak amplitude and reported that beyond age 3 there is only a slight relationship between age and changes in resonant frequencies. Both investigations showed wide variabil-

ity in results and cautioned for the need for individual ear resonance measures. Of very recent debate, however, has been the issue of using average transformation values rather than individually derived values (Byrne & Upfold, 1991; Mueller, 1989). As Byrne and Upfold point out, if one client exhibits a higher external ear resonant peak than is typical, then sounds will have to be amplified to a higher level in that frequency range to achieve the same *insertion* gain values. Instead, the authors continue, we should be thinking of *transmission* gain, or the increase in the aided signal level relative to the unaided level, using an in situ gain rather than an insertion gain target. Byrne and Upfold conclude that "insertion gain versus transmission gain is a complex issue that requires further thought and if prescriptions were made in transmission gain, then there should be no correction for individual differences in ear canal resonance" (p. 40).

The real-ear-to-coupler transformation, as a function of age, has also been investigated. It has long been documented (Bergman & Bentler, 1990; Bruel, Frederiksen, & Rasmussen, 1976; Hawkins et al., 1990; Sachs & Burkhard, 1972) that more sound pressure may be generated in an occluded ear canal than in the standard 2-cc coupler. For example, if the hearing aid manufacturer reports than a particular model has a high-frequency average output of 120 dB

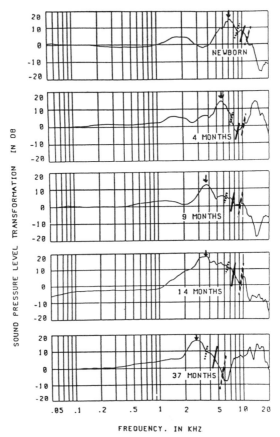

Figure 5.6. Diffuse field to ear canal transformation for a newborn, and 4-, 9-, 14-, and 37-month-old children. [Reprinted with permission from Kruger, B., An update on the external ear resonance in infants and young children. *Ear Hear.*, 85, 74–81 (1987).]

SPL in a 2-cc coupler, one might assume that the output in an average ear may be 10 dB higher. For small children that difference may be even higher! Feigin et al. (1989) obtained ear canal sound pressure levels for 31 children from the ages of 4 weeks to 5 years. Twenty-one adult subjects, ages 17 through 48, served as controls. Using a constant 10-mm depth insertion of the probe tube from the ear canal entrance, the output was measured in each ear canal for 11 pure tones presented with insert earphones. The output of the insert earphone at each of the 11 frequencies was measured and the coupler-to-real-ear differences computed. As shown in Figure 5.7, at all frequencies, the real-ear-to-coupler difference for the children exceeded that measured for adults. It was further noted by these investigators that the transformation values decrease as a function of age, as shown in Figure 5.8, and could be predicted to fall within

1 SD of the adult mean values by age 7.7. The clinician must always be cognizant of the probability that output from a prescribed hearing aid on a young child will be higher than that shown on the manufacturer's specification sheets, and the clinician must use caution in determining appropriate SSPL90 values. Obviously, excessive output can cause further deterioration of hearing; yet, unduly limiting the output will reduce the child's dynamic range of listening and may result in excessive distortion if the hearing aid is continually operated in saturation.

One issue that may never be resolved involves the choice of speech spectrum used for setting gain and output. Obviously, the primary goal of any amplification system should be to make the speech signal audible; logically, one should be able to assume that the chosen target speech spectrum is representative of what the child ac-

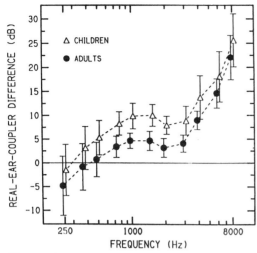

Figure 5.7. Real-ear-to-coupler difference (in dB) measured as a function of frequency (in Hz) for children and adult subjects. Error bars represent ±1SD from the mean. [Reprinted with permission from Feigin, J., Kopun, J., Stelmachowicz, P., and Gorga, M. Probe-tube microphone measures of ear-canal sound pressure levels in infants and children. *Ear Hear.*, 10, 254–258 (1989).]

tually hears. What are the characteristics of that speech signal? As Olsen, Hawkins, and Van Tasell (1987) have pointed out, the particular speech spectrum used depends on the sex, age, and vocal effort of the talker; the choice of speech material; the length of the sampled interval (and whether silent intervals between words were included in the measurement); and distance and azimuth of the microphone relative to the talker. Stelmachowicz (1991b) has attempted to describe speech spectra in more typical parent-child positions. For example, the intensity difference from the typical 1-meter distance from the talker to the ear position for a child placed at the mother's shoulder has been shown to be as much as 15 to 20 dB. Stelmachowicz points out that for adults we can expect level effects, due to the proximity of talker and listener, but that distance is typically greater, not lesser, as it may be with a child placed on the shoulder or cradled in the arms of the talker/parent. As a result, the spectrum at the child's ear may look very different (Fig. 5.9). Because the overall speech level to the microphone of the small child's hearing aid may be in excess of 70 to 80 dB, it is likely that the hearing aid will often be operating in sat-

uration, a strong argument in favor of some form of compression to avoid high levels of distortion at the output. Recall that in their DSL fitting strategy, Seewald et al. (1991a) reached a compromise in spectrum by averaging male/female/child 30-cm reference values with that spectrum obtained at the ear level of a child (refer back to Fig. 5.3).

BENEFIT/SUCCESS

Quantifying benefit from amplification implies a determination that the amplification characteristics have resulted in the availability of more of the speech spectrum, thus the potential for improved communication skills. Benefit from an amplification system is typically measured using probe microphone systems, functional gain measures, speech recognition measures, or some form of questionnaire or inventory. Often in a clinical setting, the audiologist attempts to explain the overall benefit of a hearing aid in terms of how much it improves the audibility of speech sounds. Seewald et al. (1992) compared two commonly used methods of estimating the sensation level of amplified speech: *(1)* the soundfield aided audiogram approach and *(2)* an approach using a probe mic system. Soundfield aided thresholds are used clinically to provide an aided audiogram, or measured thresholds in a sound field obtained while wearing the desired amplification system. A frequent misconception of those employing this method of determining hearing aid benefit is that a hearing aid improves thresholds, but this is not the case. Incoming signals are amplified; the child's thresholds are not changed. In fact, because of the nonlinear characteristics of some hearing aids, providing functional gain measures may indicate more gain than the child is actually receiving for moderate input signals. This is due to the fact that in the aided condition, soundfield aided thresholds are often obtained using low SPL levels, whereby in a typical communicative setting, higher input may activate an input compression circuit, resulting in less usable gain than was indicated by the functional gain measure. Seewald et al. (1989) compared the sensation level (SL) of speech obtained by soundfield functional gain mea-

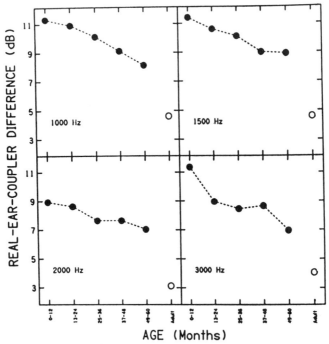

AGE (Months)

Figure 5.8. Real-ear-to-coupler difference (in dB) measured as a function of age (in months). Open circles represent adult means at each frequency. [Reprinted with permission from Feigin, J., Kopun, J., Stelmachowicz, P., and Gorga, M. Probe-tube microphone measures of ear-canal sound pressure levels in infants and children. *Ear Hear.*, 10, 254–258 (1989).]

sures to that obtained with a probe microphone measure of insertion gain. "For 74% of all comparisons, the soundfield aided audiogram approach produced higher SL estimates than the electroacoustic approach by more than 15 to 20 dB" (p. 145). The authors suggest caution in providing aided information to parents and/or educators that may, in fact, overpredict hearing levels and abilities. Hearing aids using some input compression circuitry will provide differing gain dependent on the level of the input stimulus. In fact, use of an "SPL-ogram," as shown in Figure 5.10, may be a better indicator of the audibility range in question than an aided audiogram representation. The thresholds remain in the same (actual measured) location; the speech spectrum is shifted according to the amount of gain provided by the hearing aid.

More objective attempts to measure hearing aid benefit have been suggested, such as use of acoustic reflex thresholds (ART) and auditory evoked responses (AER) including auditory brainstem response (ABR), middle latency response (MLR), and 40-Hz event-related potentials (ERPs). Mueller and Grimes (1987) review these approaches, noting that their usefulness lies in the fact that they are objective rather than subjective measures of hearing aid benefit. In view of the increasing use of probe microphone systems, however, such objective tests are currently used more for threshold determination than in pediatric hearing aid evaluation.

Successful use of amplification suggests that the child for whom a particular amplification strategy has been chosen is indeed using the available information successfully in communicative attempts. For the profoundly hearing-impaired child, the options for sensory input may include vibrotactile stimulation, cochlear implantation, or more traditional acoustic stimulation via an analogue hearing aid. The audiologist must balance the need to find the best sensory aid for the child—as soon as possible—with the need to give the child enough time to show proof of successful use

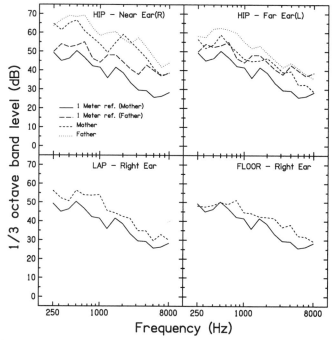

Figure 5.9. Speech spectra obtained at ear level of a 5-month-old child in various positions relative to adult talker (Mother/Father). Measuring microphone was placed at Near Ear (R), Far Ear (L), Right or Left Ear, as indicated in the figure. Reference condition refers to spectrum obtained 1 meter from Mother/Father talker and is shown for comparison.

[Reprinted with permission from Stelmachowicz, P., (1991) *Current Issues in Pediatric Amplification.* In J.A. Feigin and P.G. Stelmachowicz (Eds.) Pediatric Amplification: Proceedings of the 1991 National Conference. Published by Boys Town National Research Hospital, Omaha.]

of that benefit (this is covered in more detail in Chapter 15). For many children an unresolvable question remains: What constitutes an adequate trial period? Degree, configuration, etiology, onset, cognitive abilities, and other factors may affect the length of time it takes to adjust to, and derive benefit from, an amplification system. In view of the differing degrees of intervention employed, establishing any guidelines becomes impossible. In addition, "the time course of auditory perceptual learning can vary from one hour to one year, depending on the task, the complexity of the sounds, and the level of stimulus uncertainty under which the tasks are learned" (Watson, 1980, p. 96). With this issue comes the question of the need for auditory training or the choice of aural rehabilitation strategies to enhance the newly provided information. It is beyond the scope of this chapter to outline such remediation strategies, but we assume that the advantageously deafened child has more potential for the new perceptual learning tasks confronting him or her.

Output Limitation

The saturation sound pressure level (SSPL) of a hearing aid refers to the maximum output of a hearing aid regardless of the input level. Related to the SSPL of any amplification system are the concerns of *(1)* creating additional hearing loss as a result of overexposure or overamplification and *(2)* exceeding the threshold of discomfort for the hearing aid user. It is often not clear to the clinician that exceeding the threshold of discomfort might cause additional hearing loss (although the hearing aid may get yanked) and levels of overamplification might not cause discomfort! Yet, both issues need careful consideration.

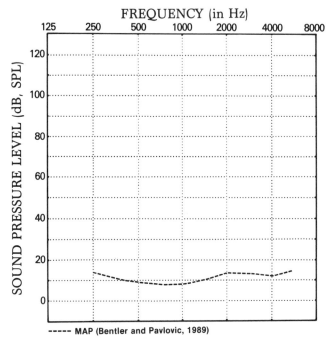

Figure 5.10. Example of an "SPL-ogram" (a term coined by Seewald, 1991b) showing the sound pressure level (dB SPL) at the eardrum as measured with a probe microphone system as a function of frequency. (Normal audiometric thresholds as measured at the eardrum shown by Bentler and Pavlovic, 1989.)

With children, setting appropriate output levels is especially critical. Often young children cannot express that a hearing aid is allowing some incoming sounds to "hurt"; parents may react to any rejection as being caused by other factors, such as stubbornness or anxiety. Obtaining thresholds of discomfort in young children is often impossible because of the cognitive level required to complete the task (Kawell, Kopun, & Stelmachowicz, 1988; Macpherson et al., 1991), and "observing the level which elicits the eye blink reflex" (Liden & Harford, 1985) generally is not acceptable. In an attempt to address this need, Kawell et al. (1988) designed a procedure to be used with children 7 years and older, using a methodology adapted from Hawkins et al. (1987). The following instructions, along with the labeled drawing (shown in Fig. 5.11), were presented:

We're going to see how loud this hearing aid makes sound. You will hear some whistles and I want you to tell me how loud the whistle is. When the sounds are "Too Loud," this is where you want the hearing aid to stop and you do not want the sounds to get any louder.

Now, for every whistle, tell me how loud it sounds (p. 136).

Data were obtained in a sound field with warble tone stimuli for 20 hearing-impaired subjects (7 to 14 years of age) wearing high-output BTE-style hearing aids. Their results indicated that thresholds of discomfort could be obtained reliably from children as young as 7 years of age. Comparing the results obtained using a similar procedure for 20 hearing-impaired adults showed no systematic differences in mean thresholds of discomfort (or standard deviations) for the two groups. Stuart, Durieux-Smith, and Stenstrom (1991) reported similar success with the Kawell et al. procedure; however, their method used an insert earphone coupled to the child's own earmold delivery system. According to the authors, using this form of coupling eliminates the potential error of soundfield measures and provides for output values that can be directly compared to hearing aid SSPL90 specifications. A limitation in the maximum linear output of the insert earphones was noted, however.

Macpherson et al. (1991) attempted to develop a procedure with cognitive and

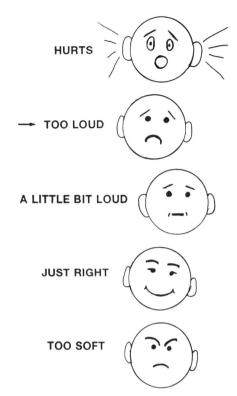

HURTS

→ TOO LOUD

A LITTLE BIT LOUD

JUST RIGHT

TOO SOFT

Figure 5.11. Verbal and pictorial representation of the loudness categories used with children 7 to 14 years of age. [Reprinted with permission from Kawell, M.E., Kopun, J.G., and Stelmachowicz, P.G., Loudness discomfort levels in children. *Ear Hear.*, 9(3), 133–136 (1988).]

language requirements appropriate for younger children. Their procedure uses four initial training tasks to teach the concept of "too much"; a fifth task is then used to obtain thresholds of discomfort under supraaural earphones for pure tones at octave frequencies, although any stimulus type would be appropriate. Refer to Appendix 5.2 for specific procedural directions. These investigators were attempting to match the task demands to the conceptual abilities of the child. Piagetian literature suggests that beginning around the age of 5 or 6, children can begin to recognize equivalencies between two distinct orderings of magnitude (Ginsburg & Opper, 1969). They point out that "children younger than age six (may) have not yet developed the cognitive ability to order different magnitudes of loudness stimuli as required in the Kawell et al. procedure" (Macpherson et al., 1991, p. 184). In fact, while 5-year-old normal hearing

subjects were able to perform the task with fair reliability, younger children with mental age levels below 5 years were not.

For younger or less cooperative children, more objective alternatives have been suggested for obtaining discomfort levels, including attempting to make predictions of discomfort based on recordings of ABR responses (Gorga, 1988; Howe & Decker, 1984; Pratt & Sohmer, 1977), acoustic reflex measures (Greenfield, Wiley, & Block, 1985; Margolis & Popelka, 1975; Ritter, Johnson, & Northern, 1979), and degree of hearing loss (Cox, 1985; Dillon, Chew & Deans, 1984; Hawkins et al., 1987; Kamm, Dirks, & Mickey, 1978; Kawell, Kopun, & Stelmachowicz, 1988; Ross & Seewald, 1988). Results have been inconclusive.

Issues of stimulus type, psychophysical method, and manner of presentation for determining discomfort levels have been discussed in great detail (Beattie & Sheffler, 1981; Cox, 1983; Cox & Sherbecoe, 1983; Hawkins, 1980; Morgan & Dirks, 1974). Of particular concern to the clinician should be the validation of the resultant SSPL90 settings. If the hearing aid is adjusted appropriately to match some threshold of discomfort contour based on frequency-specific stimuli, it would be expected that the child would not experience discomfort with any level of input. Some typical clinical procedures such as jiggling of keys or banging on the examination table may give a rough estimate of the validity of the settings, but probe microphone validation procedures may provide the most accurate assessment. Regardless of the procedure implemented, frequency-specific discomfort measures should be obtained and the hearing aid output set just below those levels. Validation should be accomplished using frequency-specific input signals as well. Stelmachowicz (1991b) points out that to check SSPL90 settings using a wide-band or speech-weighted noise may give an inaccurate picture of the maximum output of the hearing aid. As shown in Figure 5.12, SSPL90 curves obtained for a swept pure-tone input stimulus suggest possible output levels that are 15 to 20 dB higher than those obtained from the same hearing aid using a speech-weighted complex noise. Although the overall rms output would agree with the high-frequency SSPL90 obtained with a

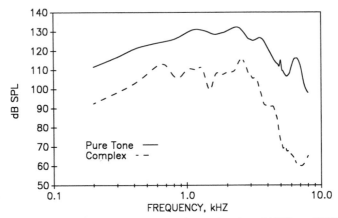

Figure 5.12. Comparison of 2-cc coupler output from a hearing aid (Oticon E38P) obtained in response to 90-dB inputs of complex and pure-tone stimuli.

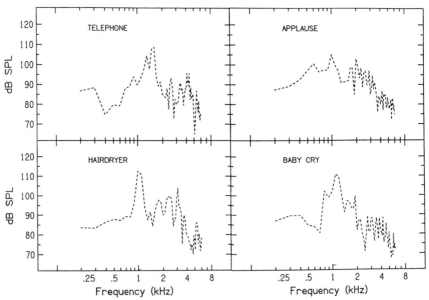

Figure 5.13. Two-cubic-centimeter coupler output of a broadband hearing aid (Phonak Audinet PPC-L) in response to applause, a baby's cry, telephone ringing, and hair dryer. [Reprinted with permission from Stelmachowicz, P., Clinical issues related to hearing-aid maximum output. In G. Studebaker, F. Bess, and L. Beck (Eds.), *The Vanderbilt Hearing Aid Report II.* Parkton, MD: York Press, Inc. (1991).]

pure-tone input, the output at any one frequency for the complex stimulus appears to be lower. It may not be obvious to the clinician that the broadband input may underestimate the output level that would be realized with other environmental inputs. Stelmachowicz (1991b) measured the output obtained from a hearing aid with a variety of environmental inputs, each presented at 90 db SPL, as shown in Figure 5.13. It is obvious that each stimulus type

results in areas of peak output that may be closer to the swept pure-tone levels than to the complex estimates of SSPL90. While measures of gain (difference in unaided and aided condition) may be accurately obtained with a wide-band complex, validation of maximum output necessitates use of a pure-tone input so that the maximum possible output in any frequency region can be compared to the discomfort threshold at the same frequency. In this way, complex environmental stimuli such as those shown in Figure 5.13 will not exceed discomfort even in those peak frequency regions.

Until a protocol is developed that results in reliable, valid measures of discomfort in very young children, a conservative—yet realistic—approach must be taken in setting hearing aid maximum output. If hearing aids are too conservatively limited, the child may be listening to all incoming information with the aid in saturation. The DSL and MSU fitting strategies prescribe relatively conservative maximum output levels based on degree of loss, whereas many of the other procedures require that additional measures be taken. Matkin (1986) has suggested the following 2-cc values for output: 110 dB SPL for "mild" losses, 120 dB SPL for "moderate" loss, and no more than 125 dB for a profound loss. More recently, he has revised those values to account for the age of the child, because of the size of the ear canal: 100 dB plus one-fourth the hearing loss at 1000 Hz, 2000 Hz, and 4000 Hz minus 5 dB for a preschooler or 10 dB for an infant or toddler (Matkin in Bebout, 1989). Based on the Sachs and Burkhard (1972) transformation data, those values at the eardrum may be 10 dB higher in the upper frequency range. In recent years the increased implementation of probe microphone systems has provided a means to determine output levels at the eardrum of the amplified child.

Effect on Residual Hearing

For over 50 years there has been concern as to the possibility of hearing aid use causing additional hearing impairment (Berry, 1939; Holmgren, 1940). Since the first studies of overamplification have appeared in the literature, there has been little consensus as to what constitutes "safe" output levels. Although reports of changes in hearing that can be directly attributed to hearing aid usage are relatively rare (Hawkins, 1982; Macrae, 1985; Mills, 1975), the literature is replete with evidence of the potential harm (Bellefleur & Van Dyke, 1968; Darbyshire, 1976; Hine, 1975; Jerger & Lewis, 1975; Markides, 1980; Markides & Ayree, 1978; Naunton, 1957; Rintelmann & Bess, 1988).

Of more current debate is the issue of sensory deprivation of the *unaided* ear. This "late-onset auditory deprivation" (Silman, Gelfand, & Silverman, 1984) may be manifested in reduced speech recognition scores in the unaided ear of unilaterally or bilaterally hearing-impaired listeners (Gatehouse, 1989a, 1989b; Gelfand, Silman, & Ross, 1987; Hood, 1990; Silverman, 1989; Stubblefield & Nye, 1989). In fact, some investigators have reported improved speech recognition scores in the aided ear as well as decreased scores in the unaided ear (Gatehouse, 1991; Markides, 1976; Markides & Aryee, 1978, 1980). The implications of these investigations for early identification and binaural aiding are portentous.

Some Style Issues

The standard rules relative to size, style, direct input capabilities, and so on still apply, despite our rapidly advancing technology. That is, regardless of how limited our audiometric information, the recommended hearing aid should have the flexibility to allow for changes in frequency response and output as further audiometric data become available. The "ideal" hearing aid for a child does not differ substantially from the "ideal" choice for an adult. (Refer to Chapter 11 for more information on basic styles and components.) A hearing aid with output and tone trimmers, strong telecoil, directional microphone, high fidelity/low distortion, and direct input capabilities should be sought for any child. Although the size of the device is frequently scrutinized for cosmetic reasons, it should be considered only in how well it fits over the smaller pinna of the child. This is especially true when the hearing aid must compete for space with eyeglasses. Behind-the-ear (BTE) style hearing aids continue to be the style of choice for children from infancy through adolescence. On a rare occasion, well-intentioned parents will press the issue of a (more discreet!) canal-style or in-the-ear (ITE) hearing aid. The ITE style is not widely used with children (Curran, 1985). The three primary limitations often encountered include *(1)* frequency of recasing; *(2)* poor telecoil response; and *(3)* no

Table 5.4
Mean Monosyllabic Word Discrimination Scores of Normal Hearing Children (Loudspeaker-Aided) and Hearing-Impaired Children. Children Listening in the High-Fidelity Condition (Loudspeaker-Aided) and Listening Through an Ear-Level Hearing Aid (Hearing Aid-Aided) for All Combinations of Reverberation Time and Message-to-Competition Ratio

Reverberation Time (sec)	Message-to-Competition Ratio in dB	Groups		
		Normal (Loudspeaker-Aided)	Hearing-Impaired (Loudspeaker-Aided)	Hearing-Impaired (Hearing Aid-Aided)
0.0	+∞	94.5	87.5	83.0
	+12	89.2	77.8	70.0
	+6	79.7	65.7	59.5
	0	60.2	42.2	39.0
0.4	+∞	92.5	79.2	74.0
	+12	82.8	69.0	60.2
	+6	71.3	54.5	52.2
	0	47.7	28.8	27.8
1.2	+∞	76.5	61.8	45.0
	+12	68.8	50.2	41.2
	+6	54.2	39.5	27.0
	0	29.7	15.3	11.2

Reprinted with permission from Finitzo-Hieber, T., and Tillman, T., Room acoustics effect on monosyllabic word discrimination ability for normal and hearing impaired children. *J. Speech Hear. Res.*, 21(3), 440–458 (1978).

provision for direct audio input. Northern and Downs (1991) point out that the child's pinna and concha may continue to grow and change in shape until the age of 9, resulting in the necessity of recasing every 3 to 5 months. The professional needs to give parents information regarding frequency and cost of recasing, need for loaner devices, and so on.

The decision relative to the choice of a directional microphone needs to be considered more often. In his review of research comparing directional microphone hearing aids to omnidirectional hearing aids, Mueller (1981, p. 19) noted that regardless of the measuring tool (electroacoustic, speech recognition measures, or listener ratings), the directional microphone hearing aid "either rated superior or equal to the omnidirectional hearing aid but never worse." Yet, he goes on to acknowledge that directional microphones are used in only 20% of BTE hearing aids, the unfortunate result of "indifference" on the part of the clinician (Mueller & Grimes, 1987).

Finally, maintaining high fidelity and low distortion may best be accomplished by use of compression circuitry, rather than peak clipping, for output control.

Occasionally, the need for a bone conduction (BC) hearing aid still arises. The child with chronic otitis media or atretic ear canals may derive great benefit from an amplification system but is not able to use the traditional earmold for reasons of hygiene or structural abnormalities. Bone conduction transducers worn with a headband and powered by a BTE-style hearing aid can be successfully recommended.

FM SYSTEMS

Auditory trainers can be construed as another "style" option. Auditory trainers or frequency modulated (FM) systems were first developed in the 1940s in an effort to provide the hearing-impaired child direct access to the teacher's voice, thus reducing the deleterious effects of background noise in reverberant classrooms (Table 5.4). The early devices were intended for severely and profoundly hearing-impaired children. They were characterized by broad and flat frequency responses and were seldom fit "to match the amplification needs of the child" (Bess & Gravel, 1981, p. 24). Current systems are composed of a teacher's (or some other talker's) microphone, often a small lapel-style wireless microphone, an FM

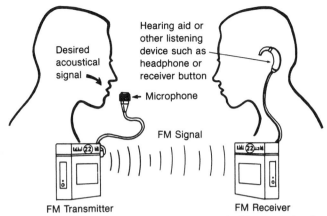

Figure 5.14. Schematic of FM transmission system. [Reprinted with permission from Compton, C.L., Assistive devices: doorways to independence. Washington, DC: Gallaudet University (1989).]

transmitter, and an FM receiver (Fig. 5.14). These portable and wireless systems are now frequently adjustable (gain and output characteristics) and typically provide signal transmission within a 300- to 600-foot radius outdoors and a 100-foot radius indoors. They operate in the 72 to 76 MHz bandwidth region originally designated by the Federal Communication Commission for "educational assistance devices for the hearing impaired" (Hammond, 1991). Thirty-two frequencies are available within that band, allowing for multiple systems to be operating at one time within a single school building.

An FM system may be coupled directly to the listener's ear via a headset or earbuds, or to a personal hearing aid in one of three manners (Fig. 5.15):

1. *Silhouette* (induction). A thin inductor that is typically shaped like a BTE hearing aid and that generates an electromagnetic field is placed under/beneath the child's hearing aid and plugged into the FM receiver. The child wears the hearing aid with the telecoil activated.
2. *Neck loop* (induction). The child wears a wire loop around the neck that generates an electromagnetic field and is plugged into the FM receiver. The hearing aid telecoil is activated.
3. *Direct audio input*. The child's own hearing aid is connected to the FM receiver using an input jack.

A number of investigators have questioned the effect of the various coupling systems on the electroacoustic characteristics of the personal hearing aid. Matkin and Olsen (1970, 1973) looked at the effect of the induction loop on hearing aid performance. They reported "undesirable" changes in performance and noted that "interference of other radio signals was periodically quite audible" (p. 77). Sung and Hodgson (1971) also reported differences in electroacoustic characteristics between microphone and telecoil modes, both in frequency response as well as total harmonic distortion levels. Other investigators (Freeman, Sinclair, & Riggs, 1980; Gladstone, 1985; Hawkins & Schum, 1985; Hawkins & Van Tasell, 1982; Thibodeau & Saucedo, 1991; Van Tasell & Landin, 1980) have demonstrated significant variability in electroacoustic measures across coupling methods. As shown in Figure 5.16 the choice of FM system as well as the choice of coupling method may have significant impact on the performance of a single hearing aid (Hawkins & Schum, 1985). The ideal arrangement, according to Hawkins (1984), includes a directional transmitting microphone in close proximity to the teacher's mouth, the FM receiver coupled via direct input to binaural hearing aids, and a user switch that allows for FM only, hearing aids only, or FM plus hearing aid function control.

Because there are currently no written standards on the measurement of the electroacoustic performance of auditory trainers, several investigators have suggested measurement protocols. Thibodeau and Saucedo (1991) suggest a coupler measure-

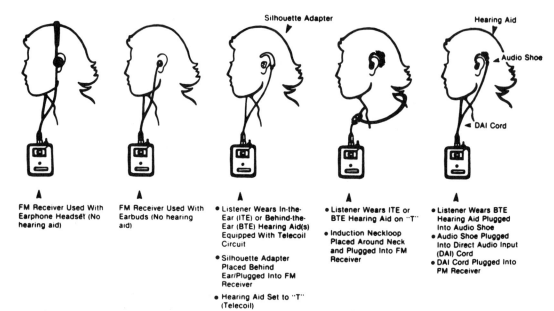

Figure 5.15. Methods of FM receiver coupling. [Reprinted with permission from Compton, C.L., Assistive devices: doorways to independence. Washington, DC: Gallaudet University (1989).]

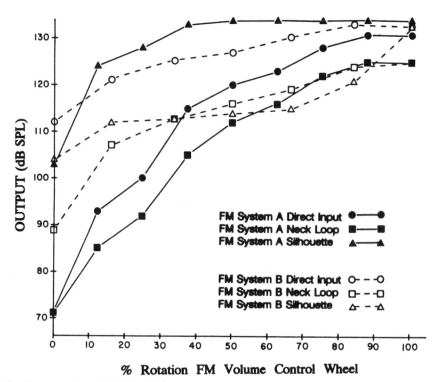

Figure 5.16. Example of variability in FM receiver volume control wheel taper curves for two FM systems when connected to a single hearing aid via direct input, neck loop, and silhouette. [Modified with permission from Hawkins, D.B., and Schum, D., Some effects of FM coupling on hearing aid characteristics. *J. Speech Hear. Disord.*, 50, 132–141 (1985).]

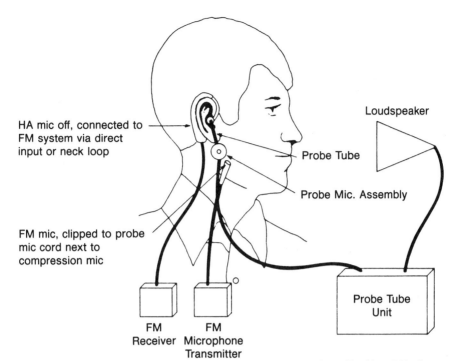

HA mic off, connected to
FM system via direct
input or neck loop

Loudspeaker

Probe Tube

Probe Mic. Assembly

FM mic, clipped to probe
mic cord next to
compression mic

Probe Tube
Unit

FM
Receiver

FM
Microphone
Transmitter

Figure 5.17. Example of arrangement to measure the real-ear response of an FM system attached to a hearing aid with an ear canal probe tube measurement device. Refer to text for explanation. [Reprinted with permission from Hawkins, D.B., Assessment of FM systems with an ear canal probe tube microphone system. *Ear Hear.*, 8, 301–303 (1987).]

ment procedure that can be carried out in most audiologic settings. The FM microphone is placed in the hearing aid test box with the transmitter outside the box. The FM receiver is attached to an HA-1 coupler via a button receiver with the measurement microphone inside the coupler.

Coupler measures of the FM system coupled to a hearing aid by way of a neck loop are more difficult because of the need for specific orientation of the hearing aid and neck loop. Thibodeau and Saucedo (1991) and Van Tasell and Landin (1980) suggest similar methods; however, each requires the use of a Knowles Electronic Manikin for Acoustic Research (KEMAR). The FM microphone is again placed inside the hearing aid test box with the FM receiver placed at KEMAR's waist, and the neck loop is hung around the neck to ensure proper orientation. The hearing aid is placed over the pinna and attached to the HA-2 coupler, supported by a "sling," with the standard tubing and performance measures taken.

Hawkins (1987) suggests that probe microphone measures of FM performance—

regardless of how they are coupled—should be taken with the child wearing the personal system. As shown in Figure 5.17, the FM microphone is placed as close as possible to the monitoring microphone of the probe system, thus allowing for controlled and consistent input to the microphone. An 80-dB input—representative of the teacher's speech level, approximately 6 inches from the transmitting microphone—is output from the loudspeaker, and performance measures are obtained. Hawkins also suggests a method for setting the FM volume control prior to taking measurements: The hearing aid is initially measured alone using a 60-dB SPL input signal. For the FM performance measure, the input signal is changed to 80 dB SPL (representative of the teacher's speech level) and the VCW is adjusted so that the output for 1000 Hz is the same as it was with the 60-dB input signal. This presupposes that the listener will have the same preferred listening level regardless of which device he or she is listening through. In view of the fact that considerable variation has been shown in performance characteristics, depending on the type of coupling employed, it must be the responsibility of the monitoring audiologist to assess accurately the appropriateness of any coupling strategy used.

One potential source of concern for FM system use in schools has not been well investigated. It has long been recognized that electromagnetic interference may affect FM use when personal or classroom loop coupling is used. Electrical outlets, fluorescent lights, and computer systems have all been shown to generate potentially disruptive electromagnetic interference (Beaulac, Pehringer, & Shough, 1989; Beck & Nance, 1989; Bevacqua et al., 1989; Carlson, 1990; Harder, 1971). With the increasing use of personal and classroom amplification systems, which often include loop coupling, the interference in the classroom setting from any of these sources may be detrimental. Although the Federal Communication Commission has developed regulations for radiated emissions from computing devices (Violette, White, & Violette, 1987), it is still unclear whether permissible levels may still interfere with hearing aid telecoil/loop function. More research is necessary in this area.

Binaural Versus Monaural Hearing

The advantages of binaural hearing have long been established. Besides the benefits of binaural summation, elimination of head shadow, and localization (discussed earlier as unilaterally hearing-impaired children's deficits), other subjective reports of "ease of listening," improved speech intelligibility in noise, spatial balance, and enhanced sound quality reports from adult hearing aid users suggest that additional subjective benefits are possible.

There is much consensus, on an intellectual or academic level, as to the desirability of providing binaural amplification to all hearing-impaired children. A number of investigators have reported advantages of binaural amplification use with children (Langford & Faires, 1973; Liden & Harford, 1985; Maxon, 1981; Mueller, 1986; North-

ern, Gabbard, & Kinder, 1990; Ross, 1977, 1980). Others have noted only situational benefits (Brooks, 1984; Grimes, Mueller, & Malley, 1981; Hawkins, 1984). Grimes, Mueller, and Malley (1981) tested 24 children (9 to 17 years of age) with synthetic speech presented in a background of multitaker noise in three aided conditions—right, left, and binaural—and at two signal-to-noise ratios. All subjects were experienced users of binaural amplification, yet for none of the subjects was the better monaural score significantly different than the binaural score at +10 dB signal-to-noise ratio; for 92% of the subjects, the scores were not significantly different even in the 0 dB signal-to-noise ratio condition. The authors caution that, in view of other reported advantages of binaural amplification (refer to Chapter 12), lack of binaural superiority in speech recognition should not be considered a sufficient reason to dismiss the option.

Obviously, the child with bilaterally symmetrical thresholds may appear to be the most likely candidate, although any child with usable hearing in each ear should be considered a potential binaural candidate. Yet, even though probe microphone measures of insertion gain may indicate that the input to each cochlea is equivalent, the assumption that the child is getting true binaural advantage cannot be made.

While a binaural fitting may be appropriate for 80% of pediatric fittings, nationally, only about 40% of children in the United States are fit with binaural amplification (Matkin in Bebout, 1989). The audiologist may refer to the cost, the limited audiologic information, the risks, parental resistance, and so on, as contraindicators; of particular interest is the current evidence of auditory deprivation in monaurally aided adults (refer to the earlier discussion).

Appropriateness of "Higher Tech" Hearing Aids

The current hearing aid market is besieged with claims of new and improved circuitry resulting in significant improvements to the hearing aid user. The "new" signal-processing schemes for noise reduction have not conclusively shown enhanced speech recognition in noisy backgrounds although, anecdotally, "ease of listening" may be improved (Bentler, 1991; Preves & Sigelman, 1989). When considering the newer programmable hearing aids, a number of options must be assessed, including advisability of remote control, multiple versus single memory, multiple versus single channel, compression parameters, and cost, to name a few. Because nearly all of the current digitally programmable hearing aids use some form of input and/or output compression, the clinician needs to understand the function and limitations of any adjustments to these parameters. Although compression in hearing aids has been scrutinized for many years (refer to entire monograph by Braida et al., 1979), it is still unclear what the optimal compression thresholds and time constants should be. Because the effect of altering release time as a function of frequency may be subtle, the clinician may have to depend on adult-derived data to direct clinical decision making. And although standardized test measures of the effect of various parametric changes may not provide evidence of setting superiority, trial periods may provide adequate feedback for appropriate changes to be made.

Perhaps the most advantageous feature of the programmable hearing aid is its flexibility. Because the diagnostic process for the pediatric client is typically ongoing and amplification cannot be postponed until a complete audiogram is obtained, the flexibility of the programmable hearing aids allows for early fitting with subsequent changes in gain and/or output. The parents are not faced with repeated purchases over the first 5 years, although the initial cost may be substantially more.

Special Applications

Diefendorf has suggested that 30 to 45% of hearing-impaired children have one or more additional disabilities (Mahon, 1987). Whether that additional disability refers to chronic middle ear effusion or some degree of mental or physical impairment, the im-

pact must be assessed for successful hearing aid use. The child with chronic or fluctuating conductive hearing loss has previously been discussed as a good candidate for amplification. The only available report of an 8-year-old with PE tubes suggests no significant change in ear canal SPL in the 250- to 6000-Hz region due to the presence of the tubes (Stelmachowitz & Seewald, 1991).

Consideration must also be given to the child with hearing impairment confounded by physical and/or mental impairments. The neurologically impaired child should not be overlooked, but rather the cognitive level should be carefully considered in the fitting stages. The terminally ill child, likewise, should be considered a potential candidate unless immediate crises deter the process. Parents may choose to deal with one impairment at a time because of the emotional and financial drain imposed. Ultimately that is their decision to make. For the physically impaired child, other considerations must be made. If the child exhibits motor impairments that may preclude control of the hearing aid's operation, in-services to teachers and caretakers must be provided in addition to orienting parents. A minimally physically impaired child may derive more benefit from a body-style hearing aid for which the controls are more easily manipulated.

Logemann and Elfenbein (in press) were concerned with the effect head and neck support systems might have on the acoustic signal arriving from different azimuths. Headrests and headwings, as used for motor-impaired wheelchair-bound individuals, were shown to affect signal level at the ear by as much as 20 dB for frequencies of 2000 and 4000 Hz. Consideration of these azimuth effects on signal transmission must be made for children placed in academic settings. Critical speech cues may be lost for signals from the rear (e.g., during classroom discussions) as a result of such unintentional sound barriers. Use of an FM system may reduce or eliminate the detrimental effects of these barriers.

Besides the uses discussed previously, auditory trainers (FM systems) have been advocated for three other unique groups: *(1)* moderate to profound hearing-impaired

Table 5.5
Suggested Components for a Training Program Designed to Teach Children Effective Monitoring Practices

Training Program
1. Instruction by audiologist
2. Instruction by THI, SLP, or others[a]
3. Establishment of age-appropriate criterion-referenced IEP goals
4. Familiarity with resources: equipment and personnel
5. Development of strategies for coping when hearing aids are nonfunctional

[a] THI, teachers of the hearing impaired; SLP, speech-language pathologists.
Reprinted with permission from Elfenbein, J. L., Bentler, R. A., Davis, J., and Niebuhr, D., Status of school children's hearing aids relative to monitoring practices. *Ear Hear.*, 9, 212–215 (1988).

preschoolers for home use; *(2)* learning disabled (LD)/auditory processing dysfunctional children for personal and soundfield use; and *(3)* school-age children with mild and/or fluctuating hearing loss.

Proponents of FM use for the first group contend that, during this critical period of language development, the improved signal-to-noise ratio will enhance language learning significantly. An additional benefit of the arrangement is encouraging parent/child acceptance of the system in a familiar background (Benoit, 1989). Opponents of FM use at home for this moderate to profound hearing-impaired group point out the unnaturalness of the stimulation and/or absence of typical environmental input when a child is using an FM system (in FM condition only) at home. Part-time use of the environmental or hearing aid microphone should alleviate some of that concern. More research is needed to determine the efficacy of such an amplification strategy.

Relative to the second group, the use of auditory trainers has also been advocated for essentially normal hearing children who have learning disabilities, attention problems, or auditory processing problems (Blake et al., 1991; Blake, Torpey, & Wertz, 1986; Loose, 1984; Willeford & Billger, 1978). In a report prepared by the Committee on Amplification for the Hearing Impaired of the American Speech-Language-Hearing Association (1991), concerns related to safety and efficacy in the use of amplification for "individuals with normal peripheral hearing" were raised. Because published articles to date on this topic have not typically provided specific information on the gain or output provided by the amplification systems, the cumulative wearing time, or the method of selection or fitting, the committee cautioned against overinterpreting the reported benefits.

Relative to the third group, the child with the fluctuating or mild hearing loss has been found to be at risk for academic achievement (Davis et al., 1986). Auditory trainers and other forms of classroom amplification have been proposed as management strategies. Careful medical and audiologic monitoring is necessary with this group as well, to ensure appropriate output limitation.

Parent Counseling

As Davis has pointed out (in Mahon, 1987), no one is more influential in the habilitative process of a hearing-impaired child than are the parents. Yet, because "parents come in all shapes and sizes when it comes to their attitudes about and their degrees of involvement" (p. 10), it is the clinician's responsibility to provide ongoing counseling to whatever degree required. It is paramount that the clinician understands the process parents pass through while learning to accept, cope, and manage the hearing impairment, regardless of its severity. Counseling is a major component of the rehabilitation amplification process. Refer to Chapter 9 for an in-depth discussion of the counseling process.

Follow-Up

While appropriate hearing aid recommendation and use constitute a major component in the pediatric rehabilitative process, it must be acknowledged that it is only one component. Besides further decision making as to speech and language remediation, auditory training, and academic placement (discussed in Chapters 6–8), the audiologist must plan for ongoing audiologic follow-up as well. It is not clear how much follow-up constitutes sufficient follow-up, but it is clear that close monitoring for threshold shifts and hearing aid function (including any classroom amplification system) is minimally required. Liden and Harford (1985) suggest that audiologic follow-up be scheduled at least every 6 to 8 weeks for the first 3 months, every 3 months until the age of 3, every 6 months until school age, and then annually. While this may be a good rule of thumb for most situations, any extenuating circumstances may require more or less frequent monitoring.

Elfenbein et al. (1988) surveyed available data over the past 20 years related to incidence of malfunction in hearing aids used by children in various settings. They found a 27 to 92% malfunction rate at any given time, depending on the particular criteria used. Of even more interest was the fact that the teachers of the hearing impaired—the individuals most likely to have responsibility for the monitoring—believed that such malfunctions rarely occur! In their own investigation of three groups of mainstreamed children, even with "conscientious parental and professional monitoring," a similar incidence of malfunction occurred. Active participation of the child may be the best available solution. As shown in Table 5.5, a training program designed to teach children effective monitoring practices should begin with the audiologist. The audiologist should provide information relative to simple monitoring tasks (such as cleaning the earmold, checking battery voltage, visual inspection) to the child as well as to the parent and teachers; this training should continue into the classroom and/or therapy room. Children should be familiarized with available resources, both equipment for monitoring their own hearing aids and contact persons for reporting malfunctions.

Summary

Although the issues surrounding amplification for the hearing-impaired child are relatively straightforward, the answers are not. As we search for better understanding of what constitutes optimal gain/output, optimal speech spectrum characteristics, and an understanding of the extent that one can generalize adult data to infants and children, we should continue to question

ourselves. Just as the diagnostic and rehabilitative processes need to be ongoing, our critical evaluation of the proposed solutions needs to be ongoing. Although we cannot make up those early years of the child's life, we should feel confident that we never stopped looking for the answers.

Acknowledgments. Preparation of this chapter was assisted by C. Colville, J. Elfenbein, J. Naumann, N. Pape, M. Robinson, and C. Sidler. Their thoughtful discussions of issues, concerns, and research needs in pediatric amplification prompted the writing of much of this chapter. A number of excellent chapters on pediatric amplification issues currently exist, and the author encourages the reader to refer to those referenced readings for further information.

References

American National Standards Institute, *American national standard methods for the calculation of the articulation index*, ANSI, S3.5. New York: American National Standards Institute (1969).

American National Standards Institute, *Specification for audiometers*, ANSI S3.6. New York: American National Standards Institute (1989).

American Speech-Language-Hearing Association, Amplification as a remediation technique for children with normal peripheral hearing. *Asha,* 33, Suppl. 3, 22–24 (1991).

Beattie, R.C., and Sheffler, M.V., Test-retest stability and effects of psychophysical methods on the speech loudness discomfort level. *Audiology,* 20, 143–156 (1981).

Beaulac, D.A., Pehringer, J.L., and Shough, L.F., Assistive listening devices: available options. *Semin. Hear.,* 10(1), 11–30 (1989).

Bebout, J.M., Pediatric hearing aid fitting: a practical overview. *Hear. J.,* 42(8), 13–20 (1989).

Beck, L., and Nance, G., Hearing aids, assistive listening devices, and telephones: issues to consider. *Semin. Hear.,* 10(1), 78–89 (1989).

Bellefleur, P.A., and Van Dyke, R.C., The effect of high gain amplification on children in a residential school for the deaf. *J. Speech Hear. Res.,* 11, 343–347 (1968).

Bender, R., and Wiig, E., Binaural hearing aids in young children. *Volta Rev.,* 62, 113–115 (1960).

Benoit, R., Home use of FM amplification systems during the early childhood years. *Hear. Instr.,* 40(3), 8–12 (1989).

Bentler, R.A., External ear resonance characteristics in children. *J. Speech Hear Disord.,* 54(2), 264–268 (1989).

Bentler, R.A., Clinical implications and limitations of current noise reduction circuitry. In G. Studebaker, F. Bess, and L. Beck (Eds.), *The Vanderbilt Hearing Aid Report II.* Parkton, MD: York Press, Inc. (1991).

Berg, F.S., Sound field FM: a new technology for the classroom. *The Clinical Connection, 1st Quarter,* 14–17 (1990).

Berger, K., Hagberg, N., and Rane, R., *Prescription of Hearing Aids.* Kent, OH: Herald Publishing Co. (1977).

Bergman, B.M., and Bentler, R.A., *Relating Hearing Aid Output to Measures of Volume and Immittance.* Paper presented at American Speech-Hearing-Language Association, Seattle (1990).

Bergman, M., Binaural hearing. *Arch. Otolaryngol.,* 66, 572–578 (1957).

Bergstrom, L., Congenital deafness. In J. Northern (Ed.), *Hearing Disorders.* Boston: Little, Brown (1976).

Berry, G., The use and effectiveness of hearing aids. *Laryngoscope,* 49, 912 (1939).

Bess, F.H., The minimally hearing-impaired child. *Ear Hear.,* 6(1), 43–47 (1985).

Bess, F.H., and Gravel, J.S., Recent trends in educational amplification. *Hear. Instru.,* 32(11), 24–29 (1981).

Bess, F.H., and Tharpe, A.M., An introduction to unilateral sensorineural hearing-impaired children. *Ear Hear.,* 7(1), 3–14 (1986).

Bevacqua, F., Cipollone, E., Morviducci, A., and Venditti, L., *Advances in Understanding of E.M. Emissions from Computing Devices.* Paper presented at the IEEE National Symposium on Electromagnetic Compatibility, Denver, CO (1989).

Blake, R., Field, B., Foster, C., Platt, F., and Wertz, P., Effect of FM auditory trainers on attending behaviors of learning-disabled children. *Lang. Speech, Hear. Serv. Schools,* 22, 111–114 (1991).

Blake, R., Torpey, C., and Wertz, P., Preliminary findings: effect of FM auditory trainers on attending behaviors of learning disabled children. Telex Communications (1986).

Braida, L.D., Durlach, N.I., Lippman, R.P., Hicks, B.L., Rabinowitz, W.M., and Reed, C.M., Hearing aids—review of past research on linear amplification, compression amplification, and frequency lowering. Washington, DC, *Asha Monograph* (1979).

Brooks, D.N., Binaural benefit—when and how much? *Scandinav. Audiol.,* 13, 237–241 (1984).

Bruel, P., Frederiksen, E., and Rasmussen, G., Investigations of a new insert earphone coupler. *Hear. Instr.,* 34, 22–25 (1976).

Byrne, D., and Cotton, S., Preferred listening levels of sensorineurally hearing-impaired listeners. *Aust. J. Audiol.,* 9(1), 7–14 (1988).

Byrne, D., and Dillon, H., The National Acoustic Laboratories (NAL) new procedure for selecting the gain and frequency response of a hearing aid. *Ear Hear.,* 7(4), 257–265 (1986).

Byrne, D., and Fifield, D., Evaluation of hearing aid fittings for infants. *Br. J. Audiol.,* 8, 47–54 (1974).

Byrne, D., Parkinson, A., and Newall, P., Hearing aid gain and frequency response requirements for the severely/profoundly hearing impaired. *Ear Hear.,* 11(1), 40–49 (1990).

Byrne, D., Parkinson, A., and Newall, P., Modified hearing aid selection procedures for severe/profound hearing loss. In G. Studebaker, F. Bess, and L. Beck (Eds.), *The Vanderbilt Hearing Aid Report II.* Parkton, MD: York Press, Inc. (1991).

Byrne, D., and Tonisson, W., Selecting the gain of hearing aids for persons with sensorineural hearing impairments. *Scand. Audiol.,* 5, 51–62 (1976).

Bryne, D., and Upfold, G., Implications of ear canal resonance for hearing aid fitting. *Sem. Hear.,* 12(1), 34–41 (1991).

Carlson, E., Corrosion concerns in EMI shielding of electronics. *Materials Performance,* 29, 76–80 (1990).

Clopton, B.M., and Silverman, M.S., Plasticity of binaural interaction. II. Critical periods and changes in midline response. *J. Neurophysiol.,* 40(6), 1275–1280 (1977).

Compton, C.L., Assistive devices: doorways to independence. Washington, DC: Gallaudet University (1989).

Cornelisse, L.E., Gagne, J-P., and Seewald, R.C., Ear level recordings of the long-term average spectrum of speech. *Ear Hear.,* 12(1), 47–54 (1991).

Cox, R.M., Using ULCL measures to find frequency/gain and SSPL90. *Hear. Instru.,* 34(7), 17–21 (1983).

Cox, R.M., Hearing aids and rehabilitation: a structural approach to hearing aid selection. *Ear Hear.,* 6(4), 226–239 (1985).

Cox, R.M., The MSU hearing instrument prescription procedure. *Hear. Instru.,* 39(1), 6–10 (1988).

Cox, R.M., and Alexander, G.C., Evaluation of an in-situ output probe-microphone method for hearing aid fitting verification. *Ear Hear.,* 11(1), 31–39 (1990).

Cox, R.M., and Moore, J.N., Composite speech spectrum for hearing aid gain prescriptions. *J. Speech Hear. Res.,* 31(1), 102–107 (1988).

Cox, R.M., and Sherbecoe, R., *Effect of Psychophysical Method on the Repeatability of Loudness Discomfort Levels.* Paper presented at the American Speech and Hearing Association Convention, Cincinnati, OH (1983).

Curran, J.R., ITE aids for children: survey of attitudes and practices of audiologists. *Hear. Instru.,* 36(4), 20–25 (1985).

Darbyshire, J.D., A study of the use of high power hearing aids by children with marked degrees of deafness and the possibility of deterioration in auditory acuity. *Br. J. Audiol.,* 10, 74–82 (1976).

Davis, J.M., Elfenbein, J.L., Schum, R., and Bentler, R.A., Effects of mild and moderate hearing impairments on language, educational, and psychosocial behavior of children. *J. Speech Hear. Disord.,* 51(1), 53–62 (1986).

Dempster, J.H., and Mackenzie, K., The resonance frequency of the external auditory canal in children. *Ear Hear.,* 11(4), 296–298 (1990).

Dennis, W., *Children of the Creche.* Century Psychology Series. New York: Prentice-Hall (1973).

Dillon, H., Chew, R., and Deans, M., Loudness discomfort level measurements and their implications for the design and fitting of hearing aids. *Aust. J. Audiol.,* 6(2), 73–79 (1984).

Dobie, R.A., and Berlin, C.I., Influence of otitis media on hearing and development. *Ann. Otol. Rhinol. Laryngol.,* 88, Suppl. 60, 48–53 (1979).

Dunn, H.K., and White, S.D., Statistical measurements on conversational speech. *J. Audiol. Soc. Am.,* 11, 278–288 (1940).

Eisen, N.H., Some effects of early sensory deprivation on later behavior: the quondam hard-of-hearing child. *J. Abnorm. Soc. Psychol.,* 65, 338 (1962).

Elfenbein, J.L., Bentler, R.A., Davis, J.M., and Niebuhr, D.P., Status of school children's hearing aids relative to monitoring practices. *Ear Hear.,* 9, 212–217 (1988).

Elssmann, S.F., Matkin, N.D., and Sabo, M.P., Early identification of congenital sensorineural hearing impairment. *Hear. J.,* 40(9), 13–17 (1987).

Evans, W.J., Webster, D.B., and Cullen, J.K., Auditory brainstem responses in neonatally sound deprived CBA/J mice. *Hear. Res.,* 10(3), 269–277 (1983).

Fabry, D.A., and Van Tasell, D.J., Evaluation of an Articulation-Index based model for predicting the effects of adaptive frequency response hearing aids. *J. Speech Hear. Res.,* 33(4), 676–689 (1990).

Feigin, J.A., Kopun, J.G., Stelmachowicz, P.G., and Gorga, M.P., Probe-tube microphone measures of ear-canal sound pressure levels in infants and children. *Ear Hear.,* 10(4), 254–258 (1989).

Festen, J.M., and Plomp, R., Speech-reception threshold in noise with one and two hearing aids. *J. Acoust. Soc. Am.,* 79(2), 465–471 (1986).

Finitzo-Hieber, T., and Tillman, T.W., Room acoustics effects on monosyllabic word discrimination ability for normal and hearing-impaired children. *J. Speech Hear. Res.,* (21)3, 440–458 (1978).

Freeman, B.A., Sinclair, J.S., and Riggs, D.E., Electroacoustic performance characteristics of FM auditory trainers. *J. Speech Hear. Disord.,* 45(1), 16–26 (1980).

French, N.R., and Steinberg, J.C., Factors governing the intelligibility of speech sounds. *J. Acoust. Soc. Am.,* 19, 90–119 (1947).

Gatehouse, S., Apparent auditory deprivation of late-onset: the effects of presentation level. *Br. J. Audiol.,* 23, 167 (1989a).

Gatehouse, S., Apparent auditory deprivation effects of late onset: the role of presentation level. *J. Acoust. Soc. Am.,* 86(6), 2103–2106 (1989b).

Gatehouse, S., *Acclimatisation to Speech.* Paper presented at the International Hearing Aid Conference, Iowa City, IA (1991).

Gelfand, S.A., Silman, S., and Ross, L., Long-term effects of monaural, binaural and no amplification in subjects with bilateral hearing loss. *Scand. Audiol.,* 16, 201–207 (1987).

Ginsburg, H., and Opper, S., *Piaget's Theory of Intellectual Development.* Englewood Cliffs, NJ: Prentice-Hall, Inc. (1969).

Gladstone, V.S., Variables affecting hearing aid telephone induction coil performance. *Hear Instru.,* 36(9), 18–21 (1985).

Gorga, M., *Clinical Applications of Auditory Evoked Potentials.* Lecture presented at the University of Iowa, Iowa City, IA (October 1988).

Greenfield, D.G., Wiley, T.L., and Block, M.G., Acoustic-reflex dynamics and the loudness-discomfort level. *J. Speech Hear. Disord.,* 50(1), 14–20 (1985).

Greenstein, J.M., Greenstein, B.B., and McConville, K., et al., *Mother Infant Communication and Language Acquisition in Infants.* New York: Lexington School for the Deaf (1976).

Grimes, A.M., Mueller, H.G., and Malley, J.D., Examination of binaural amplification in children. *Ear Hear.,* 2(5), 208–210 (1981).

Hammond, L., *FM Auditory Trainers: A Winning Choice for Students, Teachers, and Parents.* Minneapolis: Gopher State Litho Corp. (1991).

Harder, J., Digital computer systems. In R. Ficchi (Ed.), *Practical Design for Electromagnetic Compat-*

ibility. New York: Hayden Book Company, Inc., pp. 165–182 (1971).

Haskell, G.B., Functional gain. *Ear Hear.,* 8(5 Supplement), 95S–99S (1987).

Hawkins, D.B., The effect of signal type on the loudness discomfort level. *Ear Hear.,* 1(1), 38–41 (1980).

Hawkins, D.B., Overamplification: a well-documented case report. *J. Speech Hear Disord.,* 47(4), 382–384 (1982).

Hawkins, D.B., Comparisons of speech recognition in noise by mildly-to-moderately hearing-impaired children using hearing aids and FM systems. *J. Speech Hear Disord.,* 49(4), 409–418 (1984).

Hawkins, D.B., Assessment of FM systems with an ear canal probe tube microphone system. *Ear Hear.,* 8(5), 301–303 (1987).

Hawkins, D.B., Cooper, W.A., and Thompson, D.J., Comparison among SPLs in real ears, 2 cm³ and 6 cm³ couplers. *J. Am. Acad. Audiol.,* 1, 154–161 (1990).

Hawkins, D.B., and Schum, D.J., Some effects of FM-system coupling on hearing aid characteristics. *J. Speech Hear. Disord.,* 50(2), 132–141 (1985).

Hawkins, D.B., and Van Tasell, D.J., Electroacoustic characteristics of personal FM systems. *J. Speech Hear. Disord.,* 47(4), 355–362 (1982).

Hawkins, D.B., Walden, B.E., Montgomery, A., and Prosek, R.A., Description and validation of an LDL procedure designed to select SSPL90. *Ear Hear.,* 8(1), 162–169 (1987).

Hine, W.D., and Furness, H.J.S., Does wearing a hearing aid damage residual hearing? *Teacher Deaf,* 73, 261–271 (1975).

Holmgren, L., Can the hearing be damaged by a hearing aid? *Acta Otolaryngologica,* 28, 440 (1940).

Hood, J.D., Problems in central binaural integration in hearing loss cases. *Hear. Instru.,* 41, 6–11 (1990).

Howe, S.W., and Decker, T.N., Monaural and binaural auditory brainstem responses in relation to the psychophysical loudness growth function. *J. Acoust. Soc. Am.,* 76(3), 787–793 (1984).

Humes, L.E., Dirks, D.D., Bell, T.S., Ahlstrom, C., and Kincaid, G.E., Application of the Articulation Index and the Speech Transmission Index to the recognition of speech by normal-hearing and hearing-impaired listeners. *J. Speech Hear. Res.,* 29(4), 447–462 (1986).

Jerger, J.F., and Lewis, N., Binaural hearing aids: Are they dangerous for children? *Arch. Otolaryngol.,* 101, 480–483 (1975).

Kawell, M.E., Kopun, J.G., and Stelmachowicz, P.G., Loudness discomfort levels in children. *Ear Hear.,* 9(3), 133–136 (1988).

Konkle, D., and Schwartz, D., Binaural amplification: a paradox. In F.H. Bess, B.A. Freeman, and S. Sinclair (Eds.), *Amplification in Education.* Washington, DC: Alexander Graham Bell Association (1981).

Kruger, B., An update on the external ear resonance in infants and young children. *Ear Hear.,* 8(6), 333–336 (1987).

Kryter, K.D., Methods for the calculation and use of the Articulation Index. *J. Acoust. Soc. Am.,* 34, 1689–1697 (1962a).

Kryter, K.D., Validation of the Articulation Index. *J. Acoust. Soc. Am.,* 34, 1698–1702 (1962b).

Langford, S.E., and Faires, W.L., Objective evaluation of monaural vs. binaural amplification for congenitally hard-of-hearing children. *J. Aud. Res.*, 13, 263–267 (1973).

Liden, G., and Harford, E.R., The pediatric audiologist: from magician to clinician. *Ear Hear.*, 6(1), 6–9 (1985).

Logemann, J.M., and Elfenbein, J.L., Measuring the effects of head and neck support systems on signals transmitted to the ear. *Ear Hear.* (in press).

Loose, F., Learning disabled students use FM wireless systems. Telex Communications (1984).

Macpherson, B.J., Elfenbein, J.L., Schum, R.L., and Bentler, R.A., Thresholds of discomfort in young children. *Ear Hear.*, 12(3), 184–190 (1991).

Macrae, J.H., Temporary and permanent threshold shift associated with hearing aid use. *Aust. J. Aud.*, 7(2), 45–53 (1985).

Macrae, J.H., and Farrant, R.H., The effect of hearing aid use on the residual hearing of children with sensorineural deafness. *Ann. Otology*, 74, 409–419 (1965).

Mahon, W., Hearing care for infants and children. *Hear. J.*, 40, 7–10 (September 1987).

Margolis, R.H., and Popelka, G.R., Loudness and the acoustic reflex. *J. Acoust. Soc. Am.*, 58(6), 1330–1332 (1975).

Markides, A., The effect of hearing aid use on the user's residual hearing. *Scand. Audiol.*, 5, 205–210 (1976).

Markides, A., The effect of hearing aid amplification on the user's residual hearing. In E.R. Libby (Ed.), *Binaural Hearing and Amplification*, Vol. II. Chicago: Zenetron, Inc., pp. 341–355 (1980).

Markides, A., and Ayree, D.T-K., The effect of hearing aid use on the user's residual hearing: a follow-up study. *Scand. Audiol.*, 7, 19–23 (1978).

Markides, A., and Aryee, D.T-K., The effect of hearing aid use on the user's residual hearing II: a follow-up study. *Scand. Audiol.*, 9, 55–58 (1980).

Mason, D., and Popelka, G., *A Users Guide for Phase IV Hearing Aid Selection and Evaluation Program: IBM Version.* St. Louis: Central Institute for the Deaf (1982).

Matkin, N., Hearing aids for children. In W. Hodgson (Ed.), *Hearing Aid Assessment and Use in Audiologic Habilitation* (3rd ed.). Baltimore, MD: Williams & Wilkins (1986).

Matkin, N., and Olsen, W., Response of hearing aids with induction loop amplification systems. *Am. Ann. Deaf*, 115, 73–78 (1970).

Matkin, N., and Olsen, W., An investigation of radio frequency auditory training units. *Am. Ann. Deaf*, 118, 25–30 (1973).

Maxon, A.B., Binaural amplification of young children: a clinical application of Ross' Theory. *Ear Hear*, 2(5), 215–219 (1981).

McCandless, G.A., and Lyregaard, P.E., Prescription of gain/output (POGO) for hearing aids. *Hear. Instr.*, 34(1), 16–21 (1983).

Mills, J.H., Noise and children: a review of literature. *J. Acoust. Soc. Am.*, 58(4), 767–779 (1975).

Morgan, D.E., and Dirks, D.D., Loudness discomfort level under earphone and in the free field: the effects of calibration methods. *J. Acoust. Soc. Am.*, 56(1), 172–178 (1974).

Mueller, H.G., Directional microphone hearing aids: a 10 year report. *Hear. Instru.*, 32(11), 18–20 (1981).

Mueller, H.G., Binaural amplification: attitudinal factors. *Hear. J.*, 39(11), 7–10 (1986).

Mueller, H.G., Individualizing the ordering of custom hearing instruments. *Hear. Instru.*, 40(5), 18–22 (1989).

Mueller, H.G., and Grimes, A., Amplification systems for the hearing impaired. In J. Alpiner and P. McCarthy (Eds.), *Rehabilitation Audiology: Children and Adults.* Baltimore: Williams & Wilkins, pp. 115–160 (1987).

Mueller, H.B., and Hawkins, D.B., Three important considerations in hearing aid selection. In R. Sandlin (Ed.), *Handbook of Hearing Aid Amplification*, Vol. II. Boston: College Hill Press (1990).

Naunton, R.F., The effect of hearing aid use upon the user's residual hearing. *Larygoscope*, 67, 569–576 (1957).

Northern, J.L., and Downs, M.P., *Hearing in Children* (4th ed.). Baltimore: Williams & Wilkins (1991).

Northern, J.L., Gabbard, S.A., and Kinder, D.L., Pediatric considerations in selecting and fitting hearing aids. In R.E. Sandlin (Ed.), *Handbook of Hearing Aid Amplification*, Vol. II. Boston: College Hill Press (1990).

Olsen, W.O., Hawkins, D.B., and Van Tasell, D.J., Representations of the long-term spectra of speech. *Ear Hear.*, 8(Suppl. 5), 100S–108S (1987).

Pascoe, D.P., An approach to hearing aid selection. *Hear. Instru.*, 29, 12–16 (1978).

Pascoe, D.P., Clinical measurements of the auditory dynamic range and their relation to formulae for hearing aid gain. In J.H. Jensen (Ed.), *Hearing Aid Fitting: Theoretical and Practical Views.* Copenhagen: Stougaard Jensen (1988).

Pavlovic, C.V., Articulation index predictions of speech intelligibility in hearing aid selection. *Asha*, 30, 63–65 (1988).

Pavlovic, C.V., Speech spectrum considerations and speech intelligibility predictions in hearing aid evaluations. *J. Speech Hear. Disord.*, 54(1), 3–8 (1989).

Pavlovic, C.V., Speech recognition and five Articulation Indexes. *Hear. Instru.*, 42(9), 20–23 (1991).

Pavlovic, C.V., Studebaker, G.A., and Sherbecoe, R.L., An articulation index based procedure for predicting the speech recognition performance of hearing-impaired individuals. *J. Acoust. Soc. Am.*, 80(1), 50–57 (1986).

Popelka, G.R., *Program for Hearing Aid Selection and Evaluation: Phase IV.* St. Louis: Central Institute for the Deaf Publication (1983).

Popelka, G.R., The CID method: Phase IV. *Hear. Instru.*, 39(7), 15–16, 18 (1988).

Popelka, G.R., and Engebretson, A.M., A computer-based system for hearing aid assessment. *Hear. Instru.*, 34(7), 6–9, 44 (1983).

Pratt, H., and Sohmer, H., Correlations between psychophysical magnitude estimates and simultaneously obtained auditory nerve, brain stem and cortical responses to click stimuli in man. *Electroencephalogr. Clin. Neurophysiol.*, 43, 802–812 (1977).

Preves, D.A., and Sigelman, J.A., A questionnaire to evaluate signal processing hearing aids. *Hear. Instru.*, 40(11), 20–21, 24 (1989).

Rintelmann, W.F., and Bess, F.H., High-level amplification and potential hearing loss in children. In F.H. Bess (Ed.), *Hearing Impairment in Children.* Parkton, MD: York Press, pp. 278–309 (1988).

Ritter, R., Johnson, R.M., and Northern, J.L., The controversial relationship between loudness discomfort levels and acoustic reflex thresholds. *J. Am. Audiol. Soc.*, 4(4), 123–131 (1979).

Ross, M., Binaural versus monaural hearing aid amplification for hearing impaired individuals. In F.H. Bess (Ed.), *Childhood Deafness: Causation, Assessment and Management.* New York: Grune & Stratton, pp. 235–249 (1977).

Ross, M., Binaural versus monaural hearing aid amplification for hearing impaired individuals. In E.R. Libby (Ed.), *Binaural Hearing and Amplification*, Vol. 2. Chicago: Zenetron (1980).

Ross, M., and Lerman, J., Hearing aid usage and its effects upon residual hearing: a review of the literature and an investigation. *Arch. Otolaryngol.*, 86, 57–62 (1967).

Ross, M., and Seewald, R.C., Hearing aid selection and evaluation with young children. In F. Bess (Ed.), *Hearing Impairment in Children.* Parkton, MD: York Press, pp. 190–213 (1988).

Sachs, R.M., and Burkhard, M.D., Making pressure measurements in insert earphone couplers and real ears. *J. Acoust. Soc. Am.*, 51(1), 140(A) (1972).

Schum, D., and Collins, M.J., *Spectral Shaping Options for Persons with Low- or High-Frequency Sensorineural Hearing Loss.* Paper presented at the Acoustical Society of America, Indianapolis, IN (1987).

Schwartz, D.M., Lyregaard, P.E., and Lundh, P., Hearing aid selection for severe-to-profound hearing loss. *Hear. J.*, 41(2), 13–17 (1988).

Seewald, R.C., Hudson, S.P., Gagne, J-P., and Zelisko, D.L.C., Comparison of two methods for estimating the sensation level of amplified speech. *Ear Hear.*, 13(3), 142–149 (1992).

Seewald, R.C., and Ross, M., Amplification for young hearing impaired children. In M.C. Pollack (Ed.), *Amplification for the Hearing Impaired* (3rd ed.). New York: Grune & Stratton (1988).

Seewald, R.C., Ross, M., and Spiro, M.K., Selecting amplification characteristics for young hearing-impaired children. *Ear Hear.*, 6(1), 48–53 (1985).

Seewald, R.C., Zelisko, D.L.C., Ramji, K., and Jamieson, D.G., *Computer Assisted Implementation of the DSL Approach: Version 3.0.* Poster presentation at the International Hearing Aids Conference, Iowa City, IA (1991a).

Seewald, R.C., Zelisko, D.L.C., Ramji, K., and Jamieson, D.G., *DSL (Version 3.0) Users Manual.* London, Ontario: The University of Western Ontario (1991b).

Shah, C.P., Chandler, D., and Dale, R., Delay in referral of children with impaired hearing. *Volta Rev.*, 80(4), 206–215 (1978).

Shaw, E.A.G., Transformation of sound pressure level from the free field to the eardrum in the horizontal plane. *J. Acoust. Soc. Am.*, 56(6), 1848–1861 (1974).

Shaw, E.A.G., and Vaillancourt, M.M., Transformation of sound-pressure level from the free field to the eardrum presented in numerical form. *J. Acoust. Soc. Am.*, 78(3), 1120–1123 (1985).

Silman, S., Gelfand, S.A., and Silverman, C.A., Late-onset auditory deprivation: effects of monaural versus binaural hearing aids. *J. Acoust. Soc. Am.*, 76(5), 1357–1362 (1984).

Silverman, C.A., Auditory deprivation. *Hear. Instru.*, 40(9), 26–32 (1989).

Silverman, C.A., and Silman, S., Apparent auditory deprivation from monaural amplification and recovery with binaural amplification: two case studies. *J. Am. Acad. Audiol.* (in press).

Silverman, M.S., and Clopton, B.M., Plasticity of binaural interaction: I. Effect of early auditory deprivation. *J. Neurophysiol.*, 40(6), 1266–1274 (1977).

Simmons, F.B., Diagnosis and rehabilitation of deaf newborns. Part II. *Asha*, 22, 475 (1980).

Skinner, M., *Hearing Aid Evaluation.* Englewood Cliffs, NJ: Prentice-Hall (1988).

Stelmachowicz, P.G., Current issues in pediatric amplification. In J.A. Feigin and P.G. Stelmachowicz (Eds.), *Pediatric Amplification: Proceedings of the 1991 National Conference*, pp 1–17. Published by Boys Town National Research Hospital, Omaha.

Stelmachowicz, P.G., Clinical issues related to hearing-aid maximum output. In G. Studebaker, F. Bess, and L. Beck (Eds.), *The Vanderbilt Hearing Aid Report II.* Parkton, MD: York Press, Inc. (1991b).

Stelmachowicz, P.G., and Seewald, R.C., Probe-tube microphone measures in children. *Semin. Hear.*, 12(1), 62–72 (1991).

Stuart, A., Durieux-Smith, A., and Stenstrom, R., Probe tube microphone measures of loudness discomfort levels in children. *Ear Hear.*, 12(2), 140–143 (1991).

Stubblefield, J., and Nye, C., Aided and unaided time-related differences in word discrimination. *Hear. Instru.*, 40(9), 38–43, 78 (1989).

Sung, R.J., and Hodgson, W.R., Performance of individual hearing aids utilizing microphone and induction coil input. *J. Speech Hear. Res.*, 14(2), 365–371 (1971).

Tees, R.C., The effects of early auditory restriction in the rat on adult duration discrimination. *J. Aud. Res.*, 7, 195–207 (1967).

Thibodeau, L.M., and Saucedo, K.A., Consistency of electroacoustic characteristics across components of FM systems. *J. Speech Hear. Res.*, 34(3), 628–635 (1991).

Van Tasell, D.J., and Landin, D.P., Frequency response characteristics of FM mini-loop auditory trainers. *J. Speech Hear. Disord.*, 45(2), 247–258 (1980).

Violette, J., White, D., and Violette, M., *Electromagnetic Compatibility Handbook.* New York: Van Nostrand Reinhold (1987).

Watson, C.S., Time course of auditory perceptual learning. *Ann. Otol. Rhinol. Laryngol.*, 89 (Suppl. 74), 96–102 (1980).

Webster, D.B., and Webster, M., Neonatal sound deprivation affects brain stem auditory nuclei. *Arch Otolaryngol.*, 103(7), 392–396 (1977).

Webster, D.B., and Webster, M., Effects of neonatal conductive hearing loss on brain stem auditory nuclei. *Ann. Otol. Rhinol. Laryngol.*, 88(5), 684–688 (1979).

Willeford, J., and Billger, J., Auditory perception in children with learning disabilities. In J. Katz (Ed.), *Handbook of Clinical Audiology* (2nd ed.). Baltimore: Williams & Williams, pp. 410–425 (1978).

APPENDIX 5.1 DSL Selection Approach for Children (Version 3.0)

The following material is reprinted with permission from Seewald, R.C., Zelisko, D.L.C., Ramji, K., and Jamieson, D.G., *DSL (Version 3.0) Users Manual*. London, Ontario: The University of Western Ontario (1991).

Threshold (dB HL)	\multicolumn{9}{c}{Frequency (Hz)}								
	250	500	750	1000	1500	2000	3000	4000	6000
DESIRED SENSATION LEVELS (dB)[a]									
0	47	53	53	48	46	46	43	40	30
5	41	48	49	44	42	43	40	38	27
10	36	44	44	41	39	40	37	35	24
15	32	40	41	38	37	38	35	33	22
20	28	36	37	35	34	35	33	31	20
25	25	33	34	33	32	33	31	29	19
30	23	30	32	31	30	31	30	27	17
35	20	28	30	29	29	30	28	26	16
40	18	26	28	28	27	28	27	24	15
45	17	24	26	26	26	27	25	23	14
50	16	22	24	25	25	25	24	22	13
55	14	21	23	24	23	24	23	21	12
60	13	19	22	22	22	23	22	19	11
65	13	18	20	21	21	21	21	18	10
70	12	17	19	20	20	20	19	17	9
75	11	16	18	18	19	18	18	15	8
80	10	14	17	17	17	16	16	14	7
85	8	13	15	15	16	15	15	12	5
90	7	12	14	13	14	13	13	11	3
95	5	10	12	11	12	11	11	9	0
100	3	8	10	9	10	8	8	7	–
105	–	6	7	6	7	5	5	5	–
110	–	4	5	4	4	2	2	3	–
DESIRED REAL-EAR MAXIMUM SPL (dB)[b] (REAR 90)									
0	94	102	101	99	99	100	100	98	97
5	94	102	101	99	99	101	100	99	97
10	94	102	101	100	100	102	101	100	98
15	95	103	102	101	100	103	102	101	98
20	95	103	102	101	101	104	103	102	99
25	96	104	103	103	102	105	105	103	100
30	97	105	104	104	104	106	106	104	101
35	99	106	106	105	105	108	108	106	103
40	100	107	107	107	107	110	110	108	105
45	102	109	109	109	109	112	112	109	106
50	104	111	110	110	111	114	114	111	108
55	106	113	112	112	113	116	116	113	111

Threshold (dB HL)	Frequency (Hz)								
	250	500	750	1000	1500	2000	3000	4000	6000
60	109	115	114	114	115	118	118	115	113
65	111	117	117	117	117	120	120	118	115
70	114	119	119	119	119	122	123	120	117
75	117	121	121	121	121	124	125	122	120
80	120	123	123	123	123	126	127	124	122
85	123	126	125	125	125	128	129	126	124
90	126	128	127	127	127	130	130	128	125
95	129	130	129	129	129	131	132	130	127
100	132	131	131	130	131	133	133	132	128
105	–	133	132	131	132	134	135	133	–
110	–	134	134	133	133	135	136	135	–

DESIRED IN SITU GAIN (dB)[c]

0	1	2	3	1	4	11	14	13	6
5	1	2	3	2	5	12	16	15	8
10	1	3	4	4	7	15	18	18	10
15	2	4	5	6	10	17	21	20	13
20	3	5	7	9	12	20	24	23	16
25	5	7	9	12	15	23	27	26	19
30	7	9	11	15	18	26	30	30	23
35	10	12	14	18	22	29	34	33	27
40	13	15	17	21	25	32	38	37	31
45	17	18	20	25	29	36	41	40	35
50	20	21	24	28	32	40	45	44	39
55	24	25	28	32	36	43	49	48	43
60	28	28	31	36	40	47	53	52	47
65	32	32	35	39	44	50	57	55	51
70	36	36	39	43	48	54	60	59	55
75	41	40	42	47	51	57	64	63	59
80	44	43	46	50	55	61	67	66	62
85	48	47	50	54	58	64	71	70	66
90	52	50	53	57	62	67	74	73	69
95	55	54	56	60	65	70	76	76	71
100	58	57	59	62	67	72	79	79	73
105	–	60	62	65	70	75	81	81	–
110	–	62	64	67	72	77	83	85	–

TARGET SOUND FIELD AIDED THRESHOLDS (dB HL)[d]

0	0	0	0	0	0	0	0	0	0
5	5	5	5	5	5	5	4	4	4
10	10	10	9	8	8	7	7	7	7
15	14	14	13	11	11	10	9	9	9
20	18	18	16	14	13	12	11	11	11
25	21	21	19	16	15	14	13	13	13
30	24	24	22	18	17	16	15	15	14
35	26	26	24	20	19	18	16	16	16
40	28	28	26	21	20	20	18	18	17
45	29	29	28	23	22	21	19	19	18
50	31	31	29	24	23	22	20	20	18
55	32	32	30	26	24	24	21	21	19

Threshold (dB HL)	Frequency (Hz)								
	250	500	750	1000	1500	2000	3000	4000	6000
60	33	33	32	27	25	25	23	23	20
65	34	34	33	28	27	27	24	24	21
70	35	35	34	29	28	28	25	25	22
75	35	35	36	31	29	30	27	27	23
80	37	37	37	32	31	31	28	28	25
85	38	38	38	34	32	33	30	30	27
90	39	32	40	36	34	35	32	31	29
95	41	41	42	38	36	37	34	33	31
100	43	43	44	40	38	40	36	35	34
105	–	–	46	43	41	42	39	37	–
110	–	–	49	46	43	45	42	39	–

[a] The values presented in this table assume a real-ear unaided response (REUR) approximating published average adult values (Shaw & Vaillancourt, 1985). Furthermore, if audiometric data have been collected using the Etymotic ER3A insert earphone (in dB HL), the above values assume an average adult real-ear to coupler difference (Sachs & Burkhard, 1972).

[b] The values presented in this table assume a real-ear unaided response (REUR) approximating published average adult values (Shaw & Vaillancourt, 1985). Furthermore, if audiometric data have been collected using the Etymotic ER3A insert phones (in dB HL), the above values assume an average adult real-ear to coupler difference (Sachs & Burkhard, 1972).

[c] The values presented in this table assume a real-ear unaided response (REUR) approximating published average adult values (Shaw & Vaillancourt, 1985). Furthermore, if audiometric data have been collected using the Etymotic ER3A insert phones (in dB HL), the above values assume an average adult real-ear to coupler difference (Sachs & Burkhard, 1972).

[d] The values presented in this table assume the following MAF values in dB SPL, for average normal hearing sensitivity (i.e., 0 dB HL): 15.5 dB SPL at 250 Hz, 8.1 dB SPL at 500 Hz, 3.8 dB SPL at 750 Hz, 3.4 dB SPL at 1000 Hz, 1.4 dB SPL at 1500 Hz, 0.3 dB SPL at 2000 Hz, −3.5 dB SPL at 3000 Hz, −3.7 dB SPL at 4000 Hz, −3.1 dB SPL at 6000 Hz.

APPENDIX 5.2   *Testing with Five Tasks* [a]

All testing is to be done with the subject seated in a sound-treated booth. A toy traffic light is located on a table in front of the child. The traffic light is a yellow 12″ × 8″ × 8″ wooden box containing a red light bulb in the upper half and a green light bulb in the lower half. The lights are operated by a single pull, double throw light switch connected to the side of the box.

Task 1: Stop/Go

"We will play a game. I will be first. You will be second. Watch. Green light—time to go. Red light—time to stop." The car is pushed and stopped accordingly by clinician. "Now it's your turn." The clinician changes the light from green to red, and vice versa, until the child is able to stop and start the car appropriately.

Task 2: Water

The clinician pours water into a glass and says, "More water—green light." At the point at which the water fills the glass to its brim, he/she says, "No more—time to stop—red light," and changes the light to red. The child is then given a turn to change the light to red when the glass is full (poured by clinician). The clinician instructs, "No more—time to stop—you make the light red."

Task 3: Bears

The clinician drops small plastic bears in his/her hand. The clinician says, "More—green light." At the point at which bears begin to overflow the hand, the clinician says, "No more—time to stop—red light," and changes the light to red. The child is then given a turn to change the light to red at the point the bears begin to overflow (dropped by clinician). The clinician instructs, "No more—time to stop—you make the light red."

Task 4: Weights

The clinician holds a measuring cup with one hand at approximately chest height and drops weights into it. The clinician says, "More—green light." At the point at which the weights become too heavy to hold (i.e., the cup cannot be held at chest height and need to be placed on the table), he/she says, "No more—time to stop—red light," and changes the light to red. The child is then given a turn to change the light to red when he/she can no longer hold the weights (weights put in the cup by the clinician). The clinician instructs, "No more—time to stop—you make the light red."

Task 5: TDs

"Now, the same thing with beeps. Listen through these (earphones). More beeps—green light. No more—time to stop—you make the light red."

To convert TDs in HL (re: 6-cm^3 coupler) to real-ear SPL values, correction factors for each TD should be obtained individually by measuring the difference between a 70-dB HL pure-tone signal (re: audiometer dial) at each of the test frequencies and the sound pressure level (SPL) measured at the tympanic membrane. MAPC values (Bentler & Pavlovic, 1989) are then subtracted from the differences for the final 6-cc-to-real-ear correction factor values. More recently, it has been suggested that using insert earphones may result in more accurate estimation of these discomfort thresholds. Since insert earphones are calibrated in a 2-cc coupler, the TDs obtained with their use can easily be corrected for SPL using appropriate reference threshold values.

---

[a]Reprinted (in condensed form) with permission from Macpherson, B.J., Elfenbein, J.L., Schum, R.L., and Bentler, R.A., Thresholds of discomfort in young children. *Ear Hear.*, 12(3), 184–190 (1991).

6

Assessment and Intervention with Preschool Hearing-Impaired Children

MARY PAT MOELLER, M.S., ARLENE EARLEY CARNEY, Ph.D.

Clinicians serving hearing-impaired children have faced many new challenges in recent years. Federal legislation (PL 99–457, c.f. Roush & McWilliam, 1991) for early intervention has required reconceptualization of professional roles. Traditional service delivery models have been supplanted by transdisciplinary teams. Instead of teaching and directing parents, clinicians seek to develop balanced partnerships with them. Interventions previously targeted at mother and child now focus on family systems and broad family needs.

Technological advances have resulted in the availability of a wide array of sensory communication devices, such as tactile aids and cochlear implants, providing new options for families to consider in their decision-making processes. Increased appreciation for American Sign Language and deaf cultural perspectives have raised questions and controversies about selection of signs for use with young deaf children (Schick, 1990). Parents of young hearing-impaired children face complex decisions.

Professionals who work with young hearing-impaired children face a similar set of complex decisions and a bewildering array of management choices. They must learn to change their roles relative to families, to educate themselves about changes in tech-nology, and to discover the new perspectives available concerning the traditional areas of language, speech, and auditory skills. The purpose of this chapter is to provide a broad overview of the necessary components of effective assessment and intervention with young hearing-impaired children in three areas: language, auditory skills, and speech.

Language Evaluation and Intervention with Preschool Hearing-Impaired Children

Shifts in theoretical views of language and learning have resulted in replacement of didactic language intervention methods with holistic approaches delivered in functionally appropriate contexts. Parents previously were guided to bombard the child with language input (e.g., "talk, talk, talk to your hearing-impaired child"). Currently, parents are assisted in using conversational strategies (e.g., "turntake, recast, and storytell") to develop nurturing interactions with the hearing-impaired child. Social interaction within the family has been viewed as a critical foundation for acquisition of language and literacy. This has led to the adoption of functionalistic and family-centered models of intervention. Importantly, children are not viewed as passive recipients of adult input but as active constructors of meaning. Clinicians are challenged to develop activities that promote the negotiation of meaning between interactants (Wells, 1981).

These changes and challenges bring with them an increased appreciation for the need to view and treat children within the ecological system of the family (Ensher, 1989, Fitzgerald & Fischer, 1987; Simmons-Martin & Rossi, 1990; Sparks, 1989; Trout & Foley, 1989). Furthermore, they speak to the need for the clinician to assume a role of coach, partner, or collaborator in the learning process with the child and family. In a coach or partner role, the clinician respects the strengths the child and family bring to the task of learning and helps them build on this foundation.

In this chapter, strategies for evaluation that are ecologically valid and intervention models that recognize the central role of relationships in language acquisition will be explored. Two language intervention models will be described: *(1)* a collaborative problem-solving approach to parent/infant programming and *(2)* a cognitively oriented preschool program, in which the clinician serves in the role of coach. Evaluation strategies that support these intervention models will be discussed. Following the language intervention section, specific attention will be given to assessment and intervention in the areas of auditory learning and phonological development.

INTERVENTION WITH INFANTS AND FAMILIES: A COLLABORATIVE, PROBLEM-SOLVING APPROACH

PL 99–457 requires that programs implement family-centered models, where parents take an active role in decision making for their child. Although these mandates seem logical and ideal, they are difficult to implement in practice. Parents often feel powerless (Luterman, 1991) and uninformed in the face of many decisions they must make about their young hearing-impaired child. In such circumstances they may feel willing to abdicate to well-meaning professionals the responsibility of making choices. This can be especially detrimental

if the expert guidance reflects strong philosophical biases that are inconsistent with the needs of the child. In the worst case scenario, such guidance carries promises of success. The picture is complicated further by the fact that tools for objectively evaluating infants within the family system are often inadequate or lacking. This is especially problematic in view of the increasing incidence of multiple handicaps and consequent escalating need for individualized, objective evaluation. Professionals need to actively problem solve with families. Bailey (1987, p. 64) stresses that "problem-solving is an important skill in any professional, yet it can be counterproductive if applied too early in a goal-setting endeavor, especially if done for the clients rather than with them."

In response to these concerns, a team of professionals from Boys Town National Research Hospital and the Omaha Public Schools developed a collaborative, problem-solving approach to the management of hearing-impaired infants and their families (Moeller & Condon, in press; Moeller, Coufal, & Hixson, 1990). In this approach, parents of newly identified children are enrolled in a diagnostically oriented parent/infant program for a period of 6 months to 1 year, where a primary goal is to help families gain the information they need to make informed decisions about their child's needs. This educational process is accomplished through a partnership, where the parents and professional conduct a series of experiments to discern what strategies and methods are most successful for the individual child and family. The success-oriented diagnostic teaching approach is based on the Parent Intervention Method, described by Schuyler and Ruschmer (1987). This program, called the Diagnostic Early Intervention Program (DEIP), has five specific objectives (Moeller & Condon, in press):

1. To support families in understanding and coping with the child's hearing impairment
2. To guide families in stimulation of the child's language, auditory, and phonological skills in the contexts of natural interactions and routines

3. To assist families in developing an objective information base to support decision making and goal selection
4. To gain a comprehensive understanding of the family and child needs through a discovery-oriented teaching process and transdisciplinary evaluations
5. To provide a mechanism for longitudinal monitoring of the decision-making process and its efficacy

Objective evaluation of intervention outcome is accomplished in part through language sample analysis and use of formal evaluation instruments. Particularly useful to this process are recently developed communicative scales (listed below) that incorporate parental observations and noninvasive, naturalistic techniques.

1. *Assessing Linguistic Behaviors* (ALB) (Olswang et al., 1987). These infant observational scales include five subsections: *(a)* cognitive antecedents to word meanings, *(b)* communicative intentions, *(c)* play behaviors, *(d)* language comprehension, and *(e)* language expression and phonological development scales. The nondirective, observational tasks are illustrated on a videotape, which can be used for examiner training. Samples of normally developing infants are used to train coders.
2. *Communication and Symbolic Behavior Scales* (CSBS) (Wetherby & Prizant, 1990). This scale includes a caregiver questionnaire that surveys parents' observations of the child's presymbolic and early symbolic communicative behaviors. The second portion of the assessment involves videotaping of the infant during playful interactions with the parents and examiner. The videotape is later scored, using scales of Communication (Functions, Means, Reciprocity, and Social/Affective Signaling) and Symbolic Behavior (Verbal and Nonverbal).
3. *MacArthur Communicative Development Inventory* (Dale & Thal, 1989). This inventory of early lexical attainments relies on parent report, in a manner similar to parent diary studies. Checklists prompt parents to recall whether the child understands and/or produces a range of early appearing words from varied semantic classes. Because young children often have difficulty demonstrating optimal or usual performance in a structured clinical setting, this tool recruits useful observations from the home setting. The infant scale is designed for use with 8- to 16-month-old infants. The scale also appraises use of actions and gestures. A form for toddlers is designed for use between 16 and 30 months of age. A hearing-impaired child's vocabulary size can be compared to normative data collected on 659 infants and 1130 toddlers with normal hearing (Fenson et al., 1991).

Once a family has enrolled in DEIP, a variety of professionals become involved in contributing to the development of an information base. The goal is to gain a holistic perspective of needs through collaborative consultation (Moeller & Condon, in press). Transdisciplinary team members, along with the family, monitor the child's development across primary developmental domains (e.g., social, cognitive, fine and gross motor, medical, audiologic, parent/infant interaction). Yet, a highly useful source of data for decision making comes from the careful monitoring of intervention outcomes. Diagnostic questions are continually posed and outcomes are evaluated, based on the child's and family's responses. Clinicians working with a family are responsible for documenting for the team whether methods used with the child and family are bringing about the desired change. These data are obtained from pre-post intervention comparisons, from use of criterion-referenced measures (like those reported above), and from the coding of response patterns across intervention sessions (Moeller et al., 1990).

Family members and clinicians view themselves as partners in a discovery process. Parents and professionals collaboratively design a series of experiments to gather desired information, develop or enhance desired behaviors, or resolve problems (Moeller & Condon, in press; Schuyler & Ruschmer, 1987). The professional supports the parents in describing their observations, evaluating the outcomes, and planning the next step in the joint discovery process. A brief case review illustrates this process.

M.'s parents participated in DEIP when their daughter was 3 years of age, because of concerns for her learning rate. M. had a profound, bilateral hearing loss and was enrolled in an auditory/oral parent/child program. The child's teacher had reassured M.'s parents that her progress was fine. Yet, the parents felt that they lacked a reference point for determining whether her rate of development was adequate. They indicated that they understood little of her speech and that she had fewer than 50 words in her vocabulary. The family was devoted, however, to continued pursuit of auditory-oral development for their daughter. Together with the clinician they selected five focus goals that were meaningful to them as a family. They agreed to emphasize these goals regularly and to objectively evaluate the outcome. After several months of intensive exposure to systematic opportunities, M. made no change relative to family-selected goals. The clinician and parents decided to attempt a next step in the experimental process. The same five goals were emphasized, but signs were used to support M.'s acquisition of language skills. M. achieved the stated goals rapidly. The parents were enthusiastic about her success. As they focused on her progress, the decision to use signs was less threatening and more a calculated choice. The parents continued to advocate for M.'s oral skill attainment. Later in their discovery process, they chose intervention with a cochlear implant and continued to participate in monitoring the outcome of their efforts. They reported to their clinician later, "Had you told us we needed to switch to total communication when she was initially struggling, we could not have accepted that. We appreciated the time we were given to look at the problem objectively and to discover routes together that would lead to success. Time was important in adjusting our perspectives."

Through the partnership relationship with team members, parents take an active role in creation of the Individual Family Service Plan (IFSP). Family members participating in DEIP discover that an appropriate program must consider their child's and family's unique needs. Participation in the ongoing discovery process helps parents make informed decisions based on an understanding of how the child functions.

Earlier in this chapter, the authors discussed the importance of adults taking on a role as "coach." This principle applies to the guidance parents receive in the infant program. Several studies from child language acquisition confirm that the interaction between parent and child provides the child with a predictable referential context that makes language meaningful. The rate of language acquisition by young children has been found to be positively correlated with the extent to which parent language is contingent or responsive to their child's verbal and nonverbal behaviors (Barnes et al., 1983; Masur, 1982; Tomasello & Farrar, 1986). Directiveness on the part of caregivers is negatively related to the development of language in infants (Tomasello, Mannie, & Kruger, 1986; Tomasello & Todd, 1983). Earlier reports have suggested that hearing parents of young deaf children have been intrusive, directive, and overly controlling in their interactions (Meadow et al., 1981; Wedell-Monnig & Lumley, 1980). It is possible that some directive styles were related to intervention models, where parents were advised to *teach* their deaf infants.

Contemporary strategies (see Fitzgerald & Fischer, 1987; Simmons-Martin & Rossi, 1990) encourage clinicians and parents to develop a responsive rather than a directive style with hearing-impaired infants. The training program of the Hanen Early Language Resource Centre, *It Takes Two to Talk* (Manolson, 1985), is a particularly good example of a program that guides parents in a responsive, communicatively appropriate manner. Clinical experience also suggests that many parents have a good sense of supportive interaction styles prior to intervention. Skilled clinicians first act as keen and nonjudgmental observers. They identify strengths in the interaction and then support the continuation of these behaviors as the parents adjust to the difficult situation they face. Such an approach is respectful of parental expertise and the primacy of the parental roles in the child's development. Trout and Foley (1989) emphasize that family-centered approaches respect the diversity and developmental nature of parenthood. Clinicians are challenged to appreciate a diverse range of parenting styles and to acknowledge that parenthood itself is a developmental process wherein the best prepared struggle at times.

PRESCHOOL PROGRAMMING: A COGNITIVELY ORIENTED FRAMEWORK FOR LANGUAGE ENHANCEMENT

A primary goal of preschool language intervention is to help children become effective conversational interactants (Hoskins, 1990). In addition, preschool children are in the process of developing the language foundations for literacy (Westby, 1985). Thus, preschool programs have a role in preliteracy development. Miller (1990) defines literacy in ways different from traditional conceptualizations. She describes literacy attainment as "learning ways of thinking that allow cultural participation . . . that allow language users to analyze, synthesize, criticize, contrast, reason and argue" (p. 3). This definition of literacy encompasses cognitive, social, and linguistic attainments.

Researchers have documented that language and literacy behaviors are learned in the context of rich social interactions (Bates, 1979; Halliday, 1975; Snow, 1977; Wells, 1981). To achieve the goals of conversational competence and preliteracy skill attainment requires an integrated focus on social, cognitive, and linguistic skills in naturalistic contexts (Blank & Marquis, 1987; Hoskins, 1990). Conversational competence requires reliance on skills in each of these domains. Consider the example of a 4-year-old, Daniel, who was up past his bedtime, yet wanted a bedtime story. His mother said, "There's no time for a story. You have to be up early tomorrow for soccer." Daniel responded by finding a book with only a few pages. He said, enthusiastically, "Mommy, I've got it. Let's read this book. See? It's really short." Daniel focused immediately on the key point of contention, limited time. His mother replied, "Sorry, Daniel. You need to get to bed." Daniel tried a second strategy, which drew on social knowledge. "Mommy," he said, "You didn't read to me yesterday either" (the guilt trip approach). This strategy also did not succeed, so Daniel tried one more socially oriented strategy. "*Please*, mommy," he emphatically stressed. "I'll be your best friend." It is striking to see that a normally developing 4-year-old already has the cognitive and social sophistication to come up with three clever approaches to persuading his mother to his own viewpoint. Language function is intricately tied to cognitive and social attainments. This awareness compels the authors to recommend cognitively oriented language development approaches, because they use rich, functional contexts and simultaneously promote language, thinking, and social skills.

The selection of cognitively oriented language intervention methods has been motivated by several premises, supported by current developmental theories. These are summarized in Table 6.1.

Components of a Cognitively Oriented Approach

Cognitively oriented approaches share several common features. The authors' conceptualizations of key features of this approach are described in Table 6.1. Although the approach is eclectic, its foundations were heavily influenced by a Cognitively Oriented Curriculum designed for early childhood education by the High/Scope Educational Research Foundation (Hohmann, Banet, & Weikart, 1979; Weikart et al., 1971). The authors have adapted this developmental curriculum for use with hearing-impaired preschoolers. Adaptations were particularly necessary in the following areas:

1. Because of the language-learning needs of hearing-impaired children, attention has been given to developing content units that support children's expansion of schemata. Yoshinaga-Itano and Downey (1986) point out that hearing-impaired children often have gaps or incomplete world/word knowledge. They stress the need to help children expand their knowledge of scripts and schemata as a basis for comprehension of conversation and written texts. Later in this chapter, strategies for developing schema-based units will be discussed.

2. Some creative manipulation of discourse has been required to obligate the use of targeted language structures and

Table 6.1
Components of a Cognitively Oriented Approach to Language Intervention

Theoretical Premise	Strategy Components	References
Contemporary views of learners emphasize the *active* nature of the learning process. Children *construct* meaning as they form and test out hypotheses.	Experiences are designed to provoke mentally active participation; to encourage children to explore, question, and make discoveries.	Wells & Nicholls, 1985; Stone, 1980; Weikart et al., 1971; Bruner, 1975; Rogers et al., 1975; Piaget & Inhelder, 1969
Acquisition of knowledge structure (schemata and scripts) guides comprehension of discourse and print. Vocabulary learning is enhanced when children "anchor" a new word to existing knowledge.	Content units and teaching strategies are designed to expand children's word and world knowledge. Associative learning strategies help children link new with established concepts.	Pearson, 1984; Kail & Leonard, 1986; Yoshinaga-Itano & Downey, 1986
Language acquisition is facilitated when adults use a collaborative rather than a directive style. Semantic contingency to literacy-related behaviors is related to literacy attainment.	Clinicians use open-ended strategies of *(1)* presenting or capitalizing on problems; *(2)* asking divergent questions; *(3)* commenting to expand children's discoveries; *(4)* commenting on children's preliteracy observations.	Barnes et al., 1983; Masur, 1982; Tomasello & Farrar, 1986; Wells & Nicholls, 1985; Weikart et al., 1971; Snow, 1983; Grammatico & Miller, 1974
As a child's language matures, discourse demands become increasingly decontextualized and less tied to immediate contexts or perceptions. This process of decontextualization is important to literacy attainment.	Implementation of a classroom discourse model supports gradual and systematic "upping of the ante" in semantic abstraction. Social routines such as Plan-Do-Recall help children develop personal narrative skills (beginning decontextualized language use).	Blank, Rose, & Berlin, 1978; Westby, 1985; Hohmann, Banet, & Weikart, 1979

(continued)

give children sufficient, appropriate practice with targeted forms/functions. Two clinicians participate in a team-teaching situation in a group intervention setting. This allows the adults to use the powerful strategy of interactive modeling. (Interactive models have been particularly necessary with signing children who see only one primary signer at home. These children need multiple opportunities to see language used interactively in order to understand social language rules.) Clinicians create functional contexts for eliciting target behaviors and then use strategies such as semantically contingent expansions and visual and verbal scaffolds. Scaffolding (Bruner, 1978) refers to techniques adults use to reduce task complexity or support the child's effort. This might include increasing nonlinguistic support to allow the child to concentrate on the linguistic demands of the task. The clinicians also hold children accountable for representative language behaviors and routinely "up the ante." These strategies are known to enhance both language and preliteracy skills (Snow, 1983).

3. Perhaps because of reduced exposure, some hearing-impaired children are significantly delayed in the acquisition of verbal question-asking behaviors. Yet, question asking is an essential skill children use in making sense out of their world. Thus, the authors found it critical to enhance the curriculum by integrating a model of classroom discourse that would strengthen children's question-responding and question-asking skills

Table 6.1 *(continued)*
Components of a Cognitively Oriented Approach to Language Intervention

Theoretical Premise	Strategy Components	References
Interactive models in rich social contexts may aid children's ability to formulate and respond to questions. Question asking is a critical tool for active learners/hypothesis testers.	Adults verbalize their own curiosities, inferences, and discoveries; they make implicit knowledge *explicit* and scaffold children's attempts to express questions. These strategies are incorporated during storytelling and other functional routines.	Constable & van Kleeck, 1985; Yoshinaga-Itano & Downey, 1986; Snow, 1983
Systematic daily routines support children's ability to predict and plan upcoming events and to recall about past activities. Classroom time starts to be understood as a series of predictable events.	Daily routines capitalize on opportunities to plan and predict upcoming events; to learn and express time relations; and to reflect on past experiences. These activities are also relevant to the process of distancing language from immediate context.	Hohmann, Banet, & Weikart, 1979; Westby, 1985
Key experiences, based on characteristics of preoperational thinkers, can serve as a framework from which clinicians can extend and broaden opportunities. Key experiences may build a foundation for later logical thinking.	Curricular design (based in High/Scope principles) provides systematic exposure to key experiences in the areas of classification, seriation, number concepts, spatial relations, and time concepts.	Hohmann, Banet, & Weikart, 1979; Moeller, Osberger, & Morford, 1985; Moeller & McConkey, 1984
Effective parents recognize their role in supporting and encouraging children's self-activated learning. Parents and children often engage in rich social interactions, where there is shared negotiation of meaning.	Family members are given opportunities to learn to use open-ended and thought-provoking strategies with their children during natural, daily routines.	Wells & Nicholls, 1985

(Blank, Rose, & Berlin, 1978). Clinicians also explicitly verbalize their own thinking process to model for children how they can express their own natural curiosity.

4. Family members are critical to the success of intervention methods. When rich discourse occurs at home, children are accustomed to exploring the meaning of events around them and are in an ideal position to take advantage of rich experiences presented to them at school. Within a total communication program, weekly family classes support the parental role by focusing on signing skills, language facilitation strategies, and positive parenting techniques.

Hearing-impaired children represent a heterogeneous group, requiring individualized management. Ongoing evaluation of the child's emerging cognitive, linguistic, and social skills is critical to the process of individualization of the curriculum. The next section briefly addresses evaluation strategies that uniquely support curriculum objectives.

Evaluation Strategies

The following assessment materials and strategies are particularly suited to identifying children's cognitive/linguistic development. Information obtained is useful in goal setting and progress monitoring.

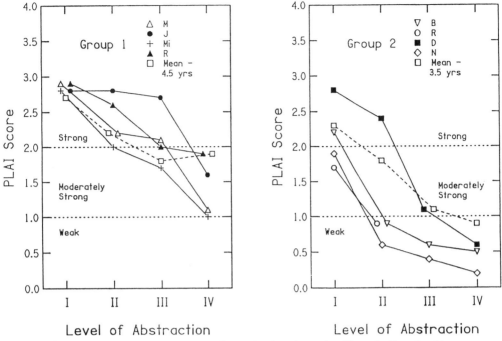

Figure 6.1.   Posttest results for eight deaf preschoolers (ages 4 to 5) on the Preschool Language Assessment Instrument compared to mean scores for children age 3.5 and 4.5.

1. *Child Assessment Record* (CAR) (High/Scope Press, 1987: 600 North River Street, Ypsilanti, MI 48198; 313–485–2000). The High/Scope curriculum contains forms that allow clinicians/teachers to record daily objective observations of children's responses across key experience areas (e.g., representation, seriation, classification, number, space, time, social). This objective record helps the interventionist track progress but is also critical for planning future sessions.

2. *Preschool Language Assessment Instrument* (PLAI) (Blank et al., 1978). This instrument evaluates children's understanding of questions posed on four distinct levels of semantic abstraction, from simple to abstract. Simple level questions (Level I) require that children apply language to what they see in the immediate context (e.g., What is that?). Level II questions require children to selectively focus on features of what they see (e.g., What is happening here?). At Level III, children must restructure their perceptions to respond (e.g., Find the things that are not … ; What will happen next?). Level IV requires the child to reason—to predict, explain, or find a logical solution. This requires the child to go beyond immediate context and perceptions.

This assessment tool has been easily adapted to use with hearing-impaired children. A picture is provided with most of the prompts, which is helpful in establishing the topic for the young hearing-impaired child, amid several topical shifts. Clinicians use the assessment results to determine what levels of question are straightforward for the child, which are emerging, and which are too complex. The clinician then provides numerous opportunities for the child to respond to tasks and questions at levels appropriately challenging for the individual child. The assessment strategy can also be used to monitor change in response to long-term intervention. Figure 6.1 shows the results from a class of seven profoundly hearing-impaired preschoolers who participated in the intervention program. Four of the eight children (represented by group 1) approximated the response levels of hearing age-mates at the posttest interval. All of the children demonstrated developmental patterns of responses.

3. *Spontaneous language sampling.* Spontaneous language sampling is a vital component of the evaluation battery. Children's emergence of personal narrative skills is tracked by taking dictation during recall and sharing time routines. These samples are analyzed using Systematic Analysis of Language Transcripts (SALT) (Miller & Chapman, 1983).

4. *Observational checklist during play.* Social behaviors are often reflected in children's play. Westby's (1980) play scale offers a structured observational checklist for evaluation of social, cognitive, and language skills during symbolic play.

5. *Task analysis.* One of the most valuable assessment tools is the astute clinician, who continually analyzes tasks and responses during intervention. Skilled clinicians constantly ask, "Is there something about this task that is preventing the child from attending to the concept? How can I restructure the learning situation to enhance his or her performance?" Skilled clinicians are also able to determine the basis of children's responses. For example, the clinician may ask, "Did John respond to that question on the basis of linguistic cues, or did he predict the correct response because of situational context? Perhaps I can manipulate the number of context cues available and see how this influences his responses." Systematically applied task analysis is fundamental to the process of individualization.

Language Intervention Strategies

In this final section, each of the characteristics of the cognitively oriented language intervention program will be discussed and illustrated. In some cases, contrasts with traditional lesson designs will be used to clarify strategies. Strategies for planning activities that emphasize key experiences and units that support expansion of schemata will also be addressed.

Active Learning. Experiential language learning has been commonplace for years in preschool programs for hearing-impaired children. Clinicians commonly believe in the importance of real experiences for language expansion. Clinicians and teachers often believe that as long as children are handling materials, they are engaged in active learning. Yet, manipulation of objects and materials is only one of the components of active learning. Thompkins (1986) describes several additional ingredients of active learning. They are:

1. *Opportunities to make choices.* The children decide what to do with the materials.

2. *A variety of materials.* An abundant supply of materials allows children to manipulate and transform objects in a variety of ways. Provision of varied materials also creates opportunities for using specific reference in requesting (e.g., "I need that middle-size hammer. The big one is too heavy for me").

3. *Language use.* The child is encouraged to express his or her unique approaches or solutions to problems.

4. *Support.* Adults and peers support the child's solutions and encourage problem solving and creativity.

A few additional ingredients of active learning have been identified, based on clinical experience with hearing-impaired children.

5. *Disequilibrium.* Clinicians can contrive opportunities for active learning by providing materials that violate expectations or that can be used or transformed to produce unexpected results. For example, one clinician generated considerable group chatter and problem solving by presenting a bulb (nasal syringe) pump, a balloon pump, and a bicycle tire pump. The children were fascinated to discover the variety of ways they could inflate balloons and were delighted with opportunities to predict the shape and size the balloon would take. These children were collaborating in discoveries and were not just physically active. They were mentally active as they made comparisons and negotiated what to try next.

6. *Collaborative problems.* Children develop independence as they become decision makers and problem solvers (Thompkins, 1986). Throughout the

preschool day there are opportunities to let children negotiate solutions to problems. "Oh, it has started to rain. We are disappointed that we can't go out. Who has ideas for what we can do instead?" (The clinician draws illustrations of each of the children's suggestions, and the group decides what to do.)

Active learning often means events are child directed, but adults are important collaborators. Often, adults are instigators of problems (Hohmann et al., 1979). At other times, adults are opportunists. They see a situation where two children are struggling with a problem, and they offer a suggestion to support the children's solution. For example, two boys were playing in preschool, pretending to drive together on a bus. Their pretend bus repeatedly collapsed because the block used for the seat was not long enough for the two of them. They made repeated attempts to sit together and were not succeeding. The adult, acting as coach, made an observation. "I notice your seat is not long enough, is it? I wonder what you could use?" With this focusing prompt, the boys were off to secure a longer block and succeeded in solving the problem.

Schema-Based Content Units. It is common for preschool programs for hearing-impaired children to organize the presentation of content with thematic units. This accepted practice is typically viewed as a mechanism for providing sufficient exposure to key concepts and words related to the theme. According to Yoshinaga-Itano and Downey (1986), such units would be even more useful for hearing-impaired children if they focused on expanding schemata. Schemata are defined as "organized representations of a person's knowledge about some concept, action, or event" (Kintsch, 1974, p. 374). Schemata are usually highly elaborate networks of information. They often change as a result of new input. Children with normal hearing gain much world knowledge through incidental exposure. Through natural language exposure they gain not just words but interrelationships between words, ideas, and experiences. When new ideas are encountered, they are easily linked to existing notions. A word like "Michelangelo" at one time referred only to a painter. Today children may recognize this word as a Ninja turtle or a computer virus. Yoshinaga-Itano and Downey (1986) emphasize that hearing-impaired children often have less access to incidental learning and may lack appreciation for links among concepts or schemata. They note that hearing-impaired children need vocabulary intervention approaches that help them build networks of meanings, and elaboration of word associations in memory. The children need to understand associational links among concepts and how concepts can be embedded. Too often, vocabulary teaching programs concentrate on memorization of specific, isolated words. When words and concepts are unelaborated in memory, children have difficulty retaining or accessing them for language use (Kail & Leonard, 1986). Furthermore, hearing-impaired children, because of limited exposure, may only know stereotypical notions for a concept. They may need explicit exposure to exceptions (Yoshinaga-Itano & Downey, 1986).

Clinicians attempting to apply schema-based interventions in the classroom find it helpful to think broadly about the thematic concept before creating lesson plans. An activity like dyeing Easter eggs (suggested by a team member) can be linked to a myriad of concepts. Intervention team members can challenge themselves to visually map out these relationships prior to lesson planning so that they will consider a variety of possible routes of exposure as they seek to expand children's knowledge structures. The dyeing of Easter eggs is a custom related to a holiday. This holiday is celebrated by many but may not be celebrated by all class members (Teach exceptions, not just stereotypes [Yoshinaga-Itano & Downey, 1986]). Easter eggs are decorated, like trees, houses, and packages are at this & other holidays. Real Easter eggs are hard-boiled, but they can also be made of plastic or chocolate. Easter eggs can be dyed; clothing and hair are dyed, too; tie dye is a recent fad. Eggs are not always hard-boiled. They can be fixed many ways (which can be explored at snack time). Contrasts could include omelets, scrambled eggs (Remember the Scrambler ride at the park? How did the children scramble to find their seats?), and sunny side up (Where do the children think that name comes from? Make observations/comparisons with the sun). Eggs are dairy foods; they come from farms, or stores, or the farmer's market.

This brainstorming of relationships and interconnections could go on for a long time. The process of brainstorming forces staff to consider what organizing concepts relate to words and what associations are relevant priorities to teach. The process leads them to consider all the possibilities and often generates multiple experiential ideas. Direct experiences are supported by use of children's literature and play activities, where the concepts and experiences are represented. For example, after a trip to the pet store, the children re-created the pet store in their classroom for several days in a row. They problem-solved what materials to use for cages, which animals their store would and would not carry, and what types of grooming and food products they would need to keep for customers. They sent customers to the vet for advice on pet illness and read many children's books about pets and their antics with their owners.

One day during planning time, a thematic unit on bird migration was suggested. Although it was fall, and this was a fall experience, the staff found it difficult to elaborate this unit concept. This led the group to develop guidelines for unit selection. When designing a schema-based unit, they ask themselves the following questions.

1. Can material from the proposed unit be actively experienced and manipulated by the children?
2. How close is the content to the child's own experience? Will the child be able to draw on world knowledge and previous experience as he or she encounters this context?
3. How does the content relate to the child's communicative needs? Will this content promote dialogue among class participants?
4. Does the unit lend itself to generalization across units and experiences?
5. Which key experiences can be reinforced in manipulative activities?
6. Can children's literature be exploited to further expand this notion? Can implied inferences be made explicit during reading time?

Classroom Discourse and Daily Routines Support Narrative Development. As described in the evaluation section, implementation of a preschool classroom discourse model (Blank et al., 1978) allows clinicians to systematically challenge children to respond to questions of gradually increasing abstraction. When applied in a context of social interaction, question-response behaviors are often scaffolded by scriptal knowledge and nonlinguistic support. One particularly effective social routine provides opportunities to emphasize questioning skills and personal narrative development. This process-oriented daily routine of the High/Scope curriculum is called plan–do–recall. This strategy centers around goal-oriented play experiences. During the planning phase, the clinician helps children learn to make and express choices about what they will play today. Guided questioning helps children extend and elaborate the plan. Table 6.2 illustrates the planning discourse that occurred between a clinician and two children (a 4-year-old and a 5-year-old). The clinician uses semantically contingent remarks to support the child's ideas. Her questions serve to help the child elaborate and specify the plan. Visual strategies, like planning boards, help children expand their plans even further. Two boys in the preschool were observed to plan days ahead. Once the process of planning was highly familiar and they realized they would always be allowed to act on their choices, they began to negotiate future plans (e.g., "Save the ladder and you and me can be firemen again on Monday, okay?).

After the planning phase, children engage in interactive play. Teachers support the play by asking thought-provoking questions, verbalizing observations to promote thinking, and instigating problems. Adults serve as play partners, supporting children's ideas and imagination. Adults also help children follow their plan, perhaps through reminders (e.g., "Remember, Jeremy, you said you wanted to play at the water table second. Is this still your plan, or did you change your mind?"). As children learn to follow through with their plans they gain confidence in creating mental plans and in predicting what will happen. Adults also help children learn strategies for joint prob-

Table 6.2

Transcripts of Planning and Recall Discourse Between Teacher/Clinician (T) and Child (C)

Planning	Recall
4-year-old	
T: OK, Russell, it's your turn to plan. C: I play house area car and key. T: OK. Quiet voice while thinking. Can you tell me again with your voice? C: Play keys. T: Keys! Where will you drive? C: Wagon. T: Oh, with a wagon. Where will you *drive*? to the zoo or . . . C: To pond. T: To the pond! What will you do at the pond? C: Feed ducks. T: Feed ducks. Have fun. Let's put your symbol up here.	T: Russell. I see you have some keys. Tell us what you did with those. C: I drive pond . . . feed ducks . . . oh! fire. T: You drove to the pond to feed the ducks *and then* there was a fire? C: Yeah. A big fire and then bad smoke. I die. T: You died? Oh my.
5-year-old	
T: Jeremy, you are next. Tell us your plan. C: I will build a fire station with four beds and two firetrucks. T: Okay Jeremy, who will you play with? C: With Kathy. T: And do you know where your fire station will be in the room? In the pit or . . . C: Pit . . . /pit . . . or I will be a shark fourth. T: What about fourth? C: I will be a shark and Mary Pat will be fishing. T: Oh, you mean after you play fire station, you will fish? C: Yes, and I will be the shark. T: How will you move to show you are a shark? C: Swim. T: Swim? On your back? . . . How will you move? C: On my stomach (represents motion). T: On your stomach? Good idea. OK, have fun.	T: Hi, Jeremy. What did you do today? C: I played with M.P. and Kathy. T: Tell me where you played with them. C: I played in the pit with one big shark. T: Tell me what you did to the shark. C: I tied the shark up! T: How did the shark feel? C: Sad! T: Oh, what else do you want to tell us? C: I played fireman and my house was on fire.

lem solution and negotiation of play schemes (e.g., "Joe, Matt wants you to play birthday party. What will you need?").

Recall time follows the play period. Again, clinician questioning is used to help children relay an immediate past event (what happened during play). Table 6.2 also illustrates transcripts from the recall period.

The advantage of recall time is that it places children in a situation where they can distance from the immediate context just slightly, by explaining what has recently happened during their play time. The samples of recall discourse in Table 6.2 illustrate the interactive nature and discourse functionality of this process.

Early in the year, children may only be able to point to a play area to express a plan, or show how a toy was used to recall. It is the repeated daily exposure to this social routine that strengthens the children's narrative participation. By the end of the year, they anticipate the clinician's scaffolding questions and include extra content in their personal narratives before it is even requested. Considering the importance of narrative to conversational and literacy success, this process is viewed as a priority in the program.

Use of routines gives children comfort and predictability. Across various preschool schedules, there are often many commonalities in the routines to which children are exposed. However, there are some additional unique ways in which cognitively oriented curricula exploit daily routines.

For example, in a traditional classroom, preschoolers are often seen around a calendar at opening time. Statements like "Today is Tuesday" may be memorized. In a cognitively oriented curriculum framework, the calendar is replaced by a 5-day timeline, representing the current school week. The block representing "today" has several visual cues representing events that will occur today. Children are encouraged to predict what is going to happen based on these cues (e.g., "Does anyone have ideas about what we will do with the drink box?" One child hypothesized, "Have grape juice for snack"; a second guessed that it would become the body of a car, like it had during an earlier craft activity). Opening time often includes a discussion of the weather chart. In traditional classrooms a child goes to the window to check the weather status. In the cognitively oriented program, children are supported in making observations based on recall of their immediate past experience (e.g., "Jon, I see you have shorts on today and so does Mandy. What does that tell you about the weather? What was it like out there?").

Snack time routines can also be fruitful for recall and discussion opportunities. In some preschool classrooms the authors have observed ritualized use of requests (e.g., "I want a cookie"; "I want more juice"). By offering snack choices, request language can be expanded. This is espe-cially true when a nonfavored choice is contrasted with favored ones. The authors have been known to provoke debates about delicious versus disgusting foods on presentation of broccoli as a snack choice. The children are surprised to discover that some people actually enjoy this vegetable. The children and clinicians keep charts at the snack table representing foods we've enjoyed and foods we didn't like. These charts help children recall and make associations when new foods are introduced. Clinicians also prompt children to recall by making observations (e.g., the clinician says, "Hmmm. This tastes salty. Can anyone remember what else we have had that was salty? Yes, chips and peanuts were salty. Jim, what can you tell me about all of these [makes simple drawing for scaffold]?" Jim, who is working on conjoining, replies, "Pretzels and peanuts and chips are salty"). Snack time can also be ideal for exploring concepts. One day the clinician presented various fruits, and the children explored for seeds. The avocado seed was a major surprise. In observing its solid and smooth attributes, one boy described it as, "like a bowling ball, but littler."

Daily routines, then, are capitalized on to help children predict, recall, summarize, and solve problems. When routines are consistent, children have concrete opportunities to establish concepts of time. The next classroom examples illustrate how routines are capitalized on to facilitate expansion of language structure in functionally appropriate contexts. The clinician manipulates routines in ways that obligate the child's use of certain functions and structures.

Example 1

Child: "What time play?"
Adult: "Oh, you are wondering . . .When is playtime?" (contingent expansion) "I'm not sure. Go ask Kathy." (functional use prompt)
Child: "Kathy. When is playtime?" (goes to Kathy)
Kathy: "Right after snack, Josh. That's when."

Example 2

Adult: Places unfamiliar object on table and waits for reaction.
Child: Looks curiously at adult.

Adult:	"Lynn, you wonder what that's for. Maybe Beki knows."
Lynn:	"Beki, what's that thing for?"
Beki:	"I don't know."
Adult:	"Beki, can Victoria help?"
Beki:	"Victoria, do you know?"
Victoria:	"Nope."
Adult:	Illustrates the function of the electric stapler on paper. Children all express a desire to try it.
Adult:	"Do we have anything else that holds papers together like this? Who can find something in the art area?"
Children:	Scatter and bring back a regular stapler and tape.
Adult:	"Good thinking. Staples and tape both hold paper together. Let's try them out. Any other ideas?"
Child:	"I know!" and brings back paper clips and a rubber band. Another child gets rubber cement. A third brings yarn.
Child:	Argues that rubber band "makes paper round, not stuck."
Adult:	"Try it and show us what you find out."
Adult:	"Oh you mean the rubber band can keep these together like a tube, but they are not attached."
Child:	"Yarn can't 'tach either. See?"
Adult:	"You all have many good ideas and opinions. Let's summarize."
Class:	Develops visual chart to aid recall. Fastened paper together? Yes: No: (pictures of the objects are placed on the chart) electric stapler stapler paper clip rubber cement rubber band yarn Summary prompt: A works, but a doesn't.

Exposure to Key Experiences to Support Logical Thinking. The High/Scope curriculum (Hohmann et al., 1979) provides detailed guidelines for exposing children to key experiences in the area of representation, language, literacy, spatial concepts, classification, seriation, temporal relations, and number concepts. It is believed that regular and consistent exposure to meaningful, explorative activities in these areas will assist children in developing a foundation for later logical thinking. The High/Scope authors stress the importance of placing primary focus on only one key experience at a time. This helps children attend to the relevant stimulus dimension as they manipulate materials and concepts. Clinicians find it useful to cycle through the key experience areas, switching the main focus every 3 to 4 weeks. Table 6.3 illustrates an experiential activity (baking muffins) approached in five different ways, depending on the key experience focus. This illustrates how key experience areas can be integrated within daily routines.

Throughout these strategies, adults and children collaborate to make and express discoveries and negotiate meanings. Cognitively oriented strategies lend themselves to the provision of active learning, social interaction, and problem-solving opportunities. The authors contend that such integration will help build a foundation for later language and literacy challenges.

Auditory and Speech Skills in Hearing-Impaired Children

INTRODUCTION TO THE DEVELOPMENTAL APPROACH

The auditory and speech production skills observed in young hearing-impaired children vary widely as a function of degree of hearing loss, age of identification, age of amplification or receipt of a sensory aid, and the presence of other handicapping conditions. This chapter presents a general approach for assessing auditory and speech skills in hearing-impaired children and for providing appropriate intervention based on the evaluation results.

This approach has evolved from research findings and clinical studies and practice and has a number of underlying assumptions. The most universal of these assumptions is that all assessment and intervention for auditory and speech skills takes place in the context of overall development for each hearing-impaired child. For some hearing-impaired children, all other areas of development (e.g., motor, cognitive, social) proceed as they do for normally hearing children. Other children

Table 6.3
Examples of Experiential Activity (Baking Muffins) with Different Key Experiences as the Focus

Experiential Activity: Preparing/Baking Muffins

Key Experience Area/Goal[a]	*Activity Plan*
Classification	
Investigate and label attributes.	Purposely make variety of muffin sizes; children describe their differences.
Describe characteristics something does *not* possess.	From cooking tools available, children problem-solve what they *don't* need or what else they will need.
	Children bake one muffin without egg; discover what happens.
Seriation	
Compare (bigger, heavier, wider, etc.).	Children experiment with different tools (hand mixer, blender, wire whisk, spoon, beaters) to determine which mixes *faster* or *better*.
Arrange items in order on a dimension.	Children review/recall about experience by seriating pictures of their tools on a continuum of slow to fast.
	Children put more or less batter in some cups and weigh the outcomes to compare (heavier/lighter).
Temporal relations	
Notice, describe, and represent the order of events.	Stir a short time—explore outcome; stir a long time. Contrast outcome.
Compare time periods (e.g., short, long).	Bake muffins in oven vs. microwave. Use concrete marker (sand timer) to visualize differences in the time required.
	Use pictures of event to support recall.
	Picture of oven *but* Microwave picture
	Recall: The oven was slow but the microwave was pretty fast.
Number	
Compare the number of items in two sets.	Purposely provide too few paper cups for the muffin tin; help children explore alternate solutions (e.g., make fewer muffins; use spray oil; buy or find paper cups; make paper cups).
Compare amounts (more/less, same).	Have children determine if there are too few or too many muffins for the class; problem-solve how to resolve.
Space	
Fit things together and take them apart.	Purposely omit needed items; pose as a problem (Where can we find a can opener? Right! In the kitchen drawer!).
Experience and describe positions of things in relation to each other.	Use nested measuring cups. Experiment with which one is best for fitting the right amount of batter.
Locate items in classroom.	Provide varied muffin types to elicit specific verbal requests (I want the blueberry one in the middle, not banana).

[a] Key experience areas and objectives are taken from Hohmann et al. (1979)—c.f. for complete list.

with hearing loss are challenged in a number of additional areas. What is interrupted for all these children with significant hearing loss, however, is the normal progression of auditory perceptual and speech production development.

A second important assumption is that auditory and speech skills are highly integrated and represent input and output functions of oral language. Consequently, assessment and intervention strategies in these areas should reflect this critical integration of language, speech, and listening. A third assumption is that visual cues from lipreading are an integral part of normal speech perception and production as well and are not specific to hearing-impaired listeners. Even at 4 months of age, normal infants are able to link the appropriate facial image with the auditory signal they hear (Kuhl & Meltzoff, 1982). A fourth assumption is that performance variability is an inherent property of the population of hearing-impaired children due to their heterogeneity. Consequently, individual differences and individual programming will occur necessarily. A fifth assumption is that training in auditory and speech skills is an important part of curricula for hearing-impaired children in both auditory/oral and total communication programs, regardless of their degree of hearing loss or the sensory aid (e.g., hearing aid, tactile aid, or cochlear implant) they use. Consequently, both assessment and intervention strategies need to be designed in a flexible and comprehensive manner.

In the remaining sections of the chapter, normal auditory and speech development will be discussed, along with the impact of hearing loss in these areas. Assessment and intervention for auditory and speech skills will be addressed individually and then as an integrated system.

AUDITORY PERCEPTUAL DEVELOPMENT: NORMAL AND INTERRUPTED

In a review article of general perceptual development for all sensory systems, Aslin and Smith (1988) proposed three levels of perceptual development: the sensory primitive level, the perceptual representation level, and the cognitive/linguistic level. During the course of normal development, children pass through each of these stages from less to more complex perceptual abilities.

The first level, the development of the sensory primitive, refers to the manner in which the sensory system, here the auditory system, actually transforms the incoming physical signal into a pattern of stimulation received by the child. This stimulation pattern changes with age, even for children with normal hearing, until adulthood (Olsho et al., 1988; Schneider, Trehub, & Thorpe, 1991). The detection of sound would occur at this level. The second level, the development of perceptual representations, is an intermediate level in which the child uses the pattern of sensory stimulation to form some type of complex neural code. Research in normal infant speech perception has provided ample evidence that complex aspects of speech, such as contrasts between voiced/ voiceless consonants, vowel, and pitch changes, can be perceived at very early stages of development (Eilers, Wilson, & Moore, 1977; Eimas et al., 1971; Kuhl, 1979, 1983). This level addresses the perception of speech but at a prelinguistic, more global level. The ability to discriminate a wide range of sound differences would occur at this level. The third level of this model deals with the higher order representations, those at the cognitive/linguistic level, in which perceptual representations have been mapped onto meaningful units such as words. The ability to recognize words and to comprehend utterances by listening only would occur at this level. Even for children with normal hearing, enormous changes continue to occur at this level throughout childhood and adolescence.

If a child has a significant hearing loss, this model of auditory perceptual development will be altered, sometimes dramatically. Because of either congenital or adventitious damage to the auditory system, the sensory primitive level is disrupted. The pattern of direct stimulation received from the physical stimulus is changed, with the outcome that an inappropriate or limited input is sent to the perceptual representation level. As a result, auditory speech perception may be underdeveloped or even absent, depending on the degree of hearing loss. The impoverished output of the perceptual representation level is directed to the cognitive/linguistic level, with the consequence that the ability to understand oral language by listening alone may be somewhat difficult to impossible, again depending on the degree of the hearing loss.

For most hearing-impaired children, the level of higher order representations does develop, sometimes in a delayed fashion, with the help of early and intensive intervention. However, it may be the visual modality that provides either part or all of the basic sensory primitives and perceptual representations to the cognitive/linguistic level for these children. For hearing-impaired children trained in an auditory/oral approach, these initial visual inputs come from lipreading combined with listening. For children trained in a total communication approach, the higher order representations are based on sign input along with lipreading and listening.

Auditory perceptual development is further affected when sensory aids are introduced to the hearing-impaired child. Amplification from traditional hearing aids, or input from tactile aids or cochlear implants, affects the sensory primitive level most directly, with indirect and long-term effects on the cognitive/linguistic levels, which may be difficult to assess.

Assessment and Auditory Perceptual Development

For a number of years, clinicians have used assessment models based on the comprehensive approach described by Erber (1982). Four levels of hearing were addressed: *(1)* detection, *(2)* discrimination, *(3)* recognition, *(4)* and comprehension. Tasks were designed that addressed some aspect of hearing. Stimuli varied as well and could be suprasegmentals, syllables, words, phrases, or sentences.

Even for the stage of parent/infant programming (up through age 2), Moeller (1984) described the integration of informal tasks addressing the first three of these levels of hearing into ongoing evaluations. This informal battery was called the Functional Auditory Skills Test (FAST). In cooperation with families, the tester would present a number of planned environmental and speech stimuli to the child to see how skills formally assessed in a test-booth situation transfer over to real situations.

While this traditional approach has been a valuable one, the perceptual development model described by Aslin and Smith (1988) assists in the formulation of some newly focused diagnostic questions for the assessment of auditory skills in hearing-impaired children. Traditionally, the evaluation of auditory skills in young hearing-impaired children has been directed at two main areas: *(1)* the measurement of unaided and aided detection thresholds for pure-tone stimuli as well as for speech stimuli and *(2)* the measurement of word recognition ability in either forced-choice or open-set contexts. The latter portion of the assessment was frequently omitted or compromised by the delays and/or gaps in lexical knowledge frequently observed in this population (Moeller, McConkey, & Osberger, 1983; Moeller, Osberger, & Eccarius, 1986). Poor word recognition scores may have been a reflection of poor speech perception, a limited vocabulary, or both. The traditional approach focused on auditory task rather than on developmental level of auditory perceptual ability. Consequently, both formal and informal tests derived from this traditional approach appeared to be shaped by the tasks used most frequently in adult tests. In terms of the Aslin and Smith model, this traditional approach addressed the sensory primitive level and the cognitive/linguistic level, while bypassing perceptual representations completely.

A comprehensive assessment for young hearing-impaired children should integrate aspects of Erber's (1982) model at each of the three developmental levels described by Aslin and Smith (1988). Many existing tests can be placed into the developmental framework. A summary of currently available assessment tools as well as the level of auditory development addressed is provided in Table 6.4.

Standard behavioral detection tasks for pure-tone and speech stimuli, as well as electrophysiological assessment procedures, address the level of the sensory primitive. In addition, both the phoneme detection task for vowels, continuants, and fricatives from the Glendonald Auditory Screening Procedure (GASP) (Erber, 1982) and the Ling Five-Sound Test (Ling & Ling, 1978) fall into this category. In all these behavioral tasks, patients are simply asked to tell whether a stimulus is present or absent. In both behavioral and electrophysiological tasks, stimuli may be acoustically simple or complex.

More recently, some assessment procedures have begun to focus on the level of perceptual representation. These procedures have addressed attributes of sound in general and of speech in particular. The change/no-change procedure, first described by Sussman and Carney (1989), presents a string of nonsense syllables to the child on each test trial. On a no-change trial, all syllables in the string are identical (e.g., /ba ba ba ba ba ba/). On a change trial, the first half of the syllables in the string are identical to each other (e.g., /ba ba ba/), followed by a second set of contrasting syllables (e.g., /da da da/). The child's task is to indicate whenever he or she hears a change by performing a simple motor act,

Table 6.4
Assessment Procedures Directed at the Three Levels of Auditory Perceptual Development

Perceptual Level	Assessment Procedure	Reference
Sensory primitive	Behavioral pure-tone detection tasks	Boothroyd, 1982; Diefendorf, 1988; Martin, 1987
	Electrophysiological procedures for detection	Gorga et al., 1989
	Phoneme detection GASP	Erber, 1982
	Ling Five-Sound Test	Ling & Ling, 1978
Perceptual representation	Change/no-change procedure	Sussman & Carney, 1989
	SCIPS	Osberger et al., 1991
	THRIFT	Boothroyd et al., 1988
	ESP Low Verbal Pattern Perception	Geers & Moog, 1989
Cognitive/ linguistic level	PBK words: open-set word recognition	Haskins, 1949
	WIPI: closed-set word recognition	Ross & Lerman, 1970
	NUCHIPS: closed-set word recognition	Elliott & Katz, 1980
	Minimal pairs: closed-set word recognition	Robbins et al., 1988
With perceptual representation	MTS: closed-set word recognition	Erber & Alencewicz,
	ANT: closed-set word recognition	1976
	GASP: closed-set word recognition	Erber, 1980
	ESP: standard version	Erber, 1982
With visual cues added	HAVE: closed-set word recognition	Geers & Moog, 1988
	PSI: closed-set word and phrase recognition	Renshaw et al., 1988
		Jerger et al., 1980
		Jerger et al., 1981
	Common Phrases	Osberger et al., 1991

such as putting a checker in a rack. No response is made on a no-change trial. Some children prefer using the labels "same" and "different" as responses, although use of a linguistic label is not necessary. Any speech contrasts may be used, including suprasegmental contrasts (such as short versus long) or segmental contrasts (such as /ba/ versus /da/). The change/no-change procedure uses a simple discrimination task to address differences in acoustic stimuli and is not affected by the linguistic abilities of the child tested.

Osberger et al. (1991) described an additional new procedure addressing the level of perceptual representations called the Screening Inventory of Perception Skills (SCIPS). In this task, children are asked to listen for a target word amid a string of other words. Even though the stimuli are real words, the child is not asked to identify the word itself, just to pick it out from other competing stimuli. This test may be classified as a fixed-target recognition task rather than a word-recognition test. For one subtest, the target is a monosyllabic word

and the two foils are three-syllable words (e.g., "ball" versus "birthday cake" and "lemonade"). Other subtests have monosyllabic targets opposite bisyllabic words (e.g., "ball" versus "popcorn" and "ice cream") and other monosyllables (e.g., "ball" versus "shoe" and "cup"), and bisyllabic words versus other bisyllabic words (e.g., "baseball" versus "hot dog" and "ice cream"). The objective of this test is to determine whether a child can attend to changing suprasegmental structure in words for the first two subtests or to changing segmental structure when syllable number is kept constant for the second two subtests.

Boothroyd et al. (1988) have also described a test that addresses the perceptual representation level called the THRIFT (Three-Interval Forced-Choice Test of Speech Pattern Contrast Perception). This test uses nonsense syllables in a three-alternative forced-choice task. Two syllables are the same, and one is different. The child's task is complex discrimination; that is, he or she must indicate which interval—

one, two, or three—contains the odd stimulus. A single suprasegmental or segmental feature is assessed in each subtest (e.g., consonant voicing). However, each feature contrast is assessed in a variety of phonetic contexts; that is, voicing differences are contrasted for several different stops and fricatives with a variety of vowels. Consequently, the actual acoustic differences between stimuli vary widely for a particular feature contrast. This is a different approach than the one used in the change/no-change procedure (Sussman & Carney, 1989), where fixed acoustic differences for a speech contrast pair are maintained throughout a subtest. The approach used in the THRIFT (Boothroyd et al., 1988) is one that looks for perceptual representations at a higher feature, rather than acoustic-phonetic, level.

Finally, one subtest of the Early Speech Perception battery–Low Verbal version (Geers & Moog, 1989) addresses the level of perceptual representations. A child is presented with two play alternatives, a train on a track and a rabbit. The tester trains the child to recognize one (the train) as a continuous stimulus "aahh" and the other (the rabbit) as an interrupted stimulus "hop hop hop." Children then perform a two-alternative forced-choice listening task in which they determine whether the tester has produced the continuous or interrupted stimulus. As in other procedures discussed above, the child is asked to make a response about an attribute of the stimulus, rather than giving a specific linguistic response.

Once an assessment procedure moves to the level of word recognition, through either picture identification or word repetition, the cognitive/linguistic level is addressed. At this level, it is important for testers to recognize that a child's overall level of language development will affect his or her word recognition ability. Although every word recognition test designed for children attempts to keep vocabulary simple and controlled and may provide picture support for closed set testing, it will not be possible to avoid the lexical-gap problem and overall language delays observed generally in hearing-impaired children (Moeller et al., 1983; Moeller et al., 1986). This issue also demonstrates the critical need for more and better assessment procedures at the perceptual representation level to provide necessary intermediary information about how speech might be coded by a particular child. In a sense, if an auditory assessment contained results from both perceptual representation and word recognition measures, it would allow the tester to make some inferences about how a child actually mapped his or her complex speech perception onto a real word perception.

Traditional adult tests of word recognition always maintained a fixed syllabic model throughout testing; that is, all test words were spondees or monosyllables. Speech perception was viewed as phoneme perception within real words only (Davis & Silverman, 1978). This approach was first applied to testing children's speech perception with the introduction of the PBK word lists (Haskins, 1949), an identical model of adult tests. Children are asked to repeat phonetically balanced monosyllables in an open-set task. The test is still used today and is a critical part of most assessment batteries for children who have received cochlear implants as a clear measure of their auditory success.

Later and more recent tests used a closed-set word recognition approach in which stimuli were represented by pictures. The most commonly used of those today include the Northwestern University Children's Perception of Speech (NUCHIPS) test designed by Elliott and Katz (1980) and the Word Intelligibility by Picture Identification (WIPI) test designed by Ross and Lerman (1970). NUCHIPS provides the child with four picture alternatives, the WIPI with six alternatives. While use of pictured words provides the child with a more direct referent for responding, it limits the tester in choosing real words that can be represented easily and vary along specific consonant and vowel dimensions. As alternatives increase, control over these segmental variables tends to decrease.

In partial response to this problem, a two-alternative closed-set word recognition task, called the Minimal Pairs test, was designed by Robbins et al. (1988). The design of this test was similar to that of the Discrimination by Identification of Pairs test (DIP), described earlier by Siegenthaler and Haspiel (1966). The Minimal Pairs test presents two pictures that vary by one segmental feature for both consonant and vowel contrast pairs. Results may be scored for both word correct and feature correct. Because of its emphasis on both vowels and consonants, this is appropriate for use with severely and profoundly hearing-impaired children as well and was designed for testing children who had received cochlear implants to measure longitudinal progress.

A different approach to word recognition testing was introduced by Erber and Alencewicz (1976). They used a closed-set format with 12 words including monosyllables, trochees, and spondees, later renamed the Monosyllable-Trochee-Spondee test (MTS). Children's responses were scored two ways, both for words correct and for stress pattern correct. Erber (1982) expanded this approach in the GASP, to include some three-syllable words as well. In addition, Erber (1980) described a simplified version of the procedure using numbers as stimuli, called the Auditory Numbers test for younger, less verbal children. The same approach and stimuli from the GASP are used to assess both pattern perception and word recognition in the Early Speech Perception battery (Geers & Moog, 1989).

This technique for assessing word recognition addresses both the cognitive/linguistic level and the perceptual representation level simultaneously. That is, word recognition is assessed directly, and the inferences about auditory attributes of the word are drawn indirectly. While this combined approach has broadened clinicians' perspectives of the auditory abilities of children with severe to profound hearing losses, the approach has a somewhat narrow interpretation; that is, testers examine wholeword perception or pattern perception. The only perceptual representation considered is a suprasegmental one, in which stress pattern and syllable number are addressed. A broadened view would accept that there might be more auditory attributes and perceptual representations available to the child, including those at a more segmental level. That is, children may represent words by the phonemes beginning them or the formant structure of vowels as well.

The integration of auditory and visual cues has received varied emphasis over the years in tests directed at the cognitive/linguistic level. The WIPI provided for items to be presented in the auditory, visual, and combined modes (Ross et al., 1972). Recently, the Hoosier Auditory-Visual Enhancement test (HAVE) has been introduced in a three-alternative picture format, containing two words that are homophenous (such as "pat" and "bat") with a third rhyming but nonhomophenous foil (such as "fat") (Renshaw et al., 1988). Each test item is presented once in a combined auditory-visual mode. Children's responses are then scored two ways: *(1)* word correct, for which the child must integrate auditory and visual information, and *(2)* visual correct, for which the child must pick one of the two homophenous items.

The Pediatric Speech Intelligibility test provided for the same three modes of presentation at the word, phrase, and sentence level, using closed-set picture referents (Jerger et al., 1980; Jerger, Jerger, & Lewis, 1981). Thus, the cognitive/linguistic demands increased even more in this assessment, since children had to comprehend short utterances. Osberger et al. (1991) reported on a slightly different sentence comprehension task called the Common Phrases test. Children are first shown a variety of pictures on a single page. They are told that the tester might talk about any of these pictures shown on the page. Picture support is removed, and short sentences are said to the child in each of the three test modes: visual only, auditory only, or combined.

Many preschool children with significant hearing losses can be assessed with the procedure discussed above. Performance data are available for children as young as 4 years of age who use hearing aids, tactile aids, or cochlear implants for the change/no-change procedure, the SCIPS, the Minimal Pairs, the MTS Test, the NUCHIPS, the HAVE, and the Common Phrases test (Carney et al., 1991; Osberger et al., 1991). Data from preschool children on the Early Speech Perception battery have also been collected for these same populations, although the language level assumed for the standard version of the test is at 6 to 7 years of age (Geers & Moog, 1991). Boothroyd (1991) indicated that, because of the task demands, the THRIFT procedure may not be appropriate in its current form for hearing-impaired children below age 6 or 7, particularly if their hearing loss is severe or profound. Standardization of the NU-CHIPS was done on children as young as 4, although they did not all have significant hearing losses. Because of its language level, the WIPI has limited usefulness for preschool children with severe to profound hearing losses, but may be used for children with milder degrees of hearing loss.

Intervention and Auditory Perceptual Development

Following a comprehensive assessment of the auditory skills of a hearing-impaired child, an intervention plan can be formulated that addresses the same three levels of perceptual development. This plan should contain both long-term and short-term objectives. The clinician may direct intervention at one earlier stage of development while providing some activities from a more complex level as well. These stages are not discrete and nonoverlapping. Rather, they should be viewed as both vertical and parallel in some aspects. This is particularly true for hearing-impaired children who have received a new sensory device such as a cochlear implant for which new listening skills must be developed.

For some children, depending on their age, degree of hearing loss, or receipt of a sensory aid, the clinician may want to focus on the sensory primitive level initially. If a reliable pure-tone audiogram has been obtained behaviorally, the first step has been taken. A second critical step in intervention is the provision and maintenance of an appropriate sensory aid or hearing aid to provide the input to the sensory primitive level. A third and ongoing process is the monitoring of the child's aided and unaided results to provide the clearest picture of the daily or long-term fluctuations in the sensory primitive level.

Hearing-impaired children are faced in their daily lives with the detection of a wide range of sounds with varying temporal, intensity, and spectral characteristics that are quite different from pure tones. These stimuli should be used in regular intervention sessions to determine which of these sounds are audible or inaudible, as well as to probe

how frequently a particular child relies on his or her hearing or sensory aid for detection.

Parent report can be an invaluable source for this information as well. This has been demonstrated by Robbins, Renshaw, and Berry (1991), who described a parent questionnaire called the Meaningful Auditory Integration Scale (MAIS). On this scale, parents are asked questions in such a way that they must provide the clinician with specific examples of how their child puts on his or her hearing aid or sensory aid every day, reports its malfunctioning, detects his or her name in both quiet and noisy situations, and reports on environmental sounds he or she experiences. This type of information is useful to evaluate the effectiveness of a hearing aid; to determine candidacy for a different sensory aid, such as a cochlear implant; or to assess the long-term effectiveness of any sensory device worn.

At the perceptual representation level, intervention is directed at learning the attributes of sound. A natural bridge between these two levels is helping the child learn which objects, people, and animals make sound and which do not. A speech perception example is one in which the clinician produces an utterance with lipreading cues either with or without voice. The child's task is to determine whether the clinician used his or her voice, blending detection with sound attribute (i.e., that people use their voices to make sound).

Many auditory training curricula exist with excellent activities that can be modified or used directly to address this level of perceptual representation. These include Auditory Training (Erber, 1982), the Auditory Skills Curriculum (1978), and Developing an Approach to Successful Listening Skills (1986). Most of these curricula follow some aspect of the traditional four levels of hearing approach. However, like many assessment tools, they may be more task oriented than developmentally oriented. Consequently, the clinician may use discrimination and recognition tasks with hearing-impaired children, but the important difference is the type of stimuli and responses elicited.

For example, some important attributes of sound are temporal ones (e.g., is the sound long or short, continuous or interrupted). Other attributes may fall in the intensity area (e.g., is the sound loud or soft or comfortable) or the spectral area (e.g., is the sound lower or higher pitched than another, is it noisy or harmonic). The important focus of intervention should be to introduce these attributes in as many meaningful contexts as possible rather than fixing one attribute with one type of activity. Thus, temporal attributes are components of many environmental stimuli that hearing-impaired children see regularly, such as blenders, hair dryers, buzzers, and alarms. They are also important components of speech at the segmental, suprasegmental, and utterance level. The more actively involved children are in the manipulation of devices and their voices (as will be discussed later in the speech section), the more likely they are to understand and use the perceptual attributes to which they are exposed.

As hearing-impaired children learn more about the attributes of sound, they can combine them, using the language and thinking skills they are learning in parallel. For example, children can describe sounds as "long and loud" or "noisy and soft," whether the sounds are environmental or speech sounds. In later stages of perceptual representation learning, children can describe suprasegmental and segmental aspects of speech, as well as combining them. That is, they can perform fixed target recognition tasks such as those on the SCIPS where they listen for short words among a list of long phrases and words, or words that have a noisy sound in them, like an /s/. If the child's response patterns in intervention are limited to reports of "same" or "different" or "picture one, two, or three," it is unlikely that the newly acquired listening skills will transfer over to daily life.

The demarcation between perceptual representation and cognitive/linguistic levels is even more blurry. It is likely that clinicians will focus on both areas simultaneously for a long time, trying to determine which auditory strategies a particular hearing-impaired child uses most frequently and which are most successful.

Carney (1991a) described an intervention program and outcome with an adventitiously deafened school-age child who had received a cochlear implant after 2 years of profound deafness. At each therapy session,

this child was asked to repeat a list of words to develop open-set word recognition skills, clearly a cognitive/linguistic level goal. The child initially was unable to repeat most words and rarely guessed at unknown items. Spontaneously, she began to report that some words were two syllables or three syllables long. Syllable number was at that time a speech production focus rather than a speech perception focus. However, with no specific instructions, the child noted the similarity in both perception and production. She clearly understood an underlying perceptual representation of the target word, even though she did not recognize the word itself.

As time progressed, she was willing to repeat a word even when she did not know what it was and did not know any sign for it. Her responses were frequently correct at the suprasegmental level, with appropriate syllable number and stress pattern. They also frequently contained a number of segments that were either present in the target word or closely related acoustically. Thus, the listening goal was cognitive/linguistic, but the response occurred at the perceptual representation level. The final goal was to map that close auditory perceptual representation onto a real word for which she had a sign. To achieve mapping, a variety of closed-set detection and recognition tasks were used, with stimulus items usually selected as part of a set of categories known to the child. In that way, she would learn to sort auditory targets and their attributes as opposed to learning a few fixed items. Once that mapping was accomplished, she was considered to have achieved true open-set word recognition and true cognitive/linguistic skill. Once this level of skill is accomplished, further emphasis on perceptual representations can help children understand, for example, what types of intonation or pitch change can accompany utterances to which they listen and how that can increase utterance understanding.

The only drawback to some established auditory training curricula is their narrow application, in which hearing-impaired children are asked to listen in restricted contexts with a limited set of responses and with limited use of speech or language skills. To facilitate carryover of listening skills to everyday life, an approach such as that described by Robbins (1990) is appropriate. She describes ways in which families and professionals can incorporate better auditory abilities into routine activities. Although this approach was designed for children with cochlear implants, it is applicable for use with all hearing-impaired children as well.

SPEECH PRODUCTION DEVELOPMENT: NORMAL AND INTERRUPTED

Recent work in the area of speech development has demonstrated clearly that the babbling and early speech observed in infants has many of the same timing and segmental characteristics as that of adults (Oller, 1983; Stoel-Gammon & Cooper, 1984). In contrast to beliefs held earlier, the speech characteristics of babbling and first oral words are continuous, suggesting that early speech activity is an important precursor for oral speech success (Vihman, Ferguson, & Elbert, 1986). In addition, new evidence is emerging that suggests that the syllable, rather than the segment, is the smallest unit of speech development in its early stages, indicating that more global properties of speech may be critical (Nittrouer, Studdert-Kennedy, & McGowan, 1989; Studdert-Kennedy, 1986).

Carney (1991b) described a new approach to coding infant vocalizations. This approach is called Reduced Aspect Feature Transcription (RAFT). Each utterance is first transcribed according to its syllabic makeup. That is, a string of syllables like /ba ba ba/ would be coded as CVCVCV. Vowel-like or vocalic segments (V) are coded globally according to broad categories of vowel height (high, mid, low), vowel place (front, mid, back), and vowel resonance (full, nasal, quasi-resonant). Closant or consonant-like segments (C) are coded globally according to place of articulation (front, mid, back), manner of articulation (stop, continuant, nasal, unknown), and voicing (voiced, voiceless, unknown). The analysis of RAFT data shows how the infant uses vocal tract space and how he or she manipulates the vocal tract. Infants with normal hearing appear to go from rather neutral use of vocal tract space to more rapid expansion in the height and place dimension during the first 12 months of life, for both vowels and consonants. The

development of true adult-like syllables occurs at approximately 7 to 8 months and escalates rapidly. These data support the idea of more general syllabic development in early vocalizations.

For the purposes of this chapter, a model of speech production development may be derived that is parallel to the auditory perceptual development model of Aslin and Smith (1988). The first level would be called the production primitive level. At this level, the infant is able to control voicing for some functions other than crying or producing vegetative sounds. These vocalizations may have very few characteristics in common with later adult speech and may sound like cooing, raspberries, or nonresonant vowel-like utterances. Oller (in press) would describe these as occurring in his stages of phonation and primitive articulation, occurring between birth and approximately 4 months of age in infants with normal hearing.

The second global stage of speech development would be called the production representation level. At this level, the infant would be producing speech sounds with some of the segmental and suprasegmental characteristics of adult speech (Oller, in press; Oller & Lynch, in press). This might occur during Oller's (in press) expansion or exploratory stage and his canonical stage, extending from approximately 3 to 10 months of age. Here, infants produce syllables that are close to adult-like, but the transitions from closant to vocalic portions sound longer and more stretched out. Oller has called these marginal syllables. Infants would also produce canonical syllables, those with the timing and phonetic characteristics like those used in adult speech.

The third global stage of speech development would be called the linguistic representation level. During this first real word stage, infants would be using segmental and suprasegmental features they developed earlier through babbling in meaningful contexts. This would occur from approximately 10 through 36 months, when rapid language development occurs.

Investigators have also shown some of the dramatic delays in the onset of canonical babbling and the phonetic inventory that occur as a function of hearing loss (Oller et al., 1985; Oller & Eilers, 1988;

Stoel-Gammon & Otomo, 1986). Oller and Eilers showed that canonical babbling does occur for infants with profound hearing losses but at much later ages. Their data show no overlap between the onset of canonical babbling in their subjects with normal hearing and those with profound hearing loss.

Infants with differing degrees of hearing loss—moderate through profound—appear to maintain their neutral vocal tract space, in contrast to infants with normal hearing. As hearing loss increases, failure to expand vocal tract space increases as well (Carney, 1991). These results suggest that infants with significant hearing losses, especially those with severe to profound losses, will begin the first oral word stage with impoverished phonetic and syllabic inventories, thus establishing a pattern of speech production delays and poor speech intelligibility. Severe-to-profound hearing loss may not interfere substantially with the production primitive, when vocalizations are quite undifferentiated. However, it does appear to affect the levels of production representations and linguistic representations dramatically and over the long term. Consequently, hearing-impaired children of preschool age may demonstrate the vocalization abilities of much younger infants. That is, they may not produce canonical syllables and may have a very limited phonetic inventory because of their failure to use and manipulate the vocal tract effectively.

A number of review articles exist that describe the characteristics of the speech of hearing-impaired and deaf children and their intelligibility (Carney, 1986; Osberger & McGarr, 1982). In a study of the acoustic properties of speech of the hearing impaired, Monsen (1978) concluded that speech intelligibility is related closely to the ability of hearing-impaired children *(1)* to demonstrate the existence of some vowel space (i.e., the presence of vowels along the height and place dimensions), *(2)* to demonstrate control of timing between consonant release at the articulators and onset of glottal pulsation, and *(3)* to control the fluid motion of semivowels such as /r/, /l/, and /w/. The results of the Monsen study provide support for the RAFT approach to analyzing early productions of young pro-

foundly hearing-impaired children with significantly delayed speech (Carney et al., 1991).

Assessment and Speech Production Development

Although a number of traditional articulation tests have been used in clinical studies of the speech of hearing-impaired children, the most widely used assessment tool is that described by Ling (1976). It has two parts: *(1)* the *Phonetic Level Evaluation* and *(2)* the *Phonologic Level Evaluation*. The first level (phonetic) is a nonsense-syllable elicitation and repetition task that addresses the ability of a speaker to repeat accurate productions of target nonsense syllables. First, suprasegmental features such as loudness, duration, and pitch are assessed. Then vowel production is assessed, followed by consonant production according to manner, place, and voicing features, and finally initial and final consonant blends are assessed. The second level (phonologic) is the estimation of a phonetic inventory from a set of spontaneous utterances.

Ling's (1976) assessment addresses the level of production primitive by evaluating the voluntary control of voice initially. The remainder of the Phonetic Level Evaluation addresses the level of production representation, because only nonsense syllables are used as production targets, in single or repeated productions, alternated with other syllables, or across a range of pitches. The complexity of these production representations increases from suprasegmental targets, through vowels, simple consonants, and consonant blends. This assessment addresses the level of linguistic representation in the Phonologic Level Evaluation, which is meant to be used in parallel with the Phonetic Level Evaluation.

Ling's (1976) approach appears to follow a developmental sequence according to the model presented here. Weissler, Carney, and Johnson (1988) presented data from 30 preschoolers with normal hearing who were tested with the Phonetic Level Evaluation. They found that overall scores on the test increased with increasing age from 3 to 5 years; in addition, scores decreased gradually as the complexity of the target task increased within subjects.

Osberger et al. (1991) have chosen a different approach to sampling speech production in young deaf children who have received cochlear implants. They use a nonsense-syllable repetition task (NITS) to elicit samples of consonants in the prevocalic position and vowels with different height and place characteristics. These samples are transcribed phonetically, and phonetic inventories are tallied. To obtain speech intelligibility information at the word level, hearing-impaired children are asked to repeat words from the Minimal Pairs speech perception test. Listeners then choose which word from a pair was produced. Finally, simple sentences are elicited with toys and actions. Listeners write down what parts of the utterance they understood to obtain speech intelligibility information at the sentence level. All these measures are directed at the level of linguistic representation.

Carotta, Carney, and Dettman (1990) described an assessment procedure called the Diagnostic Speech Inventory (DSI), designed by Carotta. This approach differs from those mentioned above because target items are real words that have either a CV, VC, or CVC makeup. Test items are elicited through repetition, both immediate and delayed. In addition, test plates have manipulable pictures and objects to encourage children to produce the number of repetitions desired and to provide them with a concrete referent for their speech. The test items are directed at the level of linguistic representation.

In a longitudinal study of speech production in young hearing-impaired children, Carney et al. (1991) used the RAFT procedure to transcribe more global features of speech from samples of the DSI. For each child, a map of the use of vocal tract space was constructed from vowel productions. In addition, percentages of consonant productions at the front, mid, and back portions of the vocal tract were plotted, as were percentages of use of manner categories (stop, continuant, nasal, and unknown) and voicing categories (voiced, voiceless, and unknown). Transcriptions with RAFT also tallied the proportion of times that the child did not use his or her voice but simply used an articulatory placement. Thus, this analysis procedure addresses the first two levels of the speech development model, that of the production primitive and the production representation.

In addition to using RAFT analysis, speech tokens were transcribed with a conventional International Phonetic Alphabet (IPA) approach. Transcribers used a strict criterion to determine whether a recognizable English segment, either vowel or consonant, had been produced. Results indicated clearly that before a particular vowel was produced with any regularity, the child had to produce a number of tokens in that vocal tract area. For example, before transcribers noted any incidences of the vowel /i/ for one subject, over 50 tokens had been produced and transcribed as being high, front vowels. Of these 50 tokens, only six of them were considered good exemplars of /i/.

This approach provides new insight into the development of speech production in hearing-impaired children. It permits the analysis of subphonemic speech skills as well as providing a picture of a child's idiosyncratic speech patterns. The RAFT analysis procedure is not tied to any particular diagnostic procedure. That is, it can be used with productions from the Phonetic Level Evaluation, NITS, and so on. Its strongest feature is that it provides an immediate starting point for intervention for each child, by showing target vocal tract areas and vocal tract manipulations that should be attempted.

Intervention and Speech Production Development

As in the area of assessment, the most widely used program for speech intervention is that described by Ling (1976). In this system, speech skills and subskills are approached according to a specific order determined by Ling's model, from voluntary control of the voice through production of consonant clusters. The strength of this system lies in its consistency and its comprehensive nature. However, it assumes indirectly that all children with hearing loss develop speech and can learn speech skills in the same order. Individual differences are not considered. In addition, this approach is very segmentally oriented rather than intelligibility oriented. The assumption would be that if a child could produce each segment correctly, he or she will be readily understood. This point of view is based on the importance of speech segments as building blocks of intelligibility (Monsen, 1978).

In contrast, the RAFT procedure reveals the specific underlying production representations in the child's vocal inventory. By using the RAFT analysis procedure, clinicians may see what types of idiosyncratic patterns each child produces and may design an intervention program specifically to address that pattern. For example, one subject whose sample was transcribed with RAFT produced 72% of her total vowels in the mid-front vowel space, the place occupied by /e/, even though the actual vowels produced were not an acceptable English /e/. The same subject produced over 70% of her consonants as mid, stop, voiced consonants, the same category as /d/, although almost none of these productions was an acceptable /d/. This represents an unusual pattern of production, even for a child with a profound hearing loss. Intervention for this subject would be directed at getting the child to produce some vowel height differences first from high to low, followed by some front and back vowel differences. Vocal tract areas would be targeted rather than specific phonemes.

By using the RAFT approach as well, clinicians will not give full segmental credit for tokens that approximate /d/ but are not an acceptable /d/. Instead, the productions will be transcribed more globally as noted above. Currently, many children are credited as producing acceptable segments before they actually do, and their phonetic inventory becomes inflated. Later, when the child produces a true segment, he/she does not receive additional credit for his/her progress, even though parents and professionals have judged that progress has been made. Finally, the RAFT analysis procedure allows clinicians to work toward speech intelligibility without having to assess it directly in young preschool children who may not know all the target vocabulary pictured. Carney (1990) showed a clear relationship between the patterns observed in RAFT analyses and the measured speech intelligibility of deaf adolescents. RAFT patterns for highly intelligible speakers were

indistinguishable from those of normal target speakers. As overall speech intelligibility decreased, RAFT patterns changed consistently, so that use of vowel space decreased as did the ability to manipulate the vocal tract. Consequently, targeting acceptable RAFT patterns targets future intelligibility, even for young hearing-impaired children.

Not all hearing-impaired children have such limited speech skills that RAFT analysis is required. Children with mild and moderate hearing losses in particular may have patterns of phonological processes that are similar to those observed in children with normal hearing (Oller, Jensen, & Lafayette, 1976). If these children have already achieved a high degree of intelligibility, then continued focus on polishing the production of individual segments is appropriate.

INTEGRATING AUDITORY AND SPEECH SKILLS

It is difficult to imagine providing intervention for speech production skills without focusing on auditory skills as well. If a child has adequate residual hearing, then auditory skill and speech production training should be combined in each session. This is not a new notion but has been advocated for some time (Ling, 1978).

Similarly, training with visual and tactile cues is appropriate for children who have no residual hearing. Visual cues may include lipreading, hand cues such as those in Cued Speech, or use of a visual feedback device. Tactile cues may include those from a vibrotactile device such as a Tactaid II or VII.

The most comprehensive approach is one that uses the child's speech, language, and cognitive skills maximally while focusing on listening skills and speech development. The activities described earlier in the chapter regarding active learning, development of schemata, and so on lend themselves to incorporation of listening and speech activities. In learning at all three levels for perception and production, auditory goals can flip-flop to speech production goals simply by having the child assume the role of the speaker or "teacher," while the clinician becomes the listener or "student." This gives the child a reason to use his or her speech skills in a real context and provides more practice for the attribute of sound or word characteristic that is targeted. In addition, children can be asked to sort or categorize in listening tasks, to underscore the skills they have acquired in preschool, and to talk about what they hear, to use their expressive language skills as well.

Conclusion

The preschool years are important ones for hearing-impaired children and their families. Professionals need to provide an integrated approach to all aspects of assessment and intervention for language, speech, and listening skills that meets the needs of the children and families they serve and to provide a basis for more complex language and learning skills that follow in the school years.

References

Aslin, R.N., and Smith, L.B., Perceptual development. *Ann. Rev. Psych.*, 39, 435–473 (1988).

Auditory Skills Curriculum. North Hollywood, CA: Foreworks (1978).

Bailey, D.J., Collaborative goal setting with families: resolving differences in values and priorities for service. *Top. Early Child. Educ.*, 7(2), 59–71 (1987).

Barnes, S., Gutfreund, M., Satterly, D., and Wells, G., Characteristics of adult speech which predict children's language development. *J. Child Lang.*, 10, 65–84 (1983).

Bates, E., *The Emergence of Symbols: Cognition and Communication in Infancy.* New York, NY: Academic Press (1979).

Blank, M., and Marquis, M.A., *Directing Discourse.* Tucson, AZ: Communication Skill Builders (1987).

Blank, M., Rose, S., and Berlin, L., *The Language of Learning: The Preschool Years.* New York, NY: Grune & Stratton, pp. 8–21 (1978).

Boothroyd, A., *Hearing Impairments in Young Children.* Englewood Cliffs, NJ: Prentice-Hall (1982).

Boothroyd, A., Speech perception measures and their role in the evaluation of hearing aids performance in a pediatric population. In J.A. Feigin and P.G. Stelmachowicz (Eds.), *Pediatric Amplification: Proceedings of the 1991 National Conference.* Omaha, NE: Boys Town National Research Hospital, pp. 77–92 (1991).

Boothroyd, A., Springer, N., Smith, L., and Schulman, J., Amplitude compression and profound hearing loss. *J. Speech Hear. Res.*, 31, 362–376 (1988).

Bruner, J.S., Learning how to do things with words. In J.S. Bruner and R.A. Garton (Eds.), *Human Growth and Development.* Oxford, UK: Oxford University Press (1978).

Bruner, J.S., The ontogenesis of speech acts. *J. Child Lang.*, 2, 1–20 (1975).

Carney, A.E., Understanding speech intelligibility in the hearing impaired. *Top. Lang. Dis.*, 6, 47–59 (1986).

Carney, A.E., Reduced Aspect Feature Transcription (RAFT) as an index of speech intelligibility. *J. Acoust. Soc. Am.*, 87 (Suppl.), S89(A) (1990).

Carney, A.E., Assessment of speech perception in children with cochlear implants and tactile aids: What should the future hold? *Am. J. Otol.*, 12 (Suppl.), 201–204 (1991a).

Carney, A.E., Vocal development in hearing-impaired infants. *J. Acoust. Soc. Am.*, 90, 2296 (A) (1991b).

Carney, A.E., Carotta, C., Dettman, D., and Karasek, A., Estimating phonetic inventories in the speech of young hearing-impaired children. *Asha*, 33, 149 (A) (1991).

Carney, A.E., Osberger, M.J., Miyamoto, R.T., Karasek, A., Dettman, D.L., and Johnson, D.L., Speech perception along the sensory aid continuum: from hearing aids to cochlear implants. In J.A. Feigin and P.G. Stelmachowicz (Eds.), *Pediatric Amplification: Proceedings of the 1991 National Conference.* Omaha, NE: Boys Town National Research Hospital, pp. 93–113 (1991).

Carotta, C., Carney, A.E., and Dettman, D., Assessment and analysis of speech production in hearing-impaired children. *Asha*, 32, 59 (A) (1990).

Constable, C.M., and van Kleeck, A., From Social to Instructional Uses of Language: Bridging the Gap. Submitted for presentation at the American Speech-Language-Hearing Association Annual Convention, Washington, DC (1985).

Dale, P., and Thal, D., *MacArthur Communicative Development Inventory.* Center for Research in Language, UCSD, San Diego, CA (1989).

Davis, H., and Silverman, R.S., *Hearing and Deafness* (4th ed.). New York: Holt, Rhinehart, and Winston (1978).

Diefendorf, A., Behavioral evaluation of hearing-impaired children. In F.H. Bess (Ed.), *Hearing Impairment in Children.* Parkton, MD: York Press (1988).

Eilers, R.E., Wilson, W.R., and Moore, J.M., Developmental changes in speech discrimination in infancy. *J. Speech Hear. Res.*, 20, 766–780 (1977).

Eimas, P.D., Siqueland, E.R., Jusczyk, P.W., and Vigorito, J., Speech perception in infants. *Science*, 171, 303–306 (1971).

Elliott, L.L., and Katz, D.R., *Northwestern University Children's Perception of Speech Test (NUCHIPS).* St. Louis, MO: Auditec (1980).

Ensher, G.L., The first three years: special education perspectives on assessment and intervention. *Top. Lang. Dis.*, 10(1), 80–90 (1989).

Erber, N.P., Use of the Auditory Numbers test to evaluate speech perception abilities of hearing-impaired children. *J. Speech Hear. Dis.*, 45, 527–532 (1980).

Erber, N.P., *Auditory Training.* Washington, DC: A.G. Bell Association for the Deaf (1982).

Erber, N.P., and Alencewicz, C.M., Audiologic evaluation of deaf children. *J. Speech Hear. Dis.*, 41, 256–267 (1976).

Fenson, L., Dale, P.S., Reznick, J.S., et al. *Technical Manual for the MacArthur Communicative Devel-*

opment Inventories. San Diego, CA: San Diego State University (1991).

Fitzgerald, M.T., and Fischer, R.M., A family involvement model for hearing-impaired infants. *Top. Lang. Dis.*, 7, 1–19 (1987).

Geers, A.E., and Moog, J.S., Evaluating speech perception skills: tools for measuring benefits of cochlear implants, tactile aids, and hearing aids. In E. Owens and D.K. Kessler (Eds.), *Cochlear Implants in Young Deaf Children.* Boston: Little, Brown (1989).

Geers, A.E., and Moog, J.S., Evaluating the benefits of cochlear implants in an education setting. *Am. J. Otol.*, 12 (Suppl.), 116–125 (1991).

Goldberg Stout, G., and Van Ert Windle, J., *The Developmental Approach to Successful Listening.* Englewood, CO: Resource Point (1986).

Gorga, M.P., Kaminski, J.R., Beauchaine, K.L., Jesteadt, W., and Neely, S.T., Auditory brainstem responses from children three months to three years of age: normal patterns of response II. *J. Speech Hear. Res.*, 32, 281–288 (1989).

Grammatico, L., and Miller, S., Curriculum for the preschool deaf child. *Volta Rev.*, 79, 19–26 (1974).

Halliday, M.A.K., *Learning How to Mean.* London: Edward Arnold (1975).

Haskins, H., A phonetically balanced test of speech discrimination for children. Unpublished Masters thesis, Northwestern University, Evanston, IL (1949).

Hohmann, M., Banet, B., and Weikart, D., *Young Children in Action.* Ypsilanti, MI: High/Scope Press (1979).

Hoskins, B., Language and literacy: participating in the conversation. *Top. Lang. Dis.*, 10(2), 46–62 (1990).

Jerger, S., Jerger, J., and Lewis, S., Pediatric speech intelligibility test. II. Effect of receptive language age and chronological age. *Int. J. Ped. Otorhinolaryngol.*, 3, 101–118 (1981).

Jerger, S., Lewis, S., Hawkins, J., and Jerger, J., Pediatric speech intelligibility test. I. Generation of test materials. *Int. J. Ped. Otorhinolaryngol.*, 2, 217–230 (1980).

Kail, R., and Leonard, L., Word-finding abilities in language-impaired children. *Asha Monograph*, 25. Rockville, MD: ASHA (1986).

Kintsch, W., *The Representation of Meaning in Memory.* Hillsdale, NJ: Erlbaum (1974).

Kuhl, P.K., Speech perception in early infancy: perceptual constancy for spectrally dissimilar vowel categories. *J. Acoust. Soc. Am.*, 66, 1668–1679 (1979).

Kuhl, P.K., Perception of auditory equivalence classes for speech in early infancy. *Inf. Behav. Dev.*, 6, 263–285 (1983).

Kuhl, P.K., and Meltzoff, A., The bimodal perception of speech in infancy. *Science*, 218, 1138–1141 (1982).

Ling, D., Auditory coding and recoding: an analysis of auditory training procedures for hearing-impaired children. In M. Ross and T.G. Giolas (Eds.), *Auditory Management of Hearing-Impaired Children.* Baltimore: University Park Press (1978).

Ling, D., *Speech for the Deaf Child.* Washington, DC: A.G. Bell Association for the Deaf (1976).

Ling, D., and Ling, A.H., *Aural Habilitation.* Washington, DC: A.G. Bell Association for the Deaf (1978).

Luterman, D.M., *Counseling the Communicatively Disordered and Their Families.* Austin, TX: ProEd (1991).

Manolson, A., *It Takes Two to Talk* (2nd ed.). Toronto: Hanen Early Language Resource Centre (1985).

Martin, F.N., *Hearing Disorders in Children.* Austin, TX: ProEd (1987).

Masur, E.F., Mothers' responses to infants' object-related gestures: influences on lexical development. *J. Child Lang.*, 9, 23–30 (1982).

Meadow, K., Greenberg, M., Erting, C., and Carmichael, H., Interactions of deaf mothers and deaf preschool children: comparisons with three other groups of deaf and hearing dyads. *Am. Ann. Deaf*, 126, 454–468 (1981).

Miller, J., and Chapman, R., *Systematic Analysis of Language Transcripts.* Madison, WI: University of Wisconsin (1983).

Miller, L., The roles of language and learning in the development of literacy. *Top. Lang. Dis.*, 10(2), 1–24 (1990).

Moeller, M.P., Assessing hearing and speechreading in hearing-impaired children. In D. Sims (Ed.), *Deafness and Communication: Assessment and Training.* Baltimore: Williams & Wilkins, pp. 127–140 (1984).

Moeller, M.P., and Condon, M., A collaborative, problem-solving approach to early intervention. In J. Roush and N.D. Matkin (Eds.), *Infants and Toddlers with Hearing Loss: Identification, Assessment and Family-Centered Intervention.* Parkton, MD: York Press, Inc. (in press).

Moeller, M.P., Coufal, K., and Hixon, P., The efficacy of speech-language intervention: hearing impaired children. *Sem. Speech Lang.*, 11(4), 227–241 (1990).

Moeller, M.P., and McConkey, A.J., Language intervention with preschool deaf children: a cognitive/linguistic approach. In W.H. Perkins (Ed.), *Current Therapy of Communication Disorders.* New York, NY: Thieme-Stratton, pp. 11–25 (1984).

Moeller, M.P., McConkey, A., and Osberger, M.J., Evaluation of the communication skills of hearing-impaired children. *Audiology*, 13, 113–126 (1983).

Moeller, M.P., Osberger, M.J., and Eccarius, M., Receptive language skills. In M.J. Osberger (Ed.), *Language and Learning Skills of Hearing-Impaired Students. Asha Monograph*, 23, 41–54 (1986).

Moeller, M.P., Osberger, M.J., and Morford, J., Enhancing the communicative skills of hearing-impaired children. In J. Alpiner and P. McCarthy (Eds.), *Rehabilitative Audiology: Children and Adults.* Baltimore, MD: Williams & Wilkins (1985).

Monson, R., Toward measuring how well hearing-impaired children speak. *J. Speech Hear. Res.*, 21, 197–219 (1978).

Nittrouer, S., Studdert-Kennedy, M., and McGowan, R.S., The emergence of phonetic segments: evidence from the spectral structure of fricative-vowel syllables spoken by children and adults. *J. Speech Hear. Res.*, 32, 120–132 (1989).

Oller, D.K., Infant babbling as a manifestation of the capacity for speech. In S.E. Gerber and G.T. Mencher (Eds.), *The Development of Auditory Behavior.* New York: Grune & Stratton, pp. 221–236 (1983).

Oller, D.K., Development of vocalizations in infancy. In H. Winitz (Ed.), *Human Communication and Its Disorders* (in press).

Oller, D.K., and Eilers, R.E., The role of audition in infant babbling. *Child Develop.*, 59, 441–449 (1988).

Oller, D.K., Eilers, R.E., Bull, D.H., and Carney, A.E., Pre-speech vocalizations of a deaf infant: a comparison with normal metaphonological development. *J. Speech Hear. Res.*, 28, 47–63 (1985).

Oller, D.K., Jensen, H.T., and Lafayette, R.H., The relatedness of phonological processes of a hearing-impaired child. *J. Comm. Dis.*, 11, 97–105 (1976).

Oller, D.K., and Lynch, M.P., Infant vocalizations and innovations in infraphonology: toward a broader theory of development and disorders. In C.A. Ferguson, L. Menn, and C. Stoel-Gammon (Eds.), *Phonological Development* (in press).

Olsho, L.W., Koch, E.G., Carter, E.A., Halpin, C.F., and Spetner, N.B., Pure-tone sensitivity of human infants. *J. Acoust. Soc. Am.*, 84, 1316–1324 (1988).

Olswang, L., Stoel-Gammon, C., Coggins, T., and Carpenter, R., *Assessing Linguistic Behavior* (ALB). Seattle, WA: University of Washington Press (1987).

Osberger, M.J., and McGarr, N., Speech production characteristics of the hearing impaired. In N. Lass (Ed.), *Speech and Language: Advances in Basic Research and Practice*, Vol. 8. New York: Academic Press (1982).

Osberger, M.J., Miyamoto, R.T., Zimmerman-Phillips, S., et al., Independent evaluation of the speech perception abilities of children with the Nucleus 22-Channel cochlear implant system. *Ear Hear.*, 12 (Suppl.), 66S–80S (1991).

Pearson, P., A primer for schema theory. In R.E. Krestschmer (Ed.), *Reading and the hearing-impaired individual. Volta Rev.*, 84(5), 25–35 (1982).

Piaget, J., and Inhelder, B., *The Psychology of the Child.* London: Routledge & Kegan Paul (1969).

Renshaw, J., Robbins, A.M., Miyamoto, R.T., Osberger, M.J., and Pope, M., *Hoosier Auditory Visual Enhancement Test.* Indiana University School of Medicine, Dept. of Otolaryngology–Head and Neck Surgery (1988).

Robbins, A.M., Developing meaningful auditory integration in children with cochlear implants. *Volta Rev.*, 92, 361–370 (1990).

Robbins, A.M., Renshaw, J., and Berry, S., Evaluating meaningful auditory integration in profoundly hearing-impaired children. *Am. J. Otol.*, 12 (Suppl.), 144–150 (1991).

Robbins, A.M., Renshaw, J., Miyamoto, R.T., Osberger, M.J., and Pope, M., *Minimal Pairs Test.* Indiana University School of Medicine, Dept. of Otolaryngology–Head and Neck Surgery (1988).

Ross, M., Kessler, M., Phillips, M., and Lerman, J., Visual, auditory, and combined mode of presentations of the WIPI Test to hearing-impaired children. *Volta Rev.*, 74, 90–96 (1972).

Ross, M., and Lerman, J., A picture identification test for hearing-impaired children. *J. Speech Hear. Res.*, 13, 44–53 (1970).

Roush, J., and McWilliam, R.A., A new challenge for pediatric audiology: Public Law 99–457. *J. Am. Acad. Audiol.*, 1(4), 196–208 (1990).

Schick, B.S., Integrating the language of the school and the language of the community. In *Missouri Record*, 113, 6–7 (1990).

Schneider, B.A., Trehub, S.E., and Thorpe, L., Developmental perspectives on the localization and detection of auditory signals. *Percept. Psychophys.*, 49, 10–20 (1991).

Schuyler, V., and Rushmer, N., *Parent Infant Habilitation: A Comprehensive Approach to Working with Hearing-Impaired Infants and Toddlers and Their Families.* Portland, OR: IHR Publications (1987).

Siegenthaler, B., and Haspiel, G., *Development of Two Standardized Measures of Hearing of Speech by Children.* Cooperative Research Program, Project No. 2372, Contract OE-5-10-003. Washington, DC: U.S. Department of Health, Education, and Welfare, U.S. Office of Education (1966).

Simmons-Martin, A., and Rossi, K., *Parents and Teachers: Partners in Language Development.* Washington, DC: A.G. Bell Association for the Deaf (1990).

Snow, C.E., The development of conversations between mothers and babies. *J. Child Lang.*, 4, 1–22 (1977).

Snow, C.E., Literacy and language: relationships during the preschool years. *Harvard Ed. Rev.*, 53(2), 165–189 (1983).

Sparks, S.N., Assessment and intervention with at-risk infants and toddlers: guidelines for the speech-language pathologist. *Top. Lang. Dis.*, 10(1), 43–56 (1989).

Stoel-Gammon, C., and Cooper, J.A., Patterns of early lexical and phonological development. *J. Child Lang.*, 11, 247–271 (1984).

Stoel-Gammon, C., and Otomo, K., Babbling development of hearing-impaired and normally hearing subjects. *J. Speech Hear. Dis.*, 51, 33–41 (1986).

Stone, P., Developing thinking skills in young hearing-impaired children. *Volta Rev.*, 82(6), 345–353 (1980).

Studdert-Kennedy, M., Sources of variability in early speech development In J. Perkell and D.H. Klatt (Eds.), *Invariance and Variability in Speech Processes.* Hillsdale, NJ: Lawrence Erlbaum Assoc., pp. 58–84 (1986).

Sussman, J.E., and Carney, A.E., Effects of transition length on the perception of stop consonants by children and adults. *J. Speech Hear. Res.*, 32, 151–160 (1989).

Thompkins, M., Active learning: making it happen in your program. Extensions: High/Scope Newsletter, 1(2) (1986).

Tomasello, M., and Farrar, M.J., Joint attention and early language. *Child Dev.*, 57, 1454–1463 (1986).

Tomasello, M., Mannie, S., and Kruger, A., The linguistic environment of one to two year old twins. *Dev. Psych.*, 22, 169–176 (1986).

Tomasello, M., and Todd, J., Joint attention and lexical acquisition style. *First Lang.*, 4, 197–212 (1983).

Trout, M., and Foley, G., Working with families of handicapped infants and toddlers. *Top. Lang. Dis.*, 10(1), 57–67 (1989).

Vihman, M., Ferguson, C.A., and Elbert, M., Phonological development from babbling to speech: common tendencies and individual differences. *Appl. Psycholing.*, 7, 3–40 (1986).

Wedell-Monnig, J., and Lumley, J., Child deafness and mother-child interaction. *Child Develt.*, 51, 766–774 (1980).

Weikart, D.P., Rogers, L., Adcock, C., and McClelland D., *The Cognitively Oriented Curriculum.* Urbana, IL: University of Illinois Press (1971).

Weissler, L., Carney, A.E., and Johnson, C.J., Developmental analysis of the Ling Phonetic Level Evaluation. *Asha*, 131, 106 (A) (1989).

Wells, G., *Learning Through Interaction.* New York, NY: Cambridge University Press (1981).

Wells, G., and Nicholls, J., *Language and Learning: An Interactional Perspective.* London: Falmer Press (1985).

Westby, C., Assessment of cognitive and language abilities through play. *Lang. Speech Hear. Serv. Schools*, 3(11), 154–163 (1980).

Westby, C., Learning to talk—talking to learn: oral-literate language differences. In C.S. Simon (Ed.), *Communication Skills and Classroom Success.* San Diego, CA: College-Hill Press, pp. 181–219 (1985).

Wetherby, A., and Prizant, B., *Communication and Symbolic Behavior Scales.* San Antonio, TX: Special Press, Inc. (1990).

Yoshinaga-Itano, C., and Downey, D., A hearing-impaired child's acquisition of schemata: something's missing. *Top. Lang. Dis.*, 7(1), 45–57 (1986).

Assessment and Intervention with School-Age Hearing-Impaired Children

JOAN LAUGHTON, Ph.D., M. SUZANNE HASENSTAB, Ph.D.

Communication models for hearing-impaired children have proliferated during the 1990s and have come of age in preparation for the 21st century. The pragmatics revolution of the 1980s has provided a framework for the metalinguistic focus of the 1990s, which has, in turn, brought light to the challenges of educating hearing-impaired children in mainstream settings alongside their hearing counterparts. To actively participate in learning, students must be competent in receiving and expressing the language of the classroom.

As if the work of providing rehabilitative services for hearing-impaired children were not difficult enough, this field is subject to the same tumultuous changes that seem to be characteristic of our world in general. Where once there was solid ground, now there is shifting sand; what once was dogma may now not even be relevant; and the craft you so carefully mastered as a student is a changeling and requires updated information for its care and feeding. The authors provide you first with an overview of issues that promise or threaten to become focal points for more sweeping changes. Then a current model of each phase of auditory processing, in all its intricacies, is presented as background for a full-blown discussion of each facet of assessment and intervention. The chapter is designed to provide direction and answers where there is clarity; to pull you from any temptation to complacency by provoking reflection on issues of controversy and benign neglect; to channel as much information as possible about new tools and conceptual schemes that may aid you in your work; and finally to provide a sense of philosophical gratification for those who are interested.

Areas of Focus

This chapter focuses on the severely to profoundly hearing-impaired school-age student in any school setting, with particular emphasis on the integration of services required for effective intervention in mainstream educational settings. Defining "school age" has become muddied with the recent provisions for schooling for "preschool" children. However, the school age referred to here begins at kindergarten ages and continues through the secondary school years. Rehabilitation needs continue at postsecondary levels including vocational, technical, college, and university schooling, each bringing its own set of challenging conditions; however, these issues will be deleted from this discussion. The range of hearing loss includes the student with enough residual hearing to develop spoken language skills, as well as the functionally deaf child who uses sign language. Focus on the child with less severe or fluctuating hearing loss is detailed in Chapter 8. The areas of discussion here are based in prior evaluation of auditory functioning of the child (including the auditory peripheral mechanism and auditory processing). Attention is directed toward *(1)* specific language and speech abilities of the child, including receptive and expressive skills within the communication perspectives of pragmatics, semantics, syntax, morphology, and phonology and their impact on the *(2)* overall development of the child, including cognitive abilities and academic performance.

Scope

The scope of this chapter includes the assessment of communication, language, speech, and psychoeducational performance of school-age children with hearing disorders. Intervention should focus on integration of all the assessed areas. If assessment and intervention are not ongoing and holistic, and if the child receives a little speech training here and a little language training there without follow-up or interest across the environment, the service process becomes a parody where professionals draw their paycheck and everyone is served except the child.

Issues and Changes
A GUIDE FOR VIEWING THE CHANGING LANDSCAPE

The newly graduated communication disorders specialist, whether audiologist, speech pathologist, or educator of hearing-impaired students, emerges from the rarefied air of academia into the real world armed with the most up-to-date information that universities can offer. And veterans have likely already pledged their allegiance to documented systems of theory and practice. But now both may be in need

of a map of the terrain or a guide book, describing points of interest as well as caution. A multiplicity of forces—including technological, theoretical, political, and cultural—have converged to change the once familiar, if often conflict-ridden, landscape of rehabilitation of hearing-impaired school-age children.

TECHNOLOGIES

Technology has added new dimensions to the resolution of long-standing issues, and new issues have emerged. The multichannel cochlear implant has brought new challenges and potential to intervention efforts for profoundly hearing-impaired children. The potential is for no less than mastery of spoken language. The challenges include breaking free from old categories (e.g., Teacher: "Children who are being educated in total communication settings should continue to be educated in those settings") and fine-tuning expectations such that each child is pushed to his or her growing edge. Expectations set too low (e.g., Parent: "If my child can only hear car horns, I will be happy") short-circuit success, and expectations set too high (e.g., Parent: "He can hear now and does not need rehabilitation to start understanding and speaking in the next few weeks") foster frustration and sense of failure.

Speech, often a source of frustration for teachers and hearing-impaired students, has a new powerful friend in cochlear implants. This new technology provides the opportunity for all speech strategies and programs of the past to be successfully implemented in the present. Enhancement of auditory experience, in turn, opens a new realm of possibilities for hearing-impaired children to develop spoken language.

There has, perhaps, never been another time in history in which rehabilitative audiology in theory and practice has been more relevant or possible for hearing-impaired children. Current technology in amplification systems (hearing aids, FM systems, assistive devices), tactile devices, and cochlear implants brings a new tone to habilitation of school-age hearing-impaired children. Auditory training strategies have been used for many years, but the quality and quantity of sound now available make the task of rehabilitation more hopeful.

ASL, ESL, AND ESS

Because of the new technologies and child language theory and research, the age-old manual versus oral debate has both changed and accelerated. Instead of a dichotomy, now there is a bridge composed of American Sign Language (ASL) and English Sign Systems (ESS) instruction leading to English as a Second Language (ESL). Using second-language learning techniques, ASL and ESS can be the bases to learn ESL. The new technologies, and especially cochlear implants, now provide substantial residual hearing for oral strategies to develop auditory-based spoken language.

The modality and language issues reflect both the differences and the commonalities between interpersonal (face-to-face) and school (written and instructional) language. Further discussion is available in the native language (L 1) and English as a Second Language (L 2) literature (Paul & Quigley, 1990; Wilbur, 1987).

Deaf Versus deaf

Cultural and political shifts have given a segment of the Deaf community a new avenue to expressing the human—and specifically the Deaf human—condition. Their philosophical stance is that Deaf is a point of cultural identity rather than a disability. Deafness unites them in culture as well as language, and they should be accorded the rights of any other minority. No longer do they have to be victim to the subtle subjugation implicit in client-professional relationships. They look to the Deaf world for their role models and measure themselves against Deaf, not hearing, standards. Audiology and speech pathology students likely will have been exposed only to the deaf perspective in their training, where hearing loss is regarded as a handicap and a disability, and the primary question is what to do to rehabilitate. No doubt there are deaf students whose hearing parents want their children rehabilitated into a hearing world. But as hearing professionals assume roles in the real world and meet the Deaf perspective, it will begin to be apparent that their education has only just begun. This confrontation is the prototypical, ethical dilemma. The choice is whether, on the one hand, to open to the sometimes painful, always profound, process of self-searching, releasing old attitudes and thereby expanding professionally, or, on the other hand, to shrink from challenge and maintain the status quo in service to form at the expense of the real needs of clients.

COGNITIVE RESEARCH AND HEARING-IMPAIRED EXPERIENCE IN THE MAINSTREAM

In psycholinguistic and cognitive research, normal language acquisition is viewed as a creative process. The child actively constructs meaning rather than merely assimilating externals into the linguistic system. Meaning is shared by individuals with similar experiences and a same fundamental knowledge of a given language. This construction of personal meaning by a child makes language a creative or generative process that applies across phonologic, morphologic, semantic, syntactic, and pragmatic rule systems. Hearing-impaired children also construct meaning, but the absence or restrictions of auditory input caused by hearing loss inhibit the coding of meaning by virtue of fragmented rule systems for the linguistic components of spoken language.

The current status of education of the profoundly hearing-impaired "can be characterized as one of creative confusion" (Quigley & Paul, 1984, p. xi). The creative component has led to significant change, but there is limited information for educational practice. We have come a long way since investigators were intrigued by the deaf as a pure research sample because they had no language—or have we? The relationship between language and thought is yet unresolved. Cognition has been described as the acquisition, organization, and application of knowledge (Sternberg, 1984). So cognition includes an acquisition or encoding phase to establish cognitive structures, and cognitive processes play active roles in the initial representation of knowledge (structure). Metacognition or an individual's awareness of thinking and reasoning is a more advanced and very powerful aspect of cognitive processing. Cognition then is composed of a structural, representational level, as well as a dynamic executive level for application of knowledge (Anderson, 1985; Paul & Quigley, 1990).

METALINGUISTICS AND THE SCHOOL-AGE HEARING-IMPAIRED STUDENT

A child must have several levels of linguistic and nonlinguistic knowledge to communicate effectively. Knowledge of the rules for pragmatic, semantic, syntactic, morphologic, and phonologic use is necessary. This knowledge is reflected in comprehension and performance in communication. At another level, a child who has knowledge of these rules may discuss or reflect on language as a topic. This is metalinguistic function.

School language requires this metalinguistic competence for both spoken and written language. This level of awareness is critical because success in the academic setting can be summarized as school = language use, whether the task involves listening, speaking, or writing. Children are expected to function independently in the use of receptive language (listening, reading) and expressive language (speaking, writing) by the fourth grade in order to support learning in the content subjects (i.e., comprehend the language of math, history, and other subjects) (Laughton & Hasenstab, 1986).

School systems attempt to foster school language through language arts programs. Much of the categorical content addressed in such language arts programs may be appropriate for hearing-impaired students, but too often the programs neglect linguistic differences among children. They presuppose that all children have equal facility for mastering objectives. One child may appear to have a competent semantic-syntactic system and yet be unable to use that system in daily communication. Such a pragmatic problem will be reflected in the child's inability to accomplish communication goals. Another student may have phonological problems that mask difficulties in semantic, syntactic, and pragmatic performance. In this case, it will be necessary to probe beyond sound production. As children move through school, metalinguistic expectations increase. Students are no longer coached through the language learning process but are instead expected to use language to synthesize information and generalize new learning.

The key to understanding these individual patterns of cognition lies in processes of auditory learning, beginning long before birth and shaped and qualified during the formative years.

Auditory Learning

Auditory learning is the ability to use auditory information. It is a process that may actually begin around the 20th week of the prenatal period, once development of the auditory system is completed. Early studies and more recent evidence of fetal hearing (Birnholz & Bernacerraf, 1983; Elliot & Elliot, 1964; Johansson, Wedenberg, & Westin, 1964; Kuczwara, Birnholz, & Klodd, 1984) lead to the hypothesis that auditory experiences affect the unborn child's cognitive beginnings in the form of auditory percepts. By the time a child is born, he or she is able to make specific responses to auditory stimuli. For example, the newborn infant shows discriminatory abilities for suprasegmental features (Spring & Dale, 1977) and segmental aspects of speech (Eilers & Minifie, 1975; Eimas, 1975; Eimas & Tartter, 1979; Eisenberg, 1970, 1976; Morse, 1972). Neonates also demonstrate a preference for mother's voice and differentiate her voice from those of other females (DeCasper & Fifer, 1980). Auditory learning accelerates during infancy and early childhood. Normal auditory function permits auditory experiences that provide the child with auditory foundations necessary for the full development of cognition and spoken language.

Auditory learning involves the reception, processing, representation, recognition, and comprehension of sound. It emerges, in all its complexity, from experience with sound impinging on the auditory system. In addition, auditory learning is interactive with other sensory knowledge, and integration of sensory data helps create internal representations in the form of concepts and schema.

Auditory Processing

Once sound enters the auditory system (reception) it is analyzed and certain decisions are made regarding the specific parameters of the stimulus. This phase is auditory processing. Auditory processing is a continuum of analyses and decisions made by the auditory system about incoming auditory data (Hasenstab & Schoeny, 1982). Such analyses and decisions are interactive and interdependent and become more complex as auditory information "moves" through the system. Analytic errors and incorrect decisions at initial points will alter the entire processing composite. Discussion of analyses and resulting decisions follow (Hasenstab et al., in prep.; Hasenstab & Schoeny, 1982).

DETECTION

Awareness of the Acoustic Signal

Awareness of sound as opposed to silence is the first analysis and begins the processing of an auditory stimulus. This fundamental ability to distinguish sound from no sound is necessary for cognitive, linguistic, and psychological development (Ramsdell, 1970). Psychological implications stem from the notion that the auditory system, by virtue of its function as a monitoring system, creates a bridge between self and environmental reality (Sanders, 1977). The relationship of awareness of an auditory signal to cognitive and linguistic development is also important. Unless a child is aware that sound, whether environmental or linguistic, has occurred, ceased, or changed, higher levels of auditory processing cannot occur.

ATTENTION

Localization

Auditory attention requires a listener to prioritize and follow the growing pattern of auditory information over a period of time. Localization of sound is crucial to all attending behavior. Localization, or search behavior, relates a listener to the sound source. Once a child is aware of a sound and has made a decision that it is salient, there is motivation to determine the sound origin. Localization then is the initial step in attending analyses and links detection to more complex decisions within the processing continuum. In addition, sound localization forms the basis for decisions about figure-ground relationships and intensive concentration on the source of the stimulus.

Selective Attention

Selective attention, based on localization of sound, separates and prioritizes an auditory stimulus from other sounds within the environment. This is also called signal-to-noise perception, and based on an analysis about the importance of a particular sound, the signal becomes a figure against the background of all other sounds occurring at the same time. The auditory system is constantly bombarded with auditory stimuli. To process effectively, some priority must be established in attending behavior. It is at this point that listening occurs.

Sustained Attention

A sustaining function establishes the optimal condition of eliminating interfering stimuli in order to devote the system to the target auditory experience. Time is the essential component in sustained attention. The duration of sustained attention is usually referred to as "attention span" and is vital for focus on relevant information. The length of required attention depends on the nature of the stimulus. The importance of attention analyses and decisions lies in the fact that if information is unattended it cannot be recognized, interpreted, remembered, or applied (Garwood, 1979).

DISCRIMINATION

Auditory Differentiation

Auditory discrimination is commonly defined as the ability to distinguish between phonemes but actually constitutes the ability to make a distinction between all forms of auditory patterns. The critical analyses and decisions for differentiation of auditory input into broad categories, such as linguistic or nonlinguistic sounds, are made in this phase of the processing continuum. The listener determines aspects of a sound as meaningful versus nonmeaningful, speech versus nonspeech, and linguistic versus nonlinguistic. This processing component is the foundation for later discrimination decisions that assist in interpretation of incoming acoustic information, relevant to spoken language. A substantial amount of evidence exists indicating that speech linguistic sounds are perceived and interpreted in the left hemisphere of the cerebral cortex (Gazzanega, 1967; Geschwind, 1972; Kimura, 1961; Lenneberg, 1967). Other sounds, such as music, are processed and interpreted in the right hemisphere (Molfese, 1973). Thus, auditory differentiation is crucial to developing cognitive and communication behaviors in young children.

Acoustic Differentiation

Acoustic differentiation is necessary in determining parameters in auditory patterns. It is generally included in all listings of subcomponents of auditory processing. Differentiation between auditory patterns is based on perceptual variables, such as length, complexity, rate, structure, temporal relationships, frequency, and intensity. Acoustic differentiation permits discrimination with respect to each perceptual variable. This phase is complex and interdependent with the other discrimination analyses. Actual discrimination can take place only when the auditory pattern is compared with an internal model and categorized according to acoustic parameters.

Suprasegmental Discrimination

Suprasegmental discrimination or prosodic distinction is the analysis of pattern variation in spoken language. Pattern variations include the intonation contours of sentences and the emotive cues carried by pitch and stress variations. There is a close developmental relationship between this ability and the acquisition of pragmatics, phonology, and syntax. Suprasegmental feature discrimination in English is based on phrase, word, and syllable stress; tone or pitch variation; intonation contour or the pattern of rhythmic stress across an utterance; and timing factors such as pauses indicating word boundaries.

Segmental Discrimination

While suprasegmental discrimination concerns features that provide "quality" to speech or vocalization, segmental discrimination focuses on the differentiation of phoneme patterns. Language components of morphology and phonology, and ultimately semantics, are dependent on this discrimination analysis. The mutual interaction of suprasegmental features and phonemic aspects signals the linguistic rules that make speech meaningful to a listener.

ORGANIZATION

Auditory Retention

The concept of auditory memory receives much attention. An auditory stimulus occurs over time, and therefore, acoustic information must be held or stored as it is analyzed. The stimulus pattern is organized into units or "chunks" of information that can be reorganized and then processed cognitively and linguistically. The function of "chunking" information into units allows restructuring into larger and larger meaningful units within the capacity of the system, thereby increasing the potential of establishing continuity of input for eventual use. Retention capacity for adults is usually considered to be approximately seven units (plus or minus two) (Miller, 1956). The way in which information can be chunked depends on previous experience and requires recognition of recurrent patterns and associations of stimuli that can be redefined into more and more complex units of information. Through the chunking process, phonemes can be grouped into words, words into phrases or sentence components, and finally, sentence patterns.

Auditory Sequencing

Auditory sequencing meshes with auditory retention and specifies seriation or order of components in patterns. This is an important factor in determining meaning. It is closely related to structural rules of sentence formation. As children develop, normal shifts or reversals may be seen in word pronunciation or word order in sentences. However, persistence of these language restrictions in school-age children indicates language-processing problems (Aten, 1974). Sequencing problems can also be noted for nonlinguistic auditory stimuli. Memory behavior in this context is immediate recall for sequenced, patterned information.

Auditory Synthesis

As auditory information is received, blending or synthesis must occur. Auditory synthesis is necessary for the acoustic event to be relevant. Synthesis merges information and allows total pattern presentation for cognitive activity so that interpretation, application, comprehension, and information storage can occur. It is the summation of all processing decisions.

Auditory Representation

Auditory representation may be likened to a "picture" of a sound as it corresponds to the actual event. For example, a fire engine is represented by a siren (the sound). Children's early representations of objects, actions, and events are reflected in their imitative production of sound characteristics (sound = object). The more accurate the match between auditory reality and how it is internally represented, the better a child can function within the auditory milieu. Effective and efficient auditory learning depends on how well the auditory system is able to maintain the reality of the sound stimulus in the formation of concepts and schema.

Auditory Recognition

Recognition is knowing the sound; that is, the sound has meaning. Recognition requires a reference and is therefore based on representation. At beginning stages of auditory learning, recognition is not coupled with sound labels (next section). The sound is familiar enough for the child to attach meaning (i.e., mother's voice) even though he or she does not linguistically label it as such. Recognition depends on auditory differentiation analyses and decisions.

Auditory Symbolization and Comprehension

Hearing is the primary input modality in the development of spoken language. It is the avenue for the reception and processing of the auditory verbal language code. The sound must first be received, processed, represented, and recognized. But, spoken language also requires additional facets of auditory learning. Spoken language is an arbitrary code composed of various acoustic properties that in turn make up symbols (words) that are assigned meaning by a certain society or culture. One must be able to interpret and comprehend the code. Symbols are paired with their referents and thereby become meaningful. The linguistic symbols are thus interpreted to stand for reality and the "pictured" representation that exists cognitively. Comprehension has taken place when symbols themselves have meaning.

Deficits in Auditory Learning

Early research by Myklebust (1954) and Furth (1961) suggested that concept formation and representation strategies could be significantly altered by deficits in auditory capabilities. Restrictions and auditory fragmentation or inconsistencies in the input of auditory information, especially over time, can alter both the quantity and quality of auditory learning and thus affect cognition and language (Hasenstab, 1987).

A breakdown in any phase of auditory experience will interrupt or inhibit auditory learning. A hearing-impaired child, as a result of hearing loss, has a breakdown at the reception or acuity level. The extent of the hearing loss will affect the quality of processing analyses and decisions. If there is insufficient received "data" to be analyzed, representation does not occur; thus, auditory recognition is not possible because there is no true representation of the auditory reality. Learning for a hearing-impaired child develops with partial or absent sound characteristics. They simply do not exist. A child with an auditory-processing deficit has normal acuity. However, the system is not able to effectively analyze and make decisions regarding incoming and auditory stimuli. Incorrect decisions alter the quality of the auditory reality; therefore, information that is represented can be fragmented, inconsistent, or modified in some way. The result is that concepts and schema may be intact according to other sensory parameters but be inaccurate relative to auditory aspects. An auditory-processing deficit is most critical in its effect on a child's linguistic system. Faulty processing prohibits accurate symbolization, interpretation, and code comprehension. The extent of an auditory-processing deficit will govern the limitations imposed on a child's cognitive and linguistic capabilities.

Evaluating Auditory Learning

The evaluation of effective and efficient auditory learning in school-age children is a complex endeavor. A single test administered by one professional will not accomplish the task. Since auditory learning is a child's ability to use auditory information, evaluation of this capacity must encompass how this use operates in communication, academic areas, classroom function, and other daily life contexts. Even a child with normal hearing may pass an auditory-processing test battery administered by an audiologist and still display auditory-based deficits in academic areas and listening behavior in school. Tests are not perfect in design or format, and they are administered in contrived settings. They frequently fail to reflect real-life listening situations that children encounter daily. Comprehensive evaluation of children with suspected hearing deficits in auditory learning should include audiological and psychoeducational testing, in-depth communication analyses, and careful observation of auditory behavior in school and at home.

Auditory Learning and Children with Cochlear Implants

A new population of hearing-impaired children is entering school programs—children with cochlear implants (CI). Over 800 children between 2 and 17 years of age have received the Nucleus multichannel device. These numbers will continue to increase now that the Food and Drug Administration (FDA) has approved the use of the device in children as of June 1990.

Children with cochlear implants are far from homogeneous. Although there are specific criteria that designate candidacy for a CI (Northern et al., 1986), children vary with regard to age, onset of hearing loss, etiology, specific cognitive and communication abilities, home settings, and school experiences.

Young children with cochlear implants generally fall into three categories (Hasenstab, 1989):

Postlinguistically deafened children who lose their hearing after age 3 years, who have developed foundations of the auditory linguistic code, and who receive implants soon after the onset of deafness

Prelinguistically deafened children who lose their hearing before age 3 years and should have not fully developed foundations of the auditory linguistic code

Children who have profound congenital hearing loss

Two additional groups of school-age children also exist:

Children with progressive hearing loss

Postlinguistically deafened children who received implants 2 or more years following the onset of hearing loss

Changes in auditory learning are evident in children using cochlear implants (Staller, 1991). The first change is reception capacity. Audiograms reflect improvement in acuity levels and Speech Awareness Thresholds (SATs) as reflected in the audiograms in Figure 7.1. The initial impact on auditory processing is at detection level for most children. But children with postlinguistically acquired hearing loss or progressive deafness or those who have developed some auditory skills with amplification systems show better initial performance for attention and discrimination analyses.

Children with cochlear implants do not become children with normal auditory systems. They have developed to the age when they received their CI according to the operative function of their pre-CI auditory systems: That is, cognitive and linguistic status is a result of their prior auditory experiences. New auditory experience must be integrated into existing formal representations that have already been established and have meaning for the child. This requires relearning. Previous formats are no longer correct based on new realities.

Children with cochlear implants should be monitored carefully for changes

SUBJECT A

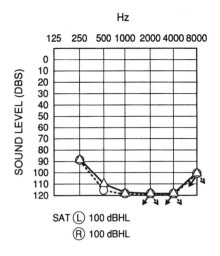

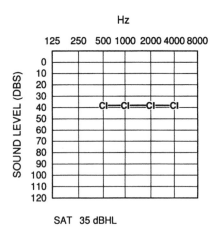

SUBJECT B

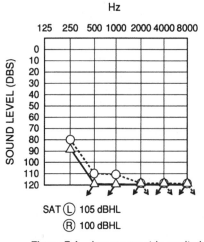

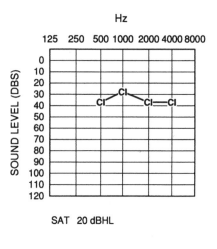

Figure 7.1. Improvement in acuity levels and SATs, for subjects A, B, C, and D.

in their auditory capabilities. However, audiological testing alone will not reflect auditory learning. In-depth communication analyses and evaluation of academic performance and cognitive strategies will indicate how the availability of new auditory experiences affect the child. Audi-tory learning is the ability to use auditory information; therefore, use becomes the focus of evaluation. Many of the same assessment tools used with other hearing-impaired students will be used with children who have cochlear implants to evaluate their abilities.

SUBJECT C

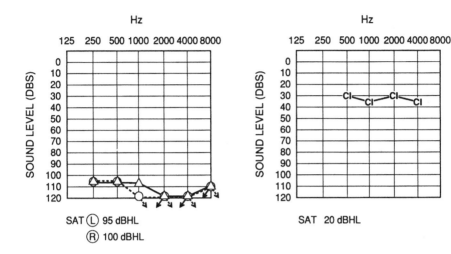

SUBJECT D

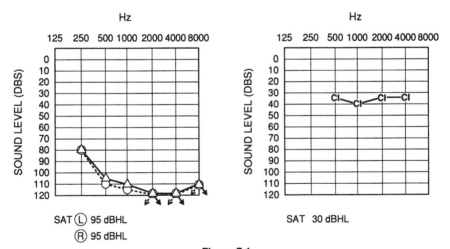

Figure 7.1

Auditory Learning/Processing and Hearing Impairment

It is axiomatic that learning language through the auditory channel results in a different kind of processing system than does any kind of visual language learning. Furthermore, the tools are now available to ensure auditory learning for most hearing-impaired children. More and more hearing-impaired children are receiving cochlear implants, and yet, like the complex amplification systems before CI, benefits may be denied by failure on the part of professionals to maximize use of the auditory channel. Whether the amplification costs $1500 or $25,000, failure to acknowledge that hearing-impaired children, like their hearing counterparts, also come with learning style preferences—including auditory preferences—renders amplification useless.

Auditory learning represents a continuum of auditory experience from detection through understanding as well as the ability to use the experience in some way (e.g., response by action, response by communication, data for concept/schema development, memory). Auditory learning requires the integrity and interface of sound detection, auditory processing, and cognition. A breakdown at any of these levels will interfere with or inhibit auditory learning. A hearing-impaired child, because of the presence of hearing loss, is affected by a breakdown at the level of detection. The degree of inhibition depends on the degree and profile of hearing loss. This is a quantity deficit. Hearing loss also exerts a qualitative deficit by restricting the ability to process auditory information accurately or efficiently. The result is that what data, if any, finally reach cognitive levels are fragmented and not a true representation of auditory experience.

Learning for hearing-impaired children is organized with partial or no sound characteristics. Hearing does not function as a fully operative avenue for learning. Deaf children are not aware that objects, actions, and events have auditory characteristics. Auditory representation at cognitive levels is necessary if children are to use auditory information. Auditory representation may be likened to a picture of a sound as it corresponds to the actual event in the environment. For example, a siren, auditorily represented, is a fire engine.

Furthermore, the ability to deal with spoken language requires a more sophisticated level of representation. A child must be able to interpret auditory information, specifically the acoustics of speech or the spoken language code, to symbolize the actual event in the environment. Thus, the spoken word, fire engine, represents the real thing (Hasenstab et al., in progress). Hearing-impaired children construct meaning, but the absence or restriction of auditory input caused by hearing loss inhibits the coding of meaning according to the rule systems for the linguistic components of spoken language.

Success in school and the weight of rehabilitation rest on a complex of interactive child- and school-centered variables that must be considered to facilitate auditory learning.

Child-Centered Variables

One of the primary variables that must be considered in planning rehabilitation for hearing-impaired children is, of course, the nature and extent of hearing loss. Factors such as degree of hearing loss, age of onset, amplification use, previous instruction, and etiology are pertinent for decisions regarding assessment and intervention. However, the hearing-impaired child is more than a set of ears that do not function to full capacity. Other variables specific to each individual child include:

Other sensory avenues	(especially vision, which is important for speech-reading, learning strategies that require spatial processing, reading)
Additional handicaps	(for example, a learning disability that combines with hearing loss to produce a more complicated processing problem)
Personality factors	(motivation, independence, self-esteem)
Learning styles	(some hearing-impaired children are able to use auditory information despite limitations imposed by hearing loss, as do hearing auditory learners)
Communication model	(what, when, how consistent)
Use of amplification	(what, when, how consistent)
Educational history	(school-age children bring baggage of earlier educational experiences, including setting, methodologies, extent, etc.)
Family factors	(parental attitudes, support, ability of the family to comply with what is necessary for the child)

Life factors   (access to services, environmental issues)

All of these variables interact to produce varying degrees and patterns of readiness for the social and academic challenges of school.

School Context Variables

More and more hearing-impaired children find themselves mainstreamed into regular classroom settings, rather than in schools for the deaf, as in the past (Moores, 1991). Although this could be an opportunity, without comprehensive services—that is, ongoing assessment and intervention—the picture not only is bleak but is an apt metaphor for the splintered worldview that may be constructed in the absence of auditory language. For example, speech therapy two times a week for 30 minutes is an exercise in futility unless integrated into a total curriculum for school-age hearing-impaired children. Without interested follow-up across the environment, it not only fails to provide any real speech training but leaves the child with yet another absurd reality to integrate into a meaningful whole.

Unfortunately, educational intervention and habilitation for hearing-impaired children are often a compromise of what is needed to optimize a child's cognitive and auditory abilities and what actually is available through the educational agency. Options vary from state to state and from school system to school system. All options are not available to all hearing-impaired children in all settings. If they were, appropriate placement would be relatively easy. However, this is not the rule. A child may attend a residential school or a day school for hearing-impaired children because there is nothing else available and not because the child requires that type of programming. Another child may receive only speech services or itinerant programming even though more intensive educational support is required, simply because such programming is all there is in the child's school system. For many hearing-impaired children, there is only one option. That option may or may not have any relationship to actual educational needs. Hearing-im-

paired children in rural areas or smaller communities or in areas without regionalized programs may be especially affected by this lack of alternatives. Generally, more populated areas present a wider continuum of services. The role of the rehabilitation specialist includes acting as an advocate for the student's receipt of all services to which he or she is entitled. Some school context variables to consider are:

Placement options   (residential school, day school, public school resource)

Support services   (speech services, language therapy, counseling, learning disabilities or other resources if additional handicaps are present)

Competencies of professionals   (teacher preparation and experience, counseling, and other competencies)

School philosophy   (general attitude toward education, toward special education, and toward hearing-impaired children)

Curricula   (regular education or specifically for hearing impaired, availability of instructional/learning materials)

Access   (to all facilities and materials available to hearing students)

The assessment process is largely a reflection and definition of the interplay of child and school variables for each individual student.

Assessment

A comprehensive assessment is essential to implement effective rehabilitation or instruction. Such an assessment must include analysis of the various contexts that constitute the child's world, as well as a complete description of the child's language, speech, and communication systems used for learning in and out of school.

As Simeonsson (1987, pp. 195–96) aptly observes about testing hearing-impaired children, "Their characteristics and needs cannot be adequately approached through traditional assessment practices. Any attempt to evaluate hearing-impaired children, therefore, mandates a thorough understanding of the methodological and procedural elements necessary to maximize the validity of assessment with this group."

The primary purpose of assessment of school-age students is to determine the nature and extent of the child's disability so that appropriate intervention and education can follow. Assessment includes formal testing, use of informal measures, and review of case history and current performance in school and other social settings. The repertoire of formal tests, with specific guidelines to administer, score, and interpret results, is sparse with respect to inclusion of hearing-impaired students in the standardization sample. These tests are norm-referenced; that is, they have a normative group for comparing a student's performance, and they yield several types of scores providing information about a student's performance relative to other students. Informal testing is often less structured and is used to determine present performance levels, student progress, and changes subsequent to direct instruction (McLoughlin & Lewis, 1990). Group and individual testing is common for hearing students, whereas individual testing is more likely necessary for hearing-impaired students. The five major purposes for assessment or administration of tests are:

1. Screening
2. Placement
3. Program planning
4. Program evaluation
5. Monitoring of individual progress (Salvia & Ysseldyke, 1988)

These purposes are valid for assessment of the performance of hearing-impaired students across communicative, language, speech, and psychoeducational domains. Assessment is necessary to extract information regarding a child's educational and auditory habilitation. Ongoing assessment provides parents and professionals with a fund of new information to expand and alter the child's program to nurture development.

GUIDELINES FOR ASSESSMENT RIGHTS

Public Law 94–142 provides clear guidelines regarding assessment of individuals with disabilities; these guidelines are relevant to the assessment of hearing-impaired individuals. Assessment must be nondiscriminatory. To that end assessment tools (tests) must be free from cultural or racial bias, must be administered in the student's language, and must not discriminate on the basis of the student's handicap. Assessment should be comprehensive and multidisciplinary and should focus on the student's specific educational needs. A single measure may not be the only basis for special educational placement, and no area of educational performance may be omitted. While hearing-impaired students may be eligible for educational services based solely on their hearing loss, they are entitled to a comprehensive evaluation that should include vision, intelligence, academic performance, communicative status, social/emotional status, motor abilities, and health.

The team of professionals evaluating the hearing-impaired student's performance should include at least one individual knowledgeable about hearing impairment. Assessment tools must be technically sound (valid and reliable) and administered by appropriately trained and experienced professionals. This may be a problematic area within the public school systems. Generally, the school psychologist and diagnostic team responsible for administration of intelligence and achievement tests have limited experience in testing significantly hearing-impaired students (Gibbins, 1989). The final aspect of assessment with respect to PL 94–142 involves rights: informed consent of parents, right to annual evaluation of progress, and reevaluation every 3 years. Most important, no student will be placed in special education unless a comprehensive assessment including evaluation of educational needs has occurred (McLoughlin & Lewis, 1990).

Communication Assessment

The assessment of a school-age student's communication performance should include language, speech, and sign language (if used). Ying (1990) describes the components of a communication evaluation as including:

1. Reception (replicate the real-life background noise expected in school settings in addition to usual audiometric testing)
2. Comprehension (include evaluation of the amount of contextual support required for understanding within classroom settings)
3. Production (acquire from spontaneous and elicited language samples)
4. Intelligibility (evaluate across increasingly complex language contexts)
5. Conversational competence (acquire from a diversity of conversational contexts)
6. Written language (acquire for analysis along with interpersonal language samples)

These areas are all critical for effective functioning in the academic mainstream. A criterion-referenced checklist that identifies the child's communication function that can be used very easily and effectively in school settings is the *Kendall Communicative Proficiency Scale* (in Thompson et al., 1987). The primary modalities used in communication should be evaluated. These include sign language readiness and proficiency, speech, and simultaneous use of sign and speech.

ASSESSMENT OF SIGN LANGUAGE PROFICIENCY

Few specific measures are available to assess this component of a school-age hearing-impaired student's functioning. However, a rating of readiness and/or proficiency should be a part of the comprehensive evaluation for those students who use or may potentially use some form of sign language. A typical assessment includes measures of:

1. Manual dexterity and ability to form the handshapes required for signing
2. Receptive recognition and expressive performance of signs (Johnson, 1988)

Some schools for deaf students such as Kendall Elementary and the Atlanta Area School for the Deaf have developed informal assessment tools for this purpose. Such tests as the *Carolina Picture Vocabulary Test* are useful receptive measures of picture sign recognition. Many of the language tests developed specifically for hearing-impaired students recommend in their directions the use of signed or spoken language in presenting the items to the student being evaluated.

Characteristics of Speech

The landmark study of speech characteristics of deaf and severely hearing-impaired students was conducted by Hudgins and Numbers (1942). Their findings indicated a pervasive impact of hearing impairment on all aspects of speech production. More current investigations, including those conducted by Markides (1967, 1980), are consistent with earlier studies and show the following customary errors:

Vowels
1. Vowel substitution
2. Vowel neutralization (substitution of schwa for vowel)
3. Vowel prolongation
4. Vowel diphthongization
5. Diphthong errors (prolongation or neutralization)

Consonants
1. Consonant omission
2. Consonant substitution
3. Consonant distortion

Suprasegmental
1. Intonation
2. Phrasing
3. Pausing
4. Rate
5. Breath control
6. Stress
7. Loudness control
8. Pitch control
9. Voice quality

Ling (1976, 1989) notes the consistency in speech errors in respiration, phonation, rate, prosody, and vowel and consonant production.

Assessment of Speech

Assessment of speech can begin in infancy and should be continued throughout the student's academic career. After early evaluation of speech skills, many deaf students are proclaimed "oral failures" and never receive quality speech instruction again. Speech is probably the area that is most neglected in the rehabilitative process. Planning and conducting a speech development program with hearing-impaired students requires understanding of speech acoustics and the specific results of hearing evaluation. While professionals frequently support total communication strategies, they often pay only lip service to speech development unless they are committed to oral education. This is truly a disadvantage for the profoundly hearing-impaired student because any use of speech provides clues to communicative partners to improve intelligibility. Speech intervention is difficult, requires incredible consistency and creativity, and is misunderstood by many professionals working with hearing-impaired students.

Assessment of speech at any age should include evaluation of speech intelligibility (sentence and longer spoken segments), word production, syllable production, single phone productions, and underlying prerequisites. Ling (1976, 1989) has prepared an organized and comprehensive program for speech assessment. The rationale for using the procedure and specific directions are provided within the Ling program.

Assessment precursors to developing a speech program include:

1. Examination of the audiogram
2. Evaluation using the Ling Five-Sound Test
3. Use of audiometric and Ling Five-Sound responses to hypothesize what is audible to the student
4. Arrangement for the best possible amplification for the child
5. Phonetic evaluation to determine the repertoire of sound production available to the student
6. Phonologic evaluation to determine the word, phrase, sentence, and conversational production skills of the student

The first step is careful examination of the audiogram to hypothesize which components of speech fall within the various octave bands paralleling the audiometric frequencies 125 to 8000 Hz. Analysis of the audiogram includes pure-tone frequency-specific information, aided responses to pure tones and speech, immitance results, and word recognition. The professional's sensitivity to what is likely to be audible to a student is crucial to developing a speech program for that child. Ling (1989) describes the speech components associated with audiometric frequencies 125 to 8000 Hz. Ling also discusses the concept of the CLEAR zone (conversational level elements in the acoustic range) of speech, which is critical to consider prior to beginning speech work. The child's hearing levels and the effects of amplification on the various intensity levels of speech received dictate appropriate earmold selection to make all significant components of speech detectable to the child (Ling, 1989, p. 69).

The Ling Five-Sound test is conducted simply using the /a, u, i, ʃ, s/ sounds, which represent the speech range acoustic information represented on the audiogram with the amplification used by the child. The test involves repeating the five sounds to the child and requesting a hand raise or spoken imitation of each of the sounds at increasing distances away from the child. This very simple test can be useful in validating the audiometric findings, in checking the hearing aid, and in the early identification of middle ear pathology. Additionally, it is useful as a hearing test for very young children or multihandicapped children who may not respond to pure-tone or speech testing in the more formal situation.

The major stages of speech acquisition described by Ling (1976, 1989) occur at phonetic and phonologic levels. Evaluation of the student's performance is conducted at each level. The phonetic level evaluated via the Phonetic Level Evaluation (Ling, 1976) includes:

1. Vocalization freely and on demand
2. Suprasegmental patterns (intensity, pitch, duration)
3. Voice control of all vowels and diphthongs
4. Manner contrasts of consonants with all vowels

5. Place contrasts of consonants with all vowels
6. Voicing contrasts of consonants with all vowels
7. Initial and final consonant blends

The phonologic evaluation uses the Phonologic Level Evaluation (Ling, 1976) and includes analogous meaningful components:

1. Vocalization as a means of communication
2. Meaningful voice patterns
3. Vowel use for word approximation
4. Voice patterns used with word production
5. Voice patterns for phrases
6. Voice patterns for sentences
7. Intelligible speech with natural voice patterns

Ling (1989) presents a hierarchy of speech acquisition that must be evaluated prior to speech program planning. After assessment a speech development plan is implemented. Ling differentiates between informal learning facilitation, which focuses on speech play for more naturalistic development of speech, and formal teaching with prompted production of specific speech targets. Both emphases are discussed in the Intervention section of this chapter.

Limited attention has been given to evaluating phonologic simplification processes of hearing-impaired students. This is a linguistic approach based in evaluation of whole words. Hearing-impaired students' phonologic processes may be evaluated using processes developed for hearing students such as the *Assessment of Phonological Processes* (Hodson, 1986) or the *Khan-Lewis Phonological Analysis* (Khan & Lewis, 1986).

Characteristics of Language

The general language learning characteristics have been reported since earliest times; however, it is only within the past 20 years that detailed descriptions of the language systems of profoundly hearing-impaired students have been compiled. The detailed longitudinal studies of the syntactic system done by Quigley and his associates have provided a base for current detailed descriptions of other language component use. Language research has been hampered by difficulties in research design, subject heterogeneity, and small numbers (Laughton & Jacobs, 1982). Additionally, because of communication differences and difficulties, much previous research was conducted by analyzing written rather than interpersonal (spoken or signed) language use.

Table 7.1 briefly summarizes the recent pragmatic, semantic, and morphologic findings of profoundly hearing-impaired children. Studies of pragmatic aspects have focused on interactions between children and a small number of adults. Early communicative intents appear to be similar to hearing children, although there may be less use of information-seeking intentional behavior. Register changes for various conversational partners appear to be intact. Conversational exchanges are not well developed. Reception and expression of clarification or repair during conversational interactions appear to reflect some differences.

Semantic development is characterized by vocabulary deficits that have been well documented. Hearing-impaired students develop vocabulary later and at a slower rate. Later they have fewer lexical items and continue to have difficulty with functional word meaning and content words. Deficits remain into adulthood. Some disagreement exists about whether there is delay in onset of semantic relations. Morphologic development has not been studied extensively, but a similar sequence of markers, with the exception of present progressive and plural markers, has been noted.

The syntactic system has been studied in greater detail. The findings of Quigley and associates (e.g., Quigley & Paul, 1984; Russell, Power, & Quigley, 1976) suggest development of the phrase structure rules by age 10 years, although as many as 30 to 40% do not achieve full use of the determiner or auxiliary systems by age 18. As contrasted, hearing students have fairly complete comprehension and production of the base of language by 7 or 8 years. Profoundly hearing-impaired students continue to have difficulty with passive structures (processing with a Subject + Verb + Object strat-

---

Table 7.1
Language Characteristics of Deaf Children

PRAGMATIC

Interaction between adults/children

Mothers (hearing) of deaf speak less with atypical intonation; give less verbal praise; use more tutorial strategies (Gross, 1970)

Mothers are more dominant and use more directives (Weddell-Monig & Lumley, 1980)

Mothers are more inflexible, controlling, didactic, disapproving (Schlesinger & Meadow, 1972)

Intents

Early communicative intents of HI exposed to oral language similar to normal hearing (Curtis, Prutting, & Lowell, 1979)

No relation of intents to communicative mode found (Greenberg, 1980)

HI (signing) show less use of heuristic or informative intents (Pien, 1985)

Conversational exchanges

Use attention-getting statements rather than simple comments about topics to enter conversations (McKirdy & Blank, 1982)

TDD topic establishment left up to adult (Johnson & Barton, 1988)

Difficulty in deciding when to enter a conversation (Brackett & Donnelly, 1982)

Clarification

HI tend to repeat rather than revise (Donnelly & Brackett, 1982)

Much delayed in responses to requests for clarification; use many nonlinguistic forms of clarification requests (Laughton, 1982–1990)

Register changes

HI child can adjust to various registers of parents by 13 months (Blennerhassett, 1984)

Preschool HI adapt registers to three different adult registers (Small, 1985)

SEMANTIC

Vocabulary

HI had 0–9 words by 18 months compared to 20–50 for hearing; similar kinds of words; TC children more vocabulary than OC (Schafer & Lynch, 1980)

By age 18 years have fourth grade reading vocabulary (DiFrancesca, 1972)

Semantic relations

Delay in onset of two-word utterances according to some investigators; others disagree; do have same sequence (Goldin-Meadow & Feldman, 1975; Skarakis & Prutting, 1977)

MORPHOLOGIC

Similar sequence to hearing with reverse development of -ing and -s (Gilman & Raffin, 1975; Raffin, Davis, & Gilman, 1978)

---

egy), relative clauses, question forms, conjunctions, and complementation into early adulthood. Pronominalization and negation are acquired in a similar sequence to hearing students but at a much slower rate.

Similarities in development of English after development of another language base give support to the ESL issue discussed earlier in this chapter. The significance of these findings illustrates the mismatch between the language systems used by profoundly hearing-impaired students and the language expectations of the school context.

Assessment of Language

It is clear that the language of hearing-impaired students is characterized by disruptions in learning across pragmatic, semantic, syntactic, and morphologic components. Assessment of hearing-impaired students' language functioning is within the purview of the speech language pathologist, who must be knowledgeable about expected language acquisition during the school-age years. (For excellent information about school-age language see Bernstein & Tiegerman, 1989; Nippold, 1988; and Ripich & Spinelli, 1985.) The language performance of profoundly hearing-impaired students has been an area of concern since the origins of their education. Recent assessment has centered about the use of naturalistic language sample analysis and the development of language tests where none existed previously. Analysis procedures have been detailed by Kretschmer and Kretschmer (1978, 1988, 1989) and others (Thompson et al., 1987). Although early approaches followed the structured or naturalistic approaches used for teaching, more recent attempts have observed the pragmatic, semantic, syntactic, morphologic, and phonologic system integration of hearing-impaired students. Additionally, several tests similar to those used for hearing students have emerged.

The comprehensive assessment of language must include all aspects of all contexts in which the child uses language (including the teacher, the curriculum, and the learning context), as well as a complete description of the student's language system (pragmatic, semantic, morphologic, syntactic, phonologic). Hearing-impaired children are similar to hearing students with language learning disruptions in that they tend to move from acting as communicative language users, trying to satisfy basic intents, to metalinguistic language users, using language to learn. Some hearing-impaired students never move successfully into the metalinguistic domain.

The "pragmatics revolution" of the 1980s (Duchan, 1988) has had a significant impact on language assessment. Much of what we know about language and how it is used has come from observing children using language in naturalistic settings. The clinician must understand normal language acquisition in order to assess the language use, content, and form of students with hearing impairment. The major assessment questions are:

1. How does the student use language to communicate in a variety of contexts? (communicative)
2. How does the student use language to learn? (metalinguistic)
3. What are the regularities in the child's language performance?
4. What are the areas that need repair?

Answers to the assessment questions may be obtained by:

1. Description of the student's language system via language sample analysis
2. Expansion of the sampled contexts with information gleaned via language tests
3. Description of the language contexts in which the student uses language

Many tests are available for hearing students to sample parts of the language system. Few exist for the hearing-impaired student. (Included in Appendix 7.1 is a list of language tests appropriate for hearing-impaired students with indication of those developed specifically for this population.) Caution is recommended in the administration of tests because of *(1)* ample documentation of poor performance by hearing-impaired students on all types of standardized tests and *(2)* the need to engage in pragmatic violations to select the correct answer on a test (Laughton & Ray, 1982; Ray, 1989). To perform successfully on most tests, a student must be metalinguistic.

Factors to consider in test administration are:

1. Rate of stimuli input and response
2. Type of input and expected response
3. Testing conditions (distractions—visual, auditory, linguistic)
4. Directions that are clear and unambiguous
5. Context that is communicative or decontextualized

The language assessment procedures described here are appropriate for students using primarily oral or total communication instruction, and there will be no specific differentiation. Coding of information for students using signed and spoken language will follow the convention described by Johnson (1988), in which all of the language and nonlinguistic information is recorded and the modality is indicated by S (speech), I (sign), or C (combined).

NATURALISTIC SETTINGS

For nearly 30 years, low structured observation has remained a favored method for the study of language. Low structured observation occurs in natural social contexts with familiar people. It is relaxed and allows the child to choose the topics. The assumption is that nonobtrusive sampling will yield the most representative language sample, unlike language tests or even more structured elicitation techniques (Lund & Duchan, 1983). Some structures such as requests may be more effectively elicited via structured elicitation techniques (Lund & Duchan, 1988).

Curriculum-based assessment (CBA) procedures provide a naturalistic school setting necessary for the school-age hearing-impaired student. This method focuses on assessment of the school language contexts as well as the student's language system before moving into intervention and literacy. The language of instruction involves learning to read and write language, talk about language, use language to learn how to do things, and use language to learn about other things. CBA uses progress in the curriculum of the local school as a measure of success in language as well as education (Nelson, 1989). This type of assessment focuses on the type of oral and written skills required by the curriculum in contrast with the skills and strategies exhibited by the student. The expected skills for future acquisition and modification in curricular expectations are a part of this type of evaluation.

Many prelingually hearing-impaired students of school age do not master the English syntactic or lexical system because of insufficient exposure auditorily. Evaluation of their abilities is analogous to English speakers taking a psychological test in Chinese after very limited study of the language. The psychological test becomes a test of language rather than one of cognitive or learning ability. During language evaluation the examiner is concerned with the child as a language user within the communication world.

Historically, language assessment of the hearing-impaired students has been accomplished rather informally by their teachers. Until recently no tests other than informal, teacher-constructed tests were available for hearing-impaired students. However, during the 1980s, with the advent of a return to language sampling in naturalistic settings and global analysis of the language used in a variety of settings by professionals working with hearing children, these formats began to be used with hearing-impaired students as well. Also, several language tests were developed to specifically address concerns about testing these children. Included among the tests developed are several tests similar to the battery for hearing children (e.g., Test of Expressive Language Ability and Test of Receptive Language Ability) and several innovative models designed to specifically address the needs of hearing-impaired children (deVilliers, 1988; Moog & Geers, 1980, 1985).

LANGUAGE SAMPLE PROCEDURES

Currently the practice of language sample analysis combined with test-oriented procedures is used to provide a picture of language functioning subsequent to language intervention. Evaluation for school-age students has become more discourse oriented, with the major discourse types being narratives (spoken or written), conversations, event descriptions, and school lessons (Lund & Duchan, 1988).

Lund and Duchan (1988) propose a "child-centered pragmatics framework" for analyzing language samples of hearing students. This involves reorganization of pragmatic, semantic, morphologic, and syntactic analysis into a pragmatic perspective that includes sensemaking, functions, and fine-tuning.

Sensemaking describes the child's sense of an event (event analysis) and asks about the student's understanding of common events rather than language knowledge. Included in event analysis are:

1. Scripts of action (events such as trips to the zoo)
2. Frames of discourse events (talking events such as conversation about zoo trip)

The procedure for analysis includes:

1. Identifying the beginning and end of events
2. Determining the child's idea of an event frame
3. Identifying the tightness of the frame
4. Determining the compatibility between partners
5. Identifying successful contexts and turns

Functionalism interprets what communicators want to achieve via their communication. This analysis includes:

1. Participant's agenda or what each wants to achieve
2. Formulation of intents (speech acts)
3. Execution of intents and agenda

Fine-tuning involves the sensitivity of the communicative partners to each others' comprehension and includes:

1. Contingency analysis
2. Interaction mode analysis (directiveness/nurturance; motherese)

This procedure is very appropriate for hearing-impaired students as detailed by Duchan (1988). The assessment procedures should include:

1. Preassessment
2. Family interview
3. Observation of child in naturalistic contexts
4. Deep testing of structure not observed in sample

5. Analyzing for structures

The language sample analysis procedure provides examples of language functioning in several settings. The sampling procedure is helpful in observing the child's move from one linguistic phase to another. Language samples from naturalistic and more structured or contrived settings provide the data. Ongoing samples provide reliability data, that is, whether any single sample is representative of the student's language knowledge and whether usage differs with contexts. The number of utterances necessary for language sample analysis is relative to the language learning level and context (Lund & Duchan, 1988). While 50 utterances have frequently been offered as appropriate, we know clinically that young hearing-impaired children may not generate 50 utterances within several settings. With older students the 50 utterances may be easily obtained, but more utterances will reflect flexibility (or lacks), as well as changes within the utterances contingent on pragmatic demands. For example, single-word utterances may be common when the examiner asks consecutive questions of the child, but longer utterances may occur when a child is engaged in event description. The specific utterances and the number selected for the analysis should reveal the strengths of the language system. Further discussion of language sample procedures is available from Lund and Duchan (1988).

The most preferred language elicitation procedures for preschool age through adult are informal conversation followed by imperatives and WH questions for elementary and secondary school-age students (Atkins & Cartwright, 1982). Other authors have observed that children's language is richer in syntax, content, and ideas when unstructured elicitation procedures are used.

SPECIFIC ELICITATION TASKS

A variety of tasks have been critiqued for use in obtaining language samples. The authors have found the following to be the most effective:

1. Spontaneous interaction (free play or interaction, conversation) can be produc-

tive. With younger children, making puppets "talk," identifying the characters, and beginning action with dialogue have been helpful. With older students, discussion of school- or age-related topics is generally more productive. There are many hearing-impaired children who do not communicate freely with a stranger in this type of setting, so a teacher or peer would elicit a more representative sample.

2. Elicited interaction may be necessary for students who are somewhat reluctant to communicate. Enticing the student to provide instruction in how to play a game often yields a representative sample.

3. Specific setups such as a role play with peers can be productive as well. A creative example includes a situation where students were directed to talk with each other about their favorite snack foods during TV watching, and their conversation was audiotaped using an unobtrusive flat microphone taped to the corner of the table (Schober-Peterson, 1988).

4. Other contexts include storytelling or use of a Viewmaster where the clinician directs the child to describe a frame and then tries to guess which one is being described.

5. Deep testing for structures that do not appear in the sample can be done by patterning, sentence completion, interview, questions for information, retells, pretend situations, or games.

The authors have found the following to be helpful in eliciting a language sample.

1. Make it real communication.
2. Sabotage the environment if necessary.
3. Avoid playing 20 Questions or single-word answers will be the product.
4. Don't anticipate the child's behavior, wants, responses; that is, don't preempt the child.
5. If possible, let someone else interact with the child while the examiner leaves the room.
6. After language sample analysis is completed, deep test for additional structures not evident in the sample.
7. For language performance in other contexts use language tests.

Analysis should extend across pragmatic, semantic, morphologic, and syntactic dimensions (phonologic will be discussed further under speech assessment in this chapter).

MLU, BROWN'S STAGE, AND TYPE-TOKEN RATIO

A morphologic mean length of utterance (MLU) is computed and serves as the entrée to the analysis system. Procedures for computing MLU are available from Chapman (in Miller, 1981). Brown's Stage is determined via both MLU and qualitative descriptors rather than MLU alone, which often inflates the Brown's Stage determination. For example, a child who has plateaued developmentally at Brown's Stage II may have a higher MLU than the expected 2.0 to 2.5 with limited development of morphologic markers (pluralization, present progressive) and determiners. Based on MLU alone, the child would qualify for Brown's Stage III but is clearly still at Brown's Stage II qualitatively. A slight modification in morphologic acquisition has been observed with hearing-impaired students using Seeing Essential English (Raffin, 1976; Raffin, Davis, & Gilman, 1978). The difference observed was that plural and past tense were apparent prior to the present progressive marker.

Type-token ratio information is also helpful in adding to the total language functioning picture. Although this procedure has been criticized as a research instrument because of variability related to sample size, it can provide helpful clinical data about the student's use of lexical items and linguistic categories. (For further description of this measure see Hess, Sefton, & Landry, 1986; Miller, 1981.)

Further analysis of language performance can be obtained through use of some of the tests developed specifically for hearing-impaired students or those modified for use by these students.

Psychoeducational Assessment

Psychoeducational assessment for handicapped children, including children with hearing loss, is necessary to determine eligibility for services, to make appropriate decisions for placement, and to establish educational and (re)habilitative objectives. The area of psychoeducational assessment for school-age children with significant hearing impairment has received less attention than identification of their language and communicative function. Yet the psychoeducational domain reflects the impact of the hearing impairment on learning within the environment in which these children are expected to compete. In some states, unlike the eligibility requirements for other handicapping conditions requiring special education, the only requirements for hearing-impaired children include audiometric evaluation, otologic evaluation, and minimal assessment of basic academic skills, expressive and receptive communication abilities, and social and emotional adjustment for developing the IEP. A psychological evaluation using instruments appropriate for hearing-impaired students is recommended but not required in some states (Georgia Department of Education Regulations and Procedures 11/01/88). Speech and language evaluation occur at least annually for hearing-impaired students, but comprehensive psychoeducational assessment may never occur during a student's school years. This state of affairs continues to present a major challenge for personnel charged with education planning. Horror stories of deaf individuals mislabeled as retarded or emotionally disturbed continue today.

Psychoeducational testing of school-age children can be arbitrarily divided into two areas: evaluation of cognitive abilities and assessment of academic performance or achievement. Tests of cognitive ability theoretically tap a child's learning potential, learning style, and problem-solving strategies. Tests of academic performance are designed to determine how well a child performs in areas such as reading, math, general information, and other content subjects. Achievement represents the knowledge and experience that a child has accumulated. Cognitive areas represent the presumed potential or learning capabilities of a child.

PSYCHOEDUCATIONAL ASSESSMENT OF HEARING-IMPAIRED CHILDREN

The purposes for assessment of hearing-impaired children are the same as for others:

1. To provide baseline information and feedback about progress
2. To identify the student's strengths and weaknesses
3. To provide an appropriate educational program with modifications as needed

The major areas of assessment include cognitive, communicative, achievement, and social-emotional functioning (Heller, 1990). Communicative assessment has been discussed previously. Additional typical psychoeducational assessment should include measures and behavior samples of:

1. Nonverbal and verbal (where possible) cognitive functioning or learning abilities
2. Achievement in reading, writing, math, and, where possible, other content academic areas
   a. See Laughton (1988)—reading
   b. See Conway (1988)—writing
3. Information-processing performance
4. Psychosocial characteristics

Current psychological assessment of hearing-impaired children has been criticized for *(1)* failure to assure that the hearing-impaired child comprehends the language and concepts used in psychological tests, *(2)* use of tests standardized on hearing children only, and *(3)* use of evaluators with limited familiarity with the language and behaviors of hearing-impaired students (Elliott, Glass, & Evans, 1987). The reader is referred to reviews of appropriate tests for this population (Bradley-Johnson & Evans, 1991; Elliott, Glass, & Evans, 1987; Simeonsson, 1987).

Psychological testing is affected by situational variables, measurement errors associated with test instruments, the personality of the evaluator, and the heterogeneity across hearing-impaired individuals (Elliott, Glass, & Evans, 1987). Differences in hearing-impaired individuals that are critical and must be considered in assessment include their language use, culture, interpreter needs, comprehension of the language of the examiner, familiarity with test instructions, and prior test-taking experiences. Testing assumes the ability to understand and communicate using the English language. Many psychological and achievement tests use complex syntax, idiomatic expressions, and awkward sentences that are not in common usage in informal spoken or signed interpersonal communication. Profoundly hearing-impaired individuals may not have the exposure to deal with this type of language use. They may have experience with oral communication only, or signing English, or ASL, or even some modified version of each language. Therefore, one would expect them to be very different in their comprehension of the language used in tests.

Cultural differences are expected across profoundly hearing-impaired populations as well. Most psychologists testing deaf students are unfamiliar with the diverse cultural aspects influencing testing of these students. These may include expectations of the assessment, appropriateness of discussing personal matters, role interaction with hearing people, and how to deal with unclear communication.

Many deaf individuals require an interpreter when the examiner is unable to sign for himself or herself. Few professionals evaluating hearing-impaired individuals are fluent in ASL or other sign systems (Sullivan & Vernon, 1979). There are no magic solutions when an interpreter is used, and many questionable practices may occur. According to many psychometrists, conceptual signing used by most interpreters to get across the message may provide too many clues to the examinee. The interpreter used for psychological testing should be trained in psychology and testing as well as sign language (Sullivan & Vernon, 1979). Even when signing for himself or herself, the examiner must continuously check to be sure the student has understood the language used.

The testing situation may not be simplified during evaluation of oral students. Many are intelligible only to professionals trained to recognize the phonetic and phonologic speech characteristics of hearing-impaired students. The typical psychological evaluator in public schools has had limited experience with profoundly hearing-impaired students using oral or total communication.

The psychological tests most commonly used to evaluate hearing-impaired students have not changed dramatically since the early 1970s (Gibbins, 1989; Levine, 1974). The WISC-R Performance Scale, the Leiter, the WAIS-R, and the Hiskey-Nebraska continue to be used most frequently. The only one of these tests that included hearing-impaired children in the original standardization sample is the Hiskey-Nebraska, which was developed specifically for hearing-impaired students. Questions of the generalizability of this test have been raised (Watson & Goldgar, 1985). The WISC-R does have hearing-impaired norms for the Performance Scale (Anderson & Sisco, 1977); however, they were developed after the fact rather than including these students in the original standardization sample. The Nonverbal Scale of the Kaufman Assessment Battery for Children (K-ABC) follows the above four tests in popularity for use with hearing-impaired students (Gibbins, 1989). Because of its ease of administration, motivation for children, and nonverbal subtest scoring, it is likely to become more popular in the future.

In spite of the clear statement in PL 94–142 requiring competent evaluators to measure hearing-impaired students' psychological abilities, few professionals are trained or experienced with these children. Of particular concern is the school psychologist performing testing of hearing-impaired children within public schools. Gibbins (1989) examined the practices of professionals providing services to hearing-impaired students. The professionals described themselves as school psychologists (77%), clinical psychologists, administrators, educational diagnosticians, and learning specialists. Eighty percent of the group indicated that their involvement with testing hearing-impaired students was only part-time, with the majority of their time dedicated to evaluation of hearing children (Gibbins, 1989). Improvement of the quality of psychological services is unlikely to occur with school psychologists who have limited experience and lack specialized training for the hearing-impaired population and who work in mostly regular educational settings that serve these students in special classes or in the continuum of mainstream settings (Gibbins, 1989).

A comprehensive assessment, although desirable, is not easily accomplished with hearing-impaired students. The interdependence of language and cognition presents difficulty in assessing intelligence without using language (Orr et al., 1987). Performance tests minimize the use of language but generally require that instructions be given using language. Being certain that students understand the task to be performed becomes complex. The Performance Scale of the WISC-R can be useful in providing an estimate of the student's general intelligence but provides little information about the individual's verbal abilities when that section of the test is not administered, as is often the case.

Psychoeducational assessment of hearing-impaired students must be accomplished within a context that provides meaningful information for educational planning. Most standardized testing requires the examinee to engage in pragmatic violations; that is, they must ignore some operating guidelines that are typically followed in interpersonal communication (Laughton & Ray, 1982; Ray, 1989). Students are removed from their usual surroundings and asked to interact with test stimuli in a structured manner that may not be generalizable to real-world interactions (Ray, 1989). Ray further comments on the lack of exploration of novel uses of stimuli afforded the child during testing. Additionally, tests are often timed without direct notification to the student during the testing. Many of these typical test conditions are likely to be unfamiliar to hearing-impaired students who are less "testwise" than most other school-age students (Ray, 1989).

The examiner is cautioned in psychoeducational testing with the hearing impaired with respect to use of:

1. Verbal tests that measure language rather than intelligence, psychosocial behavior, aptitude, or interest (Vernon, 1976; Zieziula, 1982).
2. Modifications in administration of tests including pantomime (Graham & Shapiro, 1963), visual aids (Reed, 1970), and practice items (Ray, 1976).
3. Oral communication and hearing aids, considering the adverse effect of poor speech skills on understanding (Ross, 1990); signed communication, considering the variable competencies of the student and the examiner.
4. Lack of validity of timed tests with timed responses   (Zieziula, 1982).

Whereas for hearing children, a timed test establishes an attention set that moves them efficiently through accurate responses (Vernon, 1976), hearing-impaired students typically try to finish quickly at the expense of correct work. Such a difference in response to being timed is one of a multiplicity of subtle yet substantial performance factors that inexperienced test administrators may fail to consider.

5. Group testing, because of the attention to test directions and reading level required for understanding directions (Levine, 1981; Sullivan & Vernon, 1979; Zieziula, 1982).
6. Personality assessment that may tend to identify psychological subgroups in view of the language and communication issues presented earlier.

PERSONALITY ASSESSMENT

The implications of early detection of hearing loss and optimal amplification for profoundly hearing-impaired children who develop auditory skills that allow them to function primarily in an auditory environment are that hearing-impaired children may then sample the assessment and intervention services available to any student with a disability. These students are discussed further in Chapter 8. However, students whose speech is not highly intelligible to examiners with generic special education backgrounds or whose primary language is conveyed through a signed format may not realize the comprehensive assessment and subsequent intervention guaranteed by the legislation developed for individuals with disabilities. Although the primary focus of this chapter is directed to these latter hearing-impaired students, the reader is cautioned to be sure that all hearing-impaired students, irrespective of severity of loss or relative success of the habilitation, are entitled to a comprehensive assessment prior to initiation of their habilitative programs; therefore, many of the tests and procedures will be applicable to all school-age hearing-impaired students. In spite of incredible success by the child, hearing loss is likely to interfere with communication in some interactions that occur daily. So it is likely that all students with hearing loss will need some degree of intervention. Ongoing assessment provides parents and professionals with a fund of new information to expand and alter the child's rehabilitative program to enhance development.

Intervention

The intervention phase of the rehabilitative process comes after analysis of the contexts and the repertoire of tools the school-age student brings to these contexts. The long-term goal is that the hearing-impaired child will become an independent adult (Boothroyd, 1988). Short-term goals include:

1. Well-adjusted parents
2. A child with a good self-concept
3. Reduction of the auditory deficit through amplification and auditory training
4. A child with cognitive skills commensurate with age
5. A child with language skills to accomplish communicative and cognitive needs
6. A child with speech to express language (Boothroyd, 1988)
7. A child with signs to express language

The management model then includes components suggested by Boothroyd (1988):

1. Audiologic management: hearing testing, hearing aids (or cochlear implant), hearing conservation
2. Auditory management: development of skills for auditory learning
3. Cognitive/linguistic management: developing a world schema with a symbolic system to represent it
4. Speech management: developing the motor, acoustic, phonetic, and phonologic aspects of spoken language
5. Educational management: developing the learning skills and modification of the learning contexts to facilitate learning across the curriculum
6. Social and emotional management: developing a perspective that enables active participation in the social environment with a healthy self-concept

7. Parental management: developing the skills for parents to teach and advocate for their child

Rather than differentiating the rehabilitative process from the education of hearing-impaired students, the focus in intervention is to incorporate both into an integrated model. The history of educating deaf students is rich but marked by controversy. Education for hearing-impaired students in the United States predates special education for other disability groups. The land grants for establishment of state universities also established schools for the deaf. Education of deaf students in the United States began in Hartford, Connecticut, with the establishment of the American Asylum for the Deaf and Dumb (later changed to the American School for the Deaf) in 1817. This program used the language of signs as the primary means of communication. Soon after, the establishment of the Clarke School for the Deaf in Northampton, Massachusetts, provided the option of an oral education for deaf students. To this date, disagreements continue regarding preferred methodology for communication and education of significantly hearing-impaired students. The controversy over methodology is akin to doctors prescribing penicillin to everyone who is sick. Hearing-impaired children are not homogeneous: They have different needs and therefore should have different prescriptions for habilitation.

Moores (1991) updates us on the school placement revolution, documenting the changes in the school-age hearing-impaired population in the past 5 years. He notes that fewer students are deaf (have profound losses) and that logically more children are being taught via auditory/oral-only instruction (39% of the school-age population). Simultaneous instruction using signs and speech is used with 60% of the population, with all other modes (sign only, cued speech, other) used with 1% of the population. Moores further summarized the demographics, stating that "the population of children we are serving is becoming less white and less black, less deaf, more oral and younger" (Moores, 1991, p. 307). This is, of course, reflected in educational and rehabilitative practice. In 1986 the Executive Board of the Council on Education of the Deaf (CED) affirmed the principles central to PL 94–142 to provide individualized instruction and services to hearing-impaired students of school age, noting that "no single method of instruction and/or communication (oral or total communication) or educational setting can best serve the needs of all such children" (Northcott, 1990, p. 3).

A significant aspect of the school placement revolution is that the predominance of hearing-impaired children are schooled within the public day or mainstreamed setting. The hearing-impaired students at residential schools for the deaf are the minority. Intervention then must focus on the changes brought about through this placement revolution. Public school personnel must now take very seriously their roles as case managers to implement all the communicative, educational, and other services that hearing-impaired children are entitled to in order for them to become contributing members of the mainstream community.

Ross (1990, p. ix) describes the current context for intervention for hearing-impaired students: "The core of any management program of the mainstreamed hearing-impaired child must be the regular classroom. It is the classroom teacher who is faced with the child for most of the school day." The changing map from primarily residential to primarily mainstream educational contexts has brought both new challenges and old dilemmas. The old dilemmas involve methodology (sign language or speech or combined instructional approaches), lack of a research database, appropriate school placement, community of deaf individuals, and early identification. The challenges involve methodology (use of technology to facilitate spoken language), multicultural identity, individualization based on differences, and availability of educational services based on commonalities.

Alexander Graham Bell taught deaf students to see it, say it, write it, refine it, read it, and think it (1873). As Northcott (1990) notes, the modern master teachers, Fitzgerald (1949), Buell (1934), and Groht (1958), each added a significant dimension to the art and craft of teaching hearing-impaired students. Contemporary teachers and scholars such as Kretschmer and Kretschmer (1978, 1988, 1989), Moog and Geers (1980, 1985), and Luetke-Stahlman and Luckner (1991) have interwoven the insights from the past with the findings of the present to more effectively facilitate integration of hearing-impaired students into the school community.

A primary purpose of intervention with school-age hearing-impaired students is to facilitate successful academic performance. Such success hinges on the ability to meet the requirements (comprehension and performance) for school language use. Hearing-impaired children must learn to move beyond the social and need fulfillment aspects of interpersonal communication into the realm of academic survival through communication using both spoken and written formats. In one form or another, spoken or written, language forms the foundation of the educational career for all students. Unless the linguistic rule systems are developed and used, the child will be unable to successfully meet the educational challenges of today's schools.

Assessment in itself is incomplete. It should be seen as an initial step in an intervention program and an integral part of ongoing habilitation. To provide an optimal learning environment for hearing-impaired children, assessment and educational practice must be intimately bound.

All students need effective communicative language development and metalinguistic instructional strategies to succeed in school. The role of the rehabilitative case manager is to define and locate for each hearing-impaired child all of the services he or she needs and to assist in integration of those services for the child's benefit. Intervention in speech, language, sign language, and academic areas may be necessary. The key principle that guides intervention with school-age hearing-impaired students is integration or interfacing of services. Speech therapy from the speech-language pathologist, language development from the teacher of the hearing impaired, and academic instruction from the mainstream classroom teacher will be of limited value without a clearly defined effort by all to integrate these services. Armed with all of the assessment data discussed previously in this chapter, the team should draw a map of services, grounded in ongoing assessment, that guides the student from the mechanics of communication (be it speech or sign language) through experiential and semantic expansion toward the ultimate goal of sufficient language facility for academic success. The student is likely to need speech therapy and language therapy but may also need occupational, physical, or psychological therapy; counseling; or learning disabilities remediation. Just as curriculum-based assessment has become a focus for identifying language needs for school-age students, comprehensive curriculum-based intervention that includes all aspects of school must be developed for the hearing-impaired student to learn and realize his or her potential.

Specific intervention in speech, language (interpersonal and written), audition, and academic areas becomes the domain of the speech-language pathologist, rehabilitative audiologist, and educator of hearing-impaired students. Each member of this team bears responsibility for effective integration of services as well as for the individual components of speech, language, and academics. A brief guide to each follows.

SPEECH INTERVENTION

As Northcott (1990) observes, the 1978 amendments to Title II of ESEA (Elementary and Secondary Education Act) dealing with human rights identify speaking and listening as well as reading, mathematics, and written communication as rights to which each child (including the deaf) in the U.S. public schools is entitled. This speaks to the right to comprehensive speech and language assessment and intervention services for all public school hearing-impaired students.

Facilitating intelligible speech production has been a goal since the beginning of education of hearing-impaired students. Success has not been often realized with profoundly hearing-impaired students. However, dedication to speech development and consistent strategies based in current technology have not always been a part of the speech development program. Some degree of residual hearing, amplified early, has been a consistent prerequisite for intelligible speech development. Bimodal input of vision and audition has generally resulted in superior speech reception.

Although speech development strategies have been laid out in detail in Haycock's (1972) primer on speech methods for the deaf, it has been only more recently with the development of Ling's methodology (1976, 1989) that we have seen the specifics of audiologic testing information and appropriate amplification selection brought together with known speech acoustic information to become manageable for interventionists. Speech pathologists recognize that speech development with profoundly hearing-impaired children is far from synonymous with traditional articulation therapy used with hearing students, although the newer theories of phonological processes are quite relevant to speech development with all of these students.

Intervention in speech commences at the level of breakdown identified through the speech assessment (phonetic and phonologic). Ling (1976, 1989) describes the phonetic intervention model as consisting of a hierarchy beginning with the development of suprasegmentals (intensity, duration, and frequency), continuing through vowel and diphthong development, and ending with consonant and consonant cluster development. The phonetic and phonologic intervention is implemented by informal learning or formal teaching strategies depending on the age of the child and on how long the hearing impairment has affected the child's learning (Ling, 1989). A well laid out curriculum is available for developing the phonetic component through formal teaching including:

1. Production of sound
2. Combination of consonants and vowels into syllables
3. Production of syllables rapidly and automatically
4. Alternation of syllable pairs automatically

As soon as a child is able to produce syllables automatically, it is appropriate to add the semantic or meaning component to the production. This is followed by development of words and longer spoken texts or the phonologic component of speech development. All speech-language pathologists responsible for hearing-impaired students should have the Ling materials available for use. Treatment approaches based on elimination of phonologic simplification processes should also be a part of the speech intervention. See Hodson and Paden (1991) and Edwards and Shriberg (1983).

Although no specific speech intervention is currently available for hearing-impaired students who have had cochlear implants, the Ling methodology can be used readily. The differences are likely to be that with the new processed speech ("hearing system") provided by the cochlear implant, children may not follow the hierarchy proposed by Ling in vowel and consonant development. Therefore, administration of the entire Phonetic Level Evaluation will be necessary, and targets selected for intervention may be more varied. Most other operating procedures and strategies proposed by Ling will likely maintain. More instances of "sound preferences" have been observed with CI children where they become enchanted with a specific sound and then rehearse it and use it prolifically. The use of auditory strategies that are then combined with visual strategies should be the manner of approach, as in the interpersonal communication of hearing conversational partners. The development of more specific intervention programs for CI children is underway (Tye-Murray, 1992).

LANGUAGE INTERVENTION

Historically, language development/teaching of hearing-impaired students has a rich, colorful past with remnants shaping current teaching. The analytic/synthetic methodologies have been reinterpreted into the structured/naturalistic contexts for language learning. The counterpart to the Groht and Fitzgerald teaching approaches has evolved into the metalinguistic/pragmatic focus. Current models of language intervention draw heavily on normal child language acquisition literature.

Intervention in language follows the same sequence then as language intervention with hearing students. After a comprehensive analysis, the language goals across all domains are developed and implemented within the school context. For more detailed discussion of school language intervention objectives and strategies, the reader is directed to the following references for school-age language intervention with hearing students: Bernstein and Tiegerman, 1989; Bloom and Lahey, 1978; Lahey, 1988; Rippich and Spinelli, 1985; Simon, 1985a, 1985b; Wallach and Miller, 1988. The following references are excellent resources for language intervention with hearing-impaired students: Kretschmer, 1989; Kretschmer and Kretschmer, 1978, 1988, 1989; Luetke-Stahlman and Luckner, 1991; McAnally, Rose, and Quigley, 1987; Paul and Quigley, 1990; Quigley and Kretschmer, 1982; Texas Developmental Language Centered Curriculum for Hearing Children, 1978.

Selection of language targets and strategies should be based on the language needs identified through each student's language assessment.

EDUCATIONAL INTERVENTION

The array of educational interventions available to the hearing-impaired student such as notetakers, captioning, and interpreters is discussed in Chapter 8. However, an area of concern that bears mention here as follow-up to the discussion of psychoeducational assessment is the issue of educational intervention with respect to reading, math, spelling, and the basic skills required for learning the content of school subjects. Custom has dictated that the teacher of the hearing impaired teach all content areas that cannot be readily learned in the mainstream setting. The need for collaboration and/or consultation with other professionals such as reading specialists or learning disabilities teachers should not be overlooked in the intervention phase of the process. Although not always experienced with hearing-impaired students, these professionals have much to offer in program planning.

ADDITIONAL LEARNING DIFFICULTIES

There may be instances with multihandicapped hearing-impaired students where the need for learning disabilities services is as great or greater than the need for services for hearing-impaired students. The simultaneous occurrence of additional handicapping conditions within the hearing-impaired population presents a complication to the already complex task of rehabilitating and educating hearing-impaired children. All of the major etiologies of deafness (prematurity, meningitis, Rh incompatibility, rubella, cytomegalovirus) as well as inherited deafness may be associated with other handicapping conditions (Moores, 1987, 1991; Vernon & Andrews, 1990). Because of additional conditions, as many as 25% of hearing-impaired students have multi-handicaps. There is disagreement over the definition precluding specific incidence counts; however, mental retardation, visual impairments, and learning and behavioral disabilities frequently occur with hearing impairment, making educational planning a complex venture (Moores, 1987). The current operational plan in special education for hearing students is to group these students within a "mildly handicapped" rubric, although protests from some teachers would suggest there are differences in learning styles among these children. The "learning disabled hearing impaired student" (Laughton, 1989, p. 70) has been discussed with no consensus about the characteristics demonstrated by children with this phenomenon. Suffice to say that many hearing-impaired children present additional challenges to professionals engaged in assessment and intervention, requiring multidimensional, interdisciplinary teams working in unison to provide the services necessary. Identification, assessment, and the development of intervention programs for such children are underway (Elliott & Powers, 1992; Laughton, 1992; Powers & Elliott, 1990).

A Look into the Future

As Moores (1991) observes, the revolution in education of hearing-impaired students has occurred in the shift from the residential school as primary service deliverer to the local school system and parents. The impact of this shift will be significant in the next century. Increased responsibilities will shift to local school personnel—responsibilities that include enculturation as well as rehabilitation. Whether these roles conflict or can be integrated for the benefit of the deaf and less severely hearing-impaired student is the responsibility and challenge of the rehabilitative case managers.

References

Anderson, R., Role of the reader's schema in comprehension, learning, and memory. In H. Singer and R. Ruddell (Eds.), *Theoretical Models and Processes of Reading* (3rd ed.). Newark, DE: International Reading Association, pp. 372–384 (1985).

Anderson, R., and Sisco, F., Standardization of the WISC-R performance scale for deaf children. Office of Demographics studies, Gallaudet College, Series T, No. 1 (1977).

Aten, J., Auditory memory and auditory sequencing. *Acta Symbolica*, 5, 37–65 (1974).

Atkins, C., and Cartwright, L., Preferred language elicitation procedures used in five age categories. *Asha*, 22, 321–323 (1982).

Bell, A.G., *The Sanders Reader*. Washington, DC: Alexander Graham Bell Association for the Deaf (1873).

Bernstein, D.K., and Tiegerman, E., *Language and Communication Disorders in Children*. Columbus, OH: Merrill Publishing Co. (1989).

Birnholz, J., and Bernacerraf, B., The development of human fetal hearing. *Science*, 22, 516–518 (1983).

Blennerhassett, L., Communicative styles of a 13-month-old hearing impaired child and her parents. *Volta Rev.*, 86, 217–228 (1984).

Bloom, L., and Lahey, M., *Language Development and Language Disorders*. New York: John Wiley & Sons (1978).

Boothroyd, A., *Hearing Impairments in Young Children*. Washington, DC: Alexander Graham Bell Association for the Deaf (1988).

Brackett, D., and Donnelly, J., Hearing impaired adolescents' judgments of appropriate conversational entry point. Paper presented at the meeting of the American Speech-Language-Hearing Association, Toronto (1982, November).

Bradley-Johnson, S., and Evans, L.D., *Psychoeducational Assessment of Hearing-Impaired Students*. Austin, TX: Pro-Ed (1991).

Buell, E.M., *A Companion of the Barry Five Slate System and the Fitzgerald Key*. Washington, DC: The Volta Bureau (1934).

Chapman, R., Exploring children's communicative intents. In Jon F. Miller (Ed.), *Assessing Language Production in Children: Experimental Procedures*. Baltimore, MD: University Park Press (1981).

Conway, D.F., Assessing the writing abilities of hearing-impaired children. *J. Acad. Rehabil. Audiol.*, 21 (Monograph Suppl.), 151–172 (1988).

Curtis, S., Prutting, C., and Lowell, E., Pragmatic and semantic development in young children with impaired hearing. *J. Speech Hear. Res.*, 22(3), 534–552 (1979).

DeCasper, A., and Fifer, W., Of human bonding: newborns prefer their mothers' voices. *Science*, 208, 1174–1176 (1980).

DeVilliers, P.A., Assessing English syntax in hearing-impaired children: eliciting production in pragmatically motivated situations. *J. Acad. Rehabil. Audiol.*, 21 (Monograph Suppl.), 41–71 (1988).

DiFrancesca, S., *Academic Achievement Results of a National Testing Program for Hearing-Impaired Students—United States*, Spring 1971 (Series D, No. 9). Washington, DC: Gallaudet College, Office of Demographic Studies (1972).

Donnelly, J., and Brackett, D., Conversational skills of hearing impaired adolescents: A simulated TV interview. Paper presented at the meeting of the American Speech-Language-Hearing Association, Toronto (1982, November).

Duchan, J.F., Assessing communication of hearing-impaired children: influences from pragmatics. *J. Acad. Rehabil. Audiol.*, 21 (Monograph Suppl.), 19–40 (1988).

Edwards, M.L., and Shriberg, L.D., *Phonology: Applications in Communicative Disorders.* San Diego, CA: College-Hill Press (1983).

Eilers, R., and Minifie, F., Fricative discrimination in early infancy. *J. Speech Hear. Res.*, 18, 158–167 (1975).

Eimas, P., Developmental studies of speech perception. In L. Cohen and P. Salapateck, *Infant Perception: From Sensation to Cognition.* New York: Academic Press, pp. 192–231 (1975).

Eimas, P., and Tartter, V., On the development of speech perception: mechanism analogies. *Advanced Child Develop. Behav.*, 13, 296–307 (1979).

Eisenberg, R., *Auditory Competence in Early Life.* Baltimore: University Press (1976).

Eisenberg, R., The development of hearing in man: an assessment of current status. *Asha*, 12, 119–123 (1970).

Elliot, G., and Elliot, K., Some pathological, radiological and clinical implications of the precocious development of the human ear. *Laryngoscope*, 74, 1160–1171 (1964).

Elliott, H., Glass, L., and Evans, J.W., *Mental Health Assessment of Deaf Clients.* Boston: Little, Brown (1987).

Elliott, R., and Powers, A., *Identification and Assessment of Hearing Impaired Students with Mild Additional Disabilities.* Tuscaloosa, AL: The University of Alabama (1992).

Fitzgerald, E., *Straight Language for the Deaf: A System of Instruction for Deaf Children.* Washington, DC: The Volta Bureau (1949).

Furth, H., Influence of language on the development of concept formation in deaf children. *J. Abnorm. Psychol.*, 63, 386–389 (1961).

Garwood, S., *Educating Young Handicapped Children: A Developmental Approach.* Germantown, MD: Aspen (1979).

Gazzanega, M., The split brain in man. *Scientific Am.*, 217, 24–29 (1967).

Georgia Department of Education, *Regulations and Procedures for Special Education* (1988).

Geschwind, N., The organization of language and the brain. *Science*, 17, 940–944 (1972).

Gibbins S., The provision of school psychological assessment services for the hearing impaired: a national survey. *Volta Rev.* (February/March 1989).

Gilman, L., and Raffin, M., Acquisition of common morphemes by hearing impaired children exposed to the Seeing Essential English sign system. Paper presented at the Annual Meeting of the American Speech and Hearing Association, Washington, DC (1975).

Goldin-Meadow, S., and Feldman, H., The creation of communication system: A study of deaf children of hearing parents. Paper presented to the Society for Research in Child Development, Denver, CO (April 1975).

Graham, E., and Shapiro, E., Use of the Performance Scale of the WISC with the deaf child. *J. Consult. Psychol.*, 17, 396–398 (1963).

Greenberg, M., Social interactions between deaf preschoolers and their mothers: the effects of communication method and communication competence. *Development. Psychol.*, 16, 465–474 (1980).

Groht, M.A., *Natural Language for Deaf Children.* Washington, DC: The Volta Bureau (1958).

Gross, R., Language used by mothers of deaf children and mothers of hearing children. *Am. Ann. Deaf*, 115, 93–96 (1970).

Hasenstab, S., Auditory learning and communication competence: implications for hearing impaired infants. *Sem. Hear.*, 8, 175–180 (1987).

Hasenstab, S., The multichannel cochlear implant in children. *Topics Lang. Disorders* (J. Laughton, Ed.), 9, 45–58 (1989).

Hasenstab, S., and Schoeny, Z., Auditory processing. In S. Hasenstab and J. Horner, *Comprehensive Intervention with Hearing Impaired Infants and Preschool Children.* Rockville, MD: Aspen Publications, pp. 69–89 (1982).

Hasenstab, S., Laughton, J., Cluver, L., Schoeny, Z., and Butts, M., *Auditory Learning.* White Plains, NY: Longman (in progress).

Haycock, G.S., *The Teaching of Speech.* Washington, DC: The Volta Bureau (1972).

Heller, P.J., Psycho-educational assessment. In M. Ross (Ed.), *Hearing-Impaired Children in the Mainstream.* Parkton, MD: York Press, Inc. (1990).

Hess, J.C., Sefton, K., and Landry, R., Sample size and type-token ratios for oral language of preschool children. *J. Speech Hear. Res.*, 29, 129–134 (1986).

Hodson, B.W., and Paden, E.P., *Targeting Intelligible Speech: A Phonological Approach to Remediation.* Austin, TX: Pro-ed (1991).

Hudgins, C.V., and Numbers, F., An investigation of the intelligibility of the speech of the deaf. *Genetic Psychol. Monographs*, 25, 289–392 (1942).

Johansson, B., Wedenberg, E., and Westin, B., Measurement of tone response by the human fetus. *Acta Otolaryngol.*, 57, 188–192 (1964).

Johnson, H.A., A sociolinguistic assessment scheme for the total communication student. *J. Acad. Rehabil. Audiol.*, 21 (Monograph Suppl.), 101–127 (1988).

Johnson, H., and Barton, L., TDD conversations: a context for language sampling and analysis. *Am. Ann. Deaf*, 133, 19–24 (1988).

Khan, L., and Lewis, N., *Khan-Lewis Phonological Analysis.* American Guidance Service (1986).

Kimura, D., Cerebral dominance and the perception of verbal stimuli. *Canad. J. Psychol.*, 15, 166–171 (1961).

King, C.M., and Quigley, S.P., *Reading and Deafness.* San Diego, CA: College-Hill Press (1985).

Kretschmer, R.R., and Kretschmer, L.W., Communication competence: impact of the pragmatics revolution on education of hearing impaired individuals. *Top. Lang. Disorders*, 9, 1–16 (1989).

Kretschmer, R.R., and Kretschmer, L.W., Communication competence and assessment. *J. Acad. Rehabil. Audiol.*, 21 (Monograph Suppl.), 5–17 (1988).

Kretschmer, R.R., and Kretschmer, L.W., *Language Development and Intervention with the Hearing Im-*

paired. Baltimore, MD: University Park Press (1978).

Kuczwara, L., Birnholz, J., and Klodd, D., Auditory responsiveness in the fetus. *National Student Speech, Lang. Hear. Assoc. J.*, 14, 12–20 (1984).

Lahey, M., *Language Disorders and Language Development*. New York: Macmillan (1988).

Laughton, J., The learning disabled, hearing impaired student: reality, myth, or overextension? *Top. Lang. Disorders*, 9(4), 70–79 (1989).

Laughton, J., Perspectives on the assessment of reading. *J. Acad. Rehabil. Audiol.*, 21 (Monograph Suppl.), 129–150 (1988).

Laughton J., Identification of hearing impaired children at risk for mild additional disabilities impacting on learning. In R. Elliott and A. Powers (Eds.), *Identification and Assessment of Hearing Impaired Students with Mild Additional Disabilities*. Tuscaloosa, AL: The University of Alabama (1992).

Laughton, J., and Hasenstab, S., *The Language Learning Process*. Rockville, MD: Aspen Publishers (1986).

Laughton, J., and Jacobs, J.F., A model for research methodology in language acquisition and hearing impairment. In H. Hoemann and R. Wilbur (Eds.), *Interpersonal Communication and Deaf People Monograph*, 5, Washington, DC: Gallaudet College pp. 57–101 (1982).

Laughton, J., and Ray, S., Pragmatic violations in language assessment. 2nd Annual Special Education Conference, Baton Rouge, LA (February 1982).

Lenneberg, E., *Biological Foundations of Language*. New York: John Wiley (1967).

Luetke-Stahlman, B., and Luckner, J., *Effectively Educating Students with Hearing Impairments*. New York: Longman (1991).

Levine, E., The ecology of early deafness. In *Guides to Fashioning Environments and Psychological Assessments*. New York: Columbia University Press (1981).

Levine, E.S., *The Psychology of Deafness*. New York: Columbia University Press (1974).

Ling, D., *Speech and the Hearing-Impaired Child: Theory and Practice*. Washington, DC: Alexander Graham Bell Association for the Deaf (1976).

Ling, D., *Foundations of Spoken Language for Hearing-Impaired Children*. Washington, DC: Alexander Graham Bell Association for the Deaf (1989).

Lund, N., and Duchan, J., *Assessing Children's Language in Naturalistic Contexts* (1st ed.). Englewood Cliffs, NJ: Prentice-Hall (1983).

Lund, N., and Duchan, J., *Assessing Children's Language in Naturalistic Contexts* (2nd ed.). Englewood Cliffs, NJ: Prentice-Hall (1988).

Markides, A., The speech of deaf and partially-hearing children with special reference to factors affecting intelligibility. Unpublished thesis, University of Manchester (1967).

Markides, A., Type of pure tone audiogram configuration and speech intelligibility. *J. Br. Assoc. Teachers Deaf*, 4, 125–129 (1980).

McAnally, P.L., Rose, S., and Quigley, S.P., *Language Learning Practices with Deaf Children*. San Diego, CA: College-Hill Press (1987).

McKirdy, L., & Blank, M., Dialogue in deaf and hearing preschoolers. *J. Speech Hear. Res.*, 25, 487–499 (1982).

McLoughlin, J.A., and Lewis, R.B., *Assessing Special Students*. Columbus, OH: Merrill Publishing Co. (1990).

Miller, G.A., The magical number seven, plus or minus two: some limits on our capacity for processing information. *Psycholog. Rev.*, 63, 81–97 (1956).

Miller, J., *Assessing Language Production in Children*. Baltimore, University Park Press (1981).

Molfese, D., Cerebral asymmetry in infants, children and adults: auditory evoked responses to speech and music stimuli. *J. Acoustic Soc. Am.*, 53, 363 (1973).

Moog, J.S., and Geers, A.E., *Grammatical Analysis of Elicited Language Complex Sentence Level*. St. Louis, MO: Central Institute for the Deaf (1980).

Moog, J.S., and Geers, A.E., *Grammatical Analysis of Elicited Language Simple Sentence Level*. St. Louis, MO: Central Institute for the Deaf (1985).

Moores, D., *Educating the Deaf: Psychology, Principles, and Practices* (3rd ed.). Boston, MA: Houghton Mifflin (1987).

Moores, D., The school placement revolution. *Am. Ann. Deaf*, 136(4), 307–308 (1991).

Morse, P., The discrimination of speech and non-speech stimuli in early infancy. *J. Experiment. Child Psychol.*, 14, 477–492 (1972).

Morse, P., Infant speech perception. In D. Sanders, *Auditory Perception of Speech*. Englewood Cliffs, NJ: Prentice-Hall, pp. 161–176 (1977).

Myklebust, H., *Auditory Disorders in Children*. New York: Grune & Stratton (1954).

Nelson, N.W., Curriculum-based language assessment and intervention. *Asha*, 20, 170–184 (1989).

Nippold, M.A., *Later Language Development*. Boston, MA: College-Hill Press (1988).

Northcott, W.H., Mainstreaming: roots and wings. In M. Ross (Ed.), *Hearing-Impaired Children in the Mainstream*. Parkton, MD: York Press (1990).

Northern, J., Black, O., Brimacombe, J., et al., Selection of children for cochlear implantation. *Sem. Hear.*, 7, 341–347 (1986).

Orr, F.C., DeMatteo, A., Heller, B., et al. (Eds.), *Mental Health Assessment of Deaf Clients*. Boston: Little, Brown, pp. 93–106 (1987).

Paul, P.V., and Quigley, S.P., *Education and Deafness*. White Plains, NY: Longman (1990).

Pien, D., The development of language functions in deaf infants of hearing parents. In D. Martin (Ed.), *Cognition, Education, and Deafness*, Vol. II. Washington, DC: Gallaudet College Press, pp. 30–34 (1985).

Powers, A., and Elliott, R., Preparation of students who serve hearing-impaired students with additional mild handicaps. *Teacher Education and Special Education*, 13, 200–202 (1990).

Quigley, S.P., and Kretschmer, R.E., *The Education of Deaf Children*. Baltimore, MD: University Park Press (1982).

Quigley, S.P., and Paul, P.V., *Language and Deafness*. San Diego, CA: College-Hill Press (1984).

Raffin, M., The acquisition of inflectional morphemes by deaf children using Seeing Essential English. Doctoral dissertation, University of Iowa (1976).

Raffin, M., Davis, J., and Gilman, L., Morphological acquisition of deaf children. *J. Speech Hear. Res.*, 21, 387–400 (1978).

Ramsdell, D., The psychology of the hard of hearing and deafened adult. In H. Davis and R. Silverman,

Hearing and Deafness (3rd ed.). New York: Holt, Rinehart & Winston (1970).

Ray, S., An adaptation of the WISC-R for the deaf. Sulphur, OK: Steven Ray Publishing (1976).

Ray, S., Context and the psychoeducational assessment of hearing impaired children. *Top. Lang. Disorders*, 9(4), 33–44 (1989).

Reed, M., Deaf and partially hearing children. In P. Mittler (Ed.), *The Psychological Assessment of Mental and Physical Handicap.* London: Menthen (1970).

Ripich, D.N., and Spinelli, F.M., (Eds.), *School Discourse Problems.* San Diego, CA: College-Hill Press (1985).

Ross, M., *Hearing-Impaired Children in the Mainstream.* Parkton, MD: York Press (1990).

Russell, W.K., Quigley, S.P., and Power, D.J., *Linguistics and Deaf Children: Transformational Syntax and Its Applications.* Washington, DC: Alexander Graham Bell Association for the Deaf (1976).

Salvia, J., and Ysseldyke, J., *Assessment in Special and Remedial Education.* Boston: Houghton Mifflin (1988).

Sanders, D., *Auditory Perception of Speech.* Englewood Cliffs, NJ: Prentice-Hall (1977).

Sanders, D., *Aural Rehabilitation: A Management Plan.* Englewood Cliffs, NJ: Prentice-Hall (1982).

Schafer, D., and Lynch, J., Emergent language of six prelingually deaf children. *Teach. Deaf*, 5, 94–111 (1980).

Schlesinger, H., and Meadow, K., *Sounds and Sign.* Berkeley, CA: University of California Press (1972).

Schober-Peterson, D., *The Conversational Performance of Low Achieving and Normally Achieving Third Grade Children.* Unpublished Doctoral dissertation, University of Illinois, Champaign, IL (1988).

Simeonsson, R.J., *Assessment of Hearing-Impaired Children. Psychological and Developmental Assessment of Special Children.* Boston: Allyn & Bacon (1987).

Simon, C.S., *Communication Skills and Classroom Success: Assessment of Language-Learning Disabled Students.* San Diego, CA: College-Hill Press (1985a).

Simon, C.S., *Communication Skills and Classroom Success: Therapy Methodologies for Language-Learning Disabled Students.* San Diego, CA: College-Hill Press (1985b).

Skarakis, E., and Prutting, C., Early communication: semantic functions and communicative intentions in the communication of the preschool child with impaired hearing. *Am. Ann. Deaf*, 122, 382–391 (1977).

Small, A., *Negotiating Conversation: Interactions of a Hearing Impaired Child with Her Adult Communication Partners in Language Therapy.* Unpublished Doctoral dissertation, University of Cincinnati (1985).

Spring, D., and Dale, P., Discrimination of linguistic stress in early infancy. *J. Speech Hear. Res.*, 20, 224–232 (1977).

Staller, S.J., Dowell, R.C., Beiter, A.L., and Brimacombe, J.A., Perceptual abilities of children with the Nucleus 22-Channel cochlear implant. *Ear Hear.*, 12 (Suppl.), 34–47 (1991).

Sternberg, R.J., Testing intelligence without IQ tests. *Phi Delta Kappan*, 694–698 (June 1984).

Sullivan, P., and Vernon, M., Psychological assessment of hearing-impaired children. *School Psychol. Dig.*, 8, 217–290 (1979).

Texas Education Agency, *A Developmental Language Centered Curriculum for Hearing Impaired Children.* Austin, TX: Texas Education Agency (1978).

Thompson, M., Biro, P., Vethivelu, S., Pious, C., and Harfield, N., *Language Assessment of Hearing-Impaired School Age Children.* Seattle, WA: University of Washington Press (1987).

Tye-Murray, N., *Cochlear Implants and Children: A Handbook for Parents, Teachers, and Speech and Hearing Professionals.* Washington, DC: Alexander Graham Bell Association for the Deaf (1992).

Vernon, M., Psychologic evaluation of hearing-impaired children. In L. Lloyd (Ed.), *Communication, Assessment, and Intervention Strategies.* Baltimore: University Park Press, pp. 195–223 (1976).

Vernon, M., and Andrews, J., *The Psychology of Deafness.* New York: Longman (1990).

Wallach, G.P., and Miller, L., *Language Intervention and Academic Success.* San Diego, CA: College-Hill Press (1988).

Watson, B.U., and Goldgar, D.E., A note on the use of the Hiskey-Nebraska test of learning aptitude with deaf children. *ASHA*, 16, 53–57 (1985).

Weddell-Monig, J., and Lumley, J.M., Child deafness and mother-child interactions. *Child Develop.*, 51, 766–774 (1980).

Wilbur, R.B., *American Sign Language: Linguistic and Applied Dimensions.* San Diego, CA: College-Hill Press (1987).

Ying, E., Speech and language assessment: communication evaluation. In M. Ross (Ed.), *Hearing-Impaired Children in the Mainstream.* Parkton, MD: York Press (1990).

Zieziula, F., *Assessment of Hearing-Impaired People: A Guide for Selecting Psychological, Educational, and Vocational Tests.* Washington, DC: Gallaudet University Press (1982).

APPENDIX 7.1   *Language Tests for Hearing-Impaired Students*

ALPHABETICAL LIST OF TESTS
*designed for hearing-impaired students

 1. Assessment of Children's Language Comprehension (ACLC)
 2. Bankson Language Screening test (BLST)
 3. Bare Essentials in Assessing Really Little Kids—Concept Analysis Profile Summary (BEAR-CAPS)*
 4. Boehm Test of Basic Concepts (BTBC)
 5. Bracken Basic Concept Scale (BBCS)
 6. Carolina Picture Vocabulary Test (CPVT)*
 7. Carrow Elicited Language Inventory (CELI)
 8. CID Scales of Early Communication Skills for Hearing-Impaired Children (SECS)*
 9. Communicative Intention Inventory (CII)
10. Early Language Milestones (ELM)
11. Expressive One-Word Picture Vocabulary Test (EOWPVT)
12. Expressive One-Word Picture Vocabulatory Test—Upper Extension (EOWPVT-UE)
13. Grammatical Analysis of Elicited Language (GAEL)*
14. The Illinois Test of Psycholinguistic Abilities (ITPA)
15. Interpersonal Language Skills Assessment (ILSA)
16. Maryland Syntax Evaluation Instrument (MSEI)*
17. Miller-Yoder Language Comprehension Test
18. Northwestern Syntax Screening Test (NSST)
19. Peabody Picture Vocabulary Test—Revised (PPVT)
20. Preschool Language Assessment Instrument (PLAI)
21. Receptive One-Word Picture Vocabulary Test (ROWPVT)
22. Rhode Island Test of Language Structure (RITLS)*
23. Rockford Infant Developmental Evaluation Scales (RIDES)
24. Sequenced Inventory of Communication Development (SICD)
25. SKI-HI Receptive Language Test (SKI-HI RLT)*
26. SKI-HI Language Development Scale (SKI-HI LDS)*
27. Structured Photographic Expressive Language Test—II (SPELT-II)
28. Teacher Assessment of Grammatical Structures (TAGS)*
29. Test for Auditory Comprehension of Language—Revised (TACL-R)
30. Test for Examining Expressive Morphology (TEEM)
31. Test of Expressive Language Ability (TEXLA)*
32. Test of Receptive Language Ability (TERLA)*
33. Test of Syntactic Abilities (TSA)*
34. The Word Test (TWT)
35. Total Communication Receptive Vocabulary Test (TCRVT)*
36. Vane Evaluation of Language Scale (VANE-L)

Thompson, M., Biro, P., Vethivelu, S., Pious, C., and Hatfield, N., Language assessment of hearing-impaired school age children. Seattle, WA: University of Washington Press (1987). Reprinted with permission.

TESTS LISTED ALPHABETICALLY BY AUTHOR(S)

Bankson, N.W. (1977). *Bankson Language Screening Test.* Austin, TX: Pro-Ed.

Blagden, D.M., & McConnell, N.L. (1983). *Interpersonal Language Skills Assessment.* Moline, IL: LinguiSystems, Inc.

Blank, M., Rose, S.A., & Berlin, L.J. (1978). *Preschool Language Assessment Instrument.* New York: Grune & Stratton.

Boehm, A.E. (1967, 1969, 1970, 1971). *Boehm Test of Basic Concepts.* New York: The Psychological Corporation.

Bracken, A. (1984). *Bracken Basic Concept Scale.* Columbus, OH: Charles E. Merrill.

Bunch, G.O. (1981). *Test of Expressive Language Ability.* Toronto: G.B. Services.

Bunch, G.O. (1981). *Test of Receptive Language Ability.* Toronto: G.B. Services.

Carrow-Woolfolk, E. (1974). *Carrow Elicited Language Inventory.* Allen, TX: DLM Teaching Resources.

Carrow-Woolfolk, E. (1985). *Test for Auditory Comprehension of Language—Revised.* Allen, TX: DLM Teaching Resources.

Coggins, T.E., & Carpenter, R.L. (1981). The Communicative Intention Inventory: A system for observing and coding children's early intentional communication. *Applied Psycholinguistics, 2,* 235–251.

Coplan, J. (1983). *Early Language Milestone Scale.* Tulsa, OK: Modern Education Corp.

Dunn, L.M., & Dunn, L.M. (1981). *Peabody Picture Vocabulary Test—Revised.* Circle Pines, MN: American Guidance Service.

Engen, E., & Engen, T. (1983). *Rhode Island Test of Language Structure.* Austin, TX: Pro-Ed.

Foster, R., Gidden, J.J., & Stark, J. (1972). *Assessment of Children's Language Comprehension.* Palo Alto, CA: Consulting Psychologists Press.

Gardner, M.F. (1979, 1981). *Expressive One-Word Picture Vocabulary Test.* Novato, CA: Academic Therapy Publications.

Gardner, M.F. (1983). *Expressive One-Word Picture Vocabulary Test—Upper Extension.* Novato, CA: Academic Therapy Publications.

Gardner, M.F. (1985). *Receptive One-Word Picture Vocabulary Test.* Novato, CA: Academic Therapy Publications.

Hasenstab, M.S., & Laughton, J. (1982). Bare Essentials in Assessing Really Little Kids: An approach. In M.S. Hasenstab, & J.S. Horner (Eds.), *Comprehensive intervention with hearing-impaired infants and preschool children* (pp. 204–209). Rockville, MD: Aspen Publications.

Hedrick, D., Prather, E., & Tobin, A. (1975; revised ed., 1984). *Sequenced Inventory of Communication Development.* Seattle: University of Washington Press.

Jorgenson, C., Barrett, M., Huisingh, R., & Zackman, L. (1981). *The Word Test.* Moline, IL: LinguiSystems, Inc.

Kirk, S.A., McCarthy, J.J., & Kirk, W.D. (1961, 1969). *Illinois Test of Psycholinguistic Abilities.* Urbana, IL: University of Illinois Press.

Layton, T.L., & Holmes, D.W. (1985). *Carolina Picture Vocabulary Test.* Tulsa, OK: Modern Education Corporation.

Lee, L.L. (1971). *Northwestern Syntax Screening Test.* Evanston, IL: Northwestern University Press.

Longhurst, T.M., Briery, D., & Emery, M. (1975). *SKI-HI Receptive Language Test.* Logan, UT: Project SKI-HI, Utah State University.

Miller, J.F., & Yoder, D.E. (1984). *The Miller-Yoder Test of Grammatical Comprehension: Clinical Edition.* Austin, TX: Pro-Ed.

Moog, J.S., & Geers, A.E. (1975). *CID Scales of Early Communication Skills for Hearing-Impaired Children*. St. Louis, MO: Central Institute for the Deaf.

Moog, J.S., & Geers, A.E. (1979). *Grammatical Analysis of Elicited Language*. St. Louis, MO: Central Institute for the Deaf.

Moog, J.S., & Kozak, V.J. (1983). *Teacher Assessment of Grammatical Structures*. St. Louis, MO: Central Institute for the Deaf.

Project RHISE (1979). *Rockford Infant Developmental Evaluation Scales*. Bensenville, IL: Scholastic Testing Service, Inc.

Quigley, S.P., Steinkamp, M.W., Power, D.J., & Jones, B. (1978). *Test of Syntactic Abilities*. Beaverton, OR: Dormac, Inc.

Scherer, P. (1981). *Total Communication Receptive Vocabulary Test*. Northbrook, IL: Mental Health & Deafness Resources, Inc.

Shipley, K.G., Stone, T.A., & Sue, M.B. (1983). *Test for Examining Expressive Morphology*. Tucson, AZ: Communication Skill Builders.

Tonelson, S., & Watkins, S. (1979). *The SKI-HI Language Development Scale*. Logan, UT: Project SKI-HI, Utah State University.

Vane, J.R. (1975). *Vane Evaluation of Language Scale*. Brandon, VT: Clinical Psychology Publishing Co., Inc.

Warner, E.O'H., & Kresheck, J. (1983). *Structured Photographic Expressive Language Test—II*. Sandwich, IL: Janelle Publications, Inc.

White, A.H. (1981). *Maryland Syntax Evaluation Instrument*. Sanger, TX: Support Systems for the Deaf.

Test Name *commonly used with hearing-impaired students	Target Age Group	Norm Group	Mode		Area Tested					Test Results		
			Rec.	Exp.	Lexicon (VOC.)	Morph.	Syntax	Sem. Rel.	Other	Age Equiv.	Grade Equiv.	Percentile
Assessment of Children's Comprehension (ACLC)	3 to 6 years	365 hearing children, Fla. and Vermont areas, mixed SES	X		X			X				X
Bankson Language Screening Test (BLST)	4 to 8 years	637 hearing children middle SES, Wash., DC area	X	X		X	X	X	auditory/visual perception	X		
Bare Essentials in Assessing Really Little Kids—Concept Analysis Profile Summary (BEAR-CAPS)	1–6 to 5–9 years	None	X		X			X	concepts			
Boehm Test of Basic Concepts (BTBC)	Grades K, 1, 2	9700+ hearing children, range of SES, across U.S.	X		X			X	concepts		X	
Bracken Basic Concept Scale (BBCS)	2–6 to 7–11 years	1109 hearing children across U.S. for diagnostic test; 879 hearing children across U.S. for screening test	X		X			X		X		X
Carolina Picture Vocabulary Test (CPVT)	4 to 11–6 years	767 hearing-impaired children in U.S. using manual communication	X		X					X		X

Test Name *commonly used with hearing-impaired students	Target Age Group	Norm Group	Mode		Area Tested					Test Results		
			Rec.	Exp.	Lexicon (VOC.)	Morph.	Syntax	Sem. Rel.	Other	Age Equiv.	Grade Equiv.	Percentile
Illinois Test of Psycholinguistic Abilities (ITPA)	2–7 to 10 years	962 "normal" hearing children; middle SES	X	X					psycho-linguistic skills	X	"Psycho-linguistic Age," "Psycholinguistic Quotient," and scaled scores	
Interpersonal Language Skills Assessment (ILSA)	8 to 14 years	528 hearing children; 64 learning disabled children		X					use of social language skills			percentage
*Maryland Syntax Evaluation Assessment (ILSA)	6 to 12 years	220 hearing-impaired children		X			X			Computed syntax score and sentence ratio		
Miller-Yoder Language Comprehension Test (M-Y)	4 to 8 years	172 hearing students, Madison, Wisconsin	X				X			X		
Northwestern Syntax Screening Test (NSST)	3 to 8 years	580+ hearing children	X	X			X					X
Peabody Picture Vocabulary Test (PPVT)—Revised	2 1/2 to 40 years	4200 hearing children and adolescents	X		X					X		X
Preschool Language Assessment Instrument (PLAI)	3 to 6 years	120 hearing children matched for age, sex, and SES	X	X				X	discourse skills	X		
Receptive One-Word Picture Vocabulary Test (ROWPVT)	2 to 12 years	1128 hearing children, San Francisco Bay area	X		X					X Language Standard Score and Stanine	X	
Carrow Elicited Language Inventory (CELI)	3 to 8 years	475 hearing children, middle SES		X		X	X					X

Test Name *commonly used with hearing-impaired students	Target Age Group	Norm Group	Mode		Area Tested					Test Results		
			Rec.	Exp.	Lexicon (VOC.)	Morph.	Syntax	Sem. Rel.	Other	Age Equiv.	Grade Equiv.	Percentile
*CID Scales of Early Communication Skills for Hearing Impaired Children (SECS)	2 to 8 years	372 oral hearing-impaired children	X	X	X		X	X				X
Communicative Intention Inventory (CII)	8 to 24 months	None		X					use of language			
Early Language Milestone (ELM)	0 to 3 years	191 hearing children, New York Medical Center	X	X			X	X				X
Expressive One-Word Picture Vocabulary Test (EOWPVT)	2 to 12 years	1600 hearing children, San Francisco Bay area		X	X					X		X
Expressive One-Word Picture Vocabulary Test—Upper Extension (EOWPVT-UE)	12 to 15–11 years	465 hearing children, San Francisco Bay area		X	X					X		X
*Grammatical Analysis of Elicited Language (GAEL)	5 to 9 years	200 oral hearing-impaired children from 13 oral programs; 200 hearing children		X			X					X
Rhode Island Test of Language Structure (RITLS)	5 to 17+ years	513 hearing-impaired children in east coast states; 304 hearing children, R.I.	X			X	X					X

Test Name *commonly used with hearing-impaired students	Target Age Group	Norm Group	Mode		Area Tested					Test Results		
			Rec.	Exp.	Lexicon (VOC.)	Morph.	Syntax	Sem. Rel.	Other	Age Equiv.	Grade Equiv.	Percentile
Rockford Infant Developmental Evaluation Scales (RIDES)	0 to 4 years	None	X	X	X			X	Social/Fine Motor/Gross Motor	X		
Sequenced Inventory of Communication Development (SICD)	4 months to 4 years	252 hearing children; range of SES	X	X					Communication behaviors	X Communication age		
*SKI-HI Receptive Language Test (SKI-HI RLT)	3 to 6 1/2 years	None	X		X			X				% correct
*SKI-HI Language Development Scale (SKI-HI LDS)	0 to 5 years	None	X	X					Communication behaviors	X		
Structured Photographic Expressive Language Test (SPELT-II)	4 to 9-5 years	1178 hearing children from North Central and Southern sections of U.S.		X		X	X			X		
*Teacher Assessment of Grammatical Structures (TAGS)	0 to 9+ years	None	X	X		X	X	X				
Test for Auditory Comprehension of Language—Revised (TACL-R)	3 to 10 years	1003 hearing subjects in 20 states	X		X	X	X			X		X
Test for Examining Expressive Morphology (TEEM)	3 to 8 years	500 hearing children, Fresno, California		X		X				X		

Test Name * commonly used with hearing-impaired students	Target Age Group	Norm Group	Mode		Area Tested					Test Results		
			Rec.	Exp.	Lexicon (VOC.)	Morph.	Syntax	Sem. Rel.	Other	Age Equiv.	Grade Equiv.	Percentile
*Test of Expressive Language Ability (TEXLA)	7 to 12 years	65 hearing-impaired children from Canadian Schools for the Deaf; 17 hearing children		X		X	X			X		X
*Test of Receptive Language Ability (TERLA)	7 to 12 years	92 hearing-impaired children from Canadian Schools for the Deaf; 17 hearing children	X			X	X			X		X
*Test of Syntactic Ability (TSA)	10 to 18–11 years	450 hearing-impaired children from 18 programs in U.S.	X				X			X		X
The Word Test (TWT)	7 to 12 years	467 hearing children; Milwaukee, Wisconsin		X	X			X		X		
*Total Communication Receptive Vocabulary Test (TCRVT)	3 to 12 years	77 hearing, 95 hard-of-hearing, 251 deaf children	X		X					X		
Vane Evaluation of Language Scale (VANE-L)	2-6 to 6 years	740 hearing children, New York	X	X	X	X	X	X	Auditory/visual attention			X

8

Management of Hearing in an Educational Setting

CAROL FLEXER, Ph.D.

A primary goal of audiologic management is to facilitate access to acoustic information for all children so that they can benefit from verbal communication and instruction. To the extent that a child cannot clearly hear and attend to the teacher's instruction, that child is being denied an opportunity to obtain an appropriate education.

Hearing and listening are important for all children, not just for those who have severe hearing losses. Indeed, mainstreamed classrooms are auditory-verbal environments because instructional information is presented through the speech of the teacher with the underlying assumption that children can clearly hear and attend to the teacher's voice. Hearing and listening are thus pivotal to the child's ability to profit from teacher instruction. *Hearing*, of course, refers to the anatomical and physiological status of the auditory system, and *listening* refers to the ability to attend to the sounds that the ear receives.

Audiologists face a significant challenge as they strive to provide comprehensive audiologic management for children in an educational setting. Currently, audiologic services in the schools, both diagnostic and rehabilitative, are insufficient at best (Flexer, 1990). There are less than 700 audiologists actually employed by school districts to manage the more than 8 million children in the United States who have educationally significant hearing problems (Berg, 1986a; Wilson-Vlotman & Blair, 1986). Unfortunately, only 1% of children

with hearing loss are receiving the audiologic services necessary to facilitate their academic performance. Where are the rest of these children? Because their hearing losses remain unrecognized as a major or contributing cause of their academic/behavioral/social difficulties, they may be in special education placements for children who experience learning disabilities, or behavior disorders, or multiple handicaps, or they could be struggling in regular classrooms with inadequate support services or no support at all (Davis, 1990; Ross, Brackett, & Maxon, 1991). Audiologists have a critical role in creating and maintaining a favorable learning environment for all children because if children cannot clearly hear the teacher, the entire premise of the educational system is undermined.

Educational Audiology Association: Role Definition

The Educational Audiology Association (EAA), the national professional organization for audiologists who work with children and schools, has defined an educational audiologist as "a specialist who ensures that all aspects of a child's hearing and learning are maximized in order for their educational and real life capabilities to be met" (Blair, Wilson-Vlotman, & Von Almen, 1989, p. 14). The EAA elaborates that the educational audiologist is the professional responsible for the child who experiences any type and degree of hearing difficulty, because the audiologist is knowledgeable about sound, hearing, hearing loss, amplification technology, and auditory perception. Specifically, the educational audiologist is responsible for identification, diagnosis, assessment, amplification programming that includes hearing aids and signal-to-noise ratio enhancing technology, and aural rehabilitation programming (English, 1991). Further, the audiologist is responsible for in-servicing and training staff and support personnel, parent education and support, specialist coordination, listening training, hearing conservation programming, otologic referral, and ongoing evaluations of classroom and educational functioning of children who experience any type and degree of hearing loss (Blair, Wilson-Vlotman, & Von Almen, 1989). In other words, the audiologist is the expert on hearing and listening; that role must be taken seriously in enabling children to develop academic competencies by creating and maintaining a favorable acoustic/learning environment.

Purpose

The purpose of this chapter is to provide very practical information about the audiologic services that constitute comprehensive management of hearing in an educational setting. The focus will be on facilitating academic performance and social interaction in mainstreamed classrooms for children who would be diagnosed "hard of hearing" rather than "deaf." This population of mainstreamed children with more moderate, fluctuating, or early hearing losses constitutes the majority population of children with hearing difficulties (Berg, 1991; Davis, 1990; Ross, 1991; Upfold, 1988). In addition, some children with severe and profound hearing losses have learned to be very auditory and thus function in the mainstream as children who are hard of hearing rather than as children who are deaf (McGee, 1990; Pollack, 1985). The needs of the population of children with hearing losses who are in self-contained placements are covered in Chapter 7 of this text. Accordingly, the following topics will be discussed in this chapter: the relation-

ship of hearing and hearing loss to academic performance; changing demographics of children with hearing loss; Public Laws 94–142 and 99–457 (IDEA), and Section 504 of the Rehabilitation Act of 1973 as they govern the provision of audiologic services; models of audiologic service delivery to and in schools; identification of children who need audiologic rehabilitative services; categories of audiologic rehabilitative services in schools, emphasizing the signal-to-noise ratio enhancing technology of classroom amplification; IEP and IFSP issues relative to hearing management; inservices about hearing and hearing loss for educational personnel; and the necessity of audiologists advocating for "the right to hear" for all children.

Relationship of Hearing and Hearing Loss to Academic Performance

HEARING

Before detailing the services that constitute effective hearing management in an educational setting, one must begin by discussing the nature of hearing and the relationship of hearing to academic performance. It is important to note that one of the primary reasons why comprehensive audiologic services are *not* available in most schools is because many school personnel lack basic knowledge about the critical role of hearing in the educational process (Lass et al., 1986; Luckner, 1991; Martin et al., 1988; Ross, 1991). If the primacy of hearing is not understood, audiologic suggestions for hearing management may seem superfluous to the learning process. However, as stated previously, hearing and listening form the invisible cornerstones of the educational system. Children spend a great deal of their classroom time engaged in active listening activities, so the need for all children to be able to hear clearly must not be underestimated (Berg, 1986a).

Elliott, Hammer, and Scholl (1989) documented the importance of being able to discriminate word/sound distinctions. They tested children with normal hearing and found that the ability to perform fine-grained auditory discrimination tasks (e.g., to hear "pa" and "ba" as different syllables) correctly classified nearly 80% of the primary-level children in their study either as progressing normally or as having language-learning difficulties. The authors concluded that auditory discrimination skills are associated with the development of basic academic competencies that are essential for success in school. If a child cannot "hear" phonemic distinctions, that child is at significant risk for academic failure.

The ability to discriminate the word/sound distinctions of individual phonemes is defined as *intelligibility*, whereas the ability to simply detect the presence of speech is defined as *audibility*. If, because of a hearing loss, poor classroom acoustics, and/or poor attending and listening skills, a child cannot discriminate *hair* from *chair*, for example, he or she will not learn appropriate semantic distinctions unless deliberate intervention occurs.

HEARING LOSS

The importance of hearing in the communicative and educational process tends to be profoundly underestimated because hearing loss itself is invisible; thus the effects of hearing loss are often associated with problems or causes other than hearing loss (Ross, 1991). For example, when a child cannot keep up with the pace of topic transition in a class, the cause of that child's behavior may be attributed to "slow learning" or to "attention problems" rather than to a hearing loss.

The ambiguity of hearing loss is further magnified by the tendency to erroneously categorize hearing loss into only two classifications: "normally hearing" or "deaf" (Ross & Calvert, 1984). Such dichotomous thinking rules out the necessity to consider hearing in educational programming (i.e., a child who is "deaf" can hear nothing, and the other alternative is normally hearing, so why are audiologic services needed?) and causes educators to make statements such as, "We have no children with hearing loss in our district of 75,000 children." A child with a mild to moderate hearing loss is ob-

viously not "deaf," and about 94 to 96% of the population of people with hearing loss is functionally "hard of hearing" rather than "deaf" (Ross & Calvert, 1984). The concept that hearing loss occurs along a broad continuum needs to be emphasized, as does the fact that very few persons have no hearing at all.

Any type and degree of hearing loss can present a significant barrier to the reception of instructional information in the classroom (Bess, 1985; Davis, 1990; Flexer, Wray, & Ireland, 1989; Northern & Downs, 1991).

Acoustic Filter Effect of Hearing Loss

School personnel may have difficulty understanding how even a "minimal" hearing loss can have a detrimental influence on academic performance. Hearing loss can be presented descriptively as an invisible acoustic filter that distorts, smears, or eliminates incoming sounds (Davis, 1990; Ling, 1989). The negative effects of hearing loss are apparent, but the hearing loss itself is invisible and easily ignored.

The primary negative effect of the invisible acoustic filter of hearing loss is its detrimental impact on verbal language development. If a child has a prelingual severe/profound hearing loss, then that child will not speak unless thoughtful intervention occurs (Ling, 1989). If a child cannot hear clear, consistent, intelligible sounds because of a more moderate hearing loss or because of a continuously fluctuating hearing loss, then that child's speech and language skills will probably not be clear either, unless deliberate intervention occurs (Ling, 1989).

The secondary negative consequence of the invisible acoustic filter effect of hearing loss is its destructive impact on the higher-level linguistic skills of reading and writing (Wray, Hazlett, & Flexer, 1988). If a child cannot hear clearly enough to identify word/sound distinctions, then discrete verbal language concepts probably will not develop spontaneously. If verbal language skills are spotty or deficient, then reading skills are also likely to be deficient because reading is a secondary linguistic function built on speaking (Simon, 1985). To continue further with the concept of the spiraling negative consequences of hearing loss, if a child has poor reading skills, then academic options are likely to be limited because literacy certainly is linked to academics (Wallach & Butler, 1984). The cause of this entire unfortunate chain of events is that ambiguous, invisible, underestimated, and ignored acoustic filter effect of hearing loss. The core problem of hearing loss needs to be recognized, and hearing must be accessed before intervention at the secondary levels of verbal language, reading, and academics can be effective (Ling, 1989; Ross & Giolas, 1978).

School personnel often misinterpret the cause of a child's behaviors that result from the invisible acoustic filter effect of hearing loss because the barrier to the reception of clear/intelligible speech posed by hearing loss typically is not appreciated (Ross, 1991). Speech might be audible to a child with a hearing loss, but the words probably would not be intelligible without technological intervention, especially in a classroom environment. For example, a child with even a "mild" hearing loss might hear *goes*, *showed*, and *slows*, all as *oh* or might confuse the words *invitation* and *vacation*. The words sound alike but convey totally different concepts. If the child is asked if he or she heard a teacher, the response likely would be "yes." How can a young and linguistically naive child explain or even understand that the high-intensity vowel sounds and the suprasegmental structure of the utterances were audible, but the high-frequency, low-energy morphological markers for place, tense, and plurality were not distinguishable acoustically? Thus, it is not uncommon for teachers to make statements such as, "Of course Mary has a hearing loss, but her problem is not her hearing loss. Her problem is that she has a poor vocabulary, immature language skills, and reading difficulties." Mary's problem *is* her hearing loss. Her language and reading difficulties are a result of the acoustic filter effect of her hearing loss. Until Mary's hearing is accessed through technology and she is taught to listen for those crucial word/sound distinctions, she may have limited success improving her language and reading skills.

The point is, hearing cannot be ignored or bypassed in the schemata of intervention, just as the roots of a tree cannot be ignored if fruit is expected to develop.

Computer Analogy

One helpful way to explain the potentially negative effects of any type and degree of hearing loss on academic performance is to use a computer analogy. The core concept is, *data input precedes data processing.* A child (or anybody) must have information/data in order to learn. The primary way that information is entered into the brain in a classroom is through the ears/hearing (Berg, 1987). If data are entered inaccurately, analogous to having one's fingers on the wrong keys of a computer keyboard or to having a malfunctioning keyboard, then the child will have incorrect or incomplete information to process. How can a child be expected to learn when the information that reaches the brain is deficient? Is it the brain's fault that the entered data are incomplete? Is the computer program in error if the keyboard entry is faulty? Yet, it is common for children who have inaccurate data entry to be labeled as "learning disabled," as "attention disordered," or as "hyperactive" because they behave in that fashion because of lack of access to appropriate information.

Once the keyboard is repaired or the fingers are placed on the correct keys and data are entered accurately, analogous to using amplification technology that enables a child to detect word/sound differences, what happens to all of the previously entered inaccurate and incomplete information? Does the inaccurate data automatically convert to complete and correct information? Unfortunately, we are well aware that all of the corrected data have to be reentered. Thus, the longer a child's hearing loss remains unrecognized and unmanaged, the more destructive and far-reaching are the effects of that hearing loss.

Hearing is only the necessary first step in the chain of intervention. Once hearing has been accessed through appropriate signal-to-noise ratio enhancing technology, the child will have an opportunity to discriminate word/sound distinctions as a basis for learning language, which provides an opportunity to acquire knowledge of the world. All levels of the acoustic filter effect of hearing loss need to be understood and managed. The longer a child has inaccurate data entry, the more destructive the acoustic filter effect will be on the child's overall life development. On the other hand, the more intelligible and complete the entered data are, the better opportunity the child will have to learn language, to acquire reading skills, and to develop academic competencies. Thus, comprehensive audiologic management is absolutely essential in order for a child with any type and degree of hearing loss or listening difficulty to have an opportunity to succeed in school.

Distance Hearing and Passive Learning

Another potential consequence of hearing loss that needs to be understood and audiologically managed is the concept of distance hearing or earshot. Distance hearing can be defined as the distance over which speech sounds are intelligible and not merely audible (Ling, 1989). Hearing loss of any type and degree reduces the distance over which speech sounds are intelligible, even with amplification; typically the greater the hearing loss, the greater the reduction in earshot. This reduction in distance hearing has far-reaching consequences for classroom and life performance because distance hearing is linked to passive and casual listening and learning (Ramsdell, 1978; Ross, Brackett, & Maxon, 1991).

A child with a hearing loss, even a mild or unilateral hearing loss, cannot casually or passively overhear what people are saying or the events that are occurring. Most children with normal hearing seem to absorb passively information from their surroundings. Because hearing loss presents a barrier to the casual acquisition of information, children with hearing loss often seem oblivious to environmental events that are not directed actively to them (Pollack, 1985). Thus, because of this reduction in earshot and the elimination of passive listening and learning caused by hearing loss, children with hearing loss need to be taught directly many skills and concepts that other children learn incidentally (Erber, 1982).

Further implications for reduction of distance hearing include lack of redundancy of instructional information, lack of access to social cues (Conway, 1990), and the need for a remote microphone to expand earshot (Leavitt, 1991). Because listening is necessarily an active and not a passive process for children with hearing loss, active attention must be directed to appropriate sources at all times. A young child's attention will wander many times during the school day, causing him or her to miss some or much of what is being said. Consequently, even though a good teacher understands the importance of and uses redundancy of presentation of information, a child with a hearing loss may be attending only a fraction of the time that information is reviewed. That is, children with normal hearing and attending skills will benefit from redundancy of information presented in the classroom, but a child with a hearing loss may not hear the information often enough to learn it. Lack of opportunity to benefit from the teacher's redundant delivery of instructional information is a key reason why many children with hearing losses require pre- and posttutoring of classroom information (Ross, Brackett, & Maxon, 1991). The pre- and posttutoring provides the redundancy of information that was unavailable to the child in the classroom because of a hearing loss.

Lack of redundancy can be offset partially by the use of a remote microphone, such as that of a personal FM system. The remote microphone can be placed close to the speech or sound source, thereby making information available and alleviating some of the strain and effort of constant focused and disciplined attention (Flexer & Berg, 1990).

The high *level of effort* expended by a child with a hearing loss as he or she attempts to glean information from classroom instruction must be appreciated (Ross, 1991). For example, an eighth grade boy with a moderate to severe hearing loss and excellent auditory, language, and speech skills was earning A's and B's in his mainstreamed classes. Because he was doing so well, school personnel thought that he did not need an FM unit, and he certainly was believed to require no special services such as tutoring, notetakers, or captioned instructional materials. However, further investigation revealed that this boy routinely spent 3 to 5 hours per night doing homework, trying to make up for the redundancy of information that he was being denied access to in the classroom. He had no time to participate in extracurricular activities. His peers with normal hearing spent only 1 to 2 hours per night, at most, on homework. Although children with hearing loss typically do need to exert a higher level of effort than do children with normal hearing in order to be competitive in school, this boy was expending an unnecessary amount of energy gaining information on his own that some basic accommodations could make available to him in the classroom. Appropriate hearing management would enable this eighth grade boy to use his energy for the process of learning and integrating information, rather than working so hard just to acquire the information in the first place. An interesting aside is that when the boy was asked initially how everything was progressing in school, he said, "Just fine!" When further asked if he wanted any help, he said, "No!" He had no idea that life could be any easier for him, because he had always worked so very hard in school. His perceptions were skewed. When he finally agreed to "experiment" with a personal FM system (fit with a neckloop that provided a favorable acoustic signal and was acceptable socially/visually to the boy), a student notetaker, and some review sessions with a tutor, he was shocked to discover how much easier school became for him. He actually had time for "life after school."

Assistive devices are discussed in detail in Chapter 16 of this text. Suffice it to say that assistive listening devices that expand earshot and distance hearing are invaluable for persons with hearing losses because such devices help interface the person with the environment, thereby reducing the level of effort necessary to receive information.

Another area that is affected by reduction of earshot is the learning of appropriate social skills. Much of what a child knows about how other children behave is learned through casual observation of communicative interactions, also known as eavesdropping! Children with hearing losses have a very difficult, if not impossible, time

overhearing conversations that are not directed to them (Ling, 1989). In fact, when they are very young, children with even mild hearing losses might not realize that conversations and transactions occur that do not concern them. The implication of reduction in earshot for the learning of social skills and age-appropriate behaviors is that audiologic rehabilitation often needs to include the active teaching of social skills, especially to young children.

Beware of underestimating the barrier that any type and degree of hearing loss presents to the casual acquisition of information from the environment (Ross, 1991). The audiologist needs to access hearing through technology that includes the use of a remote microphone, then make instructional and behavioral information available to the child in a meaningful and redundant fashion.

Changing Demographics of Children with Hearing Loss

Audiologic services in the schools typically have been viewed as a support service relevant for only a very small population of children who are labeled as "deaf" (Blair, 1986). While children who are deaf certainly require audiologic services, the necessity for hearing management is not limited to these few children. There are approximately 40 million school children in this country, and at least 8 million of them have some degree of hearing loss (Berg, 1986a; Ross, Brackett, & Maxon, 1982). Consequently, when a persistent mild-moderate hearing loss (greater than 15 dB HL) is recognized for the disabling condition that it is (Bess, 1985; Dobie & Berlin, 1979; Northern & Downs, 1991), children with hearing loss represent the largest single population of school children requiring special services (Hull & Dilka, 1984). According to the Iowa model of one hearing specialist, per 5000 school children we would need at least 8000 additional educational audiologists to provide the full spectrum of audiologic services in U.S. schools (Dublinske, 1971). As stated previously, the 700 audiologists currently in the schools are able to manage less than 1% of the children who need support for mainstreamed placement.

Upfold (1988) reported that the population of children with hearing loss has changed over the last few decades. Because maternal rubella and Rh incompatibility have been virtually eliminated, there are fewer children with severe-profound hearing losses and many more children with mild-moderate hearing losses who have been identified and fit with amplification. In fact, the number of children with severe-profound hearing losses is half that known 10 years ago (Upfold, 1988).

The incidence of mild-moderate hearing loss, most often caused by otitis media with effusion, may be much higher than school screenings lead us to believe (Anderson, 1991; Ross, 1991). Because hearing screening environments in schools typically have less than ideal levels of ambient noise, hearing tends to be screened at 20 to 35 dB HL (Anderson, 1991). Thus, school screenings may miss many children who are at risk for academic failure, because even a 15-dB hearing loss poses a significant problem for the young child who must learn crucial word/sound distinctions (Dobie & Berlin, 1979; Northern & Downs, 1991).

A recent prevalence study was conducted by Lundeen (1991), who tested the hearing of 38,000 school children. Unfortunately, Lundeen's data are misleading because he used the criterion of a pure tone average (PTA) of greater than 25 dB HL as constituting hearing loss. With his criterion being at least 10 dB higher than that known to pose educational problems, Lundeen found only 2.63% of children from grades 1 to 12 and 5.51% of first graders to have PTAs greater than 25 dB HL.

On the other hand, when 15 dB HL is used as the criterion for identifying an educationally significant hearing loss, the incidence increases dramatically. A study conducted in the Putnam County Ohio school district found that in the primary grades, 43% of the students failed a 15-dB HL hearing screening on any given day, and approximately 75% of the primary-level children in a class for children with learning disabilities failed a 15-dB hearing screening (Flexer, 1989). In addition, the MARRS (Mainstream Amplification Resource Room Study, National Diffusion Network Project) study on soundfield amplification found that about 30% of the children in grades 3–6 and 75% of children in primary-level classes for children with learning disabilities failed a 15-dB hearing screen (Ray, Sarff, & Glassford, 1984). Flexer, Millin, and Brown (1990) were surprised to discover that only one of the nine children with developmental disabilities in their study of soundfield amplification had thresholds of 15 dB HL or better when tested in a sound room; yet none of the children had been identified by the school as having hearing difficulties!

The point is, the incidence of educationally significant hearing loss may be underestimated tremendously, and many children with fluctuating or "minimal" hearing loss probably will not be identified by school hearing screenings. Perhaps the words "mild" and "minimal" should be avoided because such terminology implies "without consequence." A "mild" hearing loss (greater than 15 dB HL) may pose little difficulty for a linguistically mature person who has sophisticated and disciplined attending skills, but "mild" can mean academic failure for a child who is learning language and acquiring academic competencies (Oyler, Oyler, & Matkin, 1988).

Unfortunately, many schools continue to use the educational models today that might have been appropriate for the population of children with hearing loss that existed 10 to 50 years ago—children with severe to profound hearing losses who were identified rather late and did not have access to early intervention (McGee, 1990; Ross & Calvert, 1984). That is, schools often behave as if the children who will require special services for hearing loss will be "deaf." If the children are not identified as "deaf," then they are believed not to need services (Davis, 1990; Ross, 1991). Today's large population of children who are physiologically or functionally hard of hearing is a different population than existed decades ago, and they often can be accommodated through progressive hearing management in mainstreamed settings (McGee, 1990).

The audiologist has a pivotal leadership role in defining and operationalizing hearing and listening in the mainstream classroom environment for the current population of children with hearing loss.

The Laws Governing Provision of Audiologic Services

Now that the overwhelming necessity for hearing management has been presented and the largest population of children who will need services has been defined, the audiologic services required by federal law will be explored. Are there laws that support comprehensive audiologic management for *all* children with hearing loss?

There are three primary federal laws that mandate and support audiologic services for children in schools: PL 94–142; PL 99–457; and the Rehabilitation Act of 1973, Title V, Section 504, Subpart D.

PL 94–142

PL 94–142 is also known as the Education for All Handicapped Children Act of 1975. The act promotes a free and appropriate public education for all children, ages 5 through 21, who are handicapped. PL 94–142 further protects the rights of parents and guarantees due process in classification and program placement for the child. In 1990, this act was renamed the Individuals with Disabilities Education Act (IDEA).

One component of this extensive law pertains to audiology. As clarified in the Code of Federal Regulations on Education, Title 34, Section 300.13 (1986, p. 14) "audiology" includes:

1. Identification of children with hearing loss
2. Determination of the range, nature, and degree of hearing loss, including referral for medical or other professional attention for the habilitation of hearing
3. Provision of habilitative activities, such as language habilitation, auditory training, speech reading (lipreading), hearing evaluation, and speech conservation
4. Creation and administration of programs for prevention of hearing loss

5. Counseling and guidance of pupils, parents, and teachers regarding hearing loss
6. Determination of the child's need for group and individual amplification, selection and fitting of an appropriate aid, and evaluation of the effectiveness of amplification

Title 34, Section 300.5 of the code (1986, p. 12) defines "deaf" as "a hearing impairment which is so severe that the child is impaired in processing linguistic information through hearing, with or without amplification, which adversely affects educational performance." The code further defines "hard of hearing" as "a hearing impairment, whether permanent or fluctuating, which adversely affects a child's educational performance but which is not included under the definition of 'deaf' in this section" (p. 12).

Note that children with all degrees of hearing loss, permanent or fluctuating, are entitled to audiologic rehabilitative services to support their educational performance.

PL 99–457

PL 99–457, passed in 1986, reauthorizes PL 94–142 but includes mandatory free and appropriate public education for children aged 3 to 5 years by the 1991–1992 school year. PL 99–457 encourages but does not require states to provide services to infants and toddlers (birth to 3 years). Full implementation of the law includes the tenets of zero reject, nondiscriminatory evaluation, Individualized Educational Plan (IEP), education in the least restrictive environment, right to due process, and the right of parents to be involved in decision making (Roush & McWilliam, 1990).

Audiology services, as delineated in the Final Regulations for Public Law 99–457 in the Federal Register (1989), include similar assessment and rehabilitative procedures as those specified in PL 94–142:

1. Identification of children with auditory impairments, using at-risk criteria and appropriate audiologic screening techniques
2. Determination of the range, nature, and degree of hearing loss and communication functions, by use of audiologic evaluation procedures

3. Referral for medical and other services necessary for the habilitation or rehabilitation of children with auditory impairment
4. Provision of auditory training, aural rehabilitation, speech reading, listening device orientation and training, and other services
5. Provision of services for prevention of hearing loss
6. Determination of the child's need for individual amplification including selecting, fitting, and dispensing of appropriate listening and vibrotactile devices, and evaluating the effectiveness of those devices (p. 26312)

Roush and McWilliam (1990) emphasized some unresolved issues concerning audiology and PL 99–457, including the fact that the law does *not* require every child who is evaluated by a multidisciplinary team to receive an audiologic evaluation. In fact, every child who is at risk for hearing loss does not even have to be screened unless the team questions the child's hearing ability.

Audiologists must assume an active role in the implementation of the audiology portions of IDEA (Public Laws 94–142 and 99–457). It is especially critical for audiologists to expand their role definition from primarily diagnostic to include the provision of aural habilitative and rehabilitative services.

THE REHABILITATION ACT OF 1973, TITLE V, SECTION 504, SUBPART D: PRESCHOOL, ELEMENTARY, AND SECONDARY EDUCATION

This law, amended in 1978, is called the "Bill of Rights" for persons with disabilities (DuBow, Geer, & Strauss, 1992). The law specifies that no otherwise qualified person with a disability in the United States will, solely by reason of his or her disability, be excluded from participation in, be denied the benefits of, or be subjected to discrimination under any program or activity receiving federal financial assistance (these programs include schools).

Comparison of IDEA with Section 504 of the Rehabilitation Act of 1973 reveals that IDEA mandates that special education and related services are to be provided through an IEP, whereas Section 504 implies that an appropriate education could be provided through regular education *without* the development of an IEP. Some implications of this difference between the two laws are as follows:

1. There are many more children who might be eligible to receive services through Section 504 than through IDEA. That is, children might not meet the eligibility criteria for special education, but they still do not have access to a free and appropriate public education (FAPE) because of a disability, in this case, hearing problems.
2. If a child is serviced through Section 504 of the Rehabilitation Act of 1973, a school district might be obligated to use *regular education funds* to provide related services or accommodations for a child who experiences a disability.
3. For children with unilateral hearing impairments and/or other hearing, processing, or attention difficulties, the issue to be focused on when requesting services under Section 504 is *acoustic accessibility.*
4. Audiologists need to demonstrate that the child in question is being *denied an appropriate education* because he or she does not have *acoustic accessibility* to instructional and/or extracurricular information.

Communication/acoustic accessibility in school, as provided by Section 504, is *not* limited to instructional services. The following devices or situations ought to be accessible to everybody: school public address announcements, fire alarms and other warning devices, time tests, and telephone services (amplified handsets or TDD). Extracurricular activities such as athletics, transportation, health services, recreational activities, special school-sponsored clubs, school employment, and counseling also must be accessible. For example, a child with a hearing problem might also need to use an FM system for extracurricular activities.

THE AMERICANS WITH DISABILITIES ACT (ADA) OF 1990

The ADA is a landmark civil rights legislation for all persons with disabilities

(Williams, 1992). Title II applies to schools; however, most accessibility issues have already been covered by the Rehabilitation Act of 1973, Section 504. The primary addition is that the ADA provides access and removal of barriers to the general population when they come to school. For example, the following conditions would be covered by the ADA: public attendance at school-sponsored programs, parent-teacher organization meetings, and school board meetings.

Models of Service Provision

How are audiologic services to be delivered to children in schools? Five primary models have been proposed: parent referral model, school-based model, school- and community-based model, contractual agreement model, and modified school- and community-based model (ASHA, 1983; Blair, 1986; Blair, 1991; Brackett & Maxon, 1986).

PARENT REFERRAL MODEL

Within this model, identification services are provided by local school districts or the local education authority or agency (LEA), typically through a hearing screening program. Then, parents have the responsibility of arranging for additional medical or audiologic evaluations at local facilities. Following these additional evaluations, the parents report the results and recommendations back to the LEA, which then initiates intervention procedures. This model is low cost but of limited effectiveness. Parents must assume responsibility for understanding the educational impact of their child's hearing loss and, subsequently, for advocating for services for their child. Because few parents are in a position to manage their child's education, a great many of the audiologic and educational needs of children with hearing loss are overlooked in this model.

SCHOOL-BASED MODEL

This model is also known as a self-contained model because all necessary services are provided by the LEA. The audiologist is responsible for assessment, referral, intervention, coordination, follow-up, and staff development. In addition, the audiologist is a member of the interdisciplinary team serving the child. This model is under direct control of the LEA and is rather costly because of the salaries and equipment that the school must provide.

Blair (1991) reports that if an audiologist manages no more than 12,000 children, then there is a high probability that most of the needs of children with hearing loss in that district will be addressed.

SCHOOL- AND COMMUNITY-BASED MODEL

As the name implies, under this model, both the school and the community share the responsibility for providing services. Clinical assessment is usually performed in the community, and the LEA's audiologist interprets the information for the school. Good communication needs to exist between school-based and community-based audiologists for this model to be effective. Further, this model assumes that if the school cannot provide the hearing services that are necessary for the child, then the referral agency will. Unfortunately, because of lack of time and high cost, if the schools do not provide services for the child, it is unlikely that the community agency will be able to provide all that the child needs to perform in school.

CONTRACTUAL AGREEMENT MODEL

In this model, the LEA contracts with private practitioners or community service agencies for the provision of audiologic services. The nature and comprehensiveness of the contracts will vary depending on cost and perceived need. The school retains the responsibility for ensuring that services are appropriate. This model has potential for development if the contracting audiologist learns to work within the system, enhances the visibility of the profession of audiology, and personalizes the delivery of a *full spectrum* of hearing services (Sexton, 1991).

MODIFIED SCHOOL- AND COMMUNITY-BASED MODEL

In this model, the school audiologist makes referrals to private practitioners or community agencies for audiologic assessment. The information provided is then interpreted by the school audiologist, who also serves as a "hearing clinician"; the hearing clinician provides direct tutorial help to children with hearing losses. While this model has the potential of providing comprehensive services, the school audiologist's role is primarily one of direct service provision (e.g., listening training, speech training, and language and academic development), and other services provided by an audiologist are frequently absent (i.e., diagnostic audiology, hearing aid monitoring, coordination of services, classroom acoustics). These supplemental audiologic services need to be contracted out for this model to work.

Ross (1991) and Blair (1986) contend that audiologic services can be provided most effectively by school-based audiologists. Indeed, professionals on site have the best opportunity to understand and to effect change within the school system because of their physical proximity and familiarity with the political infrastructure. A potential shortfall of audiologic services that are contracted out relates to lack of knowledge about hearing and the importance of hearing evidenced by school personnel (Ross, 1991). That is, schools tend to ask audiologists for audiograms only and not for any rehabilitative services.

Thus, barriers to the successful delivery of audiologic services under any model include the school administrators' views of what the role of the audiologist should be and the audiologists' perceptions of what they can do in the school (Blair, 1991).

Identification of Children Who Need Audiologic Rehabilitative Services

Regardless of the model of audiologic service provision, how can children who need hearing management be identified? The purpose of this chapter is not to design a hearing screening/identification program. For detailed discussions about school hearing conservation, the reader is referred to ASHA (1990), Anderson (1991), and Northern and Downs (1991). Nevertheless, it must be recognized that children have to be identified before they can qualify for and receive hearing services.

Anderson (1991) has graphically represented the diagnostic and rehabilitative outcomes of an effective hearing conservation program (see Fig. 8.1). Note that both *ear* (medical) and *hearing* (educational) components of hearing loss need to be identified and thoughtfully managed. That is, the purpose of hearing screening programs is not to identify only who to send to a physician. An equally important purpose is to identify who may need educational assistance. In fact, if the identification of hearing loss is treated as primarily an educational issue rather than as a medical one, aural rehabilitation follow-up will be viewed as critical by educational personnel (Anderson, 1991).

Note that, as recommended by ASHA (1990), a key component of the identification program displayed in Figure 8.2 is a recognition of the negative impact of early, persistent hearing loss on school performance. In addition, a paper-and-pencil scale that screens for educational difficulties, the S.I.F.T.E.R., has been included.

EARLY HEARING LOSS

The importance of having access to clear acoustic events during the first year of life has been emphasized in recent literature. Leonard (1991), in a literature review of early language acquisition, summarized that even before first words emerge, infants are actively sorting out and grouping the sounds of language. In fact, by 7 months of age, infants can detect major syntactic boundaries.

The question arises, can a "mild" hearing loss, such as that associated with otitis media with effusion (OME), interfere with an infant's ability to sort out and group the sounds of language? Nozza et al. (1990) found that infants and young children who have the typical 20-dB hearing loss caused by OME suffer more negative consequences than do older children with the same degree of hearing loss. The reason for the negative consequence is that infants and young children need a more favorable signal-to-noise ratio (S/N) and better hearing sensitivity than do older children and adults in order to be able to discriminate word/sound dif-

Outcomes of a Hearing Conservation Program

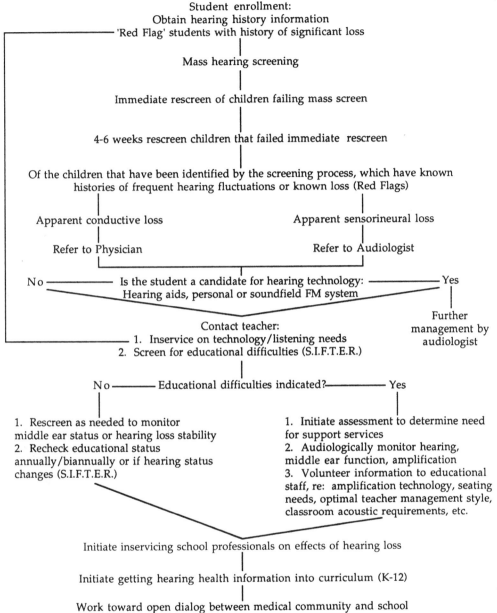

Student enrollment:
Obtain hearing history information
'Red Flag' students with history of significant loss

Mass hearing screening

Immediate rescreen of children failing mass screen

4-6 weeks rescreen children that failed immediate rescreen

Of the children that have been identified by the screening process, which have known histories of frequent hearing fluctuations or known loss (Red Flags)

Apparent conductive loss   Apparent sensorineural loss

Refer to Physician   Refer to Audiologist

No ———— Is the student a candidate for hearing technology: ———— Yes
Hearing aids, personal or soundfield FM system

Further management by audiologist

Contact teacher:
1. Inservice on technology/listening needs
2. Screen for educational difficulties (S.I.F.T.E.R.)

No ———— Educational difficulties indicated? ———— Yes

1. Rescreen as needed to monitor middle ear status or hearing loss stability
2. Recheck educational status annually/biannually or if hearing status changes (S.I.F.T.E.R.)

1. Initiate assessment to determine need for support services
2. Audiologically monitor hearing, middle ear function, amplification
3. Volunteer information to educational staff, re: amplification technology, seating needs, optimal teacher management style, classroom acoustic requirements, etc.

Initiate inservicing school professionals on effects of hearing loss

Initiate getting hearing health information into curriculum (K-12)

Work toward open dialog between medical community and school

Figure 8.1. Diagnostic and rehabilitative outcomes of an effective hearing conservation program. (Reprinted with permission of Thieme Medical Publishers, Inc., *Seminars in Hearing*.)

ferences. Therefore, children with a history of recurrent OME in their first year of life may have developed a significant auditory deficit.

One way to determine if a child has a history of early hearing loss is to have parents, during school registration, fill out a brief ear and hearing loss questionnaire, such as that depicted in Appendix 8.1. If a child is reported to have a history of early and/or continuing hearing loss or ear problems, that child is "red flagged" as a potential candidate for hearing management (Anderson, 1991). Further, information about a potential history of hearing problems would help in the interpretation of results of hearing screening and provide justification for rigorous follow-up. That is, a child who has a history of early and persistent ear and hearing problems would be at significantly greater risk for educational failure due to hearing loss than would a child who had only one or two bouts of OME later in life.

S.I.F.T.E.R.

Another key component of the hearing screening program depicted in Fig. 8.2 that would help in the identification of children who would benefit from hearing management is a formally designed teacher checklist: Screening Instrument for Targeting Educational Risk—S.I.F.T.E.R. (Anderson, 1989a). The S.I.F.T.E.R., shown in Figure 8.2, is the only instrument available to date that specifically screens the classroom performance of the child with hearing loss. The S.I.F.T.E.R. is a brief checklist filled out by the classroom teacher that asks questions about student performance in five areas: academic, attention, communication, class participation, and school behavior. There are 3 questions in each area for a total of 15 questions. The questions ask the teacher to compare the student's performance to that of his or her classmates by rating the student from 1 to 5. The teacher's ratings are then plotted on a scoring grid that shows if the student passes, fails, or has marginal performance in each of the five areas.

Matkin (1990) reported that the S.I.F.T.E.R. was effective for screening the classroom performance of children with frequent otitis media, minimal sensorineural hearing loss, and unilateral hearing loss. He has also found the S.I.F.T.E.R. useful for monitoring the classroom performance of children who have been moved from restrictive special educational programs and placed in mainstreamed settings.

The S.I.F.T.E.R. is a screening and not a diagnostic tool and as such provides only an indication of a student's areas of difficulty. Nevertheless, it is easy and fast to use and adds the critical dimension of involving the classroom teacher in the educational screening process for children with hearing loss. That is, hearing loss is not only a medical problem, and not only the audiologist's problem, but also the teacher's problem. Thus, the use of the S.I.F.T.E.R. raises teachers' awareness of some of the areas of difficulty that a child with any degree of hearing loss may experience. The S.I.F.T.E.R. also provides some justification of the need for audiologic management for the child who scores low on the instrument.

FUNCTIONAL AUDIOMETRIC INFORMATION

Regardless of their employment setting, audiologists who evaluate children need to be mindful of how hearing loss impacts school performance and, subsequently, of the necessity of providing meaningful audiologic information to the schools. "Functional" information about hearing must be included in the audiologic report to assist in the identification of children who need hearing management and educational assistance for their hearing losses. "Functional" means interpreting audiometric data for educational personnel in a fashion that includes an explanation of the speech sounds that are detectable in the classroom relative to hearing loss, distance from the sound source, and background noise.

Acoustic Phonetics and the Familiar Sounds Audiogram

The relationship between pure tones on the audiogram and the ability to detect speech sounds needs to be clarified for school personnel. That is, teachers may recognize that a child has a hearing loss, but they may not have a notion about which speech sounds are audible to the child. For example, without clarification by an audiologist, teachers are not likely to know that a "high-frequency hearing loss at 2000 Hz and 4000 Hz," by reducing access to the speech energy associated with "consonant place of production" and the /s/ morpheme, interferes significantly with the intelligibility of speech even though the child seems to "hear" the teacher.

Appendix 8.2, adapted from Ling (1989), provides a simple overview of the relationship between pure tones and speech sound detection. This table can be useful as a simple handout for teachers and parents to as-

S.I.F.T.E.R.

SCREENING INSTRUMENT FOR TARGETING EDUCATIONAL RISK

by **Karen L. Anderson,** *Ed.S., CCC-A*

STUDENT_____ TEACHER_____ GRADE_____

DATE COMPLETED_____ SCHOOL_____ DISTRICT_____

The above student is suspect for hearing problems which may or may not be affecting his/her school performance. This rating scale has been designed to sift out students who are educationally at risk possibly as a result of hearing problems.

Based on your knowledge from observations of this student, circle the number best representing his/her behavior. After answering the questions, please record any comments about the student in the space provided on the reverse side.

1. What is your estimate of the student's class standing in comparison to that of his/her classmates?	UPPER 5	4	MIDDLE 3	2	LOWER 1	**ACADEMICS** ☐
2. How does the student's achievement compare to your estimation of his/her potential?	EQUAL 5	4	LOWER 3	2	MUCH LOWER 1	
3. What is the student's reading level, reading ability group or reading readiness group in the classroom (e.g., a student with average reading ability performs in the middle group)?	UPPER 5	4	MIDDLE 3	2	LOWER 1	

4. How distractible is the student in comparison to his/her classmates?	NOT VERY 5	4	AVERAGE 3	2	VERY 1	**ATTENTION** ☐
5. What is the student's attention span in comparison to that of his/her classmates?	LONGER 5	4	AVERAGE 3	2	SHORTER 1	
6. How often does the student hesitate or become confused when responding to oral directions (e.g., "Turn to page . . .")?	NEVER 5	4	OCCASIONALLY 3	2	FREQUENTLY 1	

7. How does the student's comprehension compare to the average understanding ability of his/her classmates?	ABOVE 5	4	AVERAGE 3	2	BELOW 1	**COMMUNICATION** ☐
8. How do the student's vocabulary and word usage skills compare with those of other students in his/her age group?	ABOVE 5	4	AVERAGE 3	2	BELOW 1	
9. How proficient is the student at telling a story or relating happenings from home when compared to classmates?	ABOVE 5	4	AVERAGE 3	2	BELOW 1	

10. How often does the student volunteer information to class discussions or in answer to teacher questions?	FREQUENTLY 5	4	OCCASIONALLY 3	2	NEVER 1	**CLASS PARTICIPATION** ☐
11. With what frequency does the student complete his/her class and homework assignments within the time allocated?	ALWAYS 5	4	USUALLY 3	2	SELDOM 1	
12. After instruction, does the student have difficulty starting to work (looks at other students working or asks for help)?	NEVER 5	4	OCCASIONALLY 3	2	FREQUENTLY 1	

13. Does the student demonstrate any behaviors that seem unusual or inappropriate when compared to other students?	NEVER 5	4	OCCASIONALLY 3	2	FREQUENTLY 1	**SCHOOL BEHAVIOR** ☐
14. Does the student become frustrated easily, sometimes to the point of losing emotional control?	NEVER 5	4	OCCASIONALLY 3	2	FREQUENTLY 1	
15. In general, how would you rank the student's relationship with peers (ability to get along with others)?	GOOD 5	4	AVERAGE 3	2	POOR 1	

Copyright©1989 by
The Interstate Printers & Publishers, Inc.

Reproduction of this form, in whole or in part, is strictly prohibited.

Additional copies of this form are available in pads of 100 each from
The Interstate Printers & Publishers, Inc., Danville, Illinois 61834-0050.
ISBN 0-8134-2845-9

Figure 8.2. The S.I.F.T.E.R., as a screening tool, involves the classroom teacher in the management of hearing. (Reprinted with permission of Pro-Ed.)

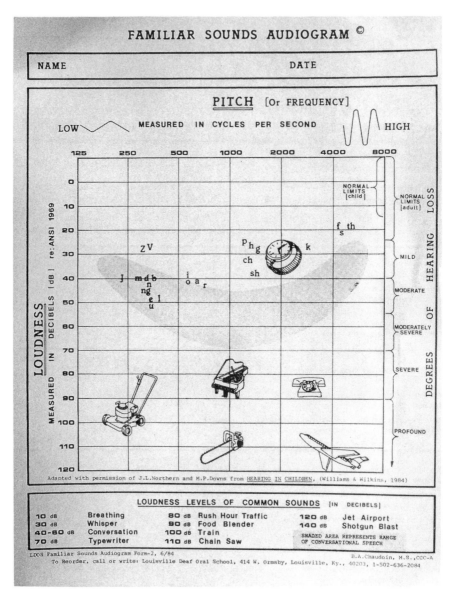

Figure 8.3. The Familiar Sounds Audiogram provides a visual representation of which speech and environmental sounds are audible with and without hearing technology. (Reprinted with permission of B.A. Chaudoin.)

sist in the explanation of the meaning of hearing loss.

Another tool that can help demystify audiometric information is the "Familiar Sounds Audiogram" (Fig. 8.3). Aided and unaided thresholds, obtained in the soundfield, can be plotted on this Familiar Sounds Audiogram. Teachers and parents benefit from the visual representation of which speech sounds the child can detect while wearing hearing aids, compared to those speech and environmental sounds

that are audible without amplification. In addition, if a child is fit with a personal FM unit (and all children with hearing loss require some form of signal-to-noise ratio [S/N] enhancing technology in the classroom), those thresholds also should be depicted on the audiogram.

Perform Word Identification Testing at 45 dB HL

By adding only two speech tests to the basic audiometric test battery, an audiologist in a clinical or school setting can provide "functional" data that can help identify children who have trouble hearing and listening in the classroom.

Word identification testing in the soundfield, aided and unaided, and when wearing a personal FM unit, ought to be conducted at the average loudness level that speech is received by the child in a favorable classroom environment—45 dB HL. If phonetically balanced (PB) words are presented at 40 dB SL under earphones only, functional information about classroom listening is not provided.

In addition, word identification testing in the soundfield, aided and unaided and when wearing a personal FM, ought to be conducted at 45 dB HL using a $+5$ S/N, which is a typical noise level in a primary-level classroom (Berg, 1987). A child might seem to hear well in the "acoustically perfect" environment of a sound room but have a great deal of difficulty hearing in a typical noisy classroom environment.

The following example illustrates the necessity of providing functional audiometric information. A 6-year-old child, audiometrically evaluated for the third time, showed the following results on testing that was performed in addition to those data typically obtained in a basic diagnostic assessment (the basic assessment revealed a mild, bilateral sensorineural hearing loss).

1. Soundfield SRT = 30 dB HL.
2. PB score at 45 dB HL in a quiet soundfield = 78%.
3. PB score at 45 dB HL at $+5$ S/N in the soundfield = 24%.
4. When tested under earphones at 40 dB SL (70 dB HL), the score was excellent: 100% for each ear.

The child in this example was having a great deal of difficulty listening in the classroom, according to his teacher, but he appeared to have no difficulty during one-to-one communication. The S.I.F.T.E.R. was completed by the teacher and resulted in low scores in all areas. The initial audiologic assessment, conducted by an audiologist who did not perform functional testing, resulted in the recommendation that no amplification of any kind was needed because the boy obtained a PB score of 100% under earphones (at 70 dB HL) and, therefore, was assumed to be able to hear

the teacher clearly. The child continued to have difficulty in the classroom, so a second audiologic opinion was obtained. The second evaluation also did not include functional soundfield information and resulted in the recommendation of binaural, mild gain in-the-ear hearing aids (ITEs). The child continued to have difficulty in the classroom and refused to wear the hearing aids because they were uncomfortable and noisy, so the parents sought a third opinion. Because hearing aids alone are not enough for classroom listening (a remote microphone placed close to the sound source is needed in the classroom to improve the S/N), the hearing aids were temporarily discontinued and a mild gain personal FM unit with Walkman earphones was recommended on a trial basis. Classroom observation of the child's listening behaviors and a teacher-completed S.I.F.T.E.R. revealed significant improvement with the FM unit. In addition, the boy willingly used the technology. Hearing aids will be coupled to the FM unit at a later time, but the boy will undoubtedly continue to benefit from S/N enhancing technology. As an aside, the child also received some academic tutoring to enable him to learn the information that he had missed previously in the classroom.

The point is, children with any type and degree of hearing loss have very complex listening needs because of the dynamic nature of their learning environments. Functional audiometric information can assist in identifying their need for hearing management.

Avoid the "Failure Model" of Identification

It must be emphasized to school personnel that the significant negative consequences of hearing loss may be *prevented* if the hearing loss is identified early, if hearing is accessed through appropriate technology, and if intervention is initiated before too much language is missed because of the filtering effect of the hearing loss. The difficulty with promoting prevention is that schools tend to allocate special services to students based on a "failure model" (Flexer, 1990). That is, technology is allotted and services provided only after children have failed one to three grades or are significantly behind their same-age peers;

services are provided too late to enable the child to "catch up" to grade level. For example, the special services of auditory skills development, language therapy, academic tutoring, and even the provision of signal-to-noise ratio enhancing technology might be authorized only after the child has failed in the mainstream without such services. Accommodations typically are not allocated to prevent failure (Blair, 1991). Audiologists need to promote a paradigm shift by emphasizing that hearing ought to be considered as a foundation for the general education of all children to prevent the necessity of special services for many children. As audiologists who want to be proactive in preventing failure, we are challenged to understand and work within regular education and not to view audiology only as a related service for a very few children.

CATEGORIES OF AUDIOLOGIC
REHABILITATIVE SERVICES

The audiologic services that a child needs are dependent on the function of the child and the demands of the learning environment. Essentially, management of hearing includes attention to all aspects of the acoustic filter effect of hearing loss, as discussed previously in this chapter. Access to acoustic events, language, reading, academics, and independent function must be facilitated. Anderson and Matkin have developed a chart that provides a general overview of the relationship of degree of long-term hearing loss to psychosocial impact and educational needs (Anderson, 1991). The chart is displayed in Figure 8.4. Note how all aspects of the acoustic filter are acknowledged.

The audiologist is the professional best able to manage the complete hearing care of a child who experiences hearing loss of any degree. Speech-language pathologists can facilitate language acquisition and teachers can teach academics, but only audiologists can assess and educationally treat hearing loss. Accordingly, the following hearing issues must be considered to enable the child with *any* degree of hearing loss to benefit from academic instruction:

1. Audiologic assessments including *functional hearing data* with and without hearing aids and assistive listening devices.
2. Fitting of amplification technologies, inclusive of S/N enhancing equipment such as personal FM units or soundfield systems, telephone amplifiers, and signal warning systems such as accommodations for fire alarms and smoke detectors.
3. Monitoring and maintaining the equipment mentioned above. How and when will the equipment be checked and managed and by whom?
4. Loaner equipment bank. Where will one be located for the school system, what equipment will be carried, and how will a student expediently access loaner equipment?
5. Provision of in-services for school personnel about hearing, hearing loss, amplification technology, and classroom management of the child with hearing loss. When and how will such in-services be conducted and by whom?
6. Auditory skills development and classroom listening. How will hearing and listening be integrated throughout the child's varied and changing learning domains with special attention to integrating listening with speech and language development and expansion?
7. Access to school instruction as appropriate for grade level, being mindful of the level of effort expended by the child and the need for redundancy of instructional information—notetakers, captioned videos and films, access to school public address (PA) announcements, assemblies and field trips, and pre- and posttutoring.
8. Assisting the child in gaining an understanding of his or her hearing loss; multiple amplification technologies; and the impact of hearing loss on personal and classroom function. Such an understanding is for the purpose of promoting the child's independent management of the learning environment. How will such individual or group counseling occur and by whom?

The IEP section of this chapter will present some examples of how the previous audiologic goals can be written in behavioral objective format.

Because, as Mark Ross has explained, the main problem with hearing loss is that one has problems hearing, the first line of audiologic management is the use of technology to access residual hearing (Ross & Giolas, 1978). Hearing is at the core of the acoustic filter; thus if acoustic events are not received, higher levels of auditory processing cannot be accessed (Ling, 1989; Madell, 1990).

ACCESS HEARING THROUGH TECHNOLOGY

Children in schools often are in demanding, degraded, and constantly changing listening situations because of noise and distance from the talker (Berg, 1987). A limitation of hearing aids is that the microphone is on the wearer who may or may not be close to the signal source. The further the microphone is from the sound source and the greater the background noise, the poorer the signal-to-noise ratio (S/N).

Signal-to-Noise Ratio

S/N is a pivotal concept relative to speech intelligibility and the justification for the use of S/N technology in addition to or instead of hearing aids in the classroom. S/N is the relationship between the primary speech or input signal and background noise. Background noise is anything and everything that interferes with the reception of the auditory signal and includes other talkers; heating or cooling systems; classroom sounds; traffic noise; computer hums; internal biological noise; televisions; playground, gym, and hall noise; wind; and so on. The more favorable the S/N (the louder the primary auditory signal relative to background sounds), the more intelligible that speech or auditory signal will be for the child. An intelligible speech signal will provide children with a better opportunity to learn the word/sound differences that underlie the development of basic academic competencies.

People with normal hearing typically require an S/N of +6 dB (speech is twice the sound pressure level of the noise) for the reception of intelligible speech. Because of internal auditory distortion, persons with any degree of hearing loss need a more favorable S/N of +20 dB; speech is approx-

imately 10 times the level of the noise (Finitzo-Hieber & Tillman, 1978). Because of reverberation, noise, and changes in teacher position, the average classroom S/N is only +4 or +5 dB and may be 0 dB, which is less than ideal even for children with normal hearing (Berg, 1986b).

RASTI

It is a well-known fact that sound is degraded as it is propagated across a space; however, the magnitude of that degradation has been difficult to determine because of difficulties relating the physical components of high-fidelity sound (dynamic range, frequency, intensity, reverberation, and S/N) to speech perception. As a result, the negative effects of a typical classroom environment on the integrity of the speech signal probably have been underestimated.

The new Bruel and Kjaer Rapid Speech Transmission Index (RASTI) system was used by Leavitt and Flexer (1991) to measure the effect of a listening environment on a speech-like signal. The RASTI signal is an amplitude-modulated broad band of noise centered at 500 Hz and 2000 Hz that is transmitted from the RASTI transmitter to the RASTI receiver (Houtgast & Steeneken, 1985). The RASTI score is a measure of the integrity of the signal as it is propagated across the classroom. A perfect reproduction of the RASTI signal at the receiver is depicted by a score of 1.0. The question investigated by Leavitt and Flexer (1991) was how much speech information is lost as the teacher's speech travels from his or her mouth to the ears of students who are seated at various locations around the classroom?

To measure the loss of critical speech information at various locations in a typical, occupied classroom, Leavitt and Flexer (1991) obtained RASTI scores at 17 different seating locations. Results showed that significant sound degradation occurred as the RASTI receiver was moved away from the RASTI transmitter. The magnitude of the loss of critical speech information was reflected by a significant decrease in RASTI scores. Even in the front-row center seat, which was the most favorable seat in the classroom, the RASTI score dropped to 0.83. In the back row, the RASTI score decreased to 0.55, reflecting a loss of 45% of

RELATIONSHIP OF
DEGREE OF LONGTERM HEARING LOSS
TO PSYCHOSOCIAL IMPACT AND EDUCATIONAL NEEDS

Degree of Hearing Loss Based on modified pure tone average (500-4000 HZ)	Possible Effect of Hearing Loss on the Understanding of Language & Speech	Possible Psychosocial Impact of Hearing Loss 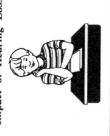	Potential Educational Needs and Programs 
NORMAL HEARING -10 - +15 dB HL	Children have better hearing sensitivity than the accepted normal range for adults. A child with hearing sensitivity in the -10 to +15 dB range will detect the complete speech signal even at soft conversation levels. However, good hearing does not guarantee good ability to discriminate speech in the presence of background noise.		
MINIMAL (BORDERLINE) 16-25 dB HL	May have difficulty hearing faint or distant speech. At 15 dB student can miss up to 10% of speech signal when teacher is at a distance greater than 3 feet and when the classroom is noisy, especially in the elementary grades when verbal instruction predominates.	May be unaware of subtle conversational cues which could cause child to be viewed as inappropriate or awkward. May miss portions of fast-paced peer interactions which could begin to have an impact on socialization and self concept. May have immature behavior. Child may be more fatigued than classmates due to listening effort needed.	May benefit from mild gain/low MPO hearing aid or personal FM system dependent on loss configuration. Would benefit from soundfield amplification if classroom is noisy and/or reverberant. Favorable seating. May need attention to vocabulary or speech, especially with recurrent otitis media history. Appropriate medical management necessary for conductive losses. Teacher requires inservice on impact of hearing loss on language development and learning.
MILD 26-40 dB HL	At 30 dB can miss 25-40% of speech signal. The degree of difficulty experienced in school will depend upon the noise level in classroom, distance from teacher and the configuration of the hearing loss. Without amplification the child with 35-40 dB loss may miss at least 50% of class discussions, especially when voices are faint or speaker is not in line of vision. Will miss consonants, especially when a high frequency hearing loss is present.	Barriers beginning to build with negative impact on self esteem as child is accused of "hearing when he or she wants to," "daydreaming," or "not paying attention." Child begins to lose ability for selective hearing, and has increasing difficulty suppressing background noise which makes the learning environment stressful. Child is more fatigued than classmates due to listening effort needed.	Will benefit from a hearing aid and use of a personal FM or soundfield FM system in the classroom. Needs favorable seating and lighting. Refer to special education for language evaluation and educational follow-up. Needs auditory skill building. May need attention to vocabulary and language development, articulation or speechreading and/or special support in reading. May need help with self esteem. Teacher inservice required.
MODERATE 41-55 dB HL	Understands conversational speech at a distance of 3-5 feet (face-to-face) only if structure and vocabulary controlled. Without amplification the amount of speech signal missed can be 50% to 75% with 40 dB loss and 80% to 100% with 50 dB loss. Is likely to have delayed or defective syntax, limited vocabulary, imperfect speech production and an atonal voice quality.	Often with this degree of hearing loss, communication is significantly affected, and socialization with peers with normal hearing becomes increasingly difficult. With full time use of hearing aids/FM systems child may be judged as a less competent learner. There is an increasing impact on self-esteem.	Refer to special education for language evaluation and for educational follow-up. Amplification is essential (hearing aids and FM system). Special education support may be needed, especially for primary children. Attention to oral language development, reading and written language. Auditory skill development and speech therapy usually needed. Teacher inservice required.

Figure 8.4. Relationship of degree of long-term hearing loss to psychosocial impact and educational needs. (Reprinted with permission of Thieme Medical Publishers, Inc., *Seminars in Hearing.*)

Degree of Hearing Loss	Possible Effect of Hearing Loss on the Understanding of Language and Speech	Possible Psychosocial Impact of Hearing Loss	Potential Educational Needs and Programs
MODERATE TO SEVERE 56-70 dB HL	Without amplification, conversation must be very loud to be understood. A 55 dB loss can cause child to miss up to 100% of speech information. Will have marked difficulty in school situations requiring verbal communication in both one-to-one and group situations. Delayed language, syntax, reduced speech intelligibility and atonal voice quality likely.	Full time use of hearing aids/FM systems may result in child being judged by both peers and adults as a less competent learner, resulting in poorer self concept, social maturity and contributing to a sense of rejection. Inservice to address these attitudes may be helpful.	Full time use of amplification is essential. Will need resource teacher or special class depending on magnitude of language delay. May require special help in all language skills, language based academic subjects, vocabulary, grammar, pragmatics as well as reading and writing. Probably needs assistance to expand experiential language base. Inservice of mainstream teachers required.
SEVERE 71-90 dB HL	Without amplification may hear loud voices about one foot from ear. When amplified optimally, children with hearing ability of 90 dB or better should be able to identify environmental sounds and detect all the sounds of speech. If loss is of prelingual onset, oral language and speech may not develop spontaneously or will be severely delayed. If hearing loss is of recent onset speech is likely to deteriorate with quality becoming atonal.	Child may prefer other children with hearing impairments as friends and playmates. This may further isolate the child from the mainstream, however, these peer relationships may foster improved self concept and a sense of cultural identity.	May need full-time special aural/oral program for with emphasis on all auditory language skills, speechreading, concept development and speech. As loss approaches 80-90dB, may benefit from a Total Communication approach, especially in the early language learning years. Individual hearing aid/personal FM system essential. Need to monitor effectiveness of communication modality. Participation in regular classes as much as beneficial to student. Inservice of mainstream teachers essential.
PROFOUND 91 dB HL or more	Aware of vibrations more than tonal pattern. Many rely on vision rather than hearing as primary avenue for communication and learning. Detection of speech sounds dependent upon loss configuration and use of amplification. Speech and language will not develop spontaneously and is likely to deteriorate rapidly if hearing loss is of recent onset.	Depending on auditory/oral competence, peer use of sign language, parental attitude, etc., child may or may not increasingly prefer association with the deaf culture.	May need special program for deaf children with emphasis on all language skills and academic areas. Program needs specialized supervision and comprehensive support services. Early use of amplification likely to help if part of an intensive training program. May be cochlear implant or vibrotactile aid candidate. Requires continual appraisal of needs in regard to communication and learning mode. Part-time in regular classes as much as beneficial to student.
UNILATERAL One normal hearing ear and one ear with at least a permanent mild hearing loss	May have difficulty hearing faint or distant speech. Usually has difficulty localizing sounds and voices. Unilateral listener will have greater difficulty understanding speech when environment is noisy and/or reverberant. Difficulty detecting or understanding soft speech from side of bad ear, especially in a group discussion.	Child may be accused of selective hearing due to discrepancies in speech understanding in quiet versus noise. Child will be more fatigued in classroom setting due to greater effort needed to listen. May appear inattentive or frustrated. Behavior problems sometimes evident.	May benefit from personal FM or soundfield FM system in classroom. CROS hearing aid may be of benefit in quiet settings. Needs favorable seating and lighting. Student is at risk for educational difficulties. Educational monitoring warranted with support services provided as soon as difficulties appear. Teacher inservice is beneficial.

NOTE: All children with hearing loss require periodic audiologic evaluation, rigorous monitoring of amplification and regular monitoring of communication skills. All children with hearing loss (especially conductive) need appropriate medical attention in conjunction with educational programming.

REFERENCES
Olsen, W. O., Hawkins, D. B., VanTassell, D. J. (1987). Representatives of the Longterm Spectrum of Speech. Ear & Hearing, Supplement 8, pp. 100-108.
Mueller, H. G. & Killion, M. C. (1990). An easy method for calculating the articulation index. The Hearing Journal, 43, 9, pp. 14-22.
Hasenstab, M. S. (1987). Language Learning and Otitis Media, College Hill Press, Boston, MA.

Adapted from: Bernero, R. J. & Bothwell, H. (1966). Relationship of Hearing Impairment to Educational Needs. Illinois Department of Public Health & Office of Superintendent of Public Instruction.
Peer Review by Members of the Educational Audiology Association, Winter 1991.

Developed by
Karen L. Anderson, Ed.S & Noel D. Matkin, Ph.D (1991)

equivalent speech intelligibility in a quiet, occupied classroom. A perfect RASTI score of 1.0 could be attained only at the 6-inch reference position.

These RASTI scores represent only the loss of speech fidelity that might be expected at the student's ear or hearing aid microphone in a quiet classroom. The negative effects that the student's central processing deficit, or hearing loss (even a minimal hearing loss), or attention/listening problem will have on speech intelligibility must be considered over and above the degraded speech signal. Even in a front-row center seat, the loss of critical speech information was substantial. Obviously, the most sophisticated of hearing aids cannot re-create those aspects of the speech signal that have been lost during transmission across the physical space.

The importance of being close to the speaker, either physically or through the use of a remote location microphone for the purpose of obtaining a complete speech signal, was demonstrated by the RASTI study. As soon as any pupil in the classroom moves farther away than 6 inches from the teacher's mouth, the speech signal begins to degrade. Data input precedes data processing. Thus, if a student does not receive a complete speech signal, that student is being denied access to instructional information.

Hearing Aids

The hearing aid typically is the primary amplification technology for children with hearing loss. The reader is referred to Chapter 5 in this book and to Maxon and Smaldino (1991) for detailed information about fitting hearing aids on young children. Nevertheless, the hearing aid alone is not enough for classroom listening because much speech fidelity is lost as the signal travels from the teacher's mouth to the hearing aid microphone on the student's ear (Leavitt & Flexer, 1991). Thus, as stated previously, a remote microphone placed close to the sound source is essential.

Personal FM Systems

The device most commonly used to enhance the S/N and to provide a complete speech signal is a personal FM system, typically coupled to a child's hearing aids through direct input or a neck loop (Hawkins & Schum, 1985; VanTasell, Mallinger, & Crump, 1986). An appropriately fit personal FM system can provide a consistent and favorable S/N: approximately +20 dB (Hawkins, 1984). Unfortunately, school personnel may be unfamiliar with personal FM systems, may be intimidated by their use, and are likely not to use FMs at the first sign of difficulty (Leavitt, 1987; Woodford, 1987). The reader is referred to Chapter 16 of this text for more information about personal FM systems. It should be noted that *mild* gain, personal FM units appear to be beneficial in improving the listening skills and attending behaviors of children who have normal hearing but who experience learning disabilities (Blake et al., 1991).

Soundfield FM Systems

Personal FM systems use wireless radio transmission to amplify the teacher's speech for each student who is wearing a receiver; soundfield units provide amplification for the entire classroom through the use of two, three, or four wall- or ceiling-mounted loudspeakers (Berg, 1987). All students in the classroom will benefit from an improved S/N of approximately +10 dB no matter where they or the teacher is positioned (Flexer, Millin, & Brown, 1990; Worner, 1988). It should be noted that +10 dB may not be enough for some children with more severe hearing losses; they may need to wear a personal FM unit tuned to the same frequency as the soundfield unit so that the teacher need wear only a single transmitter.

Rationale. Classroom public address systems have exciting promise for providing students, whether or not they have diagnosed hearing losses, with access to intelligible speech (Flexer, Millin, & Brown, 1990; Ray, Sarff, & Glassford, 1984). A 3-year study of soundfield amplification revealed the following preliminary results (Osborn, Graves, & VonderEmbse, 1989):

1. The proportion of students requiring special services decreased after 3 years with amplified classrooms.
2. Amplified kindergarten classes scored significantly higher on listening, lan-

guage, and word analysis tests than did children in unamplified classrooms.

3. According to formal classroom observations, students in amplified classrooms had better on-task behaviors than students in unamplified classrooms.
4. As reported by principals, in amplified classrooms there were fewer teacher absences due to fatigue and laryngitis.
5. Teachers in amplified kindergarten classrooms tended to use less repetition and rephrasing in their instruction.
6. The study began with 17 soundfield units; 3 years later, 47 units were in use because teachers wanted them, parents demanded that their children be placed in amplified classrooms, and administrators were convinced that student performance improved.

Another study that investigated classroom amplification was the MARRS National Diffusion Network Project (Mainstream Amplification Resource Room Study). The purpose of the study was to evaluate soundfield amplification as a means of enabling children with mild or fluctuating hearing losses to remain in the mainstream without expensive referral procedures. After the original 3-year study in Illinois, data were analyzed for three different treatments of identified target students: *(1)* those in regular classroom settings without special accommodations; *(2)* those receiving regular classroom instruction augmented by resource room instruction; and *(3)* those educated in amplified classrooms. Soundfield amplification resulted in significant improvement in academic achievement test scores for the students with "minimal" hearing losses (Ray, Sarff, & Glassford, 1984). In addition, academic gains were attained at a higher level, at a faster rate, and with less cost than gains achieved by students in the more traditional resource room model.

The logic of soundfield amplification is that, if properly adjusted, it can counteract weak teacher voice levels and ambient noise interference by *(1)* increasing the overall speech level of whoever is using the microphone, *(2)* improving the S/N, and *(3)* producing a nearly uniform speech level in the classroom that is unaffected by teacher position (Flexer, Millin, & Brown, 1990;

Ray, Sarff, & Glassford, 1984; Worner, 1988). If students receive a louder, more intact speech signal, they will be able to determine word/sound distinctions better. Indeed, Flexer, Millin, & Brown (1990) found that nine students who attended a primary-level class for children with developmental disabilities made significantly fewer errors on a word identification task when the teacher presented the words through a classroom PA system than they made when the words were presented without soundfield amplification. Informal observations made during the same study revealed that the students responded more quickly and appeared more relaxed in the amplified condition.

The advantages of soundfield amplification result from the use of a teacher-worn transmitter microphone that is positioned 4 to 6 inches from the speaker's mouth, thus avoiding the loss of critical speech elements. A second advantage is that all pupils are consistently closer to the speech source, in the form of a loudspeaker, than they could be to a mobile teacher. That is, the speech signal not only is louder when amplified through the soundfield system, but each student is closer to the signal (loudspeaker), thereby reducing the magnitude of the degradation of the speech signal as it travels across the classroom. It should be noted that a pupil could not be as close to a loudspeaker as he or she could be to a personal FM receiver that directs the sound into the ear. Therefore, a personal FM could provide a speech signal superior to that provided by a soundfield unit. To summarize, classroom amplification would facilitate the reception of a consistently more intact signal than that received in an unamplified classroom, but not as complete a signal as that received by a personal FM unit (Leavitt, 1991).

Populations. There is evidence to suggest that all children benefit from listening to an improved speech signal; however, some children seem to benefit more than others. Classroom amplification is not a replacement for all other forms of S/N technology. Rather, soundfield amplification is a new technology that will provide audiologists with more options as they address the question "How can students, with and without hearing loss, have the most efficient access to clear and complete auditory information?" The choice of sound enhancement technology is dependent on the pupil, the classroom environment, and the needs of other children in the classroom.

Based on information available to date, the following populations appear to benefit most from soundfield amplification:

1. Children with past and current histories of otitis media with effusion
2. Children with unilateral hearing losses
3. Children with minimal sensorineural hearing losses who do not wear hearing aids
4. Children with mild to moderate sensorineural hearing losses who wear hearing aids
5. Children with auditory processing or attentional difficulties but with normal peripheral hearing sensitivity
6. Preschoolers, kindergartners, and first graders with normal hearing sensitivity who are in the critical stages of developing academic competencies

Three practical advantages to appropriately installed and functioning soundfield equipment for target populations are as follows: *(1)* Classroom amplification requires no overt cooperation from the child; *(2)* the technology is not stigmatizing for any particular child; and *(3)* equipment function or malfunction is immediately obvious to everyone in the room (Anderson, 1989b).

Practical Issues.   There are many issues to evaluate when selecting classroom amplification systems or when recommending a soundfield rather than a personal FM system for a particular child, and there are few data available to guide these decisions (Flexer, 1992). Following is a list of questions that an audiologist ought to consider about classroom amplification:

1. How many loudspeakers should be installed in a given room?
2. Where should the loudspeakers be installed?
3. What is the best S/N ratio possible with the equipment?
4. What is the durability, quality, and flexibility of the equipment?
5. What is the carrier frequency for the radio signal of the unit and the potential for interference?
6. What are the number of available discrete channels within the frequency band used by the manufacturer? How many units can be installed in the same building while maintaining a good S/N within the equipment itself?
7. What is the fidelity of the unit?

Following recognition and some resolution of the equipment-related issues mentioned above comes the realization that at best, technology is simply a tool—a means to an end. The purpose of classroom amplification, or any S/N enhancing technology, is to facilitate the reception of the primary speech signal. Once students can clearly detect word/sound differences, they will have an opportunity to improve their language skills and to acquire knowledge of the world. Thus, the logical next step in the rehabilitative process concerns the student's ability to attend to the now enhanced acoustic signal—listening.

Listening Skills

Chapter 7 in this text discusses auditory learning. This chapter focuses on the student's ability to attend to verbal instruction in the classroom.

Listening in the classroom involves recognition of teacher variables, pupil variables, and environmental variables (Berg, 1987). Appendix 8.3, from Edwards (1991), is an observational tool that can be used for evaluating children with suspected listening difficulties. The form rates, on a scale of 1 to 4, overall concerns about listening, current listening strengths and weaknesses evidenced by the pupil, the child's level of awareness of his or her listening strengths and weaknesses, the child's current listening strategies, the current instructional/listening modifications employed by the teacher, and other related factors.

Children are suspected of having listening difficulties because of an early history of permanent or fluctuating hearing loss, a current history of fluctuating or permanent hearing loss, low scores on the S.I.F.T.E.R., teacher-reported concern about classroom behavior or performance, pupil-reported concerns, parent concern about classroom behaviors or performance, or functional audiometric data obtained by the audiologist that suggests that the child has difficulty hearing word/sound differences in the presence of noise.

Once the student's listening difficulties have been evaluated, Edwards (1991), (Erber (1982), and Lasky and Katz (1983) all recommend strategy teaching. That is, modifications of the listening environment, the teacher's instructional strategies, and the child's response/clarification strategies are attempted. For example, the classroom/listening environment can be modified by the use of classroom amplification, by moving the student from an open- to a closed-style classroom, and by removing external noise sources such as closing a window or a door. Teacher strategies that can be employed include developing an understanding of the student's strengths or weaknesses, talking close to the pupil either physically or through the use of a remote microphone, using the word "listen" to cue attention to verbal communication, speaking slower, drawing attention to word/sound distinctions, having the child repeat instructions, and having rest periods from listening. Child strategies include developing self-recognition of difficult and easy listening conditions, moving closer to the sound source or using S/N enhancing technology, asking the speaker to slow down or to repeat, rehearsing or reauditorializing instructions, and signaling when the information is unclear.

Specific auditory skills-building sessions, such as those discussed by Erber (1982), Estabrooks and Edwards (1986), Ling (1989), Pollack (1985), and Ying (1990), might also be necessary for a given student. Nevertheless, functional listening strategies are vital features of effective hearing management for all children with hearing loss in schools.

IEP and IFSP: How to Make Hearing Services a Reality for Children in an Educational Setting

The IEP (Individualized Education Program of PL 94–142) and IFSP (Individualized Family Service Plan of PL 99–457) are written statements designed to meet the unique needs of the family and child with a disability. An IEP is generated because a

child has been identified as being unable to derive educational benefit from the standard school curriculum. Special educational areas of need are targeted, and accommodations and special services are integrated into the child's day. An IEP is supposed to be designed to enable a child with a disability to obtain an individualized and "appropriate" education in the "least restrictive" environment.

The reason IEP issues are discussed here is because the IEP is the only ticket into the special education system of resource allocation that allows a child to receive any assistive technology, services, or strategies in school. All hearing services, including the availability, use, and maintenance of technology, listening strategies, and any other audiologic rehabilitative services must be carefully detailed on the IEP, or the school is under no obligation to provide such technology and services. The best of audiologic recommendations cannot be implemented by the school unless those recommendations are incorporated into the IEP. Therefore, the audiologist must be an active participant in the IEP process to ensure that hearing technology and services are coordinated across other goals. It is not possible for a child with any degree of hearing loss to obtain "an appropriate education" until and unless hearing is carefully and thoroughly managed (Madell, 1990; Ross, 1991).

All too often, for a child with a hearing loss, the only audiologic goal specified on the IEP is that the child must have a hearing test once a year, as if assessment is an end in itself rather than a means of determining appropriate rehabilitative services. To assist the audiologist, whether employed in a school or clinic setting, in effectively participating in the IEP, the following discussion will include the purpose of the IEP, components of an IEP, and an example of a "hearing management" objective. But first, audiologists ought to be mindful of the language used to refer to persons who experience disabilities.

PEOPLE-FIRST LANGUAGE

In recent years, much attention has been given to the rights of persons with disabilities. Efforts of many consumer groups have heightened awareness of the need for access to society and culture. Legislation and affirmative action have resulted in increasing recognition that persons with disabilities are valuable and dignified members of society; they are not "partial" people to be feared, pitied, or ignored.

The language used to refer to people with disabilities reflects attitudes and beliefs and shapes our perceptions about individuals. Beginning in 1974 with the efforts of a consumer group called "People-First," there has been an international movement to use terminology that places the individual before the disability. Therefore, instead of saying "*handicapped* person," people-first language would say, "a *person* with a disability"; instead of the term, "*hearing-impaired* person," say, "*person* with hearing loss." The person is first; the disability is second. Words with negative or demeaning connotations have been eliminated, such as *handicapped, afflicted, diseased, retarded, defective, deformed, invalid, maimed, wheelchair-bound, unfortunate, epileptic, stricken, victim,* and *insane.*

Such wording is far more than playing with semantics. People-first wording reflects the humanistic value and belief that a person is far more than a reflection of his or her disability.

PL 94–142 does not use people-first wording because it was written before recognition of the value of positive terminology.

PURPOSE OF AN IEP

The IEP, when developed and implemented as intended by the lawmakers, has a very positive function: the provision of individualized accommodations that would enable a child with special needs to obtain an "appropriate" education. Accordingly, no technology or special service can be provided for a child until those accommodations are justified and stated explicitly on the IEP. As specified in the Federal Register (1977), the IEP has a number of purposes:

1. The IEP meeting serves as a communication vehicle between parents and school personnel and enables them, as equal participants, to jointly decide on what the child's needs are, what will be provided, and what the anticipated outcomes may be.

2. The IEP itself serves as the focal point for resolving any differences between the parents and the school—first through the meeting and second, if necessary, through the procedural protections that are available to the parents.

3. The IEP sets forth in writing a commitment of resources necessary to enable a child with a disability to receive needed special education and related services.

4. The IEP is a management tool that is used to ensure that each child with a disability is provided special education and related services appropriate to his or her special learning needs.

5. The IEP is a compliance/monitoring document that may be used by monitoring personnel from each governmental level to determine whether a child with a disability is actually receiving the free appropriate public education agreed to by the parents and the school.

6. The IEP serves as an evaluation device for use in determining the extent of the child's progress toward meeting the projected outcomes. (Note: The law does not require that teachers or other school personnel be held accountable if a child with a disability does not achieve the goals and objectives set forth in his or her IEP.)

The law further specifies that the IEP is an invaluable education tool that should be fully and unreservedly used by every school in the nation with every child with a disability; that the IEP should be seen as concerning the whole child in all aspects of his or her life; that the preparation of each IEP should be an interdisciplinary effort; that every effort should be made to involve parents; and that school officials should demonstrate their understanding of the importance of the IEPs by establishing priorities, special in-service training programs, teacher schedules, and resource allocation procedures that recognize the needs involved and assure optimum results (PL 94–142, 1977).

COMPONENTS OF AN IEP

An understanding of the components of an IEP will assist the audiologist in developing appropriate and meaningful hearing-related objectives. According to PL 94–142, an IEP will include:

1. A statement of the present levels of educational performance of the child
2. A statement of annual goals, including short-term instructional objectives
3. A statement of the specific special education and all related services to be provided to the child, and the extent to which the child will be able to participate in regular education programs
4. The projected date for initiation and anticipated duration of such services
5. Appropriate objective criteria and evaluation procedures and schedules for determining, on at least an annual basis, whether short-term instructional objectives are being achieved and whether current placement is appropriate

To summarize, in a very logical fashion the IEP specifies where the child is functioning now, where you want him or her to be at the end of the year, how you are going to achieve that long-term goal, and how you can determine if in fact the goal was reached. So, for example, if the child has difficulty listening in class, the listening difficulty and present level of listening function need to be documented initially through some evaluative tool. Then a long-term listening objective needs to be formulated followed by the short-term steps necessary to reach the long-term goal. Finally, the means of evaluating progress to the "listening" goal needs to be specified. If the audiologist simply states, in the recommendations section of the audiologic assessment, that listening ought to be facilitated in class, there is no assurance that the IEP team can or will translate that recommendation into appropriate behavioral objective format for inclusion in the IEP.

Another example is the use of signal-to-noise ratio enhancing technology in all instructional settings. The use, maintenance, and monitoring of all equipment must be stated specifically and precisely in the IEP or resources may not be allocated. Once again, audiologists who are familiar with the dimensions of the IEP can be successful in the meaningful integration of technology into the child's learning environments.

EXAMPLES OF HEARING MANAGEMENT OBJECTIVES FOR AN IEP

The purpose of an IEP that is generated for a child with hearing loss who is in a mainstream classroom is to enable that child to obtain educational benefit from teacher instruction while also facilitating his or her social/emotional growth. Accordingly, the primary annual goal could read, "The child (insert name) will participate in his or her classes 100% of the time." Note that all goals and objectives are written from the child's perspective: what will the child do.

To meet the annual goal, short-term objectives must be developed as appropriate for the individual needs of the child. For example, following educational and functional audiologic assessments and classroom observations, these short-term objectives were written for a specific ninth-grader to enable him to derive educational benefit from mainstreamed classroom instruction at a reasonable level of effort (Note: this ninth-grade boy has a prelingual moderate to severe hearing loss with very good auditory, language, and speech skills. Nevertheless, he was having to expend an inordinate level of effort to keep up with the escalating demands of high school work):

1. John Smith will use his personal FM system in all classroom, field trip, and school assembly activities. (Note: John had been using his FM since kindergarten in most classroom activities, but he was not using it during assemblies or field trips. He admitted that, most of the time, he did not know what was going on during the assemblies or field trips; he just kind of tagged along. Unfortunately, prior to this IEP, John's high school teachers thought that John ought to "outgrow" his need for the FM system . . . as if John no longer needs to hear the classroom instruction that has become increasingly complex and ambiguous!)
2. John Smith will position himself favorably to receive visual information in classes, assemblies, and field trips. (Note: Favorable seating cannot substitute for FM use. The favorable seating is meant to provide redundancy of information through increased accessibil-

ity to visual reinforcement. John had typically been seated in the back of the auditorium during assemblies and often had been at the back of the line during field trips, further isolating him from the opportunity to receive information from the environment. Also note that John is expected to assume some responsibility for positioning himself favorably.)

3. John Smith will use student notetakers in all of his classes, employing either NCR paper or photocopying of the notes (Note: John had a difficult time attending simultaneously to the teacher's verbal instruction and to taking notes. His notes tended to be incomplete and he was getting frustrated.)

4. John Smith will use a caption decoder for videos that are close-captioned. (Note: The school had a caption decoder but teachers seldom thought ahead to have the decoder coupled to their video monitor when instructional materials were viewed. The teachers were employing an increasing number of media materials. The speakers on the video monitors were of such marginal quality that John could not understand the dialogue. If his FM transmitter was plugged into the "audio-out" jack of the monitor, the external speaker was turned off so that the rest of the class could not hear. Therefore, caption decoding was crucial in enabling John to benefit from the video materials. Indeed, without captioning, John was being denied access to the media events. Fortunately, most of the videos routinely used by the school could be obtained with captioning already in place.)

5. John Smith will use open-captioned films when available. (Note: The same reasoning applies to this objective as to the previous one. John could not even begin to hear intelligible speech over the clatter of the movie projector. And, many instructional films can be obtained with open captioning. As an aside, many other students in the class benefit from the redundancy of captioned media materials.)

6. John Smith will know the content of *all* school public address (PA) announcements through written distribution of morning announcements, through teacher repetition of announcements made during the day, and through notetakers who will write down all announcements. (Note: John could detect the presence of speech through the school's public address system, but the loudspeakers were of such poor quality that he could not understand what was being said. Consequently, he often did not know what was happening or what he was expected to do following a PA announcement. He reported that he typically followed the crowd and tried to figure out what would happen; he was often surprised by the outcome.)

7. John Smith will gain an understanding of hearing loss, of himself as a person who experiences hearing loss, and of himself as an advocate for appropriate accommodations. (Note: John needed to be encouraged to assume more responsibility for his hearing loss, for his amplification technology, and for structuring the environment so that he could obtain information. He wanted to attend a state college after high school, which was a reasonable expectation given his current performance and motivation. It is never too early to start preparing, academically and emotionally, for postsecondary education.)

There were other short-term objectives on John's IEP specifying how, when, and where John's amplification technology would be monitored, and by whom, inclusive of John's role in equipment management; audiologic assessments; speech/language therapy emphasizing current slang, figurative language, and words with multiple meanings (with the previous exceptions, John's overall language skills were age-appropriate); and in-services and support for John's teachers. Note that for each objective detailed on the IEP, there are procedures specifying how each objective will be met, who will carry it out, and how John's progress will be measured. The audiologist had a pivotal role in providing the understanding of hearing loss that governed the generation of these objectives.

IFSP

The IFSP (Individualized Family Service Plan) specified by PL 99–457 is similar to the IEP, with the exception that the IFSP calls for child and family goals with a strong family focus, not for only child-centered goals as does PL 94–142.

The IFSP document needs to include a comprehensive description of the child, as obtained through a multidisciplinary assessment, and the proposed intervention program. As detailed by Roush and McWilliam (1990), the components of an IFSP are:

1. The child's current status and present levels of development as determined by objective criteria
2. Family information needed for facilitating the development of the baby/child
3. Expected outcomes of the early intervention program
4. Details of the specific plan for the delivery, location, and method of payment for early intervention services
5. Other services not required by law but that are needed by the child, for example, medical services
6. Duration and dates of the specific early intervention services
7. Designation of the case manager to ensure that the IFSP is properly implemented
8. Plans for transition into the school system

Once again, an audiologist must be a key member of the team that develops an IFSP for a child who experiences hearing loss. Because hearing loss presents a significant barrier to the acquisition of information from the environment, that hearing loss must be managed and hearing accessed in order for an early intervention program to be successful.

In-services—Educating the Educators

Mark Ross (1991) has written that educating the public and school personnel about the importance of hearing and hearing loss is our profession's greatest challenge. Until the pivotal role of hearing in the educational process is recognized, audiologic services will continue to be considered tangential to learning.

As emphasized by Upfold (1988), the overwhelming majority of children with hearing loss will be educated in mainstreamed classrooms. Classroom teachers lack basic knowledge about hearing and hearing loss (Martin et al., 1988), which results in little growth in the development of educational procedures for managing children with hearing loss (Ross, 1991). Most teachers do not even know where to begin to provide appropriate instruction for children with hearing loss.

Maxon (1990) has generated an in-service model called an "Individualized In-Service Plan" (IIP). The IIP was developed because one or two in-services covering very general hearing-related issues cannot possibly meet the needs of all school personnel or of all mainstreamed children with hearing loss. Consequently, each IIP must address the unique needs of the educational personnel, the child with hearing loss, the child's peers, and the educational setting. Note that in-service training is not a one-time affair. As technology changes, and as teachers become more familiar with students with hearing loss, additional information is needed during the course of the school year.

A comprehensive in-service program ought to include the following topics (Maxon, 1990):

1. General information about psychosocial, linguistic, and educational consequences of hearing loss—as discussed in the first part of this chapter
2. Hearing aids and FM technology
3. Speech acoustics and perception
4. Classroom acoustics
5. Classroom management of the child with hearing loss to include consideration of hearing, communication, and social issues

In-service information needs to be provided to all educational personnel who have contact with the child who experiences hearing loss. In addition, the child's peers need information about hearing loss and hearing technology. It is very important to "demystify" the use and function of equipment. Once children understand why a certain piece of technology is needed, and once they have an opportunity to listen to the equipment, either through earphones or a hearing aid stethoscope, they become more accepting and less likely to ridicule the child who experiences hearing loss.

In-service training can be conducted in formal sessions and can also occur during informal encounters with school personnel. In fact, informal discussions can be even more productive than more formal instructional sessions. For example, visiting a teacher before class and asking how the FM is holding its charge, or asking if Johnny is responding more quickly now that he is wearing an FM unit, could be a more effective way of discussing FM use and function than having a formal group meeting.

Conclusion: Audiologists as Advocates for the Right to Hear for All Children

Audiologists, as professionals who are experts in the management of hearing in an educational setting, can have an enormous impact on the future of children with all types and degrees of hearing problems. Indeed, thorough and insightful audiologic management can make the difference between one child with hearing loss becoming an independent, contributing citizen and another child living life on the fringe.

The purpose of this chapter has been to impart a practical approach for the provision of comprehensive audiologic services in an educational setting. Topics ranged from a discussion of hearing and hearing loss relative to academic performance, to soundfield FM systems, to the crucial role of the IEP in the attainment of technology and services.

The ability to hear the teacher's instruction clearly is essential for a child to obtain an appropriate education. Audiologists must not underestimate the negative impact of hearing problems on classroom performance and, thus, ought not equivocate when recommending and providing comprehensive audiologic management.

References

Anderson, K.L., *Screening Instrument for Targeting Educational Risk*. Austin, TX: PRO-ED (1989a).

Anderson, K.L., Speech perception and the hard-of-hearing child. *Ed. Aud. Monograph*, 1, 15–29 (1989b).

Anderson, K.L., Hearing conservation in the public schools revisited. In C. Flexer (Ed.), Current audiologic issues in the educational management of children with hearing loss. *Sem. Hear.*, 12(4), 340–364 (1991).

ASHA Ad Hoc Committee on Extension of Audiological Services in the Schools, Audiology services in the school's position statement. *Asha*, 53–60 (May 1983).

ASHA Working Group on Acoustic Immittance Measurements and the Committee on Audiologic Evaluation, Guidelines for screening for hearing impairment and middle-ear disorders. *Asha*, 32 (Suppl. 2), 17–24 (1990).

Berg, F.S., Characteristics of the target population. In F.S. Berg, J.C. Blair, J.H. Viehweg, and A. Wilson-Vlotman (Eds.), *Educational Audiology for the Hard of Hearing Child*. New York: Grune & Stratton (1986a).

Berg, F.S., Classroom acoustics and signal transmission. In F.S. Berg, J.C. Blair, J.H. Viehweg, and A. Wilson-Vlotman (Eds.), *Educational Audiology for the Hard of Hearing Child*. New York: Grune & Stratton (1986b).

Berg, F.S., *Facilitating Classroom Listening: A Handbook for Teachers of Normal and Hard of Hearing Children*. Boston: College-Hill Press/Little, Brown (1987).

Berg, F.S., Historical perspectives of educational audiology. In C. Flexer (Ed.), Current audiologic issues in the educational management of children with hearing loss. *Sem. Hear.*, 12(4), 305–317b (1991).

Bess, F.H. The minimally hearing-impaired child. *Ear Hear.*, 6, 43–47 (1985).

Blair, J.C., Services needed. In F.S. Berg, J.C. Blair, S.H. Viehweg, and A. Wilson-Vlotman (Eds.), *Educational Audiology for the Hard of Hearing Child*. New York: Grune & Stratton (1986).

Blair, J.C., Educational audiology and methods for bringing about change in schools. In C. Flexer (Ed.), Current audiologic issues in the educational management of children with hearing loss. *Sem. Hear.*, 12(4), 318–328 (1991).

Blair, J.C., Wilson-Vlotman, A., and Von Almen, P., Educational audiologists: practices, problems, directions and recommendations. *Ed. Aud. Monograph*, 1, 2–14 (1989).

Blake, R., Field, B., Foster, C., Platt, F., and Wertz, P., Effect of FM auditory trainers on attending behaviors of learning-disabled children. *Lang. Speech, Hear. Serv. Schools*, 22, 111–114 (1991).

Brackett, D., and Maxon, A.B., Service delivery alternatives for the mainstreamed hearing-impaired child. *Lang. Speech Hear. Serv. Schools*, 17, 115–125 (1986).

Code of Federal Regulations on Education, Title 34-Education (parts 300–399). Washington, DC: U.S. Government Printing Office (1986).

Conway, L.C., Issues relating to classroom management. In M. Ross (Ed.), *Hearing-Impaired Children in the Mainstream*. Parkton, MD: York Press (1990).

Davis, J. (Ed.), *Our Forgotten Children: Hard-of-Hearing Pupils in Schools*. (2nd ed.). Bethesda, MD: Self-Help for Hard of Hearing People (1990).

Dobie, R.A., and Berlin, C.I., Influence of otitis media on hearing and development. *Ann. Otol. Rhinol. Laryngol.*, 88, 46–53 (1979).

Dublinske, S., Educational audiology. Unpublished proceedings of Conference for Hearing Clinicians. Iowa Department of Public Instruction. Iowa City: May 14, 15 (1971).

DuBow, S., Geer, S., and Strauss, K.P, *Legal Rights: The Guide for Deaf and Hard of Hearing People.* Washington, DC: Gallaudet University Press (1992).

Early intervention program for infants and toddlers with handicaps; final regulations. *Federal Register*, 54 (119), 26306–26348 (1989).

Education of handicapped children, PL 94–142 Regulations. *Federal Register*, 42 (163), August 23 (1977).

Edwards, C., Assessment and management of listening skills in school-aged children. In C. Flexer (Ed.), Current audiologic issues in the educational management of children with hearing loss. *Sem. Hear.*, 12(4), 389–401 (1991).

Elliott, L.L., Hammer M.A., and Scholl, M.E., Fine-grained auditory discrimination in normal children and children with language-learning problems. *J. Speech Hear. Res.*, 32, 112–119 (1989).

English, K., Best practices in educational audiology. *Lang. Speech Hear. Serv. Schools*, 22, 283–286 (1991).

Erber, N., *Auditory Training.* Washington, DC: The Alexander Graham Bell Association for the Deaf (1982).

Estabrooks, W., and Edwards, C., *Sure We Can Hear* (Videotape). Toronto, Canada: VOICE for Hearing-Impaired Children (1986).

Finitzo-Hieber, T., and Tillman, T., Room acoustics effects on monosyllabic word discrimination ability for normal and hearing-impaired children. *J. Speech Hear. Res.*, 21, 440–458 (1978).

Flexer, C., Turn on sound: an odyssey of soundfield amplification. *Ed. Aud. Assoc. Newsletter*, 5, 6–7 (1989).

Flexer, C., Audiological rehabilitation in the schools. *Asha*, 44–45 (April 1990).

Flexer, C., FM classroom public address systems. In M. Ross (Ed.), *FM Auditory Training Systems: Characteristics, Selection and Use.* Parkton, MD: York Press, pp. 189–210 (1992).

Flexer, C., and Berg, F.S., Beyond hearing aids: The mystical world of assistive communication devices. In C. Flexer, D. Wray, and R. Leavitt (Eds.), *How the Student with Hearing Loss Can Succeed in College: A Handbook for Students, Families, and Professionals.* Washington, DC: Alexander Graham Bell Association for the Deaf (1990).

Flexer, C., Millin, J.P., and Brown, L., Children with developmental disabilities: the effect of soundfield amplification on word identification. *Lang. Speech Hear. Serv. Schools*, 21, 177–182 (1990).

Flexer, C., Wray, D., and Ireland, J., Preferential seating is NOT enough: issues in classroom management of hearing-impaired students. *Lang. Speech Hear. Serv. Schools*, 20, 11–21 (1989).

Hawkins, D.B., Comparisons of speech recognition in noise by mildly-to-moderately hearing-impaired children using hearing aids and FM systems. *J. Speech Hear. Dis.*, 49, 409–418 (1984).

Hawkins, D.B., and Schum, D.J., Some effects of FM-system coupling on hearing aid characteristics. *J. Speech Hear Dis.*, 50, 132–141 (1985).

Houtgast, T., and Steeneken, H.J.M., The MTF concept in room acoustics and its use for estimating speech intelligibility in auditoria. *J. Acoust. Soc. Am.*, 77, 1069–1077 (1985).

Hull, R., and Dilka, K., *The Hearing-Impaired Child in School.* New York: Grune & Stratton (1984).

Lasky, E., and Katz, J., *Central Auditory Processing Disorders: Problems of Speech, Language, Learning.* Baltimore: University Park Press (1983).

Lass, N., Carlin, M., Woodford, C., et al., A survey of professionals' knowledge of and exposure to hearing loss. *Volta Rev.*, 88, 333–338 (1986).

Leavitt, R.J., Promoting the use of rehabilitation technology. *Asha*, 29, 28–31 (April 1987).

Leavitt, R.J., Group amplification systems for students with hearing impairment. In C. Flexer (Ed.), Current audiologic issues in the educational management of children with hearing loss. *Sem. Hear.*, 12(4), 380–388 (1991).

Leavitt, R., and Flexer, C., Speech degradation as measured by the rapid speech transmission index (RASTI). *Ear Hear.*, 12, 115–118 (1991).

Leonard, L.B., New trends in the study of early language acquisition. *Asha*, 43–44 (April 1991).

Ling, D., *Foundations of Spoken Language for Hearing-Impaired Children.* Washington DC: The Alexander Graham Bell Association for the Deaf (1989).

Luckner, J.L., Mainstreaming hearing-impaired students: perceptions of regular educators. *Lang. Speech Hear. Serv. Schools*, 22, 302–307 (1991).

Lundeen, C., Prevalence of hearing impairment among school children. *Lang. Speech Hear. Serv. Schools*, 22, 269–271 (1991).

Madell, J., Managing classroom amplification. In M. Ross (Ed.), *Hearing-Impaired Children in the Mainstream.* Parkton, MD: York Press (1990).

Martin, F.N., Bernstein, ME., Daly, J.A., and Cody, J.P., Classroom teachers' knowledge of hearing disorders and attitudes about mainstreaming hard-of-hearing children. *Lang. Speech Hear. Serv. Schools*, 19, 83–95 (1988).

McGee, D., Recognizing heterogeneity: increasing educational opportunities through mainstreaming. In M. Ross (Ed.), *Hearing-Impaired Children in the Mainstream.* Parkton, MD: York Press (1990).

Matkin, N.F., *Pediatric Update Conference.* Providence, RI: 6/15/90 (1990).

Maxon, A.B., Implementing an in-service training program. In M. Ross (Ed.), *Hearing-Impaired Children in the Mainstream.* Parkton, MD: York Press (1990).

Maxon, A.B., and Smaldino, J., Hearing aid management for children. In C. Flexer (Ed.), Current audiologic issues in the educational management of children with hearing loss. *Sem. Hear.*, 12(4), 365–379 (1991).

Northern, J.L., and Downs, M.P., *Hearing in Children*, 4th ed. Baltimore: Williams & Wilkins (1991).

Nozza, R.J., Rossman, R.N.F., Bond, L.C., and Miller, S.L., Infant speech-sound discrimination in noise. *J. Acoust. Soc. Am.*, 87, 339–350 (1990).

Osborn, J., Graves, L., and VonderEmbse, D., Three-year soundfield study in Putnam County, Ohio. Unpublished raw data (1989).

Oyler, R.F., Oyler, A., and Matkin, N.D., Unilateral hearing impairment: demographics and educational impact. *Lang. Speech Hear. Serv. Schools*, 19, 201–210 (1988).

Pollack, D., *Educational Audiology for the Limited Hearing Infant and Preschooler*, 2nd ed. Springfield, IL: Charles C. Thomas (1985).

Ramsdell, D.A., The psychology of the hard-of-hearing and deafened adult. In H. Davis and S.R. Silverman (Eds.), *Hearing and Deafness*, 4th ed. New York: Holt, Rinehart and Winston (1978).

Ray, H., Sarff, L.S., and Glassford, F.E., Sound field amplification: an innovative educational intervention for mainstreamed learning disabled students. *Directive Teach.*, Summer/Fall, 18–20 (1984).

Ross, M., A future challenge: educating the educators and public about hearing loss. In C. Flexer (Ed.), Current audiologic issues in the educational management of children with hearing loss. *Sem. Hear.*, 12(4), 402–414 (1991).

Ross, M., Brackett, D., and Maxon, A., *Hard of Hearing Children in Regular Schools*. Englewood Cliffs, NJ: Prentice-Hall (1982).

Ross, M., Brackett, D., and Maxon, A., *Assessment and Management of Hearing-Impaired Children in the Mainstream: Principles and Practice*. Austin, TX: Pro-Ed (1991).

Ross, M., and Calvert, D.R., Semantics of deafness revisited: total communication and the use and misuse of residual hearing. *Audiology*, 9, 127–145 (1984).

Ross, M., and Giolas, T.G. (Eds.), *Auditory Management of Hearing-Impaired Children*. Baltimore, MD: University Park Press (1978).

Roush, J., and McWilliam, R.A., A new challenge for pediatric audiology: Public Law 99–457. *J. Am. Acad. Audiol.*, 1, 196–208 (1990).

Sexton, J.E., Team management of the child with hearing loss. In C. Flexer (Ed.), Current audiologic issues in the educational management of children with hearing loss. *Sem. Hear.*, 12(4), 329–339 (1991).

Simon, C.S., *Communication Skills and Classroom Success*. San Diego, CA: College-Hill Press (1985).

Upfold, L.J., Children with hearing aids in the 1980's: etiologies and severity of impairment. *Ear Hear.*, 9, 75–80 (1988).

VanTasell, D.J., Mallinger, C.A., and Crump, E.S., Functional gain and speech recognition with two types of FM amplification. *Lang. Speech Hear. Serv. Schools*, 17, 28–37 (1986).

Wallach, G.P., and Butler, K.G. (Eds.), *Language Learning Disabilities in School Age Children*. Baltimore, MD: Williams & Wilkins (1984).

Williams, J., What do you know? What do you need to know? (ADA). *Asha*, 34, 54–78 (1992).

Wilson-Vlotman, A.L., and Blair, J.C., A survey of audiologists working full-time in school systems. *Asha*, 27, 33–38 (1986).

Woodford, C.M., Speech-language pathologists' knowledge and skills regarding hearing aids. *Lang. Speech Hear. Serv. Schools*, 18, 312–322 (1987).

Worner, W.A., An inexpensive group FM amplification system for the classroom. *Volta Rev.*, 90, 29–36 (1988).

Wray, D., Hazlett, J., and Flexer, C., Strategies for teaching writing skills to hearing-impaired adolescents. *Lang. Speech Hear. Serv. Schools.*, 19, 182–190 (1988).

Ying, E., Speech and language assessment: communication evaluation. In M. Ross (Ed.), *Hearing-Impaired Children in the Mainstream*. Parkton, MD: York Press (1990).

APPENDIX 8.1 *History of Ear and Hearing Problems*

Parent or guardian, please answer the following questions:

Child's Name _____ Birthdate _____

EAR PROBLEM = ear infection, earaches, draining ears, medicine taken for ears, doctor noticed fluid behind eardrum, hole in eardrum, etc.

	Yes	No
1. Did your child have *any* ear problems before the age of 1?	____	____
2. Has your child ever had a draining ear?	____	____
3. Approximately how many ear problems has your child had in his/her life? 0–2 ____ 3–5 ____ 6–10 ____ 10 or more ____		
4. Does your child tend to have four or more ear problems each year?	____	____
5. Has your child had an ear problem in the last 6 months?	____	____
6. Has your child ever had an ear problem that lasted 3 months or longer? (with or without medication)	____	____
7. Has anyone related to the child had many ear problems? (parents, brothers or sisters, cousins)	____	____
8. Has your child ever been seen by an ear doctor (otologist)? If yes, what doctor? _____ Mo/Yr of last visit? _____	____	____
9. Has your child ever had tubes placed in his/her eardrums? If yes, how many times? ____ At what age(s) ____	____	____
10. Does your child have: a. Frequent runny nose? b. Frequent colds or sinus infections? c. Allergies?	____	____

11. Does your child have any permanent hearing loss that you know about? (For example: deaf in one ear, can't hear high pitch sounds.) Please describe:
12. Did your child attend preschool?
13. Please write any additional comments on the back.

_____   _____
Completed by: School

_____   _____
Date completed:

Adapted from Anderson, K.L., Hearing conservation in the public schools revisited. In C. Flexer (Ed.), Current audiologic issues in the educational management of children with hearing loss. *Sem. Hear.,* 12(4), 340–364 (1991).

APPENDIX
8.2 *Speech Information Available at 250 Hz, 500 Hz, 1000 Hz, 2000 Hz, 4000 Hz*

At 250 Hz, plus or minus 1/2 octave, the following speech information is available:
1st formant of vowels /u/ and /i/
The fundamental frequency of females' and children's voices
Nasal murmur associated with the phonemes /m/, /n/, and /ng/
Male voice harmonics
Voicing cues
Suprasegmental patterns (stress, rate, inflection, intonation)

At 500 Hz, plus or minus 1/2 octave, the following speech information is available:
1st formants of *most* of the vowels
Harmonics of *all* voices (male, female, child)
Voicing cues
Nasality cues
Suprasegmentals
Some plosive bursts associated with /b/ and /d/

At 1000 Hz, plus or minus 1/2 octave, the following speech information is available:
2nd formants of back and central vowels
Important CV and VC transition information
Nasality cues
Some plosive bursts
Voicing cues
Suprasegmentals
The important acoustic cues for *manner* of articulation are available at 1000 Hz.

At 2000 Hz, plus or minus 1/2 octave, the following speech information is available:
THIS IS THE KEY FREQUENCY FOR INTELLIGIBILITY OF SPEECH
2nd and 3rd formant information for vowels
CV and VC transition information
Acoustic information for the liquids /r/ and /l/
Plosive bursts
Affricate bursts
Fricative turbulence
The important acoustic cues for *PLACE* of articulation are available at 2000 Hz.

At 4000 Hz, plus or minus 1/2 octave, the following speech information is available:
This is the key frequency for /s/ and /z/ morpheme audibility. The /s/ and /z/ phonemes are critical for language learning because they signal:

plurals	idioms	possessives	auxiliaries
3rd person	questions	copulas	past perfect

Adapted from Ling, D., Foundations of Spoken Language for Hearing-Impaired Children. Washington, DC: The Alexander Graham Bell Association for the Deaf (1989).

APPENDIX 8.3 *Evaluation of Children with Suspected Listening Difficulties*

Ranking Scale

1	2	3	4	NA
demonstrates all of the time	most of the time	some of the time	never observed	

1. *Overall Concerns about Listening*

• Doesn't understand appropriate listening expectations of the classroom	1	2	3	4
• Doesn't seem to listen	1	2	3	4
• Appears to be a good listener but work suggests misunderstandings	1	2	3	4
• Has difficulty following directions	1	2	3	4
• Follows single step commands but has difficulty with multistage commands	1	2	3	4
• Frequently asks for repetition	1	2	3	4
• Tends to quit easily when frustrated	1	2	3	4
• Impulsive—often acts before thinking	1	2	3	4
• Slow at beginning new tasks	1	2	3	4
• Doesn't complete assignments	1	2	3	4
• Has difficulty sustaining attention during oral presentations	1	2	3	4
• Watches the speaker's face for more information	1	2	3	4

2. *Current Strengths and Weaknesses*
   • The child shows appropriate listening skills:
   In a Large Group Activity:

• When activity is directed	1	2	3	4
• When activity is independent	1	2	3	4
• In the gymnasium	1	2	3	4
• The noise level has impact on the student's performance	Yes _____		No _____	

   In a Small Group Activity:

• When activity is directed	1	2	3	4
• When activity is independent	1	2	3	4
• The noise level has impact on the student's performance	Yes _____		No _____	

3. *Child's Level of Awareness of Strengths and Weaknesses*

• Generally unaware of errors in processing information and doesn't attempt to clarify	1	2	3	4
• Recognizes difficult listening situations	1	2	3	4
• Recognizes that it is difficult to understand when people talk too quickly	1	2	3	4
• Has developed preferences for certain speakers	1	2	3	4

4. *Child's Current Strategies*

• Maintains eye contact with speaker	1	2	3	4
• Will choose/request seating—close to speaker	1	2	3	4
—away from noise sources	1	2	3	4
—use of FM technology	1	2	3	4
• Will ask for repetition—in large group	1	2	3	4
—with classmates	1	2	3	4
—privately with teacher	1	2	3	4
• Will rehearse information to retain it better	1	2	3	4
• Will clarify by asking questions or paraphrasing	1	2	3	4
• Will close the classroom door	1	2	3	4

• Other strategies:

• List _____

_____

• Comments _____

_____

5. *Current Modification by the Teacher*

Environmental Modifications that Improve Listening Performance:

• Use of FM technology	1	2	3	4
• Seating close to teacher	1	2	3	4
• Seating away from constant noise sources (pencil sharpener, hallway, windows, etc)	1	2	3	4
• Seating in special areas of classroom: _____				
• Use of library/hallways for projects	1	2	3	4
• Use of headphones by the child (for noise reduction during individual work periods)	1	2	3	4

Teaching Strategies that Improve Listening Performance:

• Use of buddy system	1	2	3	4
• Writing instructions on chalkboard	1	2	3	4
• Calling child's name before initiating instructions	1	2	3	4
• Touching child on shoulder to get his/her attention	1	2	3	4
• Simplifying instructions to single steps	1	2	3	4
• Comprehension checks:				
—ask child to indicate when didn't understand	1	2	3	4
—ask child to repeat the instructions heard	1	2	3	4
—ask child to summarize instructions before work initiated	1	2	3	4
• Slowing rate of speech	1	2	3	4
• Use of breaks or rest periods from listening	1	2	3	4

6. *Other Factors of Note* {fluid build-up in the middle ear (otitis media), emotional difficulties, attention deficit disorder}:

_____

_____

_____

Reprinted with permission from Edwards, C., Assessment and management of listening skills in school-aged children. In C. Flexer (Ed.), Current audiologic issues in the educational management of children with hearing loss. *Sem. Hear.,* 12(4), 389–401 (1991).

9

The Counseling Process: Children and Parents

PATRICIA B. KRICOS, Ph.D.

Hearing-impaired children can have a profound long-term impact on their families. While the family plays a significant role in providing the context in which the hearing-impaired child will grow, either facilitating or impeding progress in a number of areas of life, so also the presence of a hearing-impaired child in a family can be expected to affect the nature and quality of family life over a number of years.

There is agreement in the field of audiology that one of the most important aspects of habilitation for hearing-impaired children is parent counseling. It is well accepted that the hearing-impaired child's chances for successful communication, academic achievement, and life satisfaction are greatly enhanced when the child's parents can emotionally accept the child and are dedicated to maximizing the child's potential. From the initial diagnosis of deafness and through the school-age years, parent counseling is a powerful habilitative tool that should receive paramount consideration from professionals who work with hearing-impaired children and their parents.

This chapter is designed to explore the numerous ways that hearing loss in children can affect the family, as well as to provide practical, relevant information to audiologists regarding the counseling process. In the first section, the influence of hearing loss on the nature of family life will be delineated, including the parents' emotional reactions to hearing impairment in their children, the impact of hearing loss on par-

ent-child interactions, family dynamics, and the critical role that parents play in intervention and on their child's overall life satisfaction. In the second section, the counseling process will be explored, including the effectiveness of counseling provided by audiologists, the importance of a family-centered intervention philosophy, counseling suggestions, and multicultural considerations.

Influence of Hearing Loss on Family Life: Emotional Reactions of Parents of Hearing-Impaired Children

The emotional reactions that parents of hearing-impaired children may experience are very similar to the reactions of individuals who have lost a loved one through death. Although in reality the parents of hearing-impaired children have not "lost" their child, they nevertheless have lost the hopes, dreams, and aspirations they once held for the child when they viewed the child as normal. Thus, they may experience grief as intense and acute as if they had lost the child through death.

Tanner (1980) provides an excellent review of the implications of loss and grief for communicative disorders specialists. He points out that while grief is an understandable reaction to loss, the patient's reaction to the loss may have significant influence on rehabilitation outcomes. Likewise, the clinician's response to the grieving parent may, in turn, have considerable impact on the patient's ultimate acceptance of the disability as well as the patient's motivation to engage in therapy. There appear to be strong interrelationships among the patient's grief, the effect of grief on potential for successful rehabilitation, and the effect of the clinician's response to the patient's grieving. Therefore, it is critical that professionals respond to the grieving process in a manner that will facilitate the patient's ultimate acceptance of the loss. When the grieving process is facilitated properly, the patient will most likely show greater improvement because energy can be directed to rehabilitation rather than being expended on psychological resolution of the loss.

The stages of grief experienced by parents of hearing-impaired children parallel the sequences of grieving described by Kubler-Ross (1969) for the dying patient and by Tanner (1980) for patients who have lost a communication function. These include denial, anger, bargaining, depression, and, ultimately, acceptance. Each of these, in addition to the frequently observed reaction of guilt, will be discussed separately.

Denial is usually one of the first reactions to any major loss and, as Kubler-Ross (1969) points out, may serve as an emotional buffer that allows the grieving person time to absorb the impact of the loss and to mobilize inner strengths to deal with it. Deafness is relatively easy to deny because it is invisible, and the parents of hearing-impaired children may deny the child's disability in a number of ways. They may reject the diagnosis of deafness, taking the child to a number of different professionals and clinics, in essence "shopping" for a more palatable professional opinion. They may accept the diagnosis but reject its permanence, expressing hopes that their child will eventually outgrow the condition or be cured of it. The impact of the diagnosis may be rejected, with parents appearing unperturbed in the face of a severe disability. These latter parents often appear to be "ideal" parents to clinicians because of their positive attitudes, and yet ultimate acceptance of the child's impairment demands confrontation with the significant impact of the child's hearing loss on almost all aspects of communicative and academic development. Parents in the denial stage may appear to clinicians to be blocking efforts to initiate the rehabilitation process. However, it should be remembered that this initial reaction to the diagnosis of deafness may provide a time for parents to search for inner strength and to accumulate information. Indeed, Tanner (1980) points out that one of the primary factors influencing the degree and duration of denial is the amount of information that the individual is given regarding the disorder. The goal for clinicians during this stage of grieving is to find ways of not merely tolerating parental denial but accepting it, while still offering, to the best of their abilities, the services the child needs. Unfortunately, parents who appear to be denying their child's hearing impairment are often viewed by clinicians as foolish and stubborn when they should be viewed as loving parents who, for the time being, cannot accept the professional's diagnosis of such a severe disability in their child.

The parents of newly diagnosed hearing-impaired children may experience guilt, which can be manifested in several ways. Some parents may express the feeling that something they did caused their child's hearing loss. Even more difficult to respond to are the parents who believe that their child's impairment is punishment for a prior sin or simply because they are not "good" people and therefore do not "deserve" an unimpaired child. According to Moses and Van Hecke-Wulatin (1981), the professional must recognize feelings of guilt as a natural process, not a psychopathology, and respond to them as such. If not condemned or responded to as foolishness, guilt will run its course and cease on its own.

Feelings of anger mark the second reaction in Kubler-Ross's (1969) stages of mourning. The parents, no longer denying the diagnosis, may be left with feelings of inner rage, which are often expressed toward family, friends, and professionals. As difficult as it may be to depersonalize the anger expressed to them in various ways, clinicians must attempt to understand the parent's anger as a normal reaction to loss and as an indication of at least partial initial acceptance of the child's disability. The clinician confronted with an angry parent must understand that the parent's anger is not necessarily a personal reaction to the clinician or to the rehabilitation program, and the clinician must avoid responding to the parent in a negative manner. Likewise, the angry parent's spouse and/or family should be counseled to ensure enhanced understanding, acceptance, and handling of the parent's frustrations.

The third stage in Kubler-Ross's (1969) grieving cycle is bargaining. In this stage the parent may bargain with clinicians, health professionals, family, God, and/or themselves. Bargaining parents, for example, may vow openly or surreptitiously to do everything requested of them by the child's clinician, and often beyond, in return for which amelioration of the child's disorder is expected. On the surface, unflagging dedication to the hearing-impaired child's welfare appears to be a commendable quality, but it might also serve as a signal that the parent is engaged in unrealistic bargaining. Although bargaining may be helpful to the parent in that it offers a little more time for resolution of the loss, long periods of bargaining may not be healthy for either the parent or the hearing-impaired child. Eventually the parent's false hopes, which accompany bargaining, will have to be acknowledged and resolved in order to achieve full acceptance of the disorder. In addition, the physical health and emotional security of parents who set unrealistic demands for themselves should be of concern to clinicians because of the eventual negative impact on the child's rehabilitation program.

Depression is the fourth stage of grieving described by Kubler-Ross (1969). The parent no longer denies the loss, no longer feels inner rage toward the loss, and may realize that bargaining attempts have failed to alleviate the problems encountered as a result of the loss. Unfortunately, clinicians may view the parent's subsequent depression as a psychopathology rather than a normal reaction within the grief cycle. A natural, very human response of clinicians who face a depressed parent is to point out that things are really not as bad as the parent views them; that the child, despite a severe impairment, is a beautiful, intelligent, personable, outgoing child; and that in view of this, the parent ought to cheer up. Other clinicians may feel uncomfortable with the parent's depression and may exert great effort to avoid acknowledging the parent's suffering. Although the clinician's reactions are understandable, the result may be to make the parent feel worse. In essence, the depressed parent's response to the clinician's well-meaning attempts to downplay the significance of the loss may be to view himself or herself as inadequate in coping with the child's problem. Thus, a vicious cycle is set up in which the depressed parent may feel even more depressed. Tanner (1980) has suggested that one of the best responses that clinicians can make to the depressed patient may be nonverbal consolation. Simply touching a parent's hand or shoulder or just listening quietly and compassionately as the parent expresses inner feelings of depression may be far more effective in helping the depressed parent than verbal attempts to cheer up the parent.

According to Kubler-Ross (1969), acceptance is both the final stage and the ultimate goal of the grieving process and may provide the first evidence that the grief has been resolved. The parent may not necessarily feel happy about his or her predicament, yet the intense feelings of denial, depression, anger, and guilt are no longer present either. The parent of a hearing-impaired child may simply accept the situation as the way things are, thus enabling energies and constructive actions to be directed to the rehabilitation program.

According to Tanner (1980), a number of studies have indicated that the typical length of time to resolve the grief that accompanies a major loss is 6 to 12 months. The acute stage in which the emotional reactions to the loss are most intense usually lasts approximately 2 months, with the persistence of acute reactions beyond a 6-month period possibly indicating that pathologic mourning patterns have developed. However, it is important for clinicians to realize that the grief that accompanies the initial diagnosis of deafness and then is resolved may reappear later. For example, the impact of the child's disability may be cyclically magnified in the parent's eyes at certain predictable occasions. When the child reaches 5 years of age, the parents may realize that this would have been the time for the child to enter a regular kindergarten, had the child not been disabled. Thus the parent's initial feelings of loss, disappointment, and depression may resurface after seemingly being dormant for a number of years. The loss of a special teacher, the onset of pubescence, the reaching of the typical age of high school graduation as well as the age for living independently, and even the parent's reaching of retirement age may trigger emotional reactions typical of the initial mourning period at the time of diagnosis. While reactions to these occasions may be more transient than initial reactions, they should be recognized by professionals and responded to in a manner that will facilitate their speedy resolution.

Although from a theoretical viewpoint these stages seem straightforward, their manifestations may actually not be quite so discernible. Clark (1990) describes a number of transformations that these emotional reactions may undergo when being expressed by parents, making it difficult to recognize when the clinician responds only to the surface of clinical exchanges. For example, a parent may have strong feelings of sorrow yet fear to express them because such a reaction might not be acceptable to the clinician and might appear to others as rejection of the child. Instead, parents may redirect the initial reaction of sorrow, putting aside their feelings of sadness, jumping into the child's rehabilitation program, signing up for three sign language classes, and giving up previously enjoyed recreational activities to make more time for the hearing-impaired child. This type of response is not necessarily negative or counterproductive, *unless* the parent is repressing the sadness. If parents cannot find an outlet for their repressed feelings of sorrow, their enthusiastic drive will be difficult to maintain. It requires a sensitive clinician to be able to encourage parents to do all that needs to be done for their child, while at the same time providing a supportive environment in which the parents can divulge their innermost feelings regarding the situation in which they now find themselves. The clinician must be alert to any repressed feelings of anxiety or sorrow that the parent may harbor, letting the parent know that the welfare of parents is as much a concern

to the clinician as the welfare of the child. Sometimes just asking the parent frankly, "How are you doing with all the demands that are now being put on you? Are you finding time for yourself, to meet your physical and emotional needs?" will let the parent know that the clinician is sensitive, empathetic, concerned, and willing to recognize the strains that are on the parent.

The previous paragraphs have emphasized the importance of recognizing the strong emotional reactions that parents of hearing-impaired children may experience. Equally important to recognize, however, is that not all parents will predictably go through these stages exactly as described. Kroth (1987) and Clark (1990) warn professionals not to make assumptions about the family's reaction to the diagnosis of hearing impairment. The degree to which these emotional reactions will be experienced will likely vary from family to family depending on a number of complex factors. These factors are described in detail by Kampfe (1989), who espouses a "model of transition" for understanding and explaining how individuals respond to life transitions. The "model of transition" emphasizes that there are a number of social status factors, experiences, and personal resources that can mediate, in very complex ways, the manner in which individuals respond to stressful events.

According to Kampfe (1989), social status factors such as the age, gender, and ethnic background of the parent can influence how a stressful event is perceived. The parent's prior experience with hearing impairment or other disabling conditions might affect, either positively or negatively, the reaction to the determination of a hearing impairment in the child. Personal resources such as personality, coping strategies, and attitudes may influence overall response to a distressful situation. We all know individuals who are rarely flappable, even under extraordinary pressures, and other, more high-strung, individuals for whom even slightly uncomfortable situations appear insurmountable. It requires no stretch of the imagination to predict that the parent who is generally optimistic and easygoing might respond differently to a hearing-impaired child than the parent who has never been able to cope well even with life's minor setbacks. Kampfe (1989) also points out a number of other personality factors that may affect the reaction of the parent: For example, whether the parent is passive, perfectionistic, sensitive to others' opinions, impatient, and so on could influence the course of adaptation to a child's hearing handicap. Other parental variables that may influence reaction to a child's deafness include the parent's educational background; income; current marital relationship; and the degree of support from spouse, other family members, social networks, and service agencies.

Beyond personal resources, Kampfe (1989) describes a host of other variables that may influence how parents progress through the emotional stages outlined previously. These variables include availability and quality of service programs; effectiveness of counselors; demands on working parents; and variables associated with the hearing loss itself, such as the type, degree, cause, and age at onset of the loss.

From this discussion, it is easy to understand the danger in overgeneralizing the stages of emotional reactions through which parents progress. Whether a parent goes through any of these stages, the manner in which the emotional state is expressed, the degree to which constructive or maladaptive strategies are adopted, and the time frame in which these emotional reactions might be experienced all depend on the complex interactions of these, and likely many more, variables. The professional is cautioned, therefore, to understand the *potential* range of emotional states that may be experienced at various times by parents, without assuming that each parent will respond in a fully predictable manner. Each parent must be approached as an individual with a unique system of personal resources, social support, and background experiences. Even the mother and father of a particular hearing-impaired individual can be expected to react to their child's impairment in markedly different ways because of their unique set of characteristics, experiences, and perceptions.

An interesting survey was conducted by Martin et al. (1987), in which the perspectives regarding parents' reactions were compared between parents and audiologists.

Both audiologists and parents of hearing-impaired children were surveyed regarding parents' initial reactions to the diagnosis of hearing loss in their children, their subsequent reactions to the hearing loss, and the amount of time needed for parents to accept the hearing loss. The parents ranked sorrow (38.5% of parents), shock (36.6%), and acceptance (36.6%) as their most common reactions to the initial diagnosis of hearing impairment in their children, whereas audiologists' most common responses to describe initial parental reactions were denial (45.7% of audiologists), sorrow (40.7%), and acceptance (40.7%). The three most common responses of parents to describe their subsequent reactions were sorrow (41.4%), feeling a need for action to be taken (35.7%), and helplessness (25.7%). Audiologists continued to rank denial (49.2%) as the most common subsequent reaction of parents, followed by acceptance (27.7%) and need for action to be taken (27.7%).

Some discrepancies between parents and audiologists were also discerned in response to the amount of time needed to accept the child's hearing loss. The majority (approximately 52%) of the parents reported that they immediately accepted the child's loss. Only approximately 4% of the audiologists agreed with this time frame. The most frequent response of audiologists was that it took 1 month (28.2%) to accept the loss, followed by 7 to 12 months (24.4%) as the time needed for acceptance.

Although in general the audiologists and parents reported a similar range of emotional reactions, there were some important differences between the two sets of respondents. The results of the study by Martin et al. suggest that audiologists tend to focus more on the denial response than on the sorrow reaction. While audiologists were perhaps more objective in assessing denial than the parents, the discrepancy between the audiologists' and parents' perceptions may indicate that we should be more aware and accepting of feelings of sadness, disappointment, depression, and grief in the parents, not just at the time of diagnosis but subsequently also. By validating, rather than ignoring, the grief that parents may experience, the audiologist may help establish a more trusting and open communication between parent and professional, thus easing the long, bumpy road toward the ultimate goal, acceptance.

In this section, it has been emphasized that the emotional responses of parents should be viewed as a normal, nonpathological human response to loss and/or disability. This section will conclude with a caveat, however. Although many parents will experience these stages in response to learning that their child is hearing impaired, and will ultimately resolve their emotional conflicts, achieving acceptance of some form, the clinician must nevertheless be aware that some parents may experience distressful feelings of anxiety and depression for which a sympathetic ear will not be enough. Harvey and Green (1990), for example, describe the psychotherapeutic treatment of a mother who was obsessed with anxiety about her deaf daughter's future. When confronted with a parent who appears to be having recurrent anxieties and fears about the hearing-impaired child's status, or with a parent whose depression seems to be interfering with most aspects of the parent's life, the clinician must make an immediate referral to a qualified mental health counselor for resolution of the emotional conflicts. When in doubt as to whether the "normal" range of emotional reactions are being experienced, or a more serious psychiatric disturbance, the clinician should assist the parent in setting up a consultation with a mental health professional who can determine whether formal psychotherapeutic intervention is warranted.

PARENT-CHILD INTERACTION

A number of authors have expressed concern regarding the detrimental effect that knowledge of a child's hearing handicap may have on the mother's communication interaction style with her child. Goss (1970) was one of the first to delineate striking differences between the verbal behavior of mothers of deaf children and mothers of hearing children. His results suggested that mothers of deaf children are less likely to use verbal praise, to ask for opinions and suggestions, and to use questions, and they are more likely to show disagreement, tension, and antagonism and to give more sug-

gestions than are mothers of hearing children. Schlesinger (1972) and Meadow, Schlesinger, and Holstein (1972) have expressed concern that parents of hearing-impaired infants may be so intent on providing language stimulation that they may fail to respond playfully and in an interactive way in communication situations with their children. Moses and Van Hecke-Wulatin (1981) have also described the problems that mothers may experience in attempting to interact playfully and positively with their hearing-impaired infants, suggesting that the mother may often have difficulty viewing her relationship with the child as being reciprocal.

Kricos (1982) found that a substantial number of nonverbal communication attempts of hearing-impaired preschoolers are ignored by their mothers. Kenworthy (1986) obtained similar results in his comparison of mothers of normal-hearing children and mothers of hearing-impaired children. He found that mothers of hearing-impaired children tended to ignore the topics of conversation initiated by the child and frequently responded inappropriately to their child's communicative attempts. While mothers of the hearing children frequently used a high number of clarification requests when their child's communication was not intelligible, the mothers of hearing-impaired children rarely requested clarification. Results of these investigations suggest that there is a need to teach parents of young hearing-impaired children to identify and respond to their children's nonverbal communication attempts. Streng and her coauthors (1978) have also emphasized that teachers, as well as parents, must attempt to achieve communicative interaction with the hearing-impaired child rather than rely on one-way didactic communication.

The results of an investigation by Plapinger and Kretschmer (1991) revealed that the conversational context in which their mother-child dyad interactions took place had a pronounced effect on the style of discourse used by the mother in communicating with her hearing-impaired child. These authors collected data from a mother and her hearing-impaired child by videotaping naturally occurring interactions in the home over a period of time. The two main styles of interacting that were identified were labeling (i.e., mother assumes a "teacher" role) and dialoguing (i.e., parent serves more as a conversational facilitator). Plapinger and Kretschmer (1991) emphasize the key role that the clinician should play in observing and analyzing parent-child interactions, and their results highlight the need for these observations to be conducted in a variety of contexts in order to obtain a more representative sample of parent-child interaction styles.

In the past decade, there has been an increased emphasis on parental involvement in early intervention programs for handicapped infants, with increasing awareness of the importance of facilitating parent-child interaction. Underlying recognition of the importance of parent-child interaction is the idea that parents' behavior with their children (handicapped or not) affects the development of the children. Beyond understanding the emotional reactions that parents of hearing-impaired children may experience, there are other aspects of parent behavior that the clinician needs to consider, particularly dimensions such as parental warmth and affection, responsiveness to communication, sensitivity to the child's interests and feelings, and encouragement of independence. Rosenberg, Robinson, and Beckman (1986) review research that indicates that very young children develop most optimally when parents respond to their needs and provide experiences that are appropriate to their developmental levels. These authors point out, however, that the presence of a handicap in a child may affect the interactions between the child and his or her parents. For example, parents of handicapped infants must cope with less feedback from their infants than do parents of children without handicaps. Because of the impact that the parents' behavior may have on the handicapped child's growth, and conversely the influence that the handicap may have on the parents' behavior, the clinician should explore the nature of parent-child interactions.

Several means of evaluating the quality of interactions and the environment that parents provide young children are described by Rosenberg et al. (1986). Although many of these measures were designed for handicapped children who are not necessarily hearing impaired, they provide guidelines for interaction dimensions that should be considered. The Maternal Behavior Rating Scale (Mahoney, Finger, & Powell, 1985) consists of 18 maternal behavior items and 4 child behavior items that are rated on a five-point scale and provide information on maternal pleasure, quantity of stimulation, and control. A similar scale is the Teaching Skills Inventory (Version 2) developed by Rosenberg and Robinson (1985). This measure evaluates areas such as maternal responsiveness, maternal instructional skills, and child interest. The HOME Inventory for Infants and Toddlers (Caldwell & Bradley, 1984) uses a checklist format to assess the quality of parent-infant (0–36 months) interaction within six areas: responsivity, acceptance, organization, play materials, parental involvement, and variety of stimulation. The Parent Behavior Progression (Bromwich, 1978) is another means of evaluating the quality of parenting provided to infants. This observation checklist assesses a number of areas such as parental enjoyment of the child, parental sensitivity/responsiveness, mutuality of interaction, developmental appropriateness of interactions, and ability to generate new developmentally appropriate activities independently. Both Cole and St. Clair-Stokes (1984) and St. Clair-Stokes and Mischook (1990) have espoused a caregiver-child interaction analysis protocol based on videotaping the hearing-impaired child and the caregiver during everyday play and communication transactions. While much of their checklist evaluates the language and conversational behaviors exhibited by the caregiver, an important area for analysis is what these authors refer to as "sensitivity to child." Items included on their checklist for this parameter include handling the child in a positive manner; pacing play and conversation at the child's tempo; following the child's interest at a particular moment; providing stimulation, activities, and play that are appropriate for the child's age and developmental stage; and encouraging and facilitating the child's play with objects and materials.

The use of measures such as these are important for understanding the quality of parent-child interaction and for designing appropriate intervention to facilitate parent-child interaction. Because there is evidence that a child's hearing handicap may alter his or her interactive capacities, thus impairing the ability to contribute to mutually enjoyable exchanges with his or her parents, and because their is evidence that parents may alter their interactions with a hearing-impaired child, this is a critical area to investigate. Measures such as those described in this section can provide guidelines for working with individual parents.

FAMILY DYNAMICS

The birth of a child typically is accompanied by feelings of joy, excitement, and anticipation about the future. In most families the birth also brings about new challenges, responsibilities, and the watchword of the final decade of the 20th century, *stress*. The addition to a family of a child with a disability may bring a number of even greater challenges, demands, and sources of anxiety. Adams and Tidwell (1989) point out that hearing impairment in particular can erode the stability of a family because of its effect on ease of communication between the parents and the child. Research into families with a handicapped child typically has focused on the emotional crisis that often accompanies the diagnosis of an impairment and the period of adjustment that may follow the diagnosis.

Even before the passage of PL 99–457, which mandates a family focus to early intervention, a trend was evident in intervention programs for young handicapped children for movement of services from a narrowly focused child-centered orientation to a more broadly based home-centered orientation. This change of focus demands a thorough understanding of the family unit, sources of support for the family, effects on various family members of the presence of a handicapped child, coping and adaptation skills exhibited by family members, and sources of stress on family life. Bernheimer, Gallimore, and Weisner (1990) stress the importance of embracing what they refer to as an ecocultural theory as a framework for designing intervention for handicapped children. Ecocultural the-

ory refers to consideration of the sociocultural environment of the child and family. Likewise, Dunst et al. (1990) enumerate the ways in which a child's development is influenced by broader-based social systems. According to their model, resources and social support that parents receive from their personal network of friends and acquaintances will influence parent well-being and health; both support and parental well-being influence family functioning; support, well-being, and family functioning influence the nature of interactions between parents and their children; and support, well-being, family functioning, and caregiver interactive styles influence child behavior and development. Correlating with these influences will be parent and family characteristics, such as age, education, socioeconomic status, and values and beliefs, along with child characteristics. The interrelationships among social support, well-being, child characteristics, and child progress were documented in the study by Dunst et al. (1990) of 47 mothers and their young handicapped children. Studies such as this highlight the need to broaden the scope and focus of our services beyond the immediate needs of the hearing-impaired child. Early intervention programs for the families of hearing-impaired children need to focus attention on a number of aspects of family functioning.

The purpose of this section, then, will be to examine the influence of the presence of a hearing-impaired child on family dynamics. The counseling suggestions offered in the second section of this chapter will be most effectively applied if viewed within the context of the total family and its needs.

Family Structure

The American family has undergone some tremendous changes in structure in the last few decades. Somers (1987) reviews a number of societal changes that may affect parenting and offers suggestions for professionals to meet the needs of families with hearing-impaired children. She points out that there has been a significant increase in the number of two-career, single-parent, and low-income families. To provide effective, relevant programming for such families will require modification of traditional programming for hearing-impaired children, which has tended to emphasize the mother as the primary source of speech and language stimulation through intensive, structured language activities in the home with the child. According to U.S. Bureau of the Census figures cited by Somers (1987), married women with young children make up most of the work force. Families who work have numerous demands, needs, and stresses that must be addressed. Finding appropriate child care for the hearing-impaired child is difficult. The author recalls trying to assist the working mother of a 2-year-old profoundly hearing-impaired child to find a daycare center that would allow her son to wear his hearing aids during the day. Apparently the daycare centers were willing to accept the child, and several even expressed interest in having their staff learn some basic sign language, but they were concerned about the possibility of the child losing or damaging his hearing aids and would not accept the responsibility for that. The mother finally placed her child in a preschool program with a warm, supportive staff, but with limited hours of operation, thus creating another strain for the family.

Somers (1987) also points out that working families will probably find it difficult to participate in home training activities, daytime conferences, or observation of their children in therapy programs. Professionals who work with hearing-impaired children will be increasingly challenged to offer flexible, creative programming to meet the needs of these families. Seal (1987) describes what she refers to as a "working parents' dream"—instructional videotapes for parents of signing deaf children. In her program for hearing-impaired children in the Department of Speech Pathology and Audiology at James Madison University, the children of working parents are videotaped during spontaneous and elicited interactions in the clinic, and the tapes, along with a narrated script that points out targeted language structures and other relevant information, are sent home with the child, along with a portable videocassette player. Creative, flexible programming such as this helps to meet the needs of modern parents confronted with innumerable demands on their time.

In many families (with one exception being the author's!), there has been a mod-ification of the traditional pattern of the mother serving as the chief home caregiver for the family. With changing roles, there is a need to recognize that fathers, more than at any time in the past, are frequently equally responsible for involvement with child care, and their needs as parents of hearing-impaired children must be recognized.

The needs of single parents are even greater than those of dual-career families. In addition to full-time work, the single parent with a hearing-impaired child must often face the challenges of raising a special needs child alone, with minimal financial, emotional, physical, or social support. It is estimated that one out of every two marriages in the United States will end in divorce and that the majority of American children will spend at least half of their childhood in a single-parent household. In 1984, one out of every five families with children under 18 (compared to 1 out of 10 in 1970) was headed by a single parent (Bristol, Reichle, & Thomas, 1987). It is estimated that, combining the incidence of divorce, widowhood, and single parenthood, 67% of American children will be raised by a single parent for at least part of their lives and that the majority of these children will spend at least 5 years in a mother-child family (Vincent & Salisbury, 1988). The composition of single-parent families has also changed significantly. Bristol et al. (1987) report that whereas in 1960 widows composed the majority of single-parent households, in 1984 only 9% of mother-child households were headed by widows, with 46% headed by divorced mothers. This change in family structure will certainly have to be recognized by professionals who work with hearing-impaired children. Somers (1987) points out that there are recurring areas of concern for single parents, including financial responsibility, physical stress, feelings of isolation, and unrelenting demands of daily child care. Sensitivity to these issues by the professional is a prerequisite to the provision of services that will be effective for the hearing-impaired child. As Bristol et al. (1987) point out, however, professionals must not assume that single-parent families are a homogeneous group in terms of needs and resources. Too much focus on the stresses and demands on single-parent families might lead to an unwarranted negative labeling of all single parents. However, it must be recognized that service delivery systems for hearing-impaired children and their families have largely been based on meeting the needs of two-parent, unemployed-mother families. Audiologists and other professionals who work with hearing-impaired children must become more sensitive to the needs of the modern American family confronted with raising a hearing-impaired child.

Finally, the special needs of low-income families must be recognized. The tremendous increase in single-parent families has been paralleled by an increase in the number of children being raised in poverty (Vincent & Salisbury, 1988). The stresses of housing, feeding, and caring for a family operating under less than adequate income may cause the needs of the hearing-impaired child to be relegated to a lesser priority than day-to-day survival. Somers (1987) highlights a number of problems that may confront low-income families with hearing-impaired children, including finding appropriate daycare, obtaining hearing health care services, maintaining hearing aids, and having transportation to needed services. Another problem is that parents may feel uneducated, underqualified, and held in low esteem by professionals.

Somers (1987) offers a number of practical suggestions for professionals who are responsible for designing intervention programs for families with hearing-impaired children. Chief among these is to consider each family as unique, with individualized programming depending on a particular family's characteristics and needs. Offering opportunities for therapy and counseling sessions during nonworking hours, helping the parents to find social support networks in the community, and providing as much information to the parents as possible, to help economize their limited time, are other suggestions.

Parents

McLinden (1990) reported the results of a study designed to examine the effects of special needs children on families, as reported by 48 mothers and 35 fathers. In this study, the children's disabilities fell into several categories, including hearing impairment. Various scales were administered to these parents to assess social support, family satisfaction, and the impact of handicapped children on family functioning. McLinden's results emphasize that it cannot be assumed that all families are similarly influenced by the presence of a child with special needs, nor for that matter that members of the same family unit will be similarly affected. McLinden delineated a number of problem areas that were cited by the mothers and fathers in her study. The top three problem areas cited by the mothers in her sample were (1) demands of caring for a child with special needs to the exclusion of time for herself (42.6% of mothers); (2) worry about the child's future (42.6%); and (3) feelings of fatigue. In contrast, the top three areas cited as problems for fathers were (1) worry about the child's future (42.9%); (2) the ability to find a reliable person to care for the child with special needs; and (3) the necessity of having a daily schedule centered around the child with special needs. McLinden noted that there were twice as many problems reported by at least 30% of mothers than by 30% of the fathers. The variability in problems experienced across families was evident by the fact that when the final data were tabulated, none of the items was cited as a problem by more than 43% of the mothers or fathers.

McLinden points out a number of implications from the results of her study. Because it was evident that almost half the mothers found the time demands of caring for a special needs child to be problematic, intervention programs may need to consider the mother's willingness and capability to contribute to her child's educational program. Rather than, with all good intentions, suggesting a myriad of ways that the parent might "work with" the child in the home, the professional may want to focus more on helping the mother to better manage her time demands. When one considers that approximately 40% of mothers in McLinden's study reported extreme fatigue, and almost one-third of fathers indicated that having the family schedule revolve around the handicapped child was problematic, it becomes evident that a focus on better management of time demands, or even at the least acknowledgment of the time demands by the professional, might be a more appropriate intervention than a list of speech and language stimulation activities. Likewise, McLinden's data suggest that both mothers and fathers frequently have concerns about their child's future. The professional, then, should seek ways to provide information to the parents about what the child's prognoses for communication and education are, what his or her future service needs might be, and information about the disability so that parents have realistic expectations for their child. McLinden emphasizes, however, the variability of problem areas cited by the mothers and fathers. Thus, the professional cannot assume what areas will be problems but must be prepared for some families to have significant concerns about their child's future, some to be troubled by the time demands of raising a special needs child, and still others to be concerned about the child's current progress in the intervention program. The two key words, then, are *sensitivity* and *flexibility*. By being sensitive to the unique needs of each family (as well as various members of that family) and willing to be flexible in designing programs to meet these needs, the professional stands a far better chance of effectively addressing the needs of hearing-impaired children and their families.

The fact that parents of hearing-impaired children may perceive a number of problem areas associated with raising a hearing-impaired child may not necessarily mean that they are at risk for development of psychiatric problems or marital difficulties, although these are frequently assumed by researchers and clinicians. A recent study by Henggeler et al. (1990) compared the emotional and marital adjustment of hearing parents of hearing-impaired children with mothers and fathers of hearing youths. It was found that parents of hearing-impaired children actually reported less psychiatric symptomatology than did parents of hearing children and that there were no differences in the marital satisfaction of parents in intact families. Granted, in addition to the emotional stressors outlined at the beginning of this chapter, parents of hearing-impaired children also have a number of other sources of stress such as special medical attention for their child, high financial costs, and time demands due to their involvement in the child's education and supervision. However, Henggeler and his coauthors found abundant evidence of family cohesion, as exemplified by emotional warmth, closeness, and sharing, which appears to have a positive influence on parental adaptation. While at the same time recognizing and being prepared for emotional and marital difficulties, the professionals also should be attuned to focusing on the positive adaptation of families of hearing-impaired youth rather than taking a deficit view of the parents and their reactions to raising a hearing-impaired child. The findings of Henggeler et al. provide evidence that parents of hearing-impaired youths adjust quite well, overall, to the many stressors of parenting a child with a hearing impairment. Similar findings evolved in a study conducted by Hanson and Hanline (1990). These authors used the Parenting Stress Index (Abidin, 1983) to document, via a 3-year longitudinal study, the stress patterns and parenting experiences of mothers of children with either Down syndrome, hearing impairment, or neurological impairment. The Parenting Stress Index (PSI) contains 101 true/false items to evaluate the parent's perception of child characteristics, parental response to the child, and judgments of the quality of life. Areas such as the child's demandingness, mood, and acceptability, as well as the parents' depression, health, spousal relationship, and role restriction, are explored via the PSI. Hanson and Hanline (1990) emphasized that their results did not yield profiles of parents who were extremely dissatisfied or unable to cope with parenting a handicapped child. They noted other factors, such as socioeconomic status, marital relationships, and personal problems, which might lead to family dysfunction. The presence of a child with a disability may result in family stress, but it may not be the only factor, or even the most significant factor, influencing the quality of parenting experiences. Likewise, Salisbury (1987) cites research that shows that mothers, single parents, parents of young children, and parents of adolescents experience high levels of stress, regardless of whether there is a handicapped child in the family.

Other Family Members

Research on the effects of a handicapped child on the family has focused primarily on how the child affects the parents. Examination of the effects on other family members has received negligible attention. Israelite (1986) cites research on siblings of children with handicaps other than hearing loss that shows pronounced individual variation in effects and experiences. Some siblings feel that having a handicapped brother or sister has a positive influence on them. Others report a more negative experience, and still others report that the presence of a handicapped child in the family had virtually no effect on their growth and development. The mothers of hearing-impaired adolescents who were interviewed by Morgan-Redshaw, Wilgosh, and Bibby (1990) also reported a range of both positive and negative influences that a hearing-impaired child may have on sibling relationships. Atkins (1987) points out a number of reasons to be concerned about the well-being and adjustment of siblings of hearing-impaired children. These include, among others:

1. Their parents, knowingly or unknowingly, being less involved with them because of time demands in meeting the needs of the hearing-impaired sibling
2. The parents' fatigue, worry, and preoccupation detracting from a satisfying interaction with the hearing siblings
3. Inquiries from friends and strangers regarding the hearing-impaired child
4. A feeling that the hearing-impaired sibling is not disciplined by the parents
5. Possible feelings of guilt and responsibility for the hearing-impaired child's handicap
6. Increased responsibilities around the home, including caretaking of the hearing-impaired sibling

Atkins (1987) points out that sibling relationships in any family, regardless of the presence or not of a hearing-impaired child, are influenced by a number of variables, including family size, birth order, gender, roles of various family members, self-perceptions, temperaments, marital harmony, parenting styles, and economic status. For families with hearing-impaired children, there will likely be other variables, such as those listed above, affecting family adjustment and sibling relationships.

Israelite (1986) investigated the effects of a hearing-impaired child on the psychological functioning of hearing-impaired siblings by comparing 14 siblings of hearing-impaired children to 14 siblings of normal-hearing children on self-reported levels of family responsibility, depression, anxiety, and self-concept. Her results revealed two primary differences between the groups, one relating to identity and the other to social self-concept. That is, the siblings of hearing-impaired children tended to define themselves not only as individuals in their own right but also as siblings of hearing-impaired children, and their social self-concept was lower than that of siblings of normal-hearing children. The two groups performed similarly on measures of family responsibility, depression, anxiety, and self-esteem. Thus, although some differences in psychological functioning were noted, they did not appear to have any pronounced negative effects on the emotional stability or overall adjustment of siblings of hearing-impaired children.

Atkins (1987) points out that we have extremely limited information about the effect of hearing-impaired children on their siblings and that intervention programs for hearing-impaired children rarely include their brothers and sisters. He suggests that sibling programs be designed to meet the needs of the entire family. These programs might include special programs that bring siblings together for practical information about hearing impairment and for sharing experiences, or routine sibling meetings at the same time group parent meetings are held.

Another often overlooked family member is the grandparent. The emotional reactions earlier described for parents of newly diagnosed hearing-impaired children are relevant, also, for grandparents. In fact, they may experience grief for their beloved grandchild as well as worry about their own child's ability to cope with the added responsibilities of raising a hearing-impaired child. Vadasy, Fewell, and Meyer (1986) reported that grandparents of handicapped children frequently experience initial feelings of sadness, and to a lesser extent, shock and anger. Most of the grandparents that they interviewed reported that they eventually accepted their grandchild's handicap, although almost half of their sample continued to express feelings of sadness long after the initial diagnosis of the child's handicap. Vadasy et al. (1986) describe one of the few structured programs for grandparents, specifically a "grandparent workshop," in which participants are offered information about their grandchild's handicap as well as opportunities for sharing concerns and experiences with other grandparents. The authors point out the valuable resources that grandparents can be within a family with a handicapped child, and advise professionals to look closely at the extended networks of families to appreciate the strengths and contributions of extended family members such as grandparents.

In this section of the chapter, a perspective on the influence of a hearing-impaired child on family functioning has been provided. As Trivette et al. (1990) point out in an excellent article on family strengths, the goal of intervention should not be viewed so much as provision of needed services by the professional as much as strengthening the functioning of families so that they will ultimately be less dependent on the professional for help. These authors espouse a shift in intervention services toward enabling and empowering families to meet the needs of their handicapped children.

Evidence of the potential influence that the family may have is provided by two studies of the effects of family environment on the progress of the hearing-impaired child. In the first, Bodner-Johnson (1986) attempted to determine the relationships between family practices and deaf children's academic skill performance in reading and mathematics. Her data clearly show the impact of family environment on the hearing-impaired child's academic performance in that deaf students who differed significantly in academic achievement also differed significantly in family environment. Family practices related to adaptation to deafness, involvement in the deaf community, and permissive rather than overprotective childrearing orientation, as well as press for achievement, were found to discriminate high- and low-level readers, while for mathematics, parents' press for achievement appeared to be the discriminatory factor.

In the second study, Warren and Hasenstab (1986) showed that of all the variables they researched, parental childrearing attitudes appeared to be the best predictors of self-concept of severely to profoundly hearing-impaired children. These authors point out that the family is typically the main source of interaction and socialization for a child, and therefore the child's relationship with the parents is vitally important for developing a positive self-concept. It is in the context of the family that a child learns about himself or herself and develops a self-concept. If the child feels unconditionally accepted, it is more likely that a positive self-concept will be developed. Given the range of emotional reactions described at the beginning of this section, it is not difficult to see how unsatisfactory resolution of the parents' grief, disappointment, and sadness could lead to unintended rejection, overprotection, and other aberrant parental responses. Warren and Hasenstab (1986) emphasize the need for professionals to focus their intervention on the total family, fostering in any means possible the development of positive childrearing practices, so that ultimately the hearing-impaired child can achieve the most optimal development in all facets of life.

The Counseling Process
EFFECTIVENESS OF COUNSELING PROVIDED BY AUDIOLOGISTS

As recognition among audiologists of the importance of parent counseling has increased in recent years, so also there have been increased reports in the literature on the effectiveness of audiologic counseling with parents of hearing-impaired children. Sweetow and Barrager (1980) attempted, via use of a questionnaire survey, to evaluate parents' views of the counseling they had received concerning hearing impairment and its ramifications. Specific areas on the questionnaire related to case history information; pretest counseling; initial audiologic evaluation; reporting of test results; referrals for educational, emotional, and financial support; hearing aid delivery; and hearing aid orientation. Results of their study suggested that parents were, for the most part, satisfied with the audiologic care provided. However, several areas of concern were expressed. The need for the audiologist to translate complicated terminology into language easily understood by the parents and the need for written information related to hearing impairment were repeatedly stressed. Many parents expressed a desire for audiologists to suggest techniques for parents to communicate with their newly identified hearing-impaired child. There was also a desire on the part of the parents to have contact with other parents of hearing-impaired children. In addition, the parents surveyed requested more frequent referrals for emotional and financial support, as well as for educational information.

Haas and Crowley (1982) also used a questionnaire format to obtain input from parents regarding their satisfaction with the delivery of hearing health information from a variety of professionals, including the family physician, pediatrician, otologist, audiologist, speech-language pathologist, deaf educator, and hearing aid dispenser. According to the respondents, the audiologist was the first referral source (56%), performed the first hearing test (53%), and confirmed the presence of the hearing loss (62%). Audiologists were rated highest in terms of incidence of participation in the diagnostic/evaluation process (91%), as well as most effective in information dissemination (72%). However, when parents were asked an open-ended question about which professional supplied the most meaningful input regarding the implications of the handicap, educators were overwhelmingly singled out for their special contributions. This may indicate that physicians and audiologists failed to supply the supportive counseling necessary for understanding the ramifications of the hearing loss.

Based on the literature and their own clinical experience, Williams and Darbyshire (1982) stated that effective management during and after the time of diagnosis is critical to the acceptance of the permanent hearing loss and subsequent involvement in rehabilitative training. In their study of parents' needs during and after the diagnosis, a 70-item questionnaire and an interview session were completed by 25 parents of hearing-impaired children who lived outside a small city in rural Ontario. The questionnaire was designed to address the following four areas of concern: *(1)* the parents' awareness of difficulties caused by hearing loss and activities to help minimize them; *(2)* reactions and steps taken to investigate the initial suspicions of hearing loss; *(3)* reactions to the diagnosis and to the professionals making the diagnosis; and *(4)* views on rehabilitative services available. The interview further probed the parents' feelings regarding existing services and the need for improvement or initiation of additional services.

Severe emotional reactions to the diagnosis of hearing impairment were reported by 80% of the responding parents. Williams and Darbyshire (1982) indicated that the parents' lack of understanding of hearing loss and its implications contributed to the severity and continuation of their emotional reactions. Eighty-four percent of the parents thought that most parents could not understand information given by the audiologist, otologist, and other specialists at the time of diagnosis. Seventy-two percent of the parents did not understand what effects the hearing loss would have on their child, and 64% did not have a realistic appreciation of the impact their child's hearing loss would have on their own lives.

A study by Martin et al. (1987) was cited earlier in this chapter, regarding the discrepancies between audiologists' and parents' viewpoints of parental reactions to hearing loss in their children. These authors also reported other data concerning the effectiveness of counseling by audiologists. The majority of the parents they surveyed stated that they received information concerning the degree of hearing loss, the functioning of the auditory mechanism, amplification, educational alternatives, and home activities. Somewhat less than half of the parents received information on speech/language development and causes of hearing loss. While the large majority of parents stated that they would have wanted to receive information on all of these topics at the time of diagnosis, 13% stated that they would have preferred no information at the time of initial diagnosis. Over 95% of the parents stated that they would have liked to receive additional information on available services, reading materials, effects of the loss on the family, coping strategies, prognosis, and information about how to meet parents of other hearing-impaired children.

The majority of parents surveyed by Martin et al. thought that they were able to understand information presented to them immediately. On the other hand, the audiologists surveyed stated that parents typically need up to a full year to understand the information that is presented to them at the time of diagnosis.

Both parents and audiologists agreed that emotional as well as informational counseling was important for parents at the time of diagnosis. For both types of counseling, the majority of parents rated the professionals (school personnel, audiologists, psychologists, and so on) who provided counseling services as being very good. Similar to the results of Haas and Crowley (1982), school personnel were singled out by parents (22%) as being the professionals who should be responsible for emotional counseling, followed by audiologists (19%). The majority of audiologists, however, stated that either an audiologist or both an audiologist and a psychologist together are the most appropriate professionals to conduct such counseling.

Both positive and negative aspects of parent-professional relationships were cited by the five mothers of hearing-impaired adolescents who were interviewed by Morgan-Redshaw et al. (1990). While many characteristics of educators and other professionals were praised, such as their devotedness to their professions, other characteristics were criticized, such as focusing on the audiogram rather than on the child and deemphasizing the family's knowledge of the child and its role in the child's intervention.

Several authors have expressed concern in recent years regarding the amount of training audiologists receive in counseling during their graduate education (McCarthy, Culpepper, & Lucks, 1986; Oyler & Matkin, 1987; Roush, 1991; Roush & McWilliam, 1990). For example, Oyler and Matkin (1987) found that fewer than one in four recently certified audiologists responding to their survey had a course in parent counseling. McCarthy et al. (1986), however, point out the difficulties of adding yet another course as a requirement in an already burgeoning masters-level program in audiology. The preservice educational needs of audiologists in the area of parent counseling, including appropriate coursework as well as supervised clinical experience, will need to be addressed in order to provide adequate services to the families of hearing-impaired children. As Roush (1991) and Roush and McWilliam (1990) point out, this area of training will be particularly crucial for successful implementation of Public Law 99–457, with its emphasis on family-centered intervention.

A FAMILY-CENTERED PERSPECTIVE OF COUNSELING

Two types of parent counseling, one focused on provision of information (sometimes referred to as content counseling) and the other dealing with the parents' personal adjustment (sometimes referred to as emotional counseling), have been cited by a number of authors (among others, Luterman, 1991; Pollack, 1978; Sanders, 1975; Stream & Stream, 1978). Information or content counseling might consist of provision of information relating to hearing aids, development of listening function, description of audiograms, and so on. Personal adjustment counseling, on the other hand, would be concerned with helping the parents adjust to having a hearing-impaired child, particularly in the emotional realm.

Flahive and White (1981) conducted a survey of audiologists regarding their perceptions and practice of parent counseling. Their respondents indicated that while they recognized and supported these two types of counseling, far more emphasis was given in practice to informational counseling. The majority of audiologists reported being satisfied with their ability to provide informational counseling, feeling less comfortable with their personal-adjustment counseling abilities. The results of Flahive and White's survey also indicated that audiologists receive less than an optimal amount of preprofessional training in counseling, particularly for personal-adjustment counseling.

Houle and Hamilton (1991) state that audiologists and speech-language pathologists will be challenged to meet the demands of PL 99–457, Part H, which shifts the target of intervention services from the child to the family. Given the mandate by PL 99–457 for dramatically increased family involvement in intervention services for handicapped infants and toddlers, as well as the increasing awareness of the importance of the family to the hearing-impaired child's overall development, it is timely to revisit the goals of parent counseling within a family-centered context. The following parent counseling goals are presented, adapted from Bromwich (1978), Dunst, Trivette, and Deal (1988), and Garwood and Fewell (1983), all of whom are renown for their work in early intervention within a family focus:

1. To promote positive child, parent, and family functioning
2. To help family members appraise their problems and needs
3. To base parent counseling and other forms of intervention on family-identified needs and priorities
4. To reduce stress and anxiety associated with parenting a hearing-impaired child
5. To identify family strengths and unique resources
6. To define means of using the family's strengths and resources within the intervention program
7. To ensure the availability and use of formal and informal social network resources and service systems for meeting family needs
8. To promote family members' sense of confidence and to reinforce the parent's perception of being the primary agent responsible for the child's intervention program and overall development
9. To promote family's abilities to acquire and use competencies and skills necessary for optimal family functioning
10. To assess the nature of parent-child interaction and to seek ways to make interactions more reciprocal and mutually satisfying

Winton and Bailey (1990) describe several current themes underlying approaches to intervention with families of handicapped children. One of these themes is family empowerment and equal partnerships with professionals. Implicit in this theme is that the family's resources and strengths should be capitalized on and incorporated into the intervention program and that families should be involved in the decision process as intervention is planned and implemented. Krauss (1990) points out that there has been an evolution in family involvement in intervention programs for handicapped children. Parental involvement used to mean assuming a passive role by acquiescing with the professional's recommendations. Family involvement then evolved to the inclusion of parents as cotherapists for their children, but professionals still directed the intervention missions. The most current approach to family involvement revolves on the concept of family empowerment, with intervention goals as well as strategies guided by parental input (Trivette et al., 1990). Of course, this shift in the family's role has and will continue to necessitate changes in the ways professionals approach families. Rather than *providing* information to families, the professional's role has shifted to *acquiring* information from families about their needs, strengths, resources, and intervention priorities. This is not in any way to suggest that intervention goals are solely left to parental preference but rather that the professional be viewed less as the "expert" and more as a "partner," with families and professionals joining in a collaborative effort to facilitate the handicapped child's development (Whitehead, Deiner, & Toccafondi, 1990; Winton & Bailey, 1990).

Trivette et al. (1990) note also that other shifts of thinking will be necessary for provision of quality family-centered intervention. The professional will need to rethink the concept that families "need to be fixed" or changed somehow; instead, professionals need to seek out and capitalize on the positive aspects of family functioning. Rather than trying to solve problems confronting a family, the professional's role should be viewed as enabling and empowering families to master problem areas in their lives.

There have been several reports in the literature recently of parents' viewpoints on what their counseling and education needs are. Summers et al. (1990) polled parents and early intervention specialists to determine priorities for program services. The most frequently mentioned theme was the need for sensitivity to families. Participants cited the need for professionals to be supportive of families' emotional needs, to be accepting and nonjudgmental, and to conduct all interactions in an unhurried atmosphere. They also mentioned the need for acknowledgment of the family as the ultimate decision maker, clear communication between parent and professional, enhanced social support for families, and acknowledgment of the diversity among families.

Interviews of parents of young children with special needs by Able-Boone, Sandall, and Frederick (1990) yielded similar suggestions. In addition, these parents emphasized their desire to become knowledgeable about their children's needs and about available services. The parents stressed the importance of being informed decision makers in their children's intervention program and recommended that professionals avoid imposing goals and home programs on parents.

A study by Bernstein and Barta (1988) was designed specifically to obtain input from parents of hearing-impaired children regarding their parent education and counseling needs and to compare parents' goals with those of professionals. Their results indicated considerable agreement between parents and professionals but highlighted the perception by parents that they wished to have more opportunity to inform the professional of their own needs as parents of hearing-impaired children.

For excellent examples of family-centered intervention programs for hearing-impaired children, the reader is directed to two books: *Parents and Teachers: Partners in Language Development*, by Simmons-Martin and Rossi (1990), and *Parent-Infant Habilitation: A Comprehensive Approach to Working with Hearing-Impaired Infants and Toddlers and Their Families*, by Schuyler and Rushmer (1987). The intervention programs described by these authors are based on parent-professional partnerships, and both of these sources contain practical suggestions for implementing a family-focused intervention program.

INFORMATION SHARING WITH PARENTS

No one enjoys being the bearer of bad tidings, and certainly no one likes being in the position of receiving bad news. Like it or not, however, audiologists are frequently called on to deliver "bad news" to parents of hearing-impaired children. Kroth (1987) believes that bad news that is delivered clearly *and* tactfully to parents is likely to be accepted more readily. The key, according to Kroth (1987), is for professionals to be sensitive to the stressful situation in which the parents are to receive information, and to strive to be an "active informer" during the counseling process. An active informer, according to Kroth, is one who shares concerns with the family of a hearing-impaired child, rather than maintaining a cool, aloof distance from the family's situation. The active informer demonstrates genuine interest in the family and seeks out the family's involvement in finding solutions to their problems. The professional conveys respect for and confidence in the family's ability to cope with their child's hearing loss, and attempts to manipulate the environment, timing of information provision, and wording of statements and questions in a manner that is sensitive to the family's needs. The active informer views himself or herself not as "the authority" but rather as "the helper."

The audiologists and parents surveyed by Martin et al. (1987) thought that it was important for audiologists to be honest, empathetic, nonjudgmental, and direct in their interactions with parents at the time of diagnosis. While the parents expressed positive regard for many aspects of the counseling process that they had experienced, they also suggested that counselors need to be more supportive listeners, to offer more realistic hope for the future, to serve more of a role as a resource for information, and to be more willing to spend time with them during counseling. Although the parents in the study by Martin et al. acknowledged that they had been given information during counseling, they thought that more detailed information would have been helpful.

An important component of counseling programs for parents of hearing-impaired children can thus be satisfied by professionals providing information to family members. Information provision can range from the formal (e.g., grandparent workshops) to the informal (conversations focused on problem areas). The current emphasis on providing information to families, according to Turnbull and Turnbull (1986), contrasts with the older focus on training parents to conduct educational programs in the home. Turnbull and Turnbull (1986) believe that the rationale for parent training evolved more from professional ideology than from parent-focused directives. Instead of conceiving of parent training as the main focus of early intervention, these authors think that the concept of "parent support" or "family support," with its emphasis on providing information to families, should be the philosophy governing program development. This new emphasis would enable families to determine their own priorities rather than following those imposed by professionals, and it would also acknowledge the needs of the entire family, not just those of the hearing-impaired child.

Numerous levels of parent/professional contact for information sharing have been described in the literature (Clark & Watkins, 1978; Northcott, 1977; Schuyler & Rushmer, 1987; Simmons-Martin & Rossi, 1990). These levels could include home visits; individual and group guidance sessions; special groups for fathers, siblings, and grandparents; individual demonstration therapy; parent/child notebooks, logs, and/or scrapbooks; and guided individual and/or group therapy observations. One of the most powerful counseling tools available to clinicians is the establishment of parent-to-parent networks. Parent discussion groups, in which the clinician serves more as a facilitator than as a leader, can be an extremely beneficial forum in which parents can share concerns, problems, and solutions as well as provide emotional bolstering on an ongoing basis. An additional strategy that can be most effective is to put the parent of a recently diagnosed hearing-impaired child into contact with one or two parents of an older deaf child, who may be regarded as "survivors" of this traumatic period. The author's experience is that parents of young deaf children are eager to solicit input from other parents who "have been there," and that parents of older hearing-impaired children are more than willing to reciprocate, being keenly aware of the fears and frustrations that accompany the diagnosis of deafness. It is also highly advisable to give parents the names and addresses of national and local parent organizations, as well as to maintain a parent lending library that is rich in appropriate reading materials.

COUNSELING THE HEARING-IMPAIRED CHILD

Much of this chapter has focused on meeting the needs of parents of recently diagnosed young hearing-impaired children. Special note must be made also of the counseling needs of hearing-impaired children, particularly adolescents. The onset of adolescence may be a turbulent period even for normal-hearing adolescents and their parents, with a lack of communication frequently perceived by both parties in parent-child dyads. It is not surprising that these difficulties may be magnified with the existence of a severe communication handicap such as deafness. It is also likely at this time that the parent's original hopes for the child's communication, academic, and social achievements may have depreciated with the realization that little time is left in which to achieve initial expectations.

Several authors have expressed concern regarding the low self-esteem of hearing-impaired children (Davis et al., 1986; Grimes & Prickett, 1988; Loeb & Sarigiani, 1986). Davis et al. (1986) conducted an extensive psychoeducational evaluation of 40 hearing-impaired children, ages 5 to 18 years, to determine the effects of hearing loss on intellectual, academic, social, and language behaviors of children. Their results highlighted the heterogeneity of hearing-impaired children, with the effects of hearing loss differing from child to child. Half the children in their study expressed concern about their abilities to make friends or to be accepted socially, as compared to only approximately 15% of hearing children that they surveyed. Many of the hearing-impaired children reported that they were teased by other children, frequently because of their hearing aids; only approximately one-third said that they would be open with their normal-hearing peers about wearing hearing aids; and many others reported spending most of their time alone. The audiologist who works with hearing-impaired children needs to be aware of these opinions when dealing with children so that the issue of hearing aid use is treated sensitively.

Loeb and Sarigiani (1986) reported similar results in their study of the self-perceptions of 250 mainstreamed hearing-impaired children between the ages of 8 and 15 years. Their research indicated that hearing-impaired children in regular classrooms report that they are not popular, that they have a hard time making friends, that they are shy around their peers, and that they do not feel accepted by their families.

The sensitive audiologist will take this diminished self-concept into consideration when interacting with hearing-impaired children and their families. There are a number of small, but important, ways that the audiologist might help nurture a positive self-concept in hearing-impaired children. One is to be circumspect about unintended messages we might be sending to hearing-impaired children as we interact with them. If we frown, look uncomfortable, or act frustrated or otherwise nonaccepting of their, in many cases, limited communication, we are reinforcing their perceptions of being inferior. If we downplay or ignore their cosmetic concerns about wearing hearing aids, we are disregarding what to them is one of the greatest sources of their social difficulties. By acknowledging their negative feelings about hearing aids, while at the same time emphasizing the social benefits of hearing aids, the audiologist might gain more trust and respect from the child and ultimately more complicity in use of the hearing aids.

Other ways that the audiologist might help bolster self-esteem might be to take every opportunity to make positive comments about any of the child's strengths (and, of course, *all* children have strengths in some area of life); to allow children to participate at least to some degree in decisions that concern them; and to encourage families to "accent the positive." Group

counseling sessions by a qualified counselor may help both deaf teenagers and their parents adjust to this often confusing period.

Finally, Meadow (1968, 1976) attributes problems in psychosocial development of deaf individuals to early childhood experiences in which negative responses may have been obtained from parents and other significant persons. In one of her many studies of the psychosocial development of deaf individuals, it was found that deaf children with deaf parents and a positive family environment had higher self-images, self-esteem, and self-confidence than deaf children with hearing parents and less positive family environments. Meadow believed that these results could be attributed to the negative reactions experienced by hearing parents in response to their child's disability. Her results highlight the need for the family focus of intervention stressed in this chapter.

MULTICULTURAL CONSIDERATIONS IN THE COUNSELING PROCESS

In this chapter, the importance of audiologists embracing a family focus to their services has been emphasized. To provide effective, relevant services to families, it will be necessary to take into account the impact of cultural diversity on family functioning and on the counseling process. This need for consideration of cultural diversity is underscored by the rapidly changing demographics in the United States. According to figures reviewed by Hanson, Lynch, and Wayman (1990), it is estimated that by the year 2000, 38% of children under 18 will be from nonwhite, non-Anglo families. As the country's demographics change, it can be expected that in many areas of the country nearly 50% of all young children will be from cultural and language groups that are different from those of most early intervention professionals. Thus, early interventionists who embrace a family-centered focus will be interacting with families whose values and practices are quite different than their own.

Cultural groups may have significantly different views of medicine and health care, in attitudes toward disability, and in child-rearing practices. The audiologist's own cultural identity, beliefs, and value systems will influence how he or she interacts with families and works with them to formulate and prioritize intervention goals. Obviously, it will be critical for audiologists who work with families of hearing-impaired children to acknowledge and respect different cultural perspectives and to learn how to work effectively with families whose views and practices are quite different from their own.

Unlike the traditional Anglo-American family, which tends to be small, nuclear, and clearly defined in family members' roles, families from other cultural backgrounds may have radically different family structures, with multiple generations living together in a single household, diverse roles among family members, and responsibilities for child care shared by all. This difference alone, coupled perhaps in some cases with the family's limited English proficiency, may necessitate the audiologist's rethinking of how best to serve the family via counseling. Prior to designing appropriate intervention goals for culturally diverse families, the audiologist needs to address a number of issues. For example, if there are language problems, how might these be circumvented? Who are the members of the hearing-impaired child's family? Who is the child's primary caregiver(s)? What are the family's beliefs about disability and causal factors of disability? What is the style of interaction among family members? What are the family's specific childrearing practices? What are the family's attitudes toward help-seeking, professionals, intervention, health, and healing?

The results of a survey of parents of Afro-American hearing-impaired children by Jones and Kretschmer (1988) hint that our present models for parent education are ineffective in teaching culturally diverse and/or lower socioeconomic status parents. Although the parents they surveyed reported a high degree of satisfaction with their children's educational program, they also reported being minimally involved with the program and unfamiliar with many of the terms, practices, and methods of teaching hearing-impaired children.

Wayman, Lynch, and Hanson (1990) caution early intervention professionals not to set up a priori expectations of family functioning for various culture groups. They point out that families within specific cultures may or may not reflect characteristics that are considered typical for that culture. Variables such as socioeconomic status, length of residence in the United States, and the degree of cultural identification may have more influence on family beliefs and style than the culture itself. Therefore, an appropriate, culturally sensitive way of approaching families would be to view each family as a unique unit that potentially may be influenced by its culture but not necessarily locked into the culture's standard characteristics.

Fischgrund, Cohen, and Clarkson (1987) and Yacobacci-Tam (1987) have discussed the provision of services to culturally diverse families with hearing-impaired children. These authors emphasize that professional sensitivity to families' cultural background will ultimately allow for more appropriate, effective services for minority hearing-impaired children and their families.

Summary

An overview has been presented of the counseling process with hearing-impaired children and their families. Audiologists have played, and will continue to play, an extremely important role in reducing the effects of hearing handicap on family functioning. An emphasis in this chapter has been given to determining and meeting family needs in counseling. This emphasis in no way suggests that audiologists abdicate their responsibilities in designing intervention programs, leaving goal determination and program implementation solely to parents. Instead, the current shift in early intervention, away from child-centered services (which in audiology have traditionally focused on the communication needs of the child) to a more family-centered perspective, is intended to enable each unique family to capitalize on its strengths in meeting the challenge of raising a hearing-impaired child. As Sass-Lehrer and Bodner-Johnson (1989) point out, the passage of PL 99–457 presents an opportunity for professionals involved with early intervention with hearing-impaired children to reevaluate current practices, resources, and models for provision of services. By responding to the challenges set forth in PL 99–457, audiologists will continue to play a key role in meeting the needs of hearing-impaired children and their families.

References

Abidin, R., *Parenting Stress Index.* Charlottesville, VA: Pediatric Psychology Press (1983).

Able-Boone, H., Sandall, S.R., and Frederick, L.L., An informed, family-centered approach to Public Law 99–457: parental views. *Top. Early Childhood Special Ed.,* 10(1), 100–111 (1990).

Adams, J.W., and Tidwell, R., An instructional guide for reducing the stress of hearing parents of hearing-impaired children. *Am. Ann. Deaf,* 134, 323–328 (1989).

Atkins, D.V., Siblings of the hearing impaired: perspectives for parents. *Volta Rev.,* 89(5), 32–45 (1987).

Bernheimer, L.P., Gallimore, R., and Weisner, T.S., Ecocultural theory as a context for the Individual Family Service Plan. *J. Early Intervention,* 14, 219–233 (1990).

Bernstein, M.E., and Barta, L., What do parents want in parent education? *Am. Ann. Deaf,* 133, 235–246 (1988).

Bodner-Johnson, B., The family environment and achievement of deaf students: a discriminant analysis. *Exceptional Children,* 52(5), 443–449 (1986).

Bristol, M.M., Reichle, N.C., and Thomas, D.D., Changing demographics of the American family: implications for single-parent families of young handicapped children. *J. Division Early Childhood,* 12(1), 56–69 (1987).

Bromwich, R., *Working with Parents and Infants: An Interactional Approach.* Austin, TX: Pro-Ed (1978).

Caldwell, B., and Bradley, R., *Home Observation for Measurement of the Environment.* Little Rock: University of Arkansas (1984).

Clark, J.G., Emotional response transformations: redirections and projections. *Asha,* 32(6), 67–68 (1990).

Clark, T., and Watkins, S., Programming for hearing impaired infants through amplification and home intervention, 3rd ed. *Project SKI-HI.* Logan, Utah: Utah State University (1978).

Cole, E.B., and St. Clair-Stokes, J., Caregiver-child interactive behaviors: a videotape analysis procedure. *Volta Rev.,* 86, 200–216 (1984).

Davis, J.M., Elfenbein, J., Schum, R., and Bentler, R.A., Effects of mild and moderate hearing impairments on language, educational, and psychosocial behavior of children. *J. Speech Hear. Dis.,* 51, 53–62 (1986).

Dunst, C.J., Trivette, C.M., and Deal, A.G., *Enabling and Empowering Families: Principles and Guidelines for Practice.* Cambridge, MA: Brookline Books (1988).

Dunst, C.J., Trivette, C.M., Hamby, D., and Pollock, B., Family systems correlates of the behavior of young children with handicaps. *J. Early Intervention,* 14(3), 204–218 (1990).

Fischgrund, J.E., Cohen, O.P., and Clarkson, R.L., Hearing-impaired children in black and hispanic families. *Volta Rev.,* 89(5), 59–68 (1987).

Flahive, M.J., and White, S.C., Audiologists and counseling. *J. Acad. Rehab. Audiol.,* 14, 274–283 (1981).

Garwood, S.G., and Fewell, R.R., *Educating Handicapped Infants: Issues in Development and Intervention.* Rockville, MD: Aspen Systems Corporation (1983).

Goss, R., Language used by mothers of deaf children and mothers of hearing children. *Am. Ann. Deaf,* 115, 93–96 (1970).

Grimes, V.K., and Prickett, H.T., Developing and enhancing a positive self-concept in deaf children. *Am. Ann. Deaf,* 133, 255–257 (1988).

Haas, W.H., and Crowley, D.J., Professional information dissemination to parents of pre-school hearing-impaired children. *Volta Rev.,* 84, 17–23 (1982).

Hanson, M.J., and Hanline, M.F., Parenting a child with a disability: a longitudinal study of parental stress and adaptation. *J. Early Intervention,* 14(3), 234–248 (1990).

Hanson, M.J., Lynch, E.W., and Wayman, K.I., Honoring the cultural diversity of families when gathering data. *Top. Childhood Special Education,* 10(1), 112–131 (1990).

Harvey, M.A., and Green, C.L., Looking into a deaf child's future: a brief treatment approach. *Am. Ann. Deaf,* 135, 364–370 (1990).

Henggeler, S.W., Watson, S.M., Whelan, J.P., and Malone, C.M., The adaptation of hearing parents of hearing-impaired youth. *Am. Ann. Deaf,* 135, 211–216 (1990).

Houle, G.R., and Hamilton, J.L., Public Law 99–457: a challenge to speech-language pathologists and audiologists. *Asha,* 33(4), 51–54 (1991).

Israelite, N.K., Hearing-impaired children and the psychological functioning of their normal-hearing siblings. *Volta Rev.,* 88(1), 47–54 (1986).

Jones, R.C., and Kretschmer, L.W., The attitudes of parents of black hearing-impaired students. *Lang. Speech Hear. Serv. Schools,* 19, 41–50 (1988).

Kampfe, C.M., Parental reaction to a child's hearing impairment. *Am. Ann. Deaf,* 134, 255–259 (1989).

Kenworthy, O., Caregiver-child interaction and language acquisition of hearing-impaired children. *Top. Lang. Disorders,* 6, 1–11 (1986).

Krauss, M.W., New precedent in family policy: Individualized Family Service Plan. *Exceptional Children,* 56(5), 388–395 (1990).

Kricos, P.B., Response of mothers to the nonverbal communication of their hearing-impaired preschoolers. *J. Acad. Rehab. Audiol.,* 15, 51–69 (1982).

Kroth, R.L., Mixed or missed messages between parents and professionals. *Volta Rev.,* 89(5), 1–10 (1987).

Kubler-Ross, E., *On Death and Dying.* New York: McMillan (1969).

Loeb, R., and Sarigiani, P., The impact of hearing impairment on self-perceptions of children. *Volta Rev.,* 88(2), 89–100 (1986).

Luterman, D.M., *Counseling the Communicatively Disordered and Their Families.* Austin, TX: Pro-Ed (1991).

Mahoney, G., Finger, I., and Powell, A., The relationship of maternal behavioral style on the developmental status of organically impaired mentally retarded infants. *Am. J. Mental Deficiency,* 90, 296–302 (1985).

Martin, F.N., George, K.A., O'Neal, J., and Daly, J.A., Audiologists' and parents' attitudes regarding counseling of families of hearing-impaired children. *Asha*, 29, 27–32 (1987).

McCarthy, P., Culpepper, N.B., and Lucks, L., Variability in counseling experiences and training among ESB-accredited programs. *Asha*, 28(9), 49–52 (1986).

McLinden, S.E., Mothers' and fathers' reports of the effects of a young child with special needs on the family. *J. Early Intervention*, 14(3), 249–259 (1990).

Meadow, K., Schlesinger, H., and Holstein, C., The developmental process in deaf preschool children: communication competence and socialization. In H. Schlesinger and K. Meadow (Eds.), *Sound and Sign: Childhood Deafness and Mental Health*. Berkeley: University of California Press (1972).

Meadow, K.P., Toward a developmental understanding of deafness. *J. Rehabil. Deaf*, 2, 1–18 (1968).

Meadow, K.P., Personality and social development of deaf persons. In B. Bolton (Ed.), *Psychology of Deafness for Rehabilitation Counselors*. Baltimore: University Park Press (1976).

Morgan-Redshaw, M., Wilgosh, L., and Bibby, M.A., The parental experiences of mothers of adolescents with hearing impairments. *Am. Ann. Deaf*, 135(4), 293–298 (1990).

Moses, K.L., and Van Hecke-Wulatin, M., The socioemotional impact of infant deafness: a counselling model. In G.T. Mencher and S.E. Gerber (Eds.), *Early Management of Hearing Loss*. New York: Grune & Stratton (1981).

Northcott, W.H., *Curriculum Guide: Hearing-Impaired Children—Birth to Three Years—and Their Parents*. Washington, DC: The Alexander Graham Bell Association for the Deaf (1977).

Oyler, R.F., and Matkin, N.D., National survey of educational preparation in pediatric audiology. *Asha*, 29(1), 27–32 (1987).

Plapinger, D., and Kretschmer, R., The effect of context on the interactions between a normally-hearing mother and her hearing-impaired child. *Volta Rev.*, 93(2), 75–85 (1991).

Pollack, M., The remediation process: psychological and counseling aspects. In J.G. Alpiner (Ed.), *Handbook of Adult Rehabilitative Audiology*. Baltimore: Williams & Wilkins (1978).

Rosenberg, S., and Robinson, C., Enhancement of mothers' interactional skills in an infant educational program. *Education Train. Mentally Retarded*, 20, 163–169 (1985).

Rosenberg, S.A., Robinson, C.C., and Beckman, P.J., Measures of parent-infant interaction: an overview. *Top. Early Childhood Special Ed.*, 6(2), 32–43 (1986).

Roush, J., Expanding the audiologist's role. *Asha*, 33(4), 47–49 (1991).

Roush, J., and McWilliam, R.A., A new challenge for pediatric audiology: Public Law 99–457. *J. Am. Acad. Audiol.*, 1, 196–208 (1990).

Salisbury, C.L., Stressors of parents with young handicapped and nonhandicapped children. *J. Division Early Childhood*, 11(2), 154–160 (1987).

Sanders, D.A., Hearing aid orientation and counseling. In M. Pollack (Ed.), *Amplification for the Hearing-Impaired*. New York: Grune & Stratton (1975).

Sass-Lehrer, M., and Bodner-Johnson, B., Public Law 99–457: a new challenge to early intervention. *Am. Ann. Deaf*, 134, 71–77 (1989).

Schlesinger, H., A developmental model applied to problems of deafness. In H. Schlesinger, and K. Meadow (Eds.), *Sound and Sign: Childhood Deafness and Mental Health*. Berkeley: University of California Press (1972).

Schuyler, V., and Rushmer, N., *Parent-Infant Habilitation: A Comprehensive Approach to Working with Hearing-Impaired Infants and Toddlers and Their Families*. Portland, OR: Infant Hearing Resource (1987).

Seal, B.C., Working parents' dream: instructional videotapes for their signing deaf child. *Am. Ann. Deaf*, 132, 386–388 (1987).

Simmons-Martin, A.A., and Rossi, K.G., *Parents and Teachers: Partners in Language Development*. Washington, DC: Alexander Graham Bell Association for the Deaf (1990).

Somers, M., Parenting in the 1980s: programming perspectives and issues. *Volta Rev.*, 89(5), 68–78 (1987).

Stream, R.W., and Stream, K.S., Counseling the parents of the hearing-impaired child. In F.M. Martin (Ed.), *Pediatric Audiology*. Englewood Cliffs, NJ: Prentice-Hall (1978).

Streng, A., Kretschmer, R., and Kretschmer, L., *Language, Learning and Deafness*. New York: Grune & Stratton (1978).

St. Clair-Stokes, J., and Mischook, M., Caregiver-child interaction analysis: theory and application. Short course presented at the 1990 Biennial International Convention of the Alexander Graham Bell Association for the Deaf, Washington, DC, July 24, 1990.

Summers, J.A., Dell'Oliver, C., Turnbull, A.P., et al., Examining the Individualized Family Service Plan process: What are family and practitioner preferences? *Top. Early Childhood Special Ed.*, 10(1), 78–99 (1990).

Sweetow, R.W., and Barrager, D., Quality of comprehensive audiological care: a survey of parents of hearing-impaired children. *Asha*, 22, 841–847 (1980).

Tanner, D.C., Loss and grief: implications for the speech-language pathologist and audiologist. *Asha*, 22, 916–928 (1980).

Trivette, C.M., Dunst, C.J., Deal, A.G., Hamer, A.W., and Propst, S., Assessing family strengths and family functioning style. *Top. Early Childhood Special Ed.*, 10(1), 16–35 (1990).

Turnbull, A.P., and Turnbull, H.R., *Families, Professionals, and Exceptionality: A Special Partnership*. Columbus, OH: Merrill (1986).

Vadasy, P.F., Fewell, R.R., and Meyer, D.J., Grandparents of children with special needs: insights into their experiences and concerns. *J. Division Early Childhood*, 10(1), 36–45 (1986).

Vincent, L.J., and Salisbury, C.L., Changing economic and social influences on family involvement. *Top. Early Childhood Special Ed.*, 8(1), 48–59 (1988).

Warren, C., and Hasenstab, S., Self-concept of severely to profoundly hearing-impaired children. *Volta Rev.*, 88(6), 289–295 (1986).

Wayman, K.I., Lynch, E.W., and Hanson, M.J., Home-based early childhood services: cultural sensitivity in a family systems approach. *Top. Early Childhood Special Ed.*, 10(4), 56–75 (1990).

Whitehead, L.C., Deiner, P.L., and Toccafondi, S., Family assessment: parent and professional evaluation. *Top. Early Childhood Special Ed.*, 10(1), 63–77 (1990).

Williams, D.M., and Darbyshire, J.O., Diagnosis of deafness: a study of family responses and needs. *Volta Rev.*, 84, 24–30 (1982).

Winton, P.J., and Bailey, D.B., Jr., Early intervention training related to family interviewing. *Top. Early Childhood Special Ed.*, 10(1), 50–62 (1990).

Yacobacci-Tam, P., Interacting with the culturally different family. *Volta Rev.*, 89(5), 46–59 (1987).

3

REHABILITATIVE AUDIOLOGY: ADULTS

10

Rehabilitative Evaluation of Hearing-Impaired Adults

JEROME G. ALPINER, Ph.D., RONALD L. SCHOW, Ph.D.

· ·

Identification of hearing loss often occurs through a screening process. Screening may lead to referral and audiometric assessment. Assessment in turn may lead to medical treatment or aural rehabilitation. A *rehabilitation evaluation* occurs in order to guide the rehabilitation process. It involves an accurate evaluation of the impact of hearing loss. If medical restoration is not feasible, most professionals consider amplification to be the treatment of choice for persons with loss of hearing. Fortunately, there has been signficant improvement in instrumentation to better help the hearing-impaired. Advanced technology has provided a variety of options, such as canal and half-shell hearing aids, multiprogrammable digital-type hearing aids, "executive" mild gain aids that may be fitted on a walk-in basis, personal FM devices, infrared receivers for watching television, telephone amplifiers of various designs, and even nonelectronic hearing aids reminiscent of the older ear trumpets. We know, however, that success is a very individual matter and that even if hearing aids and other devices may be quite beneficial for many persons, they are not like new ears. Good amplification help requires a careful rehabilitation evaluation with subsequent orientation and carefully planned follow-up procedures. Occasionally additional ther-

apy is needed, and this will require even more careful evaluation.

In assessing and evaluating hearing there are two major areas that need to be considered: One is *hearing impairment*, and the other is *hearing disability* (also called *handicap*, although consumer advocates now favor the disability term). Impairment refers to the loss of hearing as measured by pure-tone and speech thresholds. Disability refers to the effect or impact of the loss on everyday life. Hearing effects may be of a social, emotional, or occupational nature. In the United States, when hearing loss has an impact on earning a living, it is referred to as a hearing disability (AAO, 1979). (In European countries the impact on jobs is called hearing handicap) (Stephens & Hetu, 1991; WHO, 1980).

Evaluation of the handicapping effects of hearing impairment in diverse communication situations allows us to better plan and evaluate the impact of aural rehabilitation. After remediation by amplification or other strategies it is helpful to evaluate the restoration of communication function. Therefore, the audiologist needs the skill to measure human communication. Obtaining aided audiologic (hearing impairment) data is only one part of this process. Identification and assessment procedures also should be used to determine the disability caused by the auditory deficit and the deficit reduction produced by remediation. In this chapter we recommend screening and assessment, which includes both audiologic procedures and self-assessment questionnaires.

Screening and Audiometric Assessment

SCREENING

For many years there has been a guideline for screening school-age children with immittance and pure tones (ASHA, 1979, 1985). Several recent proposals have been made to facilitate screening of adults as well (ASHA, 1992). The purposes for screening are to identify those with hearing disorders who may need medical attention and also to identify those who may have hearing disabilities so that they may receive the rehabilitation they need. Therefore, a screening protocol should provide checks for medical and disability concerns. Pure-tone impairment testing usually serves as one key item in screening. However, pure-tone screening is not enough by itself and should be incorporated along with other procedures. Case history information and selective use of immittance and/or visual inspection are useful procedures in screening for hearing disorders (Schow, 1991). A screening measure of handicap or disability is also important, and in recent years some tools have been proposed for this purpose (Schow & Nerbonne, 1982; Weinstein, 1986).

AUDIOMETRIC ASSESSMENT TEST BATTERY

The initial audiologic test battery usually consists of pure-tone air and bone conduction audiometry, which will indicate the severity and frequency dimensions of hearing loss and whether the type of hearing loss is conductive, sensorineural, or mixed. Speech audiometry provides information on speech thresholds plus speech recognition at suprathreshold (comfortable hearing) levels. Relevant case history information includes time of onset of hearing loss, etiology, medical data, general communi-cation problems, and the interpretation of numerical test results.

Rehabilitation Evaluation

Following an initial audiologic assessment, the client needing aural rehabilitation will require additional testing that may be referred to as the *rehabilitation evaluation*. As part of this evaluation, consideration should be given to communication difficulties encountered in the client's environment. One good way to do this is with a self-assessment questionnaire. Evaluation of speechreading, auditory abilities, and tinnitus also is needed and will be considered in this chapter.

DISABILITY/HANDICAP/ COMMUNICATION QUESTIONNAIRES

Measures of Disability: Early Attempts

In the 1930s self-assessment was used to place persons into a category of normal hearing, and this was in turn used to set the first standard for pure-tone thresholds (Noble, 1978; USPHS, 1938). In the 1940s and 1950s an effort was made to look at social interaction through use of audiologic numeric data. Davis (1948) helped develop this procedure, which was called the Social Adequacy Index (SAI). He later reported that it was not effective and stated that we need more knowledge about the relationship between hearing and understanding connected speech. The Hearing Handicap Scale was developed in the 1960s by High, Fairbanks, and Glorig (1964). It was a pioneering effort and the first in a long line of similar questionnaires designed to measure hearing handicap or disability (Alpiner et al., 1974; Ewertsen & Birk-Nielsen, 1970; Noble & Atherley, 1970; Schein et al., 1970).

Current Status

Although communication evaluation efforts have not yet resulted in the perfect tool, they have generated a variety of evaluation methods. Several of these methods will be discussed in this chapter. A 1980 survey of American Speech-Language-Hearing Association (ASHA) audiologists revealed that only 18% were using self-as-

Table 10.1
Various Self-Assessment Questionnaires Reported as Being Used by 33% of 469 Clinically Active ASHA Audiologists[a]

Questionnaires[b]	1990 (N = 140)*	
	N	%
HHIE	50	36
HHS	34	24
Denver	32	23
HPI	21	15
SAC/SOAC	19	14
CPI	14	10
Other	27	9

[a] These were the only audiologists who reported use of self-assessment questionnaires among 469 clinically active ASHA audiologists.

[b] *Key:* HHIE: Hearing Handicap Inventory for the Elderly; HHS: Hearing Handicap Scale; Denver: Denver Scale of Communication Function; HPI: Hearing Performance Inventory; SAC: Self-Assessment of Communication; SOAC: Significant Other Assessment of Communication; CPI: Communication Profile for the Hearing Impaired.

Source: Adapted from Schow, R. L., Balsara, N., Whitcomb, C., and Smedley, T. C., Aural rehabilitation by ASHA audiologists: 1980–1990. Accepted by the American Journal of Audiology (1993).

sessment procedures at that time (Whitcomb, 1982). A survey of ASHA audiologists as of 1990, however, revealed that 33% are now using such procedures. The most used of these, according to the survey, are shown in Table 10.1

Alpiner (1992) surveyed Department of Veterans Affairs Medical Centers regarding assessment procedures used by audiologists. There were 65 responses. Only 16 medical centers were using self-assessment scales. The most frequently used procedures were the Hearing Handicap Inventory for the Elderly (HHIE), followed by the Communication Profile for the Hearing Impaired (CPHI), the Hearing Handicap Inventory for Adults (HHI-A), and the Denver. Six VA programs reported using in-house procedures. It is interesting to note, however, that 50 programs did not use any self-assessment tools.

Purposes of Self-Assessment

These and other measures that have been developed have a variety of purposes and should be used appropriately. Giolas (1990) suggested that a hearing handicap self-assessment tool can be a valuable part of the audiologist's armamentarium by telling how an individual feels about hearing loss. He also stated that audiologists could use self-assessment to translate these handicapping effects into procedures for aural rehabilitation. Other purposes for self-assessment have also been noted.

Self-assessment is really a form of case history interview, and there are a variety of uses for self-assessment questionnaires. These include screening, initial diagnostic interview and counseling, the rehabilitation evaluation, benefit measures, satisfaction, compensation, demographic uses, and others.

Screening. A self-assessment screening questionnaire can alert professionals and the hearing-impaired person to problems due to hearing loss. These questionnaires are frequently used along with case history and pure tones in screening programs. They can help form the basis for identification of hearing loss and lead to medical and audiologic referrals (Schow et al., 1991).

Diagnostic Interview/Counseling. If the client is asked to complete a self-report form prior to the diagnostic evaluation, the audiologist will have information when the person first appears in the clinic. This is particularly helpful when both the client and a significant other person complete forms, since the feelings of both can be evaluated and counseling can be planned accordingly.

Rehabilitation Evaluation. When a more extensive evaluation is undertaken, after diagnosis of the hearing loss, self-report can be a very valuable tool. This often involves the use of a longer, more detailed instrument.

Benefit Measures/Satisfaction. Audiologists are increasingly measuring self-reported improvement after remediation procedures. Most audiologists measure amplification benefits with soundfield functional gain or real-ear measures. Several self-report measures have now been devised for a parallel purpose in reporting communication improvement. In addition, ratings use or satisfaction, as for example, in hours or a simple 1–7 scale, have been used to evelute success in hearing aid fitting (Brooks, 1989; Oja & Schow, 1984; Smedley, 1990).

Compensation. The major emphasis in compensation has usually been on pure-

Table 10.2
Categories and Associated Percentage Scores for Use in Classifying HHS Performance

Category	Percentage Scores
No handicap	0–20
Slight hearing handicap	21–40
Mild-moderate hearing handicap	41–70
Severe hearing handicap	1–100

Source: Schow, R. L., and Tannahill, C., Hearing handicap scores and categories for subjects with normal and impaired hearing sensitivity. *J. Am. Audiol. Soc.*, 3: 134–139 (1977).

tone findings, but recent recommendations suggest that self-report measures may have a part in this process (Salomon & Parving, 1985).

Demographic and Research Uses. Self-report has been used in national health interview surveys and for measuring improvement in cochlear implant studies, to indicate two examples.

Screening Tools

Schow and Nerbonne (1982) were among the first to emphasize the need for a screening tool to measure the communication ability of hearing-impaired adults. The Self-Assessment of Communication (SAC) and Significant Other Assessment of Communication (SOAC) are 10-item self-assessment screening questionnaires. These items are drawn from longer diagnostic instruments. The forms for SAC and SOAC are found in Appendixes 10.1 and 10.2. Items 1 through 6 assess communication difficulties in various situations, items 7 and 8 examine the client's general feelings about the handicap, and items 9 and 10 assess the individual's perception of the attitudes of others toward hearing abilities. The SOAC contains the same 10 items but with pronoun changes so that a closely associated observer can report on the hearing status of the client. Schow and Nerbonne (1977) earlier had developed a multiple form of an assessment questionnaire to measure reports from significant others (staff members at a nursing home). Following the introduction of SAC and SOAC, Ventry and Weinstein (1983) modified a longer instrument they had developed to produce another 10-item screening procedure (HHIE-S). Both the SAC and HHIE-S have been

proposed for use in a recent ASHA document (ASHA, 1992). Weinstein (1986) described use of the HHIE-S in a screening protocol for the elderly, and Schow (1991) proposed use of SAC/SOAC in connection with an overall procedure for screening adult and elderly persons. Other screening questionnaires have been developed (Schein et al., 1970; Schow et al., 1990), and audiologists now have several screening self-assessment tools from which to choose.

Intermediate-Length Questionnaires

Hearing Handicap Scale. As noted earlier, the Hearing Handicap Scale (HHS) was one of the first self-assessment questionnaires developed. It has two forms that were standardized and one of these may be found in Appendix 10.3. Respondents use a five-point scale. One limitation of the HHS cited by its authors was that the questions are similar and designed to focus on only the softness/loudness aspect of hearing handicap. Psychological, vocational, and other problems caused by hearing loss are not considered. Despite its limitations, the HHS is still a popular tool among rehabilitative audiologists and has been a factor in encouraging additional research.

Schow and Tannahill (1977) suggested a categorical method for interpreting HHS results. In this system, scores of 0 to 20% indicate no hearing handicap, 21 to 40% a slight handicap, 41 to 70% a mild-moderate handicap, and 71 to 100% a severe handicap. They found that most candidates for hearing aids or aural rehabilitation will have scores of 41% or higher (Table 10.2). This categorical procedure is now being used with several other self-assessment questionnaires.

Hearing Measurement Scale. Another self-report procedure, the Hearing Measurement Scale (HMS) (Noble, 1972, 1978, 1979; Noble & Atherley, 1970), was devised for the assessment of handicap due to industrial noise. Although the scale was designed for use with an industrial population, the authors suggest that it could probably be used for any group of hearing-impaired persons with sensorineural disorders. The scale in its current form includes seven subcategories. There was an attempt to include all possible areas of difficulty for the individual with hearing loss.

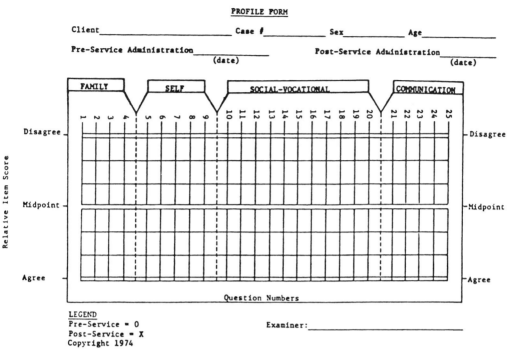

Figure 10.1. Profile form for scoring the Denver Scale of Communication Function.

The authors stressed that client reactions to hearing loss should have a definite place in an overall evaluation of each individual's problem. The HMS was devised as an interview-type technique, although a more recent self-administered version is available. They recommended the interview be tape recorded, and to increase scorer reliability, the interview can be scored by more than one clinician.

Denver Scale of Communication Function. The Denver Scale of Communication Function (Alpiner et al., 1974) was designed for use with a semantic differential-type continuum for each of 25 statements (Appendix 10.4). It examines communication function in four categories: family, self, social-vocational, and general communication experience, To encourage "first impression" responses, it was recommended that a time limit of 15 minutes be allowed for clients to complete the scale. Client responses are recorded on a form (Fig. 10.1), so that pre- and posttherapy testing compares the client with himself,

not his therapy counterparts or any other norms.

A quantified version of the Denver Scale was proposed by Schow and Nerbonne (1980) (Appendix 10.5). It is called the Quantified Denver Scale (QDS) and was used initially on 50 subjects divided into three subgroups. The degree of handicap increased as a function of greater pure-tone averages. The subjects with normal hearing had QDS scores from 0 to 15%, those with slight hearing handicap had scores of 16 to 30% and those with mild-moderate handicap had scores of 31% or greater.

McCarthy-Alpiner Scale of Hearing Handicap. The McCarthy-Alpiner Scale of Hearing Handicap (MA Scale) (McCarthy and Alpiner, 1983) (Appendix 10.6) assesses effects of adult hearing loss for an individual and also for a family member who completes a parallel form of the scale. This scale represented a pioneering effort to quantify the feelings of family members of hearing-impaired individuals. The MA Scale consists of 34 items representing psychological, social, and vocational effects of hearing loss. These items fit the proposed criteria of 0.80 correlation for test-retest at a 2-week interval and also internal consistency reliability of 0.80 or better using Cronbach's alpha method.

Several aspects emerged in connection with development of this scale: *(1)* The hearing-impaired individual may fail to accept, understand, or deal with hearing problems, whereas the family member is keenly aware of the handicapping effects; *(2)* the family member may be unable to recognize, understand, or deal with the individual's hearing impairment; *(3)* the two persons may fail to agree on the problem areas; and *(4)* any combination of the above.

A significant use of this scale relates to the counseling needs of hearing-impaired individuals *and* family members. Pollack (1978) has stated that any counseling of the hearing-impaired individual should involve the family. With this scale it is possible to systematically determine the attitudes and relationships of family members as compared to those of hearing-impaired individuals. Furthermore, family involvement can contribute to a more complete rehabilitation program for hearing-impaired persons.

This scale fulfills at least three objectives (McCarthy & Alpiner, 1983): *(1)* It provides an index of whether the organic hearing loss has manifested itself as a handicap; *(2)* it provides diagnostic data to guide the use of rehabilitative and/or hearing aid procedures; and *(3)* it provides for a detailed analysis of psychological, social, and vocational problem areas.

Other Questionnaires

The Hearing Handicap Inventory for the Elderly (HHIE) has been used on an adult population, but it is really designed for use on the elderly (see Chapter 13). A recent version of the HHIE (Newman et al., 1991) has been proposed for use with adults, the HHIA. The test-retest reliability of the HHIA was assessed on a sample of 28 hearing-impaired adults and was found to be (r = 0.97). This procedure may have potential for use with adults.

Another measurement procedure was developed by Sanders (1975). Three profile questionnaires allow rating of communicative performance in the home, occupational, and social environments. A unique feature of these scales is that they assess how often these situations occur. However, there is no specific instruction for the scoring of these scales, and they appear to be receiving very little use at present. Sanders (1975) stated that the Denver Scale and his scales may be used together to provide information about attitude and specific types of situations peculiar to a particular person's environment. For this reason, he feels these two approaches are complementary, with only a small area of overlap. Other scales may also be combined in their use.

Diagnostic Tools

Two major diagnostic tools have been developed for use with the hearing impaired. A description of each follows.

Hearing Performance Inventory. The Hearing Performance Inventory (HPI) was developed to assess hearing performance in everyday communication situations (Giolas et al., 1979). The inventory items were divided into six categories: The basic format of the HPI consists of presenting listeners with everyday situations and asking them to judge their listening performance according to a rating from 1 to 5. The original form of the inventory consisted of 158 items. The HPI has been revised three times into several shorter versions.

The 90-item revised form of the HPI was described by Lamb, Owens, and Schubert (1983) and can be administered within 20 minutes. Giolas (1983) states that the revised version can be used in most clinical settings, and the longer form will provide an additional pool of items. In the clinical scoring process, an overall percentage of difficulty is obtained by adding the numerical responses (1 to 5) for all items attempted, dividing by the number of items attempted, and multiplying by 20. Giolas (1983) stated that profiles for one or more of the sections may be generated. A comparable procedure may be followed for each section or for categories within or across sections. The HPI is not generally used in the standard audiologic test battery; rather, its greatest clinical utility is in detailed planning and assessment of rehabilitative procedures.

Weinstein (1984) discussed the advantages of the HPI. It was indicated that the

HPI has value as an assessment technique and that the items provide a description of the difficulties experienced in a wide variety of listening situations. Further, the profiles allow a convenient way of displaying responses for a rehabilitation program.

Communication Profile for the Hearing Impaired (CPHI). This profile, developed by Demorest and Erdman (1986), is also lengthy and uses 145 items that are divided into 25 scales. These different scales describe the communication performance, communication environment, communication strategies, and personal adjustment of hearing-impaired adults. Communication is assessed in a variety of environments including social situations, at home, and at work. Also, attitudes and behavior of others are assessed, as are verbal and nonverbal strategies. Personal adjustment issues include self-acceptance, acceptance of loss, anger, discouragement, stress, withdrawal, and denial. This profile was psychometrically developed through pilot use on 827 active-duty military personnel at Walter Reed Army Medical Center. The CPHI is useful when a detailed evaluation of a client is needed. Because of its psychometric refinement, it is possible to make pre- and posttherapy measurements and know when a true change has taken place. Pilot data are available on the Walter Reed population (Demorest & Erdman, 1987).

Hearing Aid User and Other Specialized Self-Report Forms

Hearing Problem Inventory. Hutton (1980) pioneered use of a questionnaire to assess dimensions of hearing aid use. This questionnaire, the Hearing Problem Inventory-Atlanta (HPI-A), was used to examine patients' perceptions of their problems and the amount of time the aids were worn. His findings included *(1)* pre- and postdata from patients receiving initial fittings and *(2)* pre- and postdata for those receiving replacement fittings.

A long history of hearing aid use was shown to substantially influence both problem perception and hearing aid use. Also, older persons reported increased problems and decreased wearing time, while employed persons had slightly higher problem scores but longer hours of hearing aid use. Pre- and postdata showed larger reductions in self-assessed problems by persons who were receiving their initial fittings as compared to experienced hearing aid users. Hearing aid wear time increased for those having their aids longer and as hearing loss increased, but wear time decreased with age of the person. Above age 55, there is a decrease in aid wear of roughly an hour per day per decade.

Hearing Aid Performance Inventory. The Hearing Aid Performance Inventory (HAPI) is another self-report procedure for measuring hearing aid benefit. It was proposed by Walden, Demorest, and Hepler (1984). This procedure involves a 64-item questionnaire that was shown to have excellent internal consistency reliability. These authors concluded that the patient's report of benefit received from the hearing aid can be used as one measure of successful hearing aid use in daily life. They identified four types of situations that can be analyzed separately: *(1)* noisy situations, *(2)* quiet situations with the speaker in proximity, *(3)* situations with reduced signal information and *(4)* situations with nonspeech stimuli. In general, they found that significantly more benefit was reported with hearing aids in quiet than in noise.

Other Hearing Aid Benefit Questionnaires. Recently, several additional questionnaires were developed for patient-assessed hearing aid benefit by Cox and her associates including the Profile of Hearing Aid Benefit (PHAB) and the Intelligibility Rating Improvement Scale (IRIS). The PHAB allows estimation of the proportion of time that certain situations presented communication problems, and the IRIS allows estimation of the proportion of speech that can be understood in various situations. Based on use with 42 hearing aid users, the PHAB did not show as much benefit as the IRIS, but it was more sensitive to different listening situations and more like other previous results (Cox, Gilmore, & Alexander, 1991).

Satisfaction and Use Reports. A variety of reports have appeared indicating the satisfaction levels of hearing aid users. Smedley (1990) provided a summary of these, which indicated that hearing aid users' satisfaction may range from 50 to 90%. In general, less than 20% are highly satisfied, and 10 to 20% tend to be strongly dissatisfied. He compared satisfaction levels on hearing aid, eyeglass, and denture users and found that hearing aid users were the least satisfied (denture 92%; eyeglass 83%; and hearing aid 71% satisfied).

Several recent reports on hearing aid use have appeared. Brooks (1989) reported on 758 hearing aid clients' use level and found that use increases with greater hearing loss and with younger ages. Use drops off dramatically above age 80. Schow et al. (1991) reported on 680 hearing aid users and found trends similar to those reported by Brooks, except that use levels were greater in the U.S. study (6 to 14 hours) compared to Brooks's study done in the United Kingdom, where hours of use ranged from 4 to 10 hours.

Hearing Performance Inventory for Severe to Profound Hearing Loss. Owens and Raggio (1984) reported the use of the Hearing Performance Inventory for Severe to Profound (HPI-SP) hearing loss. The HPI-SP may be used in connection with hearing aid use, cochlear implants, and vibrotactile use. Kaplan, Bally, and Brandt (1990) recently proposed a similar communication assessment scale for deaf adults.

Open-ended Questionnaire. Stephens (1980) proposed the use of an open-ended questionnaire in evaluating the problems of hearing-impaired patients. In this procedure the questionnaire contains the following statement: "Please make a list of the difficulties which you have as a result of your hearing loss. List these in order of importance, starting with the greatest difficulties. Write down as many as you can think of." He reported on results from the first 500 responses. There were 48% who complained of difficulty with TV/radio, 34% with general conversation, 24% with the doorbell, 23% with group conversation, 23% with speech in noise, and 20% with a telephone ring. Embarrassment was mentioned by 14%, and tinnitus was mentioned by only 8% of the respondents. Although conversation problems were not listed as often as TV/radio difficulties, they were listed first about 60% of the time, meaning they were more important, while TV/radio was listed first less than 10% of the time. Stephens encourages use of an open-ended procedure plus one of the more traditional

handicap questionnaires along with some measure of personality to look at issues such as extroversion, anxiety, and depression. He examined nearly 200 patients with personality scales and found them to be more introverted and neurotic, with pronounced elevations in the anxiety scale compared to controls. Use of the CPHI may help to evaluate some of these personality factors.

Summary

Progress has been made in the area of assessment procedures; the increasing use of self-assessment instruments by audiologists represents an improvement for both the client and the profession. Table 10.3 shows the varied dimensions that are assessed with various self-assessment questionnaires.

EVALUATION OF SPEECHREADING ABILITY
Definitions

Speechreading and *lipreading* are terms that have been used synonymously for many years. Prescod (1986) considers the terms as synonymous with the meaning, "a method of transmitting language by the visible components of oral discourse." Lipreading may be used narrowly to define the process by which a person uses the position and movement of the speaker's lips as cues (Thorn & Thorn, 1989). Speechreading may be used to describe the process by which a person uses many cues to understand ongoing speech. The cues include lipreading, facial expressions of the speaker, the residual hearing of the hearing-impaired person, and grammatical and semantic context (Walden et al., 1977). The speechreading process includes the following components: (1) listening with or without amplification; (2) recognition of gestural cues; (3) awareness of facial expressions; (4) an awareness of environmental cues; and (5) vision training (lipreading).

Montgomery and Demorest (1988) address various issues and problems regarding the assessment of speechreading. It is important to note the aspects of speechreading that need to be studied. The history of speechreading assessment is brief and reflects the clinical necessity for measuring an important mode of communication for

Table 10.3
Summary of Various Aspects Assessed in Self-Assessment Questionnaires

	HHIE	HHS	DSCF	HPI	SAC/SOAC	CPHI	M-A
Speech communication	X	X	X	X	X	X	X
General speech	X		X	X	X	X	X
Home-family			X			X	X
Vocational/work			X	X		X	X
Social	X		X	X		X	X
Individual or group	X			X			
Special communications	X	X		X	X	X	
With and without visual cues				X			
Adverse conditions		X		X		X	
Telephone/TV/radio		X		X			
Personal reactions	X		X	X	X	X	X
Response to auditory failure				X		X	
Acceptance of self/loss						X	
Hearing aid use							
Effect on activities/use	X						
Discouragement/embarrassment	X					X	
Anger/stress/anxiety	X					X	
Withdrawal/introversion	X					X	
Neuroticism							
Opinion/behavior of other			X	X	X	X	
Family relations							
Work performance							
Societal response							
Nonspeech communication		X		X	X		
Intensity/localization		X		X			
Doorbell/phone bell							
Warnings in traffic							
Related symptoms						X	
Tinnitus/fluctuations/tolerance				X			

Source: Adapted from Schow, R. L., and Gatehouse, S., Fundamental issues in self assessment of hearing. *Ear Hear.,* 11(5), 65–165 (1990).

hearing-impaired individuals. The authors of this study believe that most of the existing tests and procedures fail to meet current psychometric standards. They cite that difficulties include the failure of tests to approximate realistic communication situations, uncertainty over the most appropriate and sensitive materials to use, disagreement over the purpose of speech recognition tests in general, and continual controversy over whether it is best to test low-level perceptual skills (using nonsense words and single words) or high-level linguistic and cognitive skills (using sentences, running speech, and simulated "real situations"). Other problems include lack of correlation with other traits, measurement of change, auditory-visual integration and differences, scoring procedures, and the need for psychometric analysis. As we discuss the present situation with regard to speechreading assessment, the need for continuing research is emphasized.

Jeffers and Barley (1981) relate lipreading to a process involving three steps: *(1)* sensory reception of the motor or movement pattern, *(2)* perception of the pattern, and *(3)* association of the pattern with meaningful concepts. The lipreader receives limited visual information and must "fill in" information not received. The hearing-impaired person should strive to understand the thought or idea of the communication; it is not necessary to identify every spoken word.

Lipreading Tests

O'Neill and Oyer (1981) provided several reasons for the use of lipreading tests:

1. They are useful in the measurement of basic lipreading ability.

2. They can be used as instruments to measure the effects of lipreading training. Although one cannot always be certain of all the factors that bring about improvement, many persons will increase their skills as a result of practice.
3. They can be used in proper placement of individuals within a training program. For diagnostic purposes, it is necessary to categorize the acoustically handicapped who are excellent, average, and poor lipreaders.
4. They can be used to help decide which teaching methods, or combinations of methods, are most appropriate.

The increasing home use of VCRs allows self-instruction for improving lipreading ability. Dodd, Plant, and Gregory (1989) studied the efficacy of lipreading instruction through the use of videotaped materials. A 3-hour videocassette of nine lipreading lessons was produced. The lessons were tested over a period of 5 weeks. There was significant improvement in lipreading for those who used the videocassette programs when compared to a control group who did not. The study showed greater improvement for relatively poorer lipreaders who were cited in this study. Other studies measuring lipreading ability and subsequent improvement of from 10 to 50% have been reported (Black et al.; Oyer, 1961, 1963; Sedge & Scherr, 1979).

It is important for the client to have normal or corrected vision in order to see the visual stimuli appropriately (Thorn & Thorn, 1989). Hipskind (1989) discussed optimal conditions for presentation of visual stimuli. Live, face-to-face presentations should be conducted carefully with optimal consideration for distance (5 to 10 feet), lighting (no shadows), and viewing angle (0° to 45°). Video presentations should take into account similar considerations.

Hipskind also outlined possible limitations of lipreading tests: *(1)* absence of accompanying auditory cues; *(2)* unnatural and limited gestures; *(3)* unnatural and inappropriate facial expressions; *(4)* nonfunctional sentences; *(5)* use of a single speaker; *(6)* scored as an identification task rather than as a person's ability to perceive thoughts visually; *(7)* no differentiation between skilled and unskilled lipreaders; and *(8)* poor predictors of lipreading success. A variety of reliable lipreading tests are available, and the choice of which measuring instrument to use will probably be made according to the personal preference of the audiologist. Whether the test will be presented live or by videotape, and whether or not sound will be used, will also be at the audiologist's discretion. As indicated by Jeffers and Barley (1981), a live presentation tends to yield better scores than a video presentation. However, there are limitations to either manner of presentation. Live presentation requires considerable practice on the part of the audiologist. Items should be presented in as true-to-life a manner as possible, since in the everyday environment, this is the way in which clients ultimately receive communication.

Table 10.4 represents the percentage of respondents within groups of 140 (1980) and 77 (1990) who are using various tests for evaluating speechreading abilities. These were the only audiologists who reported speechreading tests among 371 (1980) and 469 (1990) clinically active ASHA audiologists (Schow et al., 1992).

The Denver Quick Test of Lipreading Ability (Table 10.5) is composed of 20 common, everyday expressions and scored on the basis of identification of the thought or idea of the sentence. Each sentence has a value of 5%. The Quick Test was administered live, without voice, to 40 hearing-impaired adults. Results were compared to scores for the Utley Sentence Test, presented live, without voice. Correlation between the two tests was 0.90, indicating good intertest reliability.

Erber (1977) proposed a conceptual model for the evaluation of lipreading. Although this model is designed for children, it may have clinical application for use with adults. This system previously has been used for auditory tasks. A simple matrix (Fig. 10.2) summarizes the variety of the different types of speech stimuli that can be used: speech elements, syllables, words, phrases, sentences, and connected discourse. Four response tasks are used in this matrix: detection, discrimination, recognition, and comprehension. Each box in Figure 10.2 describes the interaction between a particular type of visual speech stimulus

Table 10.4
Various Tests Used for Evaluating Speechreading

Test Used	1980 (N = 140)		1990 (N = 77)*	
	N	(%)	N	(%)
Utley	83	59	39	51
Informal	36	26	25	33
Barley	21	15	18	23
Self made	30	21	14	18
Modification of std	14	10	7	9
Keaster	6	4	3	4
Other	11	8	7	9

[a] These were the only audiologists who reported speechreading tests used among 371 (1980) and 469 (1990) clinically active ASHA audiologists.
Source: Adapted from Schow, R. L., Balsara, N., Whitcomb, C., and Smedley, T. C., Aural rehabilitation by ASHA audiologists: 1980–1990. Accepted by the American Journal of Audiology (1993).

Table 10.5
Denver Quick Test of Lipreading Ability[a]

1. Good morning.
2. How old are you?
3. I live in (state of residence).
4. I only have one dollar.
5. There is somebody at the door.
6. Is that all?
7. Where are you going?
8. Let's have a coffee break.
9. Park your car in the lot.
10. What is your address?
11. May I help you?
12. I feel fine.
13. It is time for dinner.
14. Turn right at the corner.
15. Are you ready to order?
16. Is this charge or cash?
17. What time is it?
18. I have a headache.
19. How about going out tonight?
20. Please lend me 50 cents.

[a] Devised at the University of Denver Speech and Hearing Center.

and a specific manner of response. Detection is the ability to respond differently to the presence and absence of speech articulation. Visual detection of articulatory-movements should result in the individual's orienting to the speaker's mouth for gaining more visual information as well as indicating the preserve of postdental consonants in certain vowel contexts. Discrimination requires a same-different response or the ability to perceive similarities and differences between two or more speech samples. Recognition is the ability to re-produce a visual speech stimulus by naming or identifying it in some way. Comprehension is the ability to understand the meaning of speech stimuli within an individual's language ability. The information obtained from the use of this procedure may help in planning aural rehabilitation.

Another application was suggested by Dodds and Harford (1968), who used the Utley test as part of a hearing aid evaluation. This test was used to evaluate how well clients understand sentences under visual and auditory-visual conditions. In this study, Form A of the Utley Sentence Test was presented unaided, and Form B was presented with auditory and visual cues. The latter condition resulted in greater understanding of the stimuli materials.

Bisensory Evaluation

Sometimes lipreading tests are administered in the visual-only condition. It is assumed that clients who score well in the visual-only modality have less difficulty understanding communication and should have fewer concomitant difficulties often associated with hearing loss. However, it is thought that testing in a visual-only condition is not sufficiently comprehensive for most purposes. Assessment should generally use a bisensory evaluation, allowing the client to use both visual and auditory modalities. Binnie (1973) indicated that auditory-visual scores might suggest how individuals receive person-to-person speech in general conversation situations. Because this is the general mode of communication

	SPEECH ELEMENTS	SYLLABLES	WORDS	PHRASES	SENTENCES	CONNECTED DISCOURSE
DETECTION						
DISCRIMINATION						
RECOGNITION						
COMPREHENSION						

Figure 10.2. A lipreading skills matrix for hearing impaired children. The child's visual speech perception abilities are evaluated at each level of stimulus/response complexity. These measures are used to specify goals for instruction in visual communication (Erber, 1977).

for most people, the information would be useful to the clinician in planning a realistic remediation program. Bisensory approaches are very helpful in determining how well clients perform with hearing aids. In this approach to lipreading evaluation, test materials can be presented both in a quiet condition and in the presence of different background noises, which often create major difficulties for the hearing-impaired adult. Numerous clients state that they seem to do well in one-to-one, quiet environmental situations but simply cannot understand what is being said when there is background noise. Binnie (1973) demonstrated the benefits of the bisensory approach. He stated that the level at which the best auditory-visual score is obtained may serve as the starting point for rehabilitative audiology. The data in Tables 10.6 and 10.7 show the effects of auditory and auditory-visual presentations at various sensation levels. With a combined sensory modality presentation, the contribution of visual speech cues to auditory-visual speech perception increases as the speech-to-noise ratio decreases. That is, as noise increases with respect to speech, the visual modality plays a greater role in the individual's understanding of speech. The use of audition and vision appears to result in higher scores than when either audition or lipreading is used alone.

The research cited emphasizes the need to evaluate lipreading through a bisensory approach. Because most persons perceive speech in this way, it would appear to be a realistic consideration. The work of Binnie, Montgomery, and Jackson (1974) provides substantive data for bisensory assessment. They studied 16 consonants in which five distinct homophonous categories were apparent:

1. Bilabials: /p, b, m/
2. Labiodentals: /f, v/
3. Interdentals: /θ, ʃ/
4. Rounded labials: /f, ʒ/
5. Linguals: /s, z, t, d, n, k, g/

Stimuli were presented in auditory, auditory-visual, auditory in quiet, and visual-only conditions. Signal-to-noise (S/N) ratios used for auditory and auditory-visual conditions were −18 dB, −12 dB, and −6 dB, employing a broad-band masking noise. The results of their study demonstrated that identification of consonants under noise conditions improved significantly with vision. The auditory-visual condition approaches the results of materials presented in quiet. The visual-only condition indicates the difficulties posed when relying on this modality. Table 10.8 summarizes their results.

Walden, Prosek, and Scheer (1974) found that hearing-impaired adults were able to distinguish visually within the Woodward and Barber consonant categories (1960). These consonant categories are as follows:

1. Bilabial: /p, b, m/
2. Rounded labial: /m, w, r/
3. Labiodental: /f, v/
4. Nonlabial: /t, d, n, θ, ʃ, ʃ, h, dʒ, S, z, k, n, ʒ, g/

Brannon (1961) indicates that words of less visibility are harder to lipread than words of greater visibility. His study suggests that a synthetic approach to lipreading, in which additional clues are provided, is more effective for developing lipreading ability.

Erber (1975) states that most clinical evaluations have been dominated by auditory measures, often to the exclusion of testing visual and auditory-visual capabilities. Erber's research suggests that evaluation of each client's auditory-visual per-

Table 10.6
Effect of Auditory Presentations at Various Sensation Levels[a]

Sensation Level of Presentation[b]	AUDITORY Sensorineural Loss Cases					Mean Scores for Normals
	1	2	3	4	5	
	%					%
0	30	22	20	46	42	21
8	64	40	46	86	38	59
16	74	62	60	90	54	80
24	84	84	78	94	36	94

[a] Reprinted by permission from Binnie, C.A., *J. Acad. Rehab. Audiol.*, 6, 43–53, copyright 1973, *Journal of the Academy of Rehabilitative Audiology.*

ception of speech can be helpful, since most hearing-impaired clients typically receive speech through both auditory and visual modalities during everyday communication. This means they usually watch the speaker's mouth and face to maximize perception of speech information. Auditory-visual evaluation in the clinic can give the audiologist an estimate of the patient's ability to communicate socially in this manner.

Real-life situations demand that hearing-impaired individuals understand continuous speech discourse. Clinical experience has shown that clients can perceive differences in sounds according to homophonous categories. More difficulty is encountered in understanding what is said on a day-to-day basis at work, at home, and in a variety of social situations. Clients often indicate that they experience little difficulty recognizing sounds in isolated categories in therapy. Their attempts to follow general conversation in the outside environment, however, are frustrating because the rate of the typical speaker may be either too fast or too slow, or enunciation may be poor.

Computer Applications and Lipreading

The emerging use of computers, mentioned in Chapter 1, has resulted in speechreading application. Pichora-Fuller and Benguere (1991) developed Computer-Aided Speechreading Training (CAST) for speechreading training and to further the development of assessment measures and training techniques. Our concern for this chapter is assessment. This computerized system simulates face-to-face intervention and is designed to be one component of a comprehensive aural rehabilitation program for preretirement adults with acquired mild-to-moderate hearing loss. There are eight training lessons, each focusing on a particular viseme that is practiced by a modified discourse tracking method using viseme-specific texts. Three basic speechreading skills are emphasized: visual speech perception, use of linguistic redundancy, and use of feedback between message sender and receiver. CAST lessons progress from the most visible and least variable visemes to the least visible and most variable visemes (Pichora-Fuller, 1980): /p, b, m/, /f, v/, /θ, ð/, /t, d, n, l/, /s, z/, /ʃ, ʒ, ʃ, dʒ/, /w, r/, /k, g, h, j, n/.

The CAST tracking procedure is based on face-to-face discourse tracking (DeFilippo & Scott, 1987). Compared to face-to-face discourse tracking procedures, tracking in the practice section of CAST has the advantage of allowing easy measurement and analysis of speechreading performance. This system promises to reveal more about the process of speechreading in general and about the need for and effectiveness of training for specific clients. The authors of CAST indicate that it has the advantage of regulating stimulus presentation and feedback variables that are otherwise clinician-specific and difficult to describe, replicate, or standardize.

EVALUATION OF AUDITORY RECOGNITION

Sims (1985) has indicated that criteria for selecting clients for auditory training are difficult to find in recent literature. Rubinstein and Boothroyd (1987) state that audiologists disagree about the value of formal auditory training with adventitiously hearing-impaired adults. Little scientific research exists to support it. Limited research

Table 10.7
Effect of Audio-Visual Presentations at Various Sensation Levels[a]

Sensation Level of Presentation[b]	AUDIO-VISUAL Sensorineural Loss Cases					Mean Scores for Normals
	1	2	3	4	5	
	%					%
−20	22	14	12	8	18	23
0	66	58	46	76	72	57
8	70	76	68	84	84	85
16	88	82	86	98	74	94

[a] Reprinted by permission from Binnie, C.A. *J. Acad. Rehab. Audiol.*, 6, 45–53, copyright 1973, *Journal of the Academy of Rehabilitative Audiology.*
[b] Re: Sound field SRT.

Table 10.8
Results of Stimuli Presentations Under Auditory, Auditory-Visual, Auditory in Quiet, and Visual Only Conditions[a]

Condition	Correct Response
	%
Auditory	
S/N ratio: −18	6
S/N ratio: −12	34
S/N ratio: −6	54
Auditory-visual	
S/N ratio: −18	47.7
S/N ratio: −12	83.5
S/N ratio: −6	88.7
Auditory in quiet	95
Visual only (overall)	43.2

[a] Reprinted by permission from Binnie, C.A., Montgomery, A.A., Jackson, P.L., Auditory and visual contributions to the perception of consonants. *J. Speech Hear Res.*, 17, 619–630, copyright 1974, *Journal of Speech and Hearing Research.*

may be due, in part, to the difficulty of engaging in this type of research. Some of the problems associated with this research may be due to controlling variables of stimulus materials and the time-consuming nature of these studies. Studies have been reported that do indicate improvement as a result of auditory training (Hutton, 1960; Walden et al., 1981; Watts & Pegg, 1977). Rubinstein and Boothroyd (1987) studied 20 adults with mild to moderate sensorineural hearing loss, using three tests of speech recognition: the CUNY Nonsense Syllable Test, the low predictability items of the Revised Speech Perception in Noise (RSPIN) test, and the high-predictability items of the RSPIN test. A small but statistically significant increase in speech recognition performance on the high-probability material was observed, but the effect of training methods was not significant. The authors of this study suggest that some form of training probably is appropriate. As further efforts are made in better understanding auditory training, it appears that audiologists should continue with such endeavors because of this evidence of improvement.

Word recognition or discrimination may be defined as the ability to hear and understand clearly the sounds that make up our speech and language. Many of us have encountered the classic statement, "I hear you, but I just don't understand clearly everything you say." Lack of good discrimination ability results in perceptual confusions and distortions that may inhibit or reduce the understanding of the message. This may occur whether amplification is being used or not. A hearing aid is an electronic device that can make speech sufficiently loud but not necessarily more clear. The speech signal is still being transmitted for interpretation through a damaged or degenerated auditory mechanism. Persons with discrimination problems caused by hearing loss are often frustrated by this inability to hear speach clearly. Nerbonne and Schow (1989) emphasize that an integral part of any auditory training program is the evaluation of the client's performance. They cite several reasons for assessing auditory recognition ability:

1. To determine whether auditory training appears warranted
2. To provide a basis for comparison with later performance, following a period of therapy, in order to measure the amount

of improvement in speech perception, if any, that has occurred

3. To identify specific areas of speech perception difficulties that can be concentrated on in future auditory training work.

Oyer and Frankmann (1975) indicated that the primary areas of concern regarding the need for auditory training are *(1)* confusions among various sounds due to the condition of the sensorineural hearing mechanism; *(2)* adjustment problems in the use of amplification systems due to recruitment problems; and *(3)* adjustment problems due to amplification because of speech sounding unnatural (hearing aids are not precise replacements for abnormally functioning ears). Poor auditory recognition results from sensorineural impairment. The individual with a conductive hearing loss is not usually confronted with this difficulty, since the etiology of the impairment is in the outer or middle ear. Once speech has been made sufficiently loud, it can be understood.

Owens (1978) analyzed consonant errors of hearing-impaired subjects and showed that 14 consonants caused most of the difficulty in consonant recognition. This study constitutes *(1)* a summary of auditory consonant recognition errors in a multiple-choice word format for persons with sensorineural hearing loss and *(2)* a consideration of implications for remediation. Items for this study consisted of a battery of consonant-vowel-consonant words. The initial-position consonants show lower error probabilities than their counterparts in the final position. Place errors were the most frequent, but manner errors also were noted frequently. Substitutions tended to be the same over a wide range of pure-tone configurations. Therefore, only in a few instances would the type of configuration of a given subject be of any special help in predicting those consonants that are particularly difficult to recognize. This study demonstrated that auditory recognition of consonants can be improved by training. Visual recognition errors of persons with normal hearing were consistent among consonants within visual groups. An approach directed at enhancing or sharpening of consonant recognition, per se, may contribute substantially to speech perception ability.

Another aspect of consonants as they relate to speech perception is frequency of their occurrence in everyday speech. The consonants /j, n, w, r, h, l, m/ are the most easily recognized auditorily by hearing-impaired persons. The consonants /t, d, s, k, z/, on the other hand, provide auditory as well as visual difficulty. The /s/ emerges as the most troublesome in speech perception. Along with /s/ is the cognate /z/ with /k/ close behind. Owens (1978) proposed that it might be helpful to devote part of aural rehabilitation to direct auditory training work with consonants. A variety of stimulus materials exist to ascertain an individual's recognition ability, but there is no agreement on which is best. The stimuli are presented at a level above the speech reception threshold at which the client indicates speech sounds comfortable. Words and sentences from several sources are used for auditory recognition testing (Egan, 1948; Hirsh et al, 1952; Jerger, Speaks, & Trammel, 1968; Kalikow, Stevens, & Elliott, 1977; Owens & Schubert, 1977; Tillman & Carhart, 1966). We will discuss auditory recognition assessment for purposes of therapy.

Auditory Recognition Tests

We recommend that the audiologist evaluate the client's confusion with individual sounds and general speech discourse for the purpose of planning auditory training. Sound confusions may be assessed with the monosyllabic words used in speech recognition testing. We can opt to indicate sound errors as well as whether or not a word was correctly identified. From List 1 of the 8 Northwestern University Word Test Number 6 (Tillman & Carhart, 1966), for example, the following four words were used: *bean, burn, knock,* and *moon.* Hypothetical responses might be *bean, bird, dock, mood.* While scoring, we note that /d/ is confused with /n/. Therapy would be planned to emphasize the auditory differences between the two sounds. Recognition word tests, already a part of the audiologic assessment battery, may be used. The same purpose can be accomplished with any recognition test used in an audiologic battery. Recent data in Table 10.9 indicate the most commonly used speech recognition tests in auditory rehabilitation. The first five of these are

Table 10.9
Various Materials Used for Auditory Training[a]

Material Used	1980 (N = 111)*		1990 (N = 71)*	
	N	%	N	%
LA Auditory Skills Curriculum	—	NA	32	45
CID W-22	51	46	26	37
WIPI	46	42	24	34
PB-K	44	40	18	25
NU CHIPS	—	NA	17	24
NU-6	25	23	13	18
SSI	—	NA	12	17
GASP	—	NA	11	16
SPIN	4	4	9	13
Other	33	30	21	30

[a] These were the only audiologists who reported auditory training materials among 371 (1980) and 469 (1990) clinically active ASHA audiologists.
Source: Adapted from Schow, R.L., Balsara, N., Whitcomb, C., and Smedley, T.C., Aural rehabilitation by ASHA audiologists: 1980–1990. Accepted by the American Journal of Audiology (1993).

tests developed for use on children. This indicates that much auditory training is done with children, but such materials can also be used on adults when language age or difficulty level requires easier material for an adult.

For more intensive discrimination testing between consonants, the Larson Sound Discrimination Test (Fig. 10.3) is recommended. The California Consonant Test (CCT) also allows for the identification of auditory recognition errors. List 1 of the CCT is found in Appendix 10.7.

Schwartz and Surr (1979) conducted three experiments using the CCT. The studies were designed to *(1)* determine the performance intensity function for the CCT, *(2)* compare performance scores on the CCT with those on the Northwestern University (NU) Number 6 lists, and *(3)* examine internal consistency and split-half reliability on forms 1 and 2 of the CCT. The stimuli materials consisted of CCT forms 1 and 2 and recordings of the NU Number 6. In experiment one, 12 persons with normal hearing (6 males and 6 females) and 12 males with sensorineural hearing loss composed the subjects. Word/consonant recognition was assessed with forms 1 and 2 of the CCT, which were divided into four lists of 50 words. Each subject recorded written responses on a standard answer form that was presented at increasingly higher sensation levels from 0 dB to 50 dB.

Preliminary data suggested that the CCT is particularly sensitive to the phoneme recognition difficulties of persons with high-frequency hearing loss and would be capable of differentiating between normal hearing and those with high-frequency hearing loss. In experiment two, a comparison was made of performance scores achieved on the CCT and those obtained with the NU Auditory Test Number 6 in order to further explore the assumption that the CCT is a more sensitive index of minor deficits in phoneme recognition than the NU Number 6 list for listeners with high-frequency sensorineural hearing loss. The subjects were 60 males ranging in age from 20 to 78 years. The recorded speech materials consisted of Lists 1–4, Form B of the NU 6 lists. The subjects were categorized into four groups of 15 subjects such that each was assigned to receive one of four 50-word lists in a counterbalanced fashion. The data were first analyzed for the four groups independently. The group means did not differ significantly and, therefore, the data were pooled for further examination. These data suggest that the CCT was more sensitive in differentiating among individuals with a wide range of high-frequency hearing loss than were the NU 6 lists. The majority of subjects were able to recognize the words from the NU 6 list, while the CCT list scores were more widely distributed. The third experiment mea-

Score: (Errors)

Name_____

With Aid

Date_____

Without Aid

Directions to be Given the Listener: Draw a line through the words that are pronounced to

you from each box.

Box 1 f and ch		Box 2 l and z		Box 3 l and n		Box 4 d and n		Box 5 m and l	
few	chew	lip	zip	lame	name	dot	not	mine	line
fin	chin	loan	zone	light	night	die	nigh	mast	last
filed	child	dale	daze	loan	known	deed	need	moan	loan
calf	catch	mail	maze	pail	pain	ode	own	name	nail
four	chore	hail	haze	rail	rain	did	din	home	hole

Box 6 b and m		Box 7 l and v		Box 8 k and g		Box 9 p and b		Box 10 m and v	
bill	mill	lane	vane	coal	goal	pin	bin	mice	vice
boast	most	lie	vie	came	game	pie	by	ham	have
bake	make	lace	vase	coat	goat	pole	bowl	glum	glove
robe	roam	lull	love	luck	lug	cap	cap	mine	vine
tab	tam	rail	rave	rack	rag	rope	robe	mile	vile

Box 11 n and v		Box 12 sh and f		Box 13 f and k		Box 14 f and b		Box 15 s and sh	
nice	vice	show	foe	fit	kit	fun	bun	lease	leash
nurse	verse	shore	fore	four	core	fig	big	sew	show
nine	vine	shade	fade	find	kind	cuff	cub	sigh	shy
loans	loaves	cash	calf	cliff	click	call	cab	sap	ship
lean	leave	leash	leaf	laugh	lack	graph	grab	save	shave

Box 16 p and f		Box 17 s and z		Box 18 v and f		Box 19 ch and sh		Box 20 b and d	
pour	four	ice	eyes	five	fife	chop	shop	bid	did
pile	file	seal	zeal	vase	face	chair	share	big	dig
par	far	bus	buzz	leave	leaf	watch	wash	buy	die
cap	call	lice	lies	view	few	catch	cash	rob	rod
cup	cuff	juice	Jews	loaves	loafs	cheap	sheep	robe	rode

Box 21 d and g		Box 22 t and p		Box 23 l and s		Box 24 b and v		Box 25 v and z	
doe	go	tail	pail	fine	sign	bet	vet	live	lies
date	gate	cat	cap	flat	slat	dub	dove	have	has
drove	grove	cut	cup	cuff	cuss	base	vase	rave	raise
bud	bug	tar	par	knife	nice	bigger	vigor	view	zoo
dad	gag	toll	pole	lift	list	robe	rove	wives	wise

Box 26 th and f		Box 27 t and th		Box 28 k and t		Box 29 k and p		Box 30 m and n	
thin	fin	tie	thigh	kick	tick	pike	pipe	mine	nine
thirst	first	tin	thin	kite	tight	cat	pat	new	knew
three	free	trill	thrill	code	toad	crock	crop	time	tine
thought	fought	mit	myth	shirk	shirt	cry	pry	dime	dine
thrill	frill	pat	path	park	part	coal	pole	dumb	done

Box 31 Word Endings			Box 32 th and s		Box 33 th and v	
store	stores	stored	thumb	sum	than	van
will	wills	willed	truth	truce	thy	vie
start	starts	started	path	pass	that	vat
cough	coughs	coughed	thing	sing	thine	vine
cap	caps	capped	thank	sank	loathes	loaves

Figure 10.3. Larson School Discrimination Test. (Reprinted by permission from Sanders, D.A., *Aural Rehabilitation,* Bloomington, IN: Indiana University Press, 1950.)

sured split-half reliability. The one obvious problem with the CCT is the time involved in administration of the 100 words. Two scramblings of the CCT were administered to 10 male subjects, ages 25 to 45 years, with high-frequency hearing loss. There was a high correlation between the half-tests when analyzed for the entire groups. However, because of considerable individual variances, the study did not support the use of half-lists.

In addition to assessment of individual phonemes through the auditory modality, it is also recommended that evaluation of ability to perceive continuous discourse be made. This procedure may be helpful in determining a client's auditory function with additional contextual information. The CID Everyday Speech Sentences (Davis & Silverman, 1970) is available for this purpose. These sentences are suggested for evaluation, since they represent a sample of American speech of high face validity. The 10-sentence lists are presented in Appendix 10.8. As indicated by Davis and Silverman (1970), certain important characteristics exist for these sentences:

1. The vocabulary is appropriate for adults.
2. The words appear with high frequency in one or more of the well-known word counts of the English language.
3. Proper names and proper nouns are not used.
4. Common, nonslang idioms and contractions are used freely.
5. Phonetic loading and "tongue twisting" are avoided.
6. Redundancy is high.
7. The level of abstraction is low.
8. Grammatical structure varies freely.
9. Sentence length varies.
10. Different sentence forms are used, including declarative, interrogative, imperative, and falling interrogative.

In addition to evaluating recognition ability for both individual phonemes and continuous speech discourse, the audiologist must consider any tolerance problems affecting the hearing-impaired adult. The ability to tolerate auditory stimuli at comfortable levels has significance for those clients using or needing amplification. In evaluating recognition ability, the test ma-terials should be presented in an auditory-only condition, without the use of visual cues. Emphasis in this phase of the evaluation is assessment of the auditory modality only.

Summary

Results of these evaluation procedures enable the audiologist to make some rehabilitative judgments regarding specific auditory communication deficits of the client. However, these should be seen as part of a broader effort. Oyer (1968) indicated that in a majority of cases, auditory training will not stand alone as a method of rehabilitating the hearing-impaired individual. It is part of a broad conceptual framework encompassing the entirety of aural rehabilitation.

TINNITUS EVALUATION

The National Center for Health Statistics (1967, 1980) indicates that tinnitus is a common complaint. The center reports that 32% of the population reports some form of tinnitus. According to Axelsson and Ringdahl (1989), tinnitus is uncomfortable for both the patient and the consulting physician. The reason cited is that, in most cases, there is no successful treatment to minimize treatment. We have experienced hundreds of veterans in VA medical centers who have described the problem of "noises" in their ears and the frustrations that have resulted from tinnitus: "I have difficulty sleeping at night," "The noises make me nervous," "I have difficulty hearing my family," "What can I do about this problem?" In some cases, clients have requested appointments because of tinnitus, not hearing loss.

In Sweden, the most commonly used severity grading comprises three categories (Klockhoff & Lindblom, 1967). Category 1 includes cases with intermittent tinnitus, which occasionally might be annoying and interfere with sleep. Category 2, which is common, comprises cases with continuous tinnitus much of the time, which is annoying in quiet situations and may interfere with sleep. Category 3 is the most severe degree of tinnitus; it is continuous, and the client is conscious of it all the time. It affects the ability to fall asleep and often causes the person to awake during the night. It is regarded as annoying most of the time.

Sweetow (1986) states that many audiologists seem reluctant to engage in tinnitus management with patients. It is indicated that tinnitus patients are somewhat similar to chronic pain patients in that both groups suffer from intractable symptoms. A technique that has been effectively used in helping pain patients cope with their problems is cognitive-behavioral therapy. This approach can be applied with the emphasis placed on treating the patient's reaction to tinnitus rather than the tinnitus itself. Other types of behavior modification, biofeedback, tinnitus maskers, hearing aids, and medical advisement have been of some help to a number of patients with tinnitus. It is appropriate, therefore, to evaluate the tinnitus problem and to consider management strategies that may be helpful.

Stouffer and Tyler (1990) administered a tinnitus questionnaire to 528 patients. They state that because it is not possible to eliminate tinnitus at present, we need to learn how to help patients cope with the consequences of tinnitus. Their questionnaire, the University of Iowa Tinnitus Questionnaire, is one such instrument that may be used to evaluate patients (Appendix 10.9). The results of this type of questionnaire can help audiologists to better provide tinnitus management for patients. There is an increasing awareness about tinnitus, and it appears that we do have a responsibility to do more than indicate that "many persons with hearing loss have this problem."

OVERALL TEST BATTERY

Recommendations

Information acquired from the test battery serves as a guide to planning remediation. The client's input is also important, as an estimate of the problem may provide a starting point for therapy. Although information obtained from the client is subjective, therapy based on individual problems can be initiated, avoiding a generalized remediation approach. Goldstein and Stephens (1980) have addressed rehabilitation with an evaluation that includes assessment of *(1)* communication, *(2)* associated variables like vocational and psychological, and *(3)* related conditions

such as manual dexterity. They also recommend sequencing treatment depending on attitude types. Although the sequencing is related to hearing aid attitudes, it appears that the attitude types may also apply to overall aural rehabilitation:

1. *Attitude Type I*—This implies that the patient has a strongly positive attitude toward hearing aids and audiologic care. Both auditory and psychological factors are amenable to therapeutic solutions.
2. *Attitude Type II*—This implies that there is an essentially positive attitude toward hearing aids and aural rehabilitation, but some complications are present. There may have been an unfavorable previous therapy experience or social, educational, or vocational factors that preclude the use of simple solutions. Also included in this group are clients with difficult-to-fit audiometric configurations or mild impairment in which both the client and the audiologist want assurance of benefit to warrant the cost of treatment. The authors of this study indicate that approximately two-thirds to three-quarters of clients fitted with hearing aids fit into Type I and the remainder into Type II.
3. *Attitude Type III*—This implies a fundamentally negative attitude, although there exists a shred of cooperative intent. The negative attitude toward hearing aids may arise from a variety of situations and comes in many forms. It may reflect the stigma of a hearing aid or a generalized inability to cope with change in status characteristic of different life stages.
4. *Attitude Type IV*—This implies a small group who reject hearing aids and the entire rehabilitation process. A total discharge from the therapy process is likely, but a last-ditch effort to salvage a thread of remediation potential should be attempted.

A COMPREHENSIVE SCREENING SCALE: SELF-ASSESSMENT, AUDITORY, VISUAL

Alpiner-Meline Aural Rehabilitation Screening Scale

Limited resources are available, in a screening format, that assess hearing handicap, visual ability, and auditory aptitude.

Table 10.10
Recommended Diagnostic Test Battery

Procedure	Rationale
1. *Screening* (pure tones at 25 dB, SAC/SOAC, selective use of visual inspection, immittance)	1. Quick screen to identify potential hearing problems of medical or disability/handicap nature.
2. *Audiologic assessment* (pure tone and speech audiometry)	2. Determination of type and severity of hearing loss, contribution of results to physician's diagnosis. Information on determining tolerance and recognition abilities.
3. *Rehabilitation evaluation*	3. *Rehabilitation*
a. Communication evaluation	a. Client and family member evaluation of communication.
(1) McCarthy-Alpiner Scale of Hearing Handicap (Form A and Form B)	(1) Evaluation of specific problem areas in communication situations.
(2) Other scales as deemed appropriate (HPI, CPHI, Stephens open-ended)	(2) Additional evaluation of personality and unstructured reports on communication.
(3) Denver Quick Test of Lipreading or other appropriate test	(3) Assessment of client's ability to understand visual communication. (Should be administered under visual and auditory-visual conditions.)

(4) Auditory discrimination testing:
      (a) NU Auditory Word Tests
      (b) CID Everyday Sentences
      (c) California Consonant Test
	(4) Assessment of client's ability to recognize phonemes and assessment of recognition ability of everyday speech discourse through the auditory modality.

(5) Alpiner-Meline Aural Rehabilitation Screening Scale	(5) May be used initially instead of numbers 3a(1–4).
b. Associated variables evaluation	b. Psychological, social, vocational, and educational aspects.
c. Related conditions	c. Conditions
(1) Tinnitus Questionnaire (2) Other conditions	(1) To determine if tinnitus poses communication problem.
d. Attitude evaluation	d. Assign attitude as type I, II, III, IV.

4. *Remediation*
  a. Counseling/psychosocial issues
	4. *Remediation*
	  a. Synthesis of all evaluative information and counseling efforts to assist a client to achieve as near normal communication function as possible.

b. Amplification/assistive devices	b. Determination if amplification is necessary to minimize the auditory deficit. Orientation/adjustment.
c. Communication plan of remediation	c. Speechreading and communication strategies.
d. Overall coordination	d. Working cooperatively with other medical, counseling, school, and vocational professionals.

Alpiner and Garstecki (1989) report that measures of skills related to the communication competence of hearing-impaired individuals have been given low priority in many clinical settings. Lesner (1980) speculates that possible reasons for this situation include a lack of awareness of assessment tools, time constraints in ENT clinical practices, and limited funding sources for aural rehabilitation. Alpiner, Meline, and Cotton (1991) developed a multipurpose screening scale: the Alpiner-Meline Aural Rehabilitation Screening Scale (AMAR) (Appendix 10.10a and b). To measure hearing handicap, nine items were selected from the McCarthy-Alpiner Scale of Hearing Handicap (1983); five items were chosen from the Denver Quick Test of Lipreading Ability (Alpiner, 1978); and six word-pair items were selected from the Larson Sound Discrimination Test (1950). Percentile ranks for scoring purposes were established. It was determined that individuals who scored within the 85th percentile or higher for the number of errors could be identified as those with absolute needs for aural rehabilitation. "Absolute needs" are defined as individuals who demonstrate significant difficulties in using resources, coping skills, and auditory/visual information to optimum benefit. The percentile range for "Questionable needs" for rehabilitation is the range from the 70th to the 84th percentile. These individuals demonstrate moderate difficulty. Clients who fall into the range of the 1st to 69th percentile would be unlikely to need aural rehabilitation. The AMAR scale allows us to identify problems quickly and efficiently.

Model and Tests for the Rehabilitation Process

There is no one approach. The test battery presented in Table 10.10 is recommended, although a variety of other techniques may be available to the audiologist. This outline follows the aural rehabilitation model developed by Goldstein and Stephens (1981).

References

AAO (American Academy of Otolaryngology), Guide for the evaluation of hearing handicap. *J. Am. Med. Assoc.*, 241, 2055–2059 (1979).

Alpiner, J.G., *Handbook of Adult Rehabilitative Audiology*. Baltimore, MD: Williams & Wilkins (1978).

Alpiner, J.G., Chevrette, W., Glascoe, G., Metz, M., and Olsen, B., The Denver Scale of Communication Function. Unpublished study, University of Denver (1974).

Alpiner, J.G., and Garstecki, D.C., Aural rehabilitation for adults. In R.L. Schow and M.A. Nerbonne, *Introduction to Aural Rehabilitation*. Austin, TX: Pro-Ed (1989).

Alpiner, J.G., Meline, N.C., and Cotton, A.D., An aural rehabilitation screening scale: self assessment, auditory aptitude, and visual aptitude. *J. Acad. Rehab. Audiol.* 24, 75–83 (1991).

ASHA (American Speech-Language-Hearing Association), Guidelines for acoustic immittance screening of middle-ear function. *Asha*, 21, 283–288 (1979).

ASHA, Guidelines for identification audiometry. *Asha*, 27(5), 49–53 (1985).

ASHA, Considerations in screening adults/older persons for handicapping hearing impairments. *Asha*, 81–86 (1992).

Axelsson, A., and Ringdahl, A., Tinnitus—a study of its prevalence and characteristics. *Br. J. Audiol.*, 23, 53–62 (1989).

Binnie, C.A., Bi-sensory articulation functions for normal hearing and sensorineural hearing loss patients. *J. Acad. Rehab. Audiol.*, 6, 43–53 (1973).

Binnie, C.A., Montgomery, A.A., and Jackson, P.L., Auditory and visual contributions to the perception of consonants. *J. Speech Hear. Res.*, 17, 619–630 (1974).

Black, J.W., O'Reilly, P.P., and Peck, L., Self-administered training in lipreading. *J. Speech Hear. Dis.*, 28, 183–186 (1963).

Brannon, C., Speechreading of various speech materials. *J. Speech Hear. Dis.*, 26, 348–354 (1961).

Brooks, D.N., The effect of attitude on benefit obtained from hearing aids. *Br. Soc. Audiol.*, 23, 3–11 (1989).

Cox, R.M., Gilmore, C., and Alexander, G.C., Comparison of two questionnaires for patient-assessed hearing aid benefit. *J. Am. Acad. Audiol.*, 2, 134–145 (1991).

Davis, H., The articulation area and the social adequacy index for hearing. *Laryngoscope*, 58, 761–778 (1948).

Davis, H., and Silverman, S.R., *Hearing and Deafness*. New York: Holt, Rinehart and Winston (1970).

DeFilippo, C.L., and Scott, B.L., A method for training and evaluating the reception of ongoing speech. *J. Acoust. Soc.Am.*, 63, 1186–1192 (1978).

Demorest, M.E., and Erdman, S.A., A database management system for the communication profile for the hearing impaired. *J. Acad. Rehab. Audiol.*, 17, 87–96 (1984).

Demorest M.E., and Erdman, S.A., Scale composition and item analysis of the communication profile for the hearing impaired. *J. Speech Hear. Res.*, 29, 515–535 (1986).

Demorest, M.E., and Erdman, S.A., Development of the communication profile for the hearing impaired. *JSHD*, 52, 129–142 (1987).

Dodd, B., Plant, G., and Gregory, M., Teaching lipreading: the efficacy of lessons on video. *Br. J. Audiol.*, 23, 229–238 (1989).

Dodds, E., and Harford, E., Application of a lipreading test in a hearing aid evaluation. *J. Speech Hear. Dis.*, 33, 167–173 (1968).

Egan, J.P., Articulation testing methods. *Laryngoscope*, 58, 955–991 (1948).

Erber, N.P., Auditory-visual perception of speech. *J. Speech Hear. Dis.*, 40, 481–492 (1975).

Erber, N.P., Developing materials for lipreading evaluation and instruction. *Volta Rev.*, 79, 35–42 (1977).

Ewertsen, H., and Birk-Nielsen, H., Social hearing handicap index: social handicap in relation to hearing impairment. *Audiology*, 12, 180–187 (1973).

Giolas, T.G., The self-assessment approach in audiology. *Audiology*, 3, 157–171 (1983).

Giolas, T.G., The measurement of hearing handicap revisited: a 20-year perspective. *Ear Hear.*, 11(5), 28–58 (1990).

Giolas, T.G., Owens, E., Lamb, S.H., and Schubert, E.D., Hearing performance inventory. *J. Speech Hear. Dis.*, 44, 169–195 (1979).

Goldstein, D.P., and Stephens, S.D.G., Audiological rehabilitation: management model I. *Audiology*, 20, 432–452 (1981).

High, W.S., Fairbanks, G., and Glorig, A., Scale for self-assessment of hearing handicap. *J. Speech Hear. Dis.*, 29, 215–230 (1964).

Hirsh, I.J., Davis, H., Silverman, S.R., Reynolds, E.G., Elbert, E., and Bensen, R.W., Development of materials for speech audiometry. *J. Speech Hear. Dis.*, 17, 321–337 (1952).

Hipskind, N.M., Visual stimuli in communication. In R.L. Schow and M.A. Nerbonne (Eds.), *Introduction to Aural Rehabilitation*. Austin, TX: Pro-Ed (1989).

Hutton, C.L., A diagnostic approach to combined techniques in aural rehabilitation. *J. Speech Hear. Dis.*, 25, 267–272 (1960).

Hutton, C.L., Responses to a hearing problem inventory. *J. Acad. Rehab. Audiol.*, 13, 133–154 (1980).

Jeffers, J., and Barley, M., *Speechreading (Lipreading)*. Springfield, IL: Charles C. Thomas (1981).

Jerger, J., Speaks, C., and Trammell, J.L., An approach to speech audiometry. *J. Speech Hear. Dis.*, 33, 318–328 (1968).

Kalikow, D., Stevens, K., and Elliott, L., Development of a test of speech intelligibility in noise using sentence materials with controlled word predictability. *J. Acoust. Soc. Am.*, 61, 1337–1351 (1977).

Kaplan, H., Bally, S., and Brandt, F.D., Communication strategies, attitudes, and difficulties in the prelingually deaf population. *Asha Convention Program*, 116. (1990).

Klockhoff, I., and Lindblom, U., (Dichlotride)—a critical analysis of symptoms and therapeutic effects. *Acta Otolaryngol.*, 63, 347–365 (1967).

Lamb, S.H., Owens, E., and Schubert, E.D., The revised form of the hearing performance inventory. *Ear Hear.*, 4, 152–159 (1983).

Lesner, S., Are hearing handicap scales really necessary? American Academy of Audiology National Convention, New Orleans (1990).

McCarthy, P.A., and Alpiner, J.G., An assessment scale of hearing handicap for use in family counseling. *J. Acad. Rehab. Audiol.*, 16, 256–270 (1983).

National Center for Health Statistics, Hearing levels of adults by race, region and area of residence, United States, 1960–62. *Vital and Health Statistics Publication, Series 11, No. 26.* U.S. Government Printing Office, Washington, DC (1967).

National Center for Health Statistics, Basic data on hearing levels of adults 25–74, United States, 1971–75. *Vital and Health Statistics Publication, Series 11,*

No. 215. U.S. Government Printing Office, Washington, DC (1980).

Nerbonne, M.A., and Schow, R.L., Auditory stimuli in communication. In R.L.Schow and M.A. Nerbonne (Eds.), *Introduction to Aural Rehabilitation*, Austin, TX. Pro-Ed (1989).

Newman, C.W., Weinstein, B.E., Jacobson, G.P., and Hug, G.A., Test-retest reliability of the Hearing Handicap Inventory for Adults. *Ear Hear.*, 12(5), 355–357 (1991).

Noble, W.G., The measurement of hearing handicap: a further viewpoint. *Maico Audiological Library Series*, X, 5 (1972).

Noble, W., *Assessment of Impaired Hearing: A Critique and a New Method.* Academic Press, New York (1978).

Noble, W.G., The Hearing Measurement Scale as a paper-pencil form: preliminary results. *J. Am. Audiol. Soc.*, 5, 95–106 (1979).

Noble, W.G., and Atherley, G.R.C., The Hearing Measurement Scale: A questionnaire for the assessment of auditory disability. *J. Aud. Res.*, 10, 229–250 (1970).

Oja, G., and Schow, R.L., Hearing aid evaluation based on measures of benefit, use, and satisfaction. *Ear Hear.*, 5, 77–86 (1984).

O'Neill, J.J., and Oyer, H.J., *Visual Communication for the Hard of Hearing.* Englewood Cliffs, NJ: Prentice-Hall (1981).

Owens, E., Consonant errors and remediation in sensorineural hearing loss. *J. Speech Hear. Dis.*, 43, 331–347 (1978).

Owens, E., and Raggio, M.W., *Hearing Performance Inventory for Severe to Profound Hearing Loss.* University of California (San Francisco) (1984).

Owens, E., and Schubert, E., Development of the California Consonant Test. *J. Speech Hear. Res.*, 20, 463–474 (1977).

Oyer, H.J., Teaching lip-reading by television. *Volta Rev.*, 63, 131–141 (1961).

Oyer, H.J., Auditory training—significance and usage for children and adults. In J.G. Alpiner (Ed.), *Proceedings of the Institute on Aural Rehabilitation.* University of Denver (1968).

Oyer, H.J., and Frankmann, J.P., *The Aural Rehabilitation Process.* New York: Holt, Rinehart and Winston (1975).

Pichora-Fuller, M.K., Coarticulation and lipreading (Master's thesis, University of British Columbia, 1980). Canadian Theses, 1976/77–1979/80, 2, 50023 (available from Canadian Theses on Microfiche Service, Collections Development Branch, National Library of Canada, Ottawa, K1Aon4) (1980).

Pichora-Fuller, and Benguerel, A.P., The design of CAST (Computer Assisted Instruction). *J. Speech Hear. Res.*, 34, 202–212 (1991).

Pollack, M.C., The remediation process: psychological and counseling aspects. In J.G. Alpiner (Ed.), *Handbook of Adult Rehabilitative Audiology.* Baltimore, MD: Williams & Wilkins (1978).

Prescod, S.V., *A Standard Dictionary of Audiology.* Santa Monica, California: Vanguard Institutional Publishers (1986).

Rubinstein, A., and Boothroyd, A., Effect of two approaches to auditory training on speech recognition by hearing-impaired adults. *J. Speech Hear. Res.*, 30, 153–160 (1987).

Salomon, G., and Parving, A., Hearing disability and communication handicap for compensation purposes based on self-assessment and audiometric testing. *Audiology*, 24, 135–145 (1985).

Sanders, D.A., Hearing aid orientation and counseling. In M.C. Pollack (Ed.), *Amplification for the Hearing-Impaired*. New York: Grune & Stratton (1975).

Santore, F., Tulko, C., and Keamey, A., *Communication therapy for the adult with impaired hearing. NY League Hard Hear. Rehab. Q.*, 8(1), 5–7 (1983).

Schein, J., Gentile, J., and Haase, K., Development and evaluation of an expanded hearing loss scale questionnaire. USDHEW, *National Center for Health Statistics*. Series 2, No. 37 (1970).

Schow, R.L., Considerations in selecting and validating an adult/elderly hearing screening protocol. *Ear Hear.*, 12(5), 337–348 (1991).

Schow, R.L., Fitting trends and satisfaction data on 1000+ hearing aid users. *ICRA newsletter* 4, 16 (also presented at the ICRA meeting, Zurich, Switzerland) (February 1991).

Schow, R.L., Balsara, N., Whitcomb, C., and Smedley, T.C., Aural rehabilitation by ASHA audiologists: 1980–1990. Accepted in the American Journal of Audiology (1993).

Schow, R.L., and Gatehouse, S., Fundamental issues in self-assessment of hearing. *Ear Hear.*, 11(5), 6S–16S (1990).

Schow, R.L., and Nerbonne, M.A., Assessment of hearing handicap by nursing home residents and staff. *J. Rehabil. Audiol.*, 10, 2–12 (1977).

Schow, R.L., and Nerbonne, M.A., *Introduction to Aural Rehabilitation*. Baltimore, MD: University Park Press (1980).

Schow, R.L., and Nerbonne, M.A., Communication screening profile: use with elderly clients. *Ear Hear.*, 3, 135–147 (1982).

Schow, R.L., Reese, L., and Smedley, T.C., Hearing screening in a dental setting using self assessment. *Ear Hear.*, 11(5), Supplement, 28–40 (1990).

Schow, R.L., Smedley, T.C., Brockett, J., Longhurst, T.M., and Whitaker, M., Hearing aid referral strategies based on screening of adults. *Hear. J.*, 44(9), 30–43 (1991).

Schow, R.L., and Tannahill, C., Hearing handicap scores and categories for subjects with normal and impaired hearing sensitivity. *J. Am. Audiol. Soc.*, 3, 134–139 (1977).

Schwartz, D.M., and Surr, R.K., Three experiments on the California Consonant Test. *J. Speech Hear. Dis.*, 44, 61–72 (1979).

Sedge, R.K., and Scherr, C.K., Aural rehabilitation for individuals with high frequency hearing loss. *J. Acad. Rehab. Audiol.*, 12, 47–61 (1979).

Sims, D.G., Visual and auditory training for adults. In J. Katz (ed.), *The Handbook of Clinical Audiology*. Baltimore, MD: Williams & Wilkins (1978).

Sims, D.G., Visual and auditory training for adults. In J. Katz (Ed.), *The Handbook of Clinical Audiology*. Baltimore, MD: Williams & Wilkins (1985).

Smedley, T.C., Self-assessed satisfaction levels in elderly hearing aid, eyeglass, and denture wearers. *Ear Hear.* (Suppl.), 41S–47S (1990).

Stephens, S.D.G., Evaluating the problems of the hearing impaired. *Audiology*, 19, 205–220 (1980).

Stephens, D., and Hetu, R., Impairment, disability and handicap in audiology: towards a consensus. *Audiology*, 30, 185–200 (1991).

Stouffer, J.L., and Tyler, R.S., Characterization of tinnitus patients. *J.Speech Hear. Dis.*, 55, 439–453 (1990).

Sweetow, R.W., Cognitive aspects of tinnitus patient management. *Ear Hear.*, 6, 390–396 (1986).

Thorn, F., and Thorn, S., Speechreading with reduced vision: a problem of aging. *Optical Soc. Am.*, 6, 491–499 (1989).

Tillman, T.W., and Carhart, R., An expanded test for speech discrimination utilizing CNC monosyllabic words. *Northwestern University Auditory Test No. 5, Technical Report, SAM-TR-66-55*, USAF School of Aerospace Medicine, Brooks AFB, Texas (1966).

USPHS (United States Public Health Service), Preliminary analysis of audiometric data in relation to clinical history of impaired hearing. *The National Health Survey, Hearing Study Series. Bulletin 2*, Washington, DC: Public Health Service (1938).

Ventry, I.M., and Weinstein, B.E., Identification of elderly persons with hearing problems. *Asha*, 25, 37–41 (1983).

Walden, B.E., Demorest, M.E., and Hepler, E.H., Self-report approach to assessing benefit derived from amplification. *J. Speech Hear. Res.*, 9, 91–109 (1984).

Walden, B.E., Erdman, S.E., Montgomery, A.A., Schwartz, D.M., and Prosek, R.A., Some effects of training on speech recognition by hearing impaired adults. *J. Speech Hear. Res.*, 24, 207–216 (1981).

Walden, B.E., Prosek, R.A., and Scheer, C.K., Dimensions of visual consonant perception by hearing-impaired observers. Paper presented at the annual convention of the American Speech and Hearing Association, Las Vegas (1974).

Watts, W.J., and Pegg, K.S., The rehabilitation of adults with acquired hearing loss. *Br. J. Audiol.*, 11, 103–110 (1977).

Weinstein, B.E., A review of hearing handicap scales. *Audiology*, 9, 91–109 (1984).

Weinstein, B.E., Validity of a screening protocol for identifying elderly people with hearing problems. *Asha*, 28, 41–46 (1986).

Whitcomb, C.J., A survey of aural rehabilitation services among ASHA audiologists. Unpublished manuscript, Idaho State University (1980).

WHO (World Health Organization), *International Classification of Impairments, Disabilities, and Handicaps: A Manual of Classification Relating to the Consequences of Disease*. WHO, 25–43 (1980).

Woodward, M.F., and Barber, C.G. Phoneme perception in lipreading. *J. Speech Hear. Res.*, 3, 212–222 (1960).

APPENDIX 10.1 *Self-Assessment of Communication (SAC)**

Name _____

Date _____   Raw Score _____× 2 = _____− 20 = _____× 1.25 _____%

Please select the appropriate number ranging from 1 to 5 for the following questions.
Circle only one number for each question. If you have a hearing aid, please fill out the form according to how you communicate when the hearing aid is not in use.

Various Communication Situations

1. Do you experience communication difficulties in situations when speaking with one other person? (for example, at home, at work, in a social situation, with a waitress, a store clerk, with a spouse, boss, etc.)
   1) almost never (or never)   2) occasionally (about ¼ of the time)   3) about half of the time   4) frequently (about ¾ of the time)   5) practically always (or always)

2. Do you experience communication difficulties in situations when conversing with a small group of several persons? (for example, with friends or family, co-workers, in meetings or casual conversations, over dinner or while playing cards, etc.)
   1) almost never (or never)   2) occasionally (about ¼ of the time)   3) about half of the time   4) frequently (about ¾ of the time)   5) practically always (or always)

3) Do you experience communication difficulties while listening to someone speak to a large group? (for example, at a church or in a civic meeting, in a fraternal or women's club, at an educational lecture, etc.)
   1) almost never (or never)   2) occasionally (about ¼ of the time)   3) about half of the time   4) frequently (about ¾ of the time)   5) practically always (or always)

4. Do you experience communication difficulties while participating in various types of entertainment? (for example, movies, TV, radio, plays, night clubs, musical entertainment, etc.)
   1) almost never (or never)   2) occasionally (about ¼ of the time)   3) about half of the time   4) frequently (about ¾ of the time)   5) practically always (or always)

5. Do you experience communication difficulties when you are in an unfavorable listening environment? (for example, at a noisy party, where there is background music, when riding in an auto or bus, when someone whispers or talks from across the room, etc.)
   1) almost never (or never)   2) occasionally (about ¼ of the time)   3) about half of the time   4) frequently (about ¾ of the time)   5) practically always (or always)

6. Do you experience communication difficulties when using or listening to various communication devices? (for example, telephone, telephone ring, doorbell, public address system, warning signals, alarms, etc.)
   1) almost never (or never)   2) occasionally (about ¼ of the time)   3) about half of the time   4) frequently (about ¾ of the time)   5) practically always (or always)

Feelings About Communication

7. Do you feel that any difficulty with your hearing limits or hampers your personal or social life?
   1) almost never (or never)   2) occasionally (about ¼ of the time)   3) about half of the time   4) frequently (about ¾ of the time)   5) practically always (or always)

8. Does any problem or difficulty with your hearing upset you?
   1) almost never (or never)   2) occasionally (about ¼ of the time)   3) about half of the time   4) frequently (about ¾ of the time)   5) practically always (or always)

Other people

9. Do others suggest that you have a hearing problem?
   1) almost never (or never)   2) occasionally (about ¼ of the time)   3) about half of the time   4) frequently (about ¾ of the time)   5) practically always (or always)

10. Do others leave you out of conversations or become annoyed because of your hearing?
   1) almost never (or never)   2) occasionally (about ¼ of the time)   3) about half of the time   4) frequently (about ¾ of the time)   5) practically always (or always)

* Reprinted by permission from Schow, R. L., and Nerbonne, M. A., Communication screening profile; use with elderly clients. *Ear Hear.*, **3**, 135–147 (1982).

APPENDIX
10.2 *Significant Other Assessment of Communication (SOAC)**

Name _____

Form filled out with reference to _____ (client/patient)

Relationship to client/patient _____ (for example, wife, son, friend)

Date _____ Raw Score _____ × 2 = _____ − 20 = _____ × 1.25 _____ %

Please select the appropriate number ranging from 1 to 5 for the following questions. Circle only one number for each question. If the client/patient has a hearing aid, please fill out the form according to how he/she communicates when the hearing aid is not in use.

Various Communication Situations

1. Does he/she experience communication difficulties in situations when speaking with one other person? (for example, at home, at work, in a social situation, with a waitress, a store clerk, with a spouse, boss, etc.)

   1) almost never (or never)   2) occasionally (about ¼ of the time)   3) about half of the time   4) frequently (about ¾ of the time)   5) practically always (or always)

2. Does he/she experience communication difficulties in situations when conversing with a small group of several persons? (for example, with friends or family, co-workers, in meetings or casual conversations, over dinner or while playing cards, etc.)

   1) almost never (or never)   2) occasionally (about ¼ of the time)   3) about half of the time   4) frequently (about ¾ of the time)   5) practically always (or always)

3. Does he/she experience communication difficulties while listening to someone speak to a large group? (for example, at church or in a civic meeting, in a fraternal or women's club, at an educational lecture, etc.).

   1) almost never (or never)   2) occasionally (about ¼ of the time)   3) about half of the time   4) frequently (about ¾ of the time)   5) practically always (or always)

4. Does he/she experience communication difficulties while participating in various types of entertainment? (for example, movies, TV, radio, plays, night clubs, musical entertainment, etc.).

   1) almost never (or never)   2) occasionally (about ¼ of the time)   3) about half of the time   4) frequently (about ¾ of the time)   5) practically always (or always)

5. Does he/she experience communication difficulties when in an unfavorble listening environment? (for example, at a noisy party, where there is background music, when riding in an auto or bus, when someone whispers or talks from across the room, etc.).

   1) almost never (or never)   2) occasionally (about ¼ of the time)   3) about half of the time   4) frequently (about ¾ of the time)   5) practically always (or always)

6. Does he/she experience communication difficulties when using or listening to various communication devices? (for example, telephone, telephone ring, doorbell, public address system, warning signals, alarms, etc.).

   1) almost never (or never)   2) occasionally (about ¼ of the time)   3) about half of the time   4) frequently (about ¾ of the time)   5) practically always (or always)

Feelings About Communication

7. Do you feel that any difficulty with his/her hearing limits or hampers his/her personal or social life?

   1) almost never (or never)   2) occasionally (about ¼ of the time)   3) about half of the time   4) frequently (about ¾ of the time)   5) practically always (or always)

8. Does any problem or difficulty with his/her hearing visibly upset them?

   1) almost never (or never)   2) occasionally (about ¼ of the time)   3) about half of the time   4) frequently (about ¾ of the time)   5) practically always (or always)

Other People

9. Do you or others suggest he/she has a hearing problem?

   1) almost never (or never)   2) occasionally (about ¼ of the time)   3) about half of the time   4) frequently (about ¾ of the time)   5) practically always (or always)

10. Do you or others leave him/her out of conversations or become annoyed because of his/her hearing?

   1) almost never (or never)   2) occasionally (about ¼ of the time)   3) about half of the time   4) frequently (about ¾ of the time)   5) practically always (or always)

** Reprinted by permission from Schow, R. L., and Nerbonne, M. A. Communication screening profile: use with elderly clients, Ear Hear., **3**, 135–147 (1982).*

APPENDIX 10.3 *Hearing Handicap Inventory for Adults (HHIA)*

Instructions: The purpose of the scale is to identify the problems your hearing loss may be causing you. Check Yes, Sometimes, or No for each question. Do not skip a question if you avoid a situation because of a hearing problem.

		Yes (4)	Some-times (2)	No (0)
S-1.	Does a hearing problem cause you to use the phone less often than you would like?	___	___	___
E-2.*	Does a hearing problem cause you to feel embarrassed when meeting new people?	___	___	___
S-3.	Does a hearing problem cause you to avoid groups of people?	___	___	___
E-4.	Does a hearing problem make you irritable?	___	___	___
E-5.*	Does a hearing problem cause you to feel frustrated when talking to members of your family?	___	___	___
S-6.	Does a hearing problem cause you difficulty when attending a party?	___	___	___
S-7.*	Does a hearing problem cause you difficulty hearing/ understanding coworkers, clients, or customers?	___	___	___
E-8.*	Do you feel handicapped by a hearing problem?	___	___	___
S-9.*	Does a hearing problem cause you difficulty when visiting friends, relatives, or neighbors?	___	___	___
E-10.	Does a hearing problem cause you to feel frustrated when talking to coworkers, clients, or customers?	___	___	___
S-11.*	Does a hearing problem cause you difficulty in the movies or theater?	___	___	___
E-12.	Does a hearing problem cause you to be nervous?	___	___	___
S-13.	Does a hearing problem cause you to visit friends, relatives, or neighbors less often than you would like?	___	___	___
E-14.*	Does a hearing problem cause you to have arguments with family members?	___	___	___
S-15.*	Does a hearing problem cause you difficulty when listening to TV or radio?	___	___	___
S-16.	Does a hearing problem cause you to go shopping less often than you would like?	___	___	___
E-17.	Does any problem or difficulty with your hearing upset you at all?	___	___	___
E-18.	Does a hearing problem cause you to want to be by yourself?	___	___	___
S-19.	Does a hearing problem cause you to talk to family members less often than you would like?	___	___	___
E-20.*	Do you feel that any difficulty with your hearing limits or hampers your personal or social life?	___	___	___
S-21.*	Does a hearing problem cause you difficulty when in a restaurant with relatives or friends?	___	___	___

E-22. Does a hearing problem cause you to feel depressed? _____ _____ _____

S-23. Does a hearing problem cause you to listen to TV or radio less often than you would like? _____ _____ _____

E-24. Does a hearing problem cause you to feel uncomfortable when talking to friends? _____ _____ _____

E-25. Does a hearing problem cause you to feel left out when you are with a group of people? _____ _____ _____

*Items comprising the HHIA-S.

Reprinted by permission from Newman, C.W., Weinstein, B.E., Jacobson, G.P. and Hug, G.A., Test-retest reliability of the Hearing Handicap Inventory for Adults, *Ear Hear.*, 12, 355–357 (1991).

APPENDIX 10.4   *Denver Scale of Communication Function**

Pre-Service_____   Post-Service_____

Date _____   Case No. _____

Name _____Age ___Sex___

Address _____

_____
(City)   (State)   (Zip)

Lives Alone_____In Apartment _____Retired_____
                                  (if no, specify)

Occupation _____

Audiogram (Examination Date_____Agency_____)
   Pure Tone:
          250   500   1000   2000   4000   8000   Hz

   RE __   __   __   __   __   __
                                                                      dB (re: ANSI)
   LE __   __   __   __   __   __
Speech:
   SRT   DISCRIMINATION SCORE (%)

                         Quiet   Noise (S/N =   )

   RE_____dB   RE_____

   LE_____dB   LE_____

---

* Reprinted by permission from Alpiner, Chevrette, Glascoe, Metz, and Olsen: Unpublished study, the University of Denver, © 1974.

Hearing Aid Information

Aided_____For How Long_____Aid Type_____

Satisfaction _____

EXAMINER:_____

The following questionnaire was designed to evaluate your communication ability as you view it. You are asked to judge or scale each statement in the following manner.

If you judge the statement to be *very closely related* to either extreme, please place your check mark as follows:

Agree _X_   _____   _____   _____   _____   _____   _____ Disagree

or

Agree _____   _____   _____   _____   _____   _____   _X_ Disagree

If you judge the stagement to be *closely related* to either end of the scale, please mark as follows:

Agree _____   _X_   _____   _____   _____   _____   _____ Disagree

or

Agree _____   _____   _____   _____   _____   _X_   _____ Disagree

If you judge the statement to be only slightly related to either end of the scale, please mark as follows:

Agree _____   _____   _X_   _____   _____   _____   _____ Disagree

or

Agree _____   _____   _____   _____   _X_   _____   _____ Disagree

If you consider the statement to be irrelevant or unassociated to your communication situation, please mark as follows:

Agree _____   _____   _____   _X_   _____   _____   _____ Disagree

PLEASE NOTE: Check a scale for every statement.

Put only one checkmark on each scale.

Make a separate judgment for each statement.

ALSO: You may comment on each statement in the space provided.

1. The members of my family are annoyed with my loss of hearing.
   Agree_____   _____   _____   _____   _____   _____   _____ Disagree
   Comments:
2. The members of my family sometimes leave me out of conversations or discussions.

Agree _____   _____   _____   _____   _____   _____   _____ Disagree
Comments:

3. Sometimes my family makes decisions for me because I have a hard time following discussions.
Agree _____   _____   _____   _____   _____   _____   _____ Disagree
Comments:

4. My family becomes annoyed when I ask them to repeat what was said because I did not hear them.
Agree _____   _____   _____   _____   _____   _____   _____ Disagree
Comments:

5. I am not an "outgoing" person because I have a hearing loss.
Agree _____   _____   _____   _____   _____   _____   _____ Disagree
Comments:

6. I now take less of an interest in many things as compared to when I did not have a hearing problem.
Agree _____   _____   _____   _____   _____   _____   _____ Disagree
Comments:

7. Other people do not realize how frustrated I get when I cannot hear or understand.
Agree _____   _____   _____   _____   _____   _____   _____ Disagree
Comments:

8. People sometimes avoid me because of my hearing loss.
Agree _____   _____   _____   _____   _____   _____   _____ Disagree
Comments:

9. I am not a calm person because of my hearing loss.
Agree _____   _____   _____   _____   _____   _____   _____ Disagree
Comments:

10. I tend to be negative about life in general because of my hearing loss.
Agree _____   _____   _____   _____   _____   _____   _____ Disagree
Comments:

11. I do not socialize as much as I did before I began to lose my hearing.
Agree _____   _____   _____   _____   _____   _____   _____ Disagree
Comments:

12. Since I have trouble hearing, I do not like to go places with friends.
Agree _____   _____   _____   _____   _____   _____   _____ Disagree
Comments:

13. Since I have trouble hearing, I hestitate to meet new people.
Agree _____   _____   _____   _____   _____   _____   _____ Disagree
Comments:

14. I do not enjoy my job as much as I did before I began to lose my hearing.
Agree _____   _____   _____   _____   _____   _____   _____ Disagree
Comments:

15. Other people do not understand what it is like to have a hearing loss.
Agree _____   _____   _____   _____   _____   _____   _____ Disagree
Comments:

16. Because I have difficulty understanding what is said to me, I sometimes answer questions wrong.
Agree _____ _____ _____ _____ _____ _____ _____ Disagree
Comments:

17. I do not feel relaxed in a communicative situation.
Agree _____ _____ _____ _____ _____ _____ _____ Disagree
Comments:

18. I do not feel comfortable in most communication situations.
Agree _____ _____ _____ _____ _____ _____ _____ Disagree
Comments:

19. Conversations in a noisy room prevent me from attempting to communicate with others.
Agree _____ _____ _____ _____ _____ _____ _____ Disagree
Comments:

20. I am not comfortable having to speak in a group situation.
Agree _____ _____ _____ _____ _____ _____ _____ Disagree
Comments:

21. In general, I do not find listening relaxing.
Agree _____ _____ _____ _____ _____ _____ _____ Disagree
Comments:

22. I feel threatened by many communication situations due to difficulty hearing.
Agree _____ _____ _____ _____ _____ _____ _____ Disagree
Comments:

23. I seldom watch other people's facial expressions when talking to them.
Agree _____ _____ _____ _____ _____ _____ _____ Disagree
Comments:

24. I hesitate to ask people to repeat if I do not understand them the first time they speak.
Agree _____ _____ _____ _____ _____ _____ _____ Disagree
Comments:

25. Because I have difficulty understanding what is said to me, I sometimes make comments that do not fit into the conversation.
Agree _____ _____ _____ _____ _____ _____ _____ Disagree
Comments:

APPENDIX 10.5   *Quantified Denver Scale**

Name _____   Score:
                                          Raw score:
Age _____

Date _____

	Strongly disagree				**Strongly agree**
1. The members of my family are annoyed with my loss of hearing.	1	2	3	4	5
2. The members of my family sometimes leave me out of conversations or discussions.	1	2	3	4	5
3. Sometimes my family makes decisions for me because I have a hard time following discussions.	1	2	3	4	5
4. My family becomes annoyed when I ask them to repeat what was said because I did not hear them.	1	2	3	4	5
5. I am not an "outgoing" person because I have a hearing loss.	1	2	3	4	5
6. I now take less of an interest in many things as compared to when I did not have a hearing problem.	1	2	3	4	5
7. Other people do not realize how frustrated I get when I cannot hear or understand.	1	2	3	4	5
8. People sometimes avoid me because of my hearing loss.	1	2	3	4	5
9. I am not a calm person because of my hearing loss.	1	2	3	4	5

_____

* Modified from Denver Scale of Communication Function (Alpiner *et al.*, 1974).

	Strongly disagree				Strongly agree
10. I tend to be negative about life in general because of my hearing loss.	1	2	3	4	5
11. I do not socialize as much as I did before I began to lose my hearing.	1	2	3	4	5
12. Since I have trouble hearing, I do not like to go places with friends.	1	2	3	4	5
13. Since I have trouble hearing, I hesitate to meet new people.	1	2	3	4	5
14. I do not enjoy my job as much as I did before I began to lose my hearing.	1	2	3	4	5
15. Other people do not understand what it is like to have a hearing loss.	1	2	3	4	5
16. Because I have difficulty understanding what is said to me, I sometimes answer questions wrong.	1	2	3	4	5
17. I do not feel relaxed in a communicative situation.	1	2	3	4	5
18. I don't feel comfortable in most communication situations.	1	2	3	4	5
19. Conversations in a noisy room prevent me from attempting to communicate with others.	1	2	3	4	5
20. I am not comfortable having to speak in a group situation.	1	2	3	4	5
21. In general, I do not find listening relaxing.	1	2	3	4	5
22. I feel threatened by many communication situations due to difficulty hearing.	1	2	3	4	5
23. I seldom watch other people's facial expressions when talking to them.	1	2	3	4	5
24. I hesitate to ask people to repeat if I do not understand them the first time they speak.	1	2	3	4	5
25. Because I have difficulty understanding what is said to me, I sometimes make comments that do not fit into the conversation.	1	2	3	4	5

APPENDIX 10.6 *McCarthy-Alpiner Scale of Hearing Handicap (M-A Scale)**

by
Patricia McCarthy, Ph.D
and
Jerome G. Alpiner, PhD.
FORM A

NAME: _____DATE: _____

AGE: _____SEX: _____TIME: _____

OCCUPATION: _____PHONE: _____

ADDRESS: _____

HEARING AID: YES _____NO _____   ONSET OF HEARING LOSS: _____

    TYPE _____

    HOW LONG _____

    SATISFACTION _____

AUDIOGRAM: DATE OF EXAMINATION _____

    EXAMINER _____

    CATEGORY OF HEARING LOSS _

RIGHT EAR

	250 Hz	500 Hz	1000 Hz	2000 Hz	4000 Hz	8000 Hz
AIR						
BONE						

LEFT EAR

	250 Hz	500 Hz	1000 Hz	2000 Hz	4000 Hz	8000 Hz
AIR						
BONE						

SPEECH RECEPTION THRESHOLD: SPEECH DISCRIMINATION:

RIGHT EAR _____dB HL   RIGHT EAR _____% @_____ dB HL

LEFT EAR _____dB HL   LEFT EAR _____% @_____ dB HL

* Copyright (1980) by Patricia McCarthy, Ph.D., V. A. Medical Center, North Chicago, IL and Jerome G. Alpiner, Ph.D., The University of Mississippi, University, MS.

DIRECTIONS

The following questionnaire will be used to help audiologists understand what it is like to have a hearing loss and the effects of a hearing loss on your life. You are asked to give your reaction to each of the statements included in the questionnaire. For example, you might be given this statement:

People avoid me because of my hearing loss.

_____	_____	____X____	_____	_____
ALWAYS	USUALLY	SOMETIMES	RARELY	NEVER

You are asked to mark your reaction to the statement with an X on the appropriate space. Please mark every item with only one answer as seen in the example.

In marking your answer, please keep in mind that ALWAYS means at all times or on all occasions. USUALLY refers to generally, commonly or ordinarily. SOMETIMES means occasionally or on various occasions. RARELY refers to seldom or infrequently. NEVER means not ever or at no time.

If you are not presently employed, please respond "N/A" for not applicable.

All answers will be kept strictly confidential and used only to help audiologists to understand what it is like to have a hearing loss and the effects of hearing loss on your life.

1. I get annoyed when people do not speak loud enough for me to hear them.

_____	_____	_____	_____	_____
ALWAYS	USUALLY	SOMETIMES	RARELY	NEVER

2. I get upset if I can not hear or understand a conversation.

_____	_____	_____	_____	_____
ALWAYS	USUALLY	SOMETIMES	RARELY	NEVER

3. I feel like I am isolated from things because of my hearing loss.

_____	_____	_____	_____	_____
ALWAYS	USUALLY	SOMETIMES	RARELY	NEVER

4. I feel negative about life in general because of my hearing loss.

_____	_____	_____	_____	_____
ALWAYS	USUALLY	SOMETIMES	RARELY	NEVER

5. I admit that I have a hearing loss to most people.

_____	_____	_____	_____	_____
ALWAYS	USUALLY	SOMETIMES	RARELY	NEVER

6. I get upset when I feel that people are "mumbling".

_____	_____	_____	_____	_____
ALWAYS	USUALLY	SOMETIMES	RARELY	NEVER

7. I feel very frustrated when I can not understand a conversation.

_____	_____	_____	_____	_____
ALWAYS	USUALLY	SOMETIMES	RARELY	NEVER

8. I feel that people in general understand what it is like to have a hearing loss.

_____	_____	_____	_____	_____
ALWAYS	USUALLY	SOMETIMES	RARELY	NEVER

9. My hearing loss has affected my life in general.

_____	_____	_____	_____	_____
ALWAYS	USUALLY	SOMETIMES	RARELY	NEVER

10. I am afraid that people will not like me if they find out that I have a hearing loss.

_____	_____	_____	_____	_____
ALWAYS	USUALLY	SOMETIMES	RARELY	NEVER

11. I tend to avoid people because of my hearing loss.

_____	_____	_____	_____	_____
ALWAYS	USUALLY	SOMETIMES	RARELY	NEVER

12. People act annoyed when I cannot understand what is being said in a group conversation.

_____	_____	_____	_____	_____
ALWAYS	USUALLY	SOMETIMES	RARELY	NEVER

13. My family is patient with me when I can not hear.

_____	_____	_____	_____	_____
ALWAYS	USUALLY	SOMETIMES	RARELY	NEVER

14. Strangers react rudely when I do not understand what they say.

    ALWAYS   USUALLY   SOMETIMES   RARELY   NEVER

15. I ask a person to repeat if I do not hear or understand what he said.

    ALWAYS   USUALLY   SOMETIMES   RARELY   NEVER

16. My hearing loss has affected my relationship with my spouse.

    ALWAYS   USUALLY   SOMETIMES   RARELY   NEVER

17. I do not go places with my family because of my hearing loss.

    ALWAYS   USUALLY   SOMETIMES   RARELY   NEVER

18. Group discussions make me nervous because of my hearing loss.

    ALWAYS   USUALLY   SOMETIMES   RARELY   NEVER

19. People in general are tolerant of my hearing loss.

    ALWAYS   USUALLY   SOMETIMES   RARELY   NEVER

20. I avoid going to movies or plays because of my hearing loss.

    ALWAYS   USUALLY   SOMETIMES   RARELY   NEVER

21. I avoid going to restaurants because of my hearing loss.

    ALWAYS   USUALLY   SOMETIMES   RARELY   NEVER

22. I enjoy social situations with considerable conversation.

    ALWAYS   USUALLY   SOMETIMES   RARELY   NEVER

23. I am not interested in group activities because of my hearing loss.

    ALWAYS   USUALLY   SOMETIMES   RARELY   NEVER

24. I enjoy group discussions even though I have a hearing loss.

    ALWAYS   USUALLY   SOMETIMES   RARELY   NEVER

25. My hearing loss has interfered with my job performance.

    ALWAYS   USUALLY   SOMETIMES   RARELY   NEVER

26. I can not perform my job well because of my hearing loss.

    ALWAYS   USUALLY   SOMETIMES   RARELY   NEVER

27. My co-workers know what it is like to have a hearing loss.

    ALWAYS   USUALLY   SOMETIMES   RARELY   NEVER

28. I try to hide my hearing loss from my co-workers.

    ALWAYS   USUALLY   SOMETIMES   RARELY   NEVER

29. I do not enjoy going to work because of my hearing loss.

    ALWAYS   USUALLY   SOMETIMES   RARELY   NEVER

30. I am given credit for doing a good job at work even though I have a hearing loss.

    ALWAYS   USUALLY   SOMETIMES   RARELY   NEVER

31. I feel more pressure at work because of my hearing loss.

    ALWAYS   USUALLY   SOMETIMES   RARELY   NEVER

32. My employer understands what it is like to have a hearing loss.

    ALWAYS   USUALLY   SOMETIMES   RARELY   NEVER

33. I try to hide my hearing loss from my employer.

    ALWAYS   USUALLY   SOMETIMES   RARELY   NEVER

34. My co-workers speak loudly and clearly.

    ALWAYS   USUALLY   SOMETIMES   RARELY   NEVER

APPENDIX 10.7 *California Consonant Test**

Name_____   Date_____

List 1

Test Items

	1	GAVE ___	11	PAGE ___	21	SHIN ___	31	VALE ___	41	KIT ___
		GAME ___		PAID ___		SIN ___		DALE ___		KICK ___
		GAZE ___		PAYS ___		THIN ___		JAIL ___		KISS ___
		GAGE ___		PAVE ___		CHIN ___		BALE ___		KID ___
	2	PAIL ___	12	KICK ___	22	MUFF ___	32	PEACH ___	42	PIN ___
		SAIL ___		PICK ___		MUCH ___		PEAT ___		KIN ___
Sample Items		FAIL ___		TICK ___		MUSH ___		PEAK ___		TIN ___
		TAIL ___		THICK ___		MUSS ___		PEEP ___		THIN ___
1 BACK ___	3	CUFF ___	13	LAUGH ___	23	REACH ___	33	RACK ___	43	BUS ___
BAG ___		CUP ___		LASH ___		REAP ___		RASH ___		BUT ___
BATCH ___		CUSS ___		LASS ___		REEF ___		RAT ___		BUCK ___
BATH ___		CUT ___		LAP ___		REEK ___		RAP ___		BUFF ___
2 RICE ___	4	MUSS ___	14	SHEEP ___	24	BACK ___	34	HAG ___	44	GATE ___
DICE ___		MUCH ___		SEEP ___		BAT ___		HAD ___		BAIT ___
NICE ___		MUSH ___		CHEAP ___		BATCH ___		HAVE ___		DATE ___
LICE ___		MUFF ___		HEAP ___		BATH ___		HAS ___		WAIT ___
3 SEEN ___	5	FAKE ___	15	GAVE ___	25	TAME ___	35	TICK ___	45	LAUGH ___
SEED ___		FATE ___		GAME ___		SHAME ___		SICK ___		LASS ___
SEAL ___		FACE ___		GAGE ___		FAME ___		THICK ___		LASH ___
SEAT ___		FAITH ___		GAZE ___		SAME ___		PICK ___		LAP ___
4 BAIL ___	6	TILL ___	16	BEACH ___	26	CORE ___	36	CHAIR ___	46	HIP ___
TALE ___		CHILL ___		BEEP ___		PORE ___		CARE ___		HIT ___
SAIL ___		PILL ___		BEAK ___		TORE ___		SHARE ___		HISS ___
DALE ___		KILL ___		BEET ___		SORE ___		FAIR ___		HITCH ___
5 LEAVE ___	7	LEASE ___	17	MASS ___	27	RAGE ___	37	BEACH ___	47	HICK ___
LEASH ___		LEASH ___		MAP ___		RAISE ___		BEAK ___		SICK ___
LEAN ___		LEAF ___		MAT ___		RAVE ___		BEET ___		THICK ___
LEAGUE ___		LEAP ___		MATH ___		RAID ___		BEEP ___		CHICK ___
6 RAIL ___	8	SEEP ___	18	PATH ___	28	FILL ___	38	BEAK ___	48	LEAF ___
JAIL ___		CHEAP ___		PATCH ___		PILL ___		BEEP ___		LEASE ___
TAIL ___		SHEEP ___		PACK ___		KILL ___		BEAT ___		LEASH ___
BALE ___		HEAP ___		PAT ___		TILL ___		BEEF ___		LEAK ___
	9	FACE ___	19	GAZE ___	29	CHOP ___	39	CHEEK ___	49	CHEEK ___
		FAITH ___		GAGE ___		POP ___		CHIEF ___		CHEAP ___
		FATE ___		GAVE ___		TOP ___		CHEAT ___		CHEAT ___
		FAKE ___		GAME ___		SHOP ___		CHEAP ___		CHIEF ___
	10	BAYS ___	20	SICK ___	30	MUCK ___	40	CUP ___	50	RID ___
		BABE ___		CHICK ___		MUTT ___		CUT ___		RIB ___
		BALE ___		THICK ___		MUSS ___		CUSS ___		RIDGE ___
		BATHE ___		TICK ___		MUFF ___		CUFF ___		RIG ___

_____

* Reprinted by permission from *California Consonant Test*, Auditec of St. Louis, 330 Selma Ave., St. Louis, MO 63119.

51	THIN	___	61	TAN	___	71	THAN	___	81	MATCH	___	91	HIP	___
	TIN	___		CAN	___		VAN	___		MAT	___		HICK	___
	SIN	___		FAN	___		BAN	___		MATH	___		HIT	___
	SHIN	___		PAN	___		PAN	___		MAP	___		HISS	___
52	HIT	___	62	TORE	___	72	SHEATH	___	82	PATCH	___	92	TIN	___
	HIP	___		CORE	___		SHEEP	___		PAT	___		KIN	___
	HISS	___		PORE	___		SHEIK	___		PASS	___		PIN	___
	HITCH	___		CHORE	___		SHEET	___		PATH	___		THIN	___
53	PAYS	___	63	SIS	___	73	TAN	___	83	FAITH	___	93	CASH	___
	PAVE	___		SIP	___		PAN	___		FATE	___		CAT	___
	PAGE	___		SIT	___		CAN	___		FAKE	___		CAP	___
	PAID	___		SICK	___		FAN	___		FACE	___		CATCH	___
54	HIT	___	64	CUSS	___	74	BATCH	___	84	RID	___	94	HATCH	___
	HICK	___		CUP	___		BAT	___		RIB	___		HAT	___
	HITCH	___		CUT	___		BACK	___		RIG	___		HACK	___
	HIP	___		CUFF	___		BATH	___		RIDGE	___		HALF	___
55	SICK	___	65	RAP	___	75	PAIL	___	85	CHEAP	___	95	DIVE	___
	SIP	___		RACK	___		TAIL	___		CHEAT	___		DIED	___
	SIT	___		RASH	___		SAIL	___		CHEEK	___		DIES	___
	SIS	___		RAT	___		FAIL	___		CHIEF	___		DINE	___
56	BEET	___	66	KILL	___	76	BUG	___	86	SORE	___	96	SIN	___
	BEEP	___		PILL	___		BUDGE	___		CHORE	___		FIN	___
	BEACH	___		TILL	___		BUZZ	___		SHORE	___		THIN	___
	BEAK	___		FILL	___		BUD	___		FOR	___		SHIN	___
57	HATCH	___	67	SICK	___	77	SAIL	___	87	POP	___	97	RODE	___
	HACK	___		TICK	___		PAIL	___		TOP	___		ROBE	___
	HALF	___		PICK	___		TAIL	___		CHOP	___		ROVE	___
	HAT	___		THICK	___		FAIL	___		COP	___		ROSE	___
58	CHIN	___	68	PAGE	___	78	ROBE	___	88	MAP	___	98	BAIL	___
	SHIN	___		PAYS	___		RODE	___		MATCH	___		JAIL	___
	THIN	___		PAVE	___		ROSE	___		MATH	___		DALE	___
	PIN	___		PAID	___		ROVE	___		MAT	___		GALE	___
59	HAIL	___	69	TORE	___	79	LASS	___	89	DIES	___	99	LEAF	___
	TAIL	___		PORE	___		LAUGH	___		DIED	___		LEASE	___
	FAIL	___		CORE	___		LATCH	___		DIVE	___		LEACH	___
	SAIL	___		SORE	___		LASH	___		DINE	___		LEASH	___
60	SHUN	___	70	LEASH	___	80	FIN	___	90	PEAK	___	100	RAISE	___
	PUN	___		LEAK	___		PIN	___		PEACH	___		RAID	___
	SUN	___		LEASE	___		KIN	___		PEAT	___		RAGE	___
	FUN	___		LEAF	___		TIN	___		PEEP	___		RAVE	___

APPENDIX 10.8 *Central Institute for the Deaf (CID) Everyday Speech Sentences**

LIST A

1. Walking's my favorite exercise.
2. Here's a nice quiet place to rest.
3. Our janitor sweeps the floors every night.
4. It would be much easier if everyone would help.
5. Good morning.
6. Open your window before you go to bed!
7. Do you think that she should stay out so late?
8. How do you feel about changing the time when we begin to work?
9. Here we go.
10. Move out of the way.

LIST B

1. The water's too cold for swimming.
2. Why should I get up so early in the morning?
3. Here are your shoes.
4. It's raining.
5. Where are you going?
6. Come here when I call you!
7. Don't try go get out of it this time!
8. Should we let little children go to the movies by themselves?
9. There isn't enough paint to finish the room.
10. Do you want an egg for breakfast?

LIST C

1. Everybody should brush his teeth after meals.
2. Everything's all right.
3. Don't use up all the paper when you write your letter.
4. That's right.
5. People ought to see a doctor once a year.
6. Those windows are so dirty I can't see anything outside.
7. Pass the bread and butter please!
8. Don't forget to pay your bill before the first of the month.

---

* Reprinted by permission from Davis and Silverman: *Hearing and Deafness*, © 1970, Holt, Rinehart and Winston, Inc.

9. Don't let the dog out of the house!
10. There's a good ballgame this afternoon.

LIST D

1. It's time to go.
2. If you don't want these old magazines, throw them out.
3. Do you want to wash up?
4. It's a real dark night so watch your driving.
5. I'll carry the package for you.
6. Did you forget to shut off the water?
7. Fishing in a mountain stream is my idea of a good time.
8. Fathers spend more time with their children than they used to.
9. Be careful not to break your glasses!
10. I'm sorry.

LIST E

1. You can catch the bus across the street.
2. Call her on the phone and tell her the news.
3. I'll catch up with you later.
4. I'll think it over.
5. I don't want to go to the movies tonight.
6. If your tooth hurts that much you ought to see a dentist.
7. Put that cookie back in the box!
8. Stop fooling around!
9. Time's up.
10. How do you spell your name?

LIST F

1. Music always cheers me up.
2. My brother's in town for a short while on business.
3. We live a few miles from the main road.
4. This suit needs to go to the cleaners.
5. They ate enough green apples to make them sick for a week.
6. Where have you been all this time?
7. Have you been working hard lately?
8. There's not enough room in the kitchen for a new table.
9. Where is he?
10. Look out!

LIST G

1. I'll see you right after lunch.
2. See you later.
3. White shoes are awful to keep clean.
4. Stand there and don't move until I tell you!
5. There's a big piece of cake left over from dinner.
6. Wait for me at the corner in front of the drugstore.
7. It's no trouble at all.
8. Hurry up!

9. The morning paper didn't say anything about rain this afternoon or tonight.
10. The phone call's for you.

LIST H

1. Believe me!
2. Let's get a cup of coffee.
3. Let's get out of here before it's too late.
4. I hate driving at night.
5. There was water in the cellar after the heavy rain yesterday.
6. She'll only be gone a few minutes.
7. How do you know?
8. Children like candy.
9. If we don't get rain soon, we'll have no grass.
10. They're not listed in the new phone book.

LIST I

1. Where can I find a place to park?
2. I like those big red apples we always get in the fall.
3. You'll get fat eating candy.
4. The show's over.
5. Why don't they paint their walls some other color?
6. What's new?
7. What are you hiding under your coat?
8. How come I should always be the one to go first?
9. I'll take sugar and cream in my coffee.
10. Wait just a minute!

LIST J

1. Breakfast is ready.
2. I don't know what's wrong with the car, but it won't start.
3. It sure takes a sharp knife to cut this meat.
4. I haven't read a newspaper since we bought a television set.
5. Weeds are spoiling the yard.
6. Call me a little later!
7. Do you have change for a five-dollar bill?
8. How are you?
9. I'd like some ice cream with my pie.
10. I don't think I'll have any dessert.

APPENDIX
10.9 *University of Iowa Tinnitus Questionnaire*

Part A
(To be filled in by the patient)

1. Where is your tinnitus? (Please choose only *ONE* answer.)
   a. Left ear
   b. Right ear
   c. Both ears, equally
   d. Both ears, but worse in left ear
   e. Both ears, but worse in right ear
   f. In the head, but no exact place
   g. More in the right side of head
   h. More in the left side of head
   i. Outside of head
   j. Middle head

If you hear more than one sound or a different sound in each ear, answer the following questions with regard to the one most annoying sound.

2. Describe the most prominent *PITCH* of your tinnitus by circling *ONE* of the numbers below. Number 1 is like a *VERY LOW* pitched fog horn, and Number 10 is like a *VERY HIGH* pitched whistle.

PITCH

1	2	3	4	5	6	7	8	9	10
(VERY LOW)									(VERY HIGH)

3. When the tinnitus is there does it ever change *PITCH*?
   a. No
   b. Yes, suddenly
   c. Yes, gradually
4. Does the *PITCH* of the tinnitus vary from day to day?
   a. No
   b. Yes
5. Describe the *LOUDNESS* of your tinnitus by circling *ONE* of the numbers below. Number 1 is a *VERY FAINT* tinnitus, and Number 10 is a *VERY LOUD* tinnitus.

LOUDNESS

1	2	3	4	5	6	7	8	9	10
(VERY FAINT)									(VERY LOUD)

6. When it is there, does the tinnitus ever change *LOUDNESS*?
   a. No
   b. Yes, suddenly
   c. Yes, gradually
7. Does the *LOUDNESS* of the tinnitus vary from day to day?
   a. No
   b. Yes
8. Which of all these qualities *BEST* describes your tinnitus? (Please circle only *ONE*.)
   a. Buzzing
   b. Clanging
   c. Clicking
   d. Crackling
   e. Cricket-like
   j. Pounding
   k. Pulsing
   l. Ringing
   m. Roaring
   n. Rushing

f. Hissing
g. Humming
h. Musical note
i. Popping
o. Steam whistle
p. Throbbing
q. Whistling
r. Whooshing
s. OTHER, PLEASE SPECIFY _____

9. Does the tinnitus ever change to a completely different sound?
   a. No
   b. Yes, suddenly
   c. Yes, gradually

10. During the time you are awake, what percentage of the time is your tinnitus present? For example, 100% would indicate that your tinnitus was there all the time, and 25% would indicate that your tinnitus was there 1/4 of the time.
    _____ % Please write in a single number between 1 and 100.

11. On the average, how many days per month are you bothered by your tinnitus?
    _____ days per month (maximum = 30 days)

Since your tinnitus began, is your tinnitus *NOW*:

12. a. higher   b. lower   c. same IN PITCH   (circle a, b, or c)
13. a. louder   b. softer   c. same IN LOUDNESS   (circle a, b, or c)
14. a. higher   b. lower   c. same IN SEVERITY   (circle a, b, or c)
15. When your tinnitus first began, how many sounds was it composed of?
    _____ (number of sounds)
16. How many sounds is your tinnitus composed of *NOW*?
    _____ (number of sounds)
17. How many years have you had tinnitus?
    _____ years
18. How many years has your tinnitus really bothered you?
    _____ years
19. When you have your tinnitus, which of the following makes it *WORSE*?
    (CIRCLE ALL OF THESE THAT APPLY TO YOU.)
    a. Alcohol
    b. Being in a noisy place
    c. Being in a quiet place
    d. Changing head position
    e. Coffee/tea
    f. Constipation
    g. During your menstrual period
    h. Drugs/medicine
    i. Emotional or mental stress
    j. Food (please specify) _____
    k. Having just recently been in a noisy place
    l. Having just recently worn a hearing aid
    m. Lack of sleep
    n. Relaxation
    o. Shooting guns, rifles, etc.
    p. Smoking
    q. Sudden physical activity
    r. When you are excited
    s. When you are tired from doing physical work
    t. While you are wearing a hearing aid
    u. When you first wake up in the morning

    v. OTHER, PLEASE SPECIFY _____

    w. Nothing makes it worse.

20. Which of the following *REDUCES* your tinnitus?
(CIRCLE ALL OF THE ANSWERS THAT APPLY TO YOU.)

    a. Alcohol

    b. Being in a noisy place

    c. Being in a quiet place

    d. Coffee/tea

    e. Drugs/medicine

    f. Food (please specify) _____

    g. Having just recently been in a noisy place

    h. Having just recently been in a quiet place

    i. Listening to television or radio

    j. Sleep

    k. Smoking

    l. Wearing a hearing aid

    m. OTHER, PLEASE SPECIFY _____

    n. Nothing reduces my tinnitus.

21. What do you think originally caused your tinnitus? Select *ONE* only.

    a. Accident (please specify) _____

    b. Alcohol

    c. Drugs/medicine

    d. Food (please specify) _____

    e. Hearing loss

    f. Illness (please specify) _____

    g. Noise

    h. Smoking

    i. Surgery

    j. OTHER, PLEASE SPECIFY _____

    k. I have no idea.

22. Please write a *single* number between 0 and 100 to indicate how *ANNOYING* you find your tinnitus—a "0" would indicate that it is not annoying at all, a "100" would indicate that it is extremely annoying.

    _____ (Please write a *single* number between 0 and 100.)

23. What percentage of the time does your tinnitus interfere with your getting to sleep (0% = does not interfere; 100% = interferes every night).

    _____ (Please write a *single* number between 0 and 100.)

24. To what degree are you *DEPRESSED* by your tinnitus? (0 indicates your tinnitus does not depress you; 100 indicates you are extremely depressed by your tinnitus.)

    _____ (Please write a *single* number between 0 and 100.)

25. Do you have trouble *CONCENTRATING* because of your tinnitus? (0 indicates your tinnitus does not affect concentration; 100 indicates that your tinnitus always interferes with concentration.)

    _____ (Please write a *single* number between 0 and 100.)

26. Does your tinnitus interfere with your understanding speech? (0 indicates your tinnitus does not interfere with speech; 100 indicates your tinnitus interferes extremely with understanding speech.)

    _____ (Please write a *single* number between 0 and 100.)

27. I am concerned that my tinnitus is a symptom of a much worse disease
Yes / No

28. I am concerned that I might go deaf because of my tinnitus.
    Yes / No
29. Were you taking any medications just *BEFORE* your tinnitus began?
    a. No
    b. Yes
30. Are you taking any medications *NOW?*
    a. No
    b. Yes

Part B
(To be filled in by the audiologist)

1. Primary Diagnosis (circle only *ONE*)
   1. Noise-induced hearing loss
   2. Presbycusis
   3. Ménière's
   4. Middle-ear disorder (please specify)
   5. Retrocochlear (please specify) _____
   6. Normal hearing (please specify) _____
   7. Other (please specify) _____
   8. Unknown
2. Primary Complaint (circle only *ONE*)
   1. Hearing loss
   2. Dizziness
   3. Tinnitus
   4. Pain or headaches
   5. Other (please specify) _ _____
3. Hearing Thresholds

	Left Ear			Right Ear	
	1000 Hz	4000 Hz		1000 Hz	4000 Hz
1. ___ dB HL		2. ___ dB HL	3. ___ dB HL		4. ___ dB HL

APPENDIX 10.10a *Alpiner-Meline Aural Rehabilitation (AMAR) Screening Scale*

ADMINISTRATION INSTRUCTIONS

INTRODUCTION

The Alpiner-Meline Aural Rehabilitation Screening Scale (AMAR) is designed to identify adults who may need aural rehabilitation. The AMAR allows identification of problems related to hearing loss in three categories: (a) self assessment, (b) visual aptitude, and (c) auditory aptitude.

APTITUDE

1. The scale should be administered in a quiet room. Items are presented in an interview format.
2. Each subtest is scored independently. Part I, Self Assessment has nine items rated in terms of five possible responses: ALWAYS, USUALLY, SOMETIMES, RARELY, and

NEVER. For all of the items, (except number five), ALWAYS refers to maximum negative response possible, that is, a problem exists. For item five, NEVER REFERS TO THE MAXIMUM NEGATIVE RESPONSE.

A problem is indicated when the response is either ALWAYS, USUALLY, or SOMETIMES. For number five, a problem is counted for either NEVER, RARELY, or SOMETIMES. The possible number of problems for Part I can range from 0 to 9. Problems are designated by a minus sign.

3. The five visual aptitude sentences are presented face to face at a distance of three to five feet, with a normal to slow articulatory rate and no voice. Client's oral responses are scored on the basis of whether or not the client identifies the thought or idea of the stimulus sentence. Minus signs are circled for sentences not identified.

4. For auditory aptitude, six CVC or CV items are presented. For each of the six items, the examiner asks the client to circle one of two words. The word is presented live voice in a quiet room at a distance of five feet. A perforated 5×8 card is held three inches from the examiner's mouth so that no visual cues can be received by the client. The minus sign is circled for each incorrect response.

5. AMAR scores are calculated as the total number of problems indicated on the test form.

6. Total time required for administration, scoring, and interpretation is approximately 15 minutes.

7. Scoring (according to present norms):
   00–10 PROBLEMS = NO NEED FOR AURAL REHABILITATION
   11–13 PROBLEMS = QUESTIONABLE NEED
   14–20 PROBLEMS = ABSOLUTE NEED

REFERENCE: Alpiner, J.G., Meline, N.C., and Cotton, A.D., An Aural Rehabilitation Screening Scale: Self Assessment, Auditory Aptitude, and Visual Aptitude. *J. Acad. Rehabilitative Audiology, 24, 1991.*

APPENDIX 10.10b *Alpiner-Meline Aural Rehabilitation (AMAR) Screening Scale*

Name: _____

Birthday: _____ Age: _____ SSN: _____

Hearing Aid Status (Circle one):
    NONE ITE BODY BONE EYEGLASS MONAURAL BINAURAL

Number of Years of hearing aid use: _____

Occupation: _____

Audiologist: _____ Date of Screening: _____

PART I: Self Assessment of Hearing Handicap

(Choose One)
A = Always   U = Usually   S = Sometimes   R = Rarely   N = Never

1. I feel like I am isolated from things because of my hearing loss.   A U S R N   + −

2. I feel very frustrated when I can not understand a conversation.   A U S R N   + −

3. My hearing loss has affected my life.   A U S R N   + −

4. I tend to avoid people because of my hearing loss.	A U S R N	+	−
5. People in general are tolerant of my hearing loss.	A U S R N	+	−
6. My hearing loss has affected my relationship with my spouse.	A U S R N	+	−
7. I try to hide my hearing loss from my co-workers.	A U S R N	+	−
8. My hearing loss has interfered with job performance.	A U S R N	+	−
9. I feel more pressure at work because of my hearing loss.	A U S R N	+	−

PART I PROBLEMS _____

PART II: Visual Aptitude

1. Good morning. .... + −
2. How old are you? .... + −
3. I live in (state of residence). .... + −
4. I only have a dollar. .... + −
5. There is somebody at the door. .... + −

PART II PROBLEMS _____

PART III: AUDITORY APTITUDE

1. FEW	CHEW..	+	−
2. FIT	KIT...	+	−
3. THIN	FIN...	+	−
4. THUMB	SUM...	+	−
5. TIE	THIGH	+	−
6. KICK	TICK..	+	−

PART III PROBLEMS _____

00–10 Problems = NO NEED
11–13 Problems = QUESTIONABLE NEED
14–20 Problems = ABSOLUTE NEED

TOTAL AMAR PROBLEMS _____

Jerome G. Alpiner, Ph.D., Nannette C. Meline, M.S., Amy D. Cotton, M.C.D.
VA Medical Center, Birmingham, Alabama (1990)

11

Hearing Aid Selection and Assessment

H. GUSTAV MUELLER, Ph.D., ALISON M. GRIMES, M.A.

One of the greatest challenges faced by the clinical audiologist is the selection and assessment of a specific amplification system for a given individual. Appropriate amplification forms the basis of the rehabilitation program for an individual with impaired hearing. Inadequate or inappropriate amplification will impede or doom the rehabilitation process even as it begins. It is important, therefore, to consider carefully in detail the hearing aid candidate himself or herself, the numerous characteristics of personal hearing aids, and the factors that are crucial in successfully linking the individual to the amplification device.

Changes in Hearing Aid Selection and Assessment

There have been many significant changes in hearing aid selection procedures in recent years. These changes have occurred in several areas and to a large extent have been fueled by the continued improvements in hearing aid technology.

FITTING INDIVIDUALS WHO HAVE MILD HEARING LOSS

Approximately 80% of the hearing aids sold in the United States are the in-the-ear (ITE) style, and of this total, over 20% are the even smaller in-the-canal (ITC) model (Kirkwood, 1991). The availability of smaller hearing aids, and the fact that a U.S. president used hearing aids, has encouraged more individuals with only mild hearing loss to use amplification. Consequently, hearing aid evaluation techniques have been required to adapt to this new hearing-impaired population. For example, many individuals fitted with hearing aids today have unaided speech recognition scores at or near 100%; therefore, the measurement of aided speech recognition in quiet often is not a useful evaluation procedure—unless one believes that the hearing aid will cause *reduced* speech recognition. Likewise, at one time the measurement of the patient's aided speech reception threshold (SRT) was considered a routine practice in hearing aid selection. Now, it is common to fit hearing aids to patients with unaided SRTs of 10 dB or better, and therefore, for these individuals, aided SRTs in quiet also are no longer a relevant measure.

IMPROVED HEARING AID CIRCUITRY

Advances in electronics and hearing aid circuitry also have influenced selection procedures. The ability to extend the hearing aid's frequency response into the 4000 to 6000 Hz range and beyond has encouraged measurement of this feature. Moreover, the increased use of noise reduction circuitry and automatic signal processing has necessitated the development of evaluation procedures to determine the effectiveness of these systems.

The development of digitally programmable hearing aids also is changing the way that hearing aids are selected and fitted. It is probable that by the year 2000, nearly all hearing aids dispensed will be programmable; many of these will have the capability to store four or more different programs for user selection. Selecting the appropriate electroacoustic characteristics for each unique listening situation and educating the patient concerning the use of these different programs pose new challenges for the audiologist.

POPULARITY OF CUSTOM HEARING AIDES

As previously mentioned, the majority of hearing aids fitted in the United States are custom instruments (i.e., ITE or ITC). When the behind-the-ear (BTE) hearing aid was the most popular hearing aid style, it was a common selection procedure to try two to four different hearing aids on a given patient in a single test session to determine the "best" hearing aid for that individual. It is not practical, however, to order several custom instruments for the same person. The traditional comparative hearing aid selection procedure, therefore, is difficult to implement in today's dispensing practice. Additionally, because of the smaller size of the custom instrument, there often is not room for several potentiometers allowing for gain, frequency, and power (SSPL) adjustments. Even when there is room for potentiometer placement, the range of adjustments usually is much less than available for the larger BTE instruments. Until programmable hearing aids become the standard fitting, these limitations will continue to influence the hearing aid evaluation.

The custom hearing aid style, therefore, has caused the evaluation at the time of the fitting to be more a verification process than a selection process. Much of the time and effort that once was expended at the time of the hearing aid fitting now must be redirected to the ordering process (Mueller, 1989; Mueller, 1992a).

PRESCRIPTIVE FITTING

In the 1960s and 1970s, much of the research regarding hearing aid selection concerned the differentiation of hearing aid performance using speech measures. In the past 10 to 15 years, however, a great deal of research has focused on prescriptive fitting techniques, that is, selecting the best hearing aid based on the amount of gain that it provides at given frequencies rather than selecting the hearing aid based on the patient's performance on a speech understanding task. Presently, the trend toward prescriptive fittings continues to the extent that many audiologists do not conduct any speech testing in conjunction with the fitting of hearing aids (Martin and Morris, 1989).

INSTRUMENTATION

In addition to digitally programmable systems, another major advancement in recent years in hearing aid related instrumentation is the development of the computerized probe-microphone equipment, which allows for the precise measurement of aided or unaided auditory signals in the ear canal. Prescriptive fitting techniques require verification of the hearing aid gain delivered at specific frequencies, and probe-microphone measures provide an efficient, reliable, and valid method of making these measures. This equipment, therefore, further encourages the use of prescriptive fitting procedures. Additionally, this equipment is partly responsible for taking the hearing aid selection and fitting procedure out of the test booth, as these measures can be made reliably in a mildly reverberant room. Hence, the home-visit hearing aid fitting, once scorned by degreed professionals, now can be conducted with a reasonable amount of reliability by using a portable probe-microphone system (assuming that the patient has undergone a complete audiologic evaluation in an appropriate sound-treated enclosure).

HEARING AID DELIVERY SYSTEM

Until the mid-1970s, the Code of Ethics of the American Speech and Hearing Association (ASHA) did not allow audiologists who were members to dispense hearing aids for profit. Now, the majority of ASHA-certified audiologists are involved in direct dispensing. Hearing aids, therefore, now are dispensed for profit from hospitals, private offices, and university clinics. Accordingly, the cost-effectiveness of the time expended for the hearing aid evaluation and selection process is more carefully scrutinized. Most private practice offices or hospital-based clinics do not have the luxury to conduct the 2-hour evaluations that were popular in the 1960s.

The preceding factors are not an inclusive listing but represent some of the major changes that have shaped present hearing aid selection procedures. The basic theoretical issues, and the overall process of hearing aid selection and fitting, however, have not changed significantly and can be divided into three general areas: *(1)* consideration of patient factors, *(2)* the selection of the electroacoustic characteristics of the hearing aid, and *(3)* the verification of the electroacoustic characteristics at the time of the hearing aid fitting. This chapter reviews the theoretical and clinical applications concerning these three major areas.

Prefitting Considerations

There are numerous patient factors to consider when fitting amplification to a given individual. Degree of hearing impairment, audiometric configuration, the loudness growth function, speech recognition ability, central auditory function, typical listening environment, motivation to use amplification, and other factors all have a potentially significant impact on the ultimate success of the hearing instruments. Failure to consider even a relatively minor patient factor often can result in an unsuccessful hearing aid fitting.

HEARING AID CANDIDACY

Who is a candidate for hearing aid use? This seemingly simple question is one of the most important and, unfortunately, one of the most commonly misunderstood issues in the area of hearing aid fitting. This section will focus on three of the most prominent patient factors: degree and nature of hearing loss, motivation to use hearing aids, and the effects of a central auditory processing deficit.

Degree of Hearing Loss

How much hearing loss must a person have before he or she can be considered a candidate for hearing aids? One could argue that patients are not candidates until they admit that they have a hearing handicap and seek out hearing aids of their own accord. This is the approach commonly used by general practice physicians, as this usually is the first contact the patient has concerning their communication problems. This logic may be faulty, however, as we will discuss in the section regarding patient motivation and hearing aid use. It is reasonable to believe, however, that regardless of patient motivation, it is the audiologist's responsibility to inform the patient that hearing aids are needed when the hearing loss has reached the point that the understanding of speech is impaired. Unfortunately, the commonly administered monosyllabic speech recognition scores (often obtained by presenting words at 30 to 40 dB sensation level under earphones) are a relatively poor predictor of communication difficulty, as individuals usually will continue to score within the normal range long after communication in real-life settings has suffered and hearing aids are needed.

An approach other than pure-tone or speech audiometry to determine hearing aid candidacy is to evaluate an individual's communication handicap using some type of self-assessment handicap scale. An example of this is the Hearing Handicap Index for the Elderly (HHIE) (Ventry & Weinstein, 1982). This simple 25-item test, or its 10-item short version (HHIE-S), has been used by many researchers and clinicians to document a person's perception of his or her hearing loss.

One impediment to the use of a self-assessment scale to determine hearing aid candidacy, however, is the not-uncommon situation of the "denier," that is, the patient with significant communication problems who nevertheless rates his or her handicap as being inconsequential. The use of this type of scale for determining hearing aid candidacy, without consideration of the pure-tone audiogram, will sometimes result in the failure to recommend hearing aids when in fact they might provide substantial benefit.

When the audiogram is viewed, it is useful to predict the potential handicap of a given hearing impairment by determining what proportion of the entire speech spectrum is audible to the patient. This approach requires a comparison of a patient's audiometric data to the known frequency/ intensity distribution of speech. It is helpful, therefore, to review some important aspects of the long-term spectrum of speech.

Speech Spectrum. The long-term speech spectrum has been extensively studied over the past 40 years. While it would seem logical to use a graphic representation of the average speech spectrum for hearing aid selection, this procedure is only recently becoming more commonly used. One reason for this may be that various research studies have reported conflicting data regarding the estimates of the levels and spectra of speech. Additionally, the speech spectra data often are not plotted in an audiogram format, making clinical applications somewhat cumbersome and requiring conversion procedures.

Olsen, Hawkins, and Van Tasell (1987) have published a review paper that compares many of the various calculations of the speech spectrum and provides several plottings of speech spectrum data from different studies on an audiogram format. Figure 11.1A illustrates the normal speech levels for males, females, and children based on the work of Pearsons, Bennett, and Fidell (1977). These average data show the speech spectra to be approximately 45 dB HL at 500 Hz, 30 to 40 dB HL from 1000 to 4000 Hz, and only 20 HL dB for the 6000 Hz range. Figure 11.1B is based on the work of Tyler (1979). This figure shows the intensity range of different types of speech sounds separated according to the manner of production. While the spectrum illustrated in Figure 11.1B is slightly different from that of Figure 11.1A, both figures clearly illustrate the reduction in intensity that occurs above 3000 Hz for important speech material.

The relatively low average speech spectra shown for the higher frequencies in Figure 11.1 points out several practical applications regarding hearing aid candidacy and hearing aid fittings. First, individuals with even a 30 to 40 dB impairment at 3000 to 4000 Hz have impaired speech understanding ability. Second, because these frequencies are important for speech intelligibility, it is critical that effective hearing aid gain is available in this region to make speech signals audible. Finally, because the speech

signals in this frequency range are relatively weak, even with amplification, it is often difficult to make these speech signals audible if the person has a severe hearing impairment.

Intensity Range of Speech Spectrum. When determining hearing aid candidacy—that is, whether a given hearing loss is handicapping—it is helpful to consider the range of average speech and the typical listening environments experienced by the patient. The data presented in Figure 11.1 represent average speech spectrum levels. Figure 11.2, also from the work of Pearsons et al. (1977), illustrates the variation of the speech spectrum averaged for five female talkers. It can be seen that the range between "casual" and "raised" speech is approximately 15 to 20 dB. As shown in this figure, people who are engaged in conversations using "casual-level" speech must rely on signals no more than 30 to 35 dB SPL for the frequencies above 2000 Hz (note that these values are SPL and would be less when converted to dB HL for direct comparison to the pure-tone thresholds plotted on the audiogram).

It is also important to consider the intensity of speech relative to the background noise in a particular environment. It is well known that background noise has a marked effect on speech understanding and that this effect seems to be more handicapping for the hearing impaired than for normal-hearing individuals (see Mueller & Hawkins, 1990, or Skinner, 1989 for review). One factor contributing to the speech-understanding-in-noise problem is that talkers do not typically raise their voices proportionally as the background noise increases. This relationship is shown in Figure 11.3, again taken from the work of Pearsons et al. (1977). As shown in this figure, people normally speak at 55 dB SPL for background noise up to 45 dB SPL; thus, a favorable signal-to-noise (S/N) ratio of at least +10 dB will exist. Hearing-impaired individuals usually do relatively well at a +10 dB S/N ratio if the speech spectrum has been made audible with hearing aids. The regression line in Figure 11.3, however, clearly illustrates that when the background noise becomes more intense, talkers raise their voices disproportionately. For example, when the background noise is 55 dB, av-

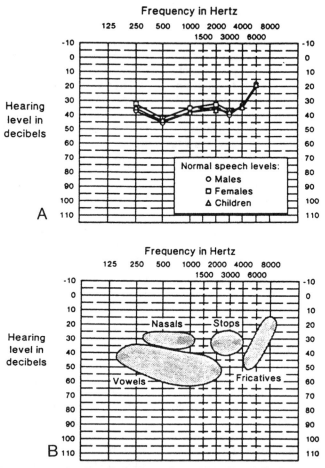

Figure 11.1. Normal speech levels (**A**) and distribution of speech sounds (**B**), both plotted in hearing level on audiogram form. (From Olsen, W., Hawkins, D., and Van Tasell, D., Representations of the long-term spectra of speech. *Ear Hear.,* 8(5), 1003–1085 [1987].)

erage speech is 61 dB (+6 dB S/N), and when the background noise reaches 65 dB, average speech is only 68 dB (+3 dB S/N). The S/N becomes 0 dB or worse when the background noise exceeds 75 dB. These data help explain the difficulties experienced by hearing-impaired people and must be considered in hearing aid selection, fitting, and postfitting counseling.

Articulation Index. Related to the preceding discussion of the relationship between the speech spectrum and an individual's hearing loss is the articulation index (AI). The AI is a calculation of what part of the total speech signal is available (audible) to the listener and is expressed in values ranging from 0.0 to 1.0. For calculation purposes, the speech signal is divided into intelligibility bands. The weighting of each band is determined by the proportion of speech energy that is provided in that band. Most of the present AI work is based on the original theory proposed by French and Steinberg (1947).

The advantage of the AI is that it provides a reasonable estimate of an individual's communication ability without conducting speech recognition testing. Given the unreliability of many speech recognition tests, and the variety of methods used to conduct these measures, it is possible that for some individuals the AI may be a better predictor of average speech understanding than the actual results of speech testing. The AI can be used in at least three different ways related to hearing aid fitting: *(1)* to determine candidacy based on the unaided AI; *(2)* to determine improvement by

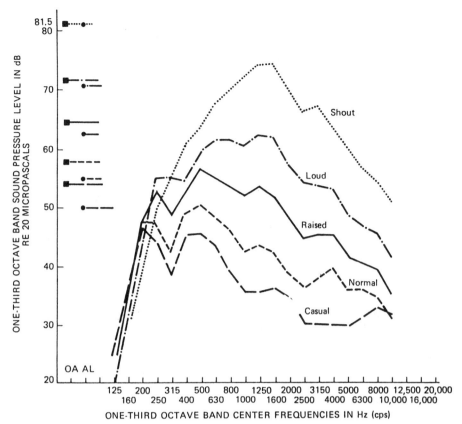

Figure 11.2 Average speech spectra for females measured at 1 meter from talker. (From Pearsons, K., Bennett, R., and Fidell, S., Speech levels in various noise environments. Project Report on Contract 68 01-2466. Washington DC, Office of Health and Ecological Effects, US. Environmental Protection Agency [1977].)

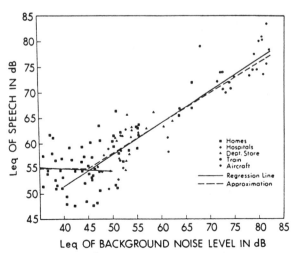

Figure 11.3 Relationship between level of speech as a function of level of background noise for five different environments. (From Pearsons, K., Bennett, R., and Fidell, S., Speech levels in various noise environments. Project Report on Contract 68 01-2466. Washington DC, Office of Health and Ecological Effects, U.S. Environmental Protection Agency [1977].)

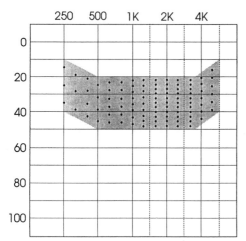

Figure 11.4 Count-the-dot audiogram for estimation of articulation index. (From Mueller, H., and Killion, M., An easy method for calculating the articulation index. *Hear. J.,* 43, 14–17 [1990].)

comparing the aided versus unaided AI; and *(3)* to help select the "best" hearing aid by comparing aided AIs from different hearing instruments.

Some researchers have divided the speech spectrum into as many as 20 bands for the purposes of AI calculation. By varying the width of these bands it is possible to assign an equal weight of 0.05 to each band. For clinical purposes, it is convenient to use bands that have the common frequencies of the clinical audiometer as their center frequency. Popelka and Mason (1987) have suggested using this approach, and they present a nine-band calculation procedure. Pavlovic (1988) also developed a simplified version of the AI calculation for clinical use. He advocated using only four frequencies (500, 1000, 2000, and 4000 Hz) and assigning equal weight to each frequency.

Another AI procedure that is relatively very simple to implement clinically has been proposed by Mueller and Killion (1990) and is based on the count-the-dot method of Cavanaugh et al. (1962). This procedure assigns different weights to each frequency band; as shown in Figure 11.4, the weighting is reflected in the density of the dots for 15 different frequency regions across the speech spectrum. One hundred dots are displayed on the chart. The AI simply is calculated by assigning 0.01 to each dot that is audible (those falling above the

threshold plot) for a given patient. Perhaps a better name for this procedure would be the *Audibility Index,* which conveniently also is *AI.* One advantage of this AI calculation method is that fluctuations in gain at 1500 and 3000 Hz, common areas for concern in the hearing aid fitting, will be accounted for in the AI calculation. Pavlovic (1991) and Humes (1991) also have developed count-the-dot methods of AI calculation.

The speech spectrum and the AI are directly related to candidacy for hearing aids. If a patient has a hearing loss that prevents audibility of the complete speech spectrum, this person is a hearing aid candidate. If a hearing aid amplifies the speech spectrum appropriately, improvement in speech understanding is probable. Regarding the general notion of using the AI in place of actual speech recognition measures, it is true that simple audibility of a speech signal does not guarantee understanding; however, as pointed out by Pascoe (1980), "it is even more true that without detection, the probabilities of correct identification are greatly diminished."

Motivation of the Patient

After an individual has been identified as a hearing aid candidate based on the degree and nature of the hearing impairment, a second consideration is the motivation of the patient to use hearing aids. Like most other prosthetic devices, hearing aids are a visible indication of a handicap and generally are associated with aging. It is not unexpected, therefore, that many individuals in need of hearing aids postpone the fitting and attempt to convince others that they can "get by" without the use of amplification. Appropriate guidance and encouragement from audiologists obviously are necessary. At least one study, however, has suggested that hearing-impaired individuals are not receiving the proper professional guidance.

The Hearing Industries Association (HIA) conducted a large survey that included 1050 hearing-impaired adults who did not own hearing aids. The survey revealed that of the persons who discussed their problem with more than one professional, only 15% reported receiving a consistent recommendation regarding whether they should use hearing aids. Hearing aid use was recommended for only 7% of these individuals, yet reportedly, the reason for the consultation was that the patient was experiencing communication problems. Specifically, for those individuals stating that they went to an "ear doctor" for an opinion, 11% were told to use hearing aids, 34% were told not to use hearing aids, and the remaining 55% reported that *no recommendation* concerning hearing aid use was given.

Is it possible that an individual who was not otherwise motivated to try hearing aids could be persuaded to do so by an audiologist? Will this person subsequently use and benefit from hearing aids? To some extent, these questions were answered by research by Mueller and Bender (1988). These authors surveyed 300 new hearing aid users 12 to 14 months after they received hearing aids to determine if the reason that they obtained hearing aids had a long-term effect on hearing aid use or benefit. Mueller and Bender reported that at the time of the original hearing aid fitting, three factors were listed most commonly by the subjects as having a "strong influence" on the decision to obtain hearing aids. These factors were communication problems (reported by 65% of the respondents), followed by encouragement from spouse (54%) and direction from a medical professional, usually an audiologist or an otolaryngologist (44%).

After the hearing aid use period of 12 to 14 months, 208 patients responded. Table 11.1 shows the distribution for these respondents for the three main factors. The "X" designator shows what factor(s) each group reported as a strong influence. For example, 43 individuals cited all three factors as a strong influence (Group A), whereas 28 respondents did not consider any of the three factors a strong influence (Group H). Of primary interest were the responses from the three groups that reported only one of the main factors as a strong influence (Groups D, F, and G). Shown in Figure 11.5 are the use and benefit ratings for these three groups. Observe that 72% of the patients in Group D report using their hearing aids more than 60% of the average day. This value is substantially larger than the other two groups and is somewhat predictable—one might expect the pa-

Table 11.1
Distribution for the Three Most Common Reasons for Obtaining Hearing Aids

Group	N	Communication Problems	Encouragement From Spouse	Direction From Professional
A	43	X[a]	X	X
B	39	X	X	
C	25	X		X
D	29	X		
E	11		X	X
F	20		X	
G	13			X
H	28			

[a] Factors marked with "X" represent "strong influence" ratings. Subjects were allowed to list more than one factor as strong influence or no factor as strong influence.
Source: McCarthy, P., Montgomery, A., and Mueller, H., Decision making in rehabilitative audiology. *J. Am. Acad. Audiol.*, 1(1), 23–30 (1990).

tientsreporting communication difficulty to use their hearing aids the most. When hearing aid benefit is examined, however, observe that Group G (encouragement from professional) has the same percent of subjects reporting the hearing aid to be "very beneficial" as Group D. It would appear, therefore, that long-term hearing aid benefit is not necessarily related to self-motivation.

The overall motivation of a patient to use hearing aids clearly is a contributing factor for successful hearing aid use. Fortunately, this factor can be influenced significantly by the advice of medical professionals. The results of the HIA survey show that this usually will be an audiologist, otolaryngologist, or family practice physician. Because nearly everyone with a hearing loss benefits from hearing aids, it is clearly important that this fact is related to the patient in a positive manner.

Central Auditory Processing Deficit

A final patient factor that can have an impact on the success of the hearing aid fitting is whether the patient has a central auditory processing deficit (CAPD). Although it is unlikely that hearing aids would be withheld from a patient because of a CAPD, it is probable that knowledge of this deficit would alter the dispenser's expecta-

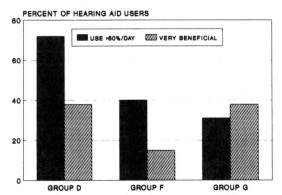

Figure 11.5 Percentage of respondents reporting greater than 60% average hearing aid use per day, and percentage of respondents rating their hearing aids as "very beneficial" for three selected groups. (See Table 11.1 for group description.) (From McCarthy, P., Montgomery, A., and Mueller, H., Decision making in rehabilitative audiology. *J. Am. Acad. Audiol.,* 1(1), 23–30 [1990].)

tions regarding hearing aid benefit and satisfaction (Davies & Mueller, 1987). In some cases, it is even possible that a different type of amplification device would be selected.

The presence of CAPD in older individuals is sometimes referred to as central presbycusis. Given that this older population comprises a large proportion of hearing aid candidates, it is relevant to ask, what is the prevalence of central presbycusis for this group? Recently, this has been studied by Stach, Spretnjak, and Jerger (1990), and these results are shown in Figure 11.6. By conducting different types of speech testing, Stach and his coworkers defined patterns of test results that identified individuals as having central presbycusis. This testing was conducted on two different samples: patients referred to the audiology clinic for routine evaluation (clinical sample) and individuals of a similar age range who simply volunteered to participate in the project (nonclinical sample). As expected, and as shown in Figure 11.6, the prevalence of CAPD is greater for the clinical sample. It is important to observe, however, that even for the nonclinical sample, CAPD occurs frequently in individuals in their sixties, and it can be expected in more than 50% of the patients over the age of 75.

Given the high prevalence noted by Stach et al. (1990), it would seem reasonable to conduct some type of central auditory speech testing prior to the hearing aid fitting to identify these individuals. The purpose of implementing this testing would be based on the notion that patients with

CAPD will experience less favorable results with hearing aids than the average patient.

One of the earliest investigations of the issues surrounding aging, central auditory dysfunction, and hearing aid use was conducted by Hayes and Jerger (1979). They reported that elderly subjects with both peripheral and central deficits perform less well with amplification than do individuals with peripheral loss alone. Hayes and Jerger noted that central auditory effects, while more pronounced in difficult listening conditions, may exist in any listening situation, limiting the overall success with hearing aids. Significantly, Hayes and Jerger noted that while a central auditory problem may limit benefit from hearing aids in some listening situations, central impairment does not preclude effective hearing aid use. They wrote that "the key is realistic counseling" (p. 40).

Stach (1990) reported on the results of a survey that measured hearing aid benefit for a group of hearing aid users matched for age and hearing loss. The subjects differed significantly, however, on their unaided performance on a central auditory speech task (the Synthetic Sentence Identification test), which caused them to be placed in either the "peripheral" or "central" group. Stach reported that the distribution of the benefit ratings from the peripheral group were centered in the "very helpful" and "often helpful" categories, whereas the ratings from the central group were more variable, and importantly, the most common rating was "no benefit."

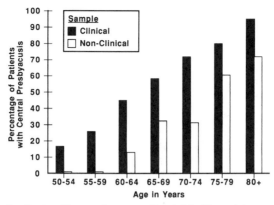

Figure 11.6   Percentage of patients with speech audiometric results consistent with central presbyacusis in clinical sample (N = 700) and nonclinical sample (N = 138) as function of age. (From Stach B., Spretnjak, M., and Jerger, J., The prevalence of central presbyacusis in a clinical population. *J. Am. Acad. Audiol.*, 1(2), 109–115 [1990].)

Similar findings to those of Stach (1990) were reported in a study by Mueller and Calkins (1988). These authors administered the Dichotic Sentence Identification (DSI) test to 135 new hearing aid users at the time that they were fitted with binaural hearing aids. Patient ratings obtained 6 to 9 months after the fitting revealed that the individuals who performed poorly on the DSI also reported less benefit and satisfaction from the hearing aids (age and hearing loss was matched for the two groups). Of interest, the "low DSI score" group reported the *greatest* use of binaural amplification.

The DSI works reasonably well for screening for CAPD with the hearing impaired, as both individual ear and double correct scores can be computed, and it is more resistant to peripheral hearing loss than most other CAP tests. The reliability of the test has been questioned, however, and this factor should be considered before categorizing a patient as having a CAPD (Cokely & Humes, 1992).

The findings from the above studies suggest that patients with CAPD may be "at risk" for poorer performance than expected with hearing aids. If these people are identified at the time of the hearing aid fitting, they can be targeted for additional aural rehabilitation and hearing aid related counseling. In some of the more severe cases, it may be necessary to take a more proactive approach and fit these individuals with assistive listening devices (ALDs) rather than traditional hearing aids (see Stach, 1990b, for a discussion of this approach).

HEARING AID STYLE

A preselection decision that relates directly to the patient's willingness to wear hearing aids is the selection of hearing aid style. In recent years, the custom hearing aid, the ITE or the ITC, has replaced the behind-the-ear (BTE) as the standard hearing aid fitting (see Mueller, 1992a, for review). This growth in custom hearing aid sales has been fueled by the demand from the consumer for a smaller, less visible hearing aid. Some audiologists have been reluctant to switch from the use of the BTE model, as they believe that the circuitry and flexibility of this style outweighs the potential cosmetic advantage of the smaller custom instrument. While there remain some definite advantages of the BTE style (e.g., direct audio input, more flexibility, more powerful telephone coil), the majority of patients can be fitted successfully, at least from an electroacoustic standpoint, with an ITE or ITC hearing aid. Whenever possible, therefore, it is probably best to allow the patient to choose the hearing aid style.

When new hearing aid users are allowed to select their hearing aid style, over 90% will choose an ITE over a BTE (Mueller & Budinger, 1990). It is often possible, however, to convince a given patient that a specific style is "really the best for you" during the prefitting counseling session. This instilled belief probably will be short-lived. Mueller et al. (1991) surveyed a group of people fitted with ITEs and a separate group of individuals fitted with BTEs. The patients had been arbitrarily placed in the ITE

Table 11.2
Hearing Aid Users' Ratings of the Other Style of Hearing Aid[a]

	Agree		Disagree	
	BTE Users	ITE Users	BTE Users	ITE Users
1. The other style of hearing aid would be less obvious to others.	94	2	2	91
2. The other style of hearing aid would cause less interference with my glasses.	94	0	2	93
3. The other style of hearing aid is more modern.	88	0	0	93
4. I would use my hearing aid(s) more if I had the other style of hearing aid.	80	0	10	91
5. The other style of hearing aid would be more comfortable to wear.	70	5	0	54
6. I would be more apt to use two hearing aids if I had the other style of hearing aids.	68	0	4	88
7. The other style of hearing aid would be easier to insert and remove.	58	14	4	68
8. The other style of hearing aid would be more stable.	46	0	0	41
9. The other style of hearing aid is more durable.	41	2	4	23
10. I could understand speech better with the other style of hearing aid.	26	2	0	51
11. The other style of hearing aid has better electronics.	24	7	0	32
12. The other style of hearing aid would have fewer repair problems.	24	0	2	22

[a] Percent BTE ($n = 52$) and ITE ($n = 43$) users responding in each category for the twelve statements. The "other style" refers to the instrument the patient was *not* fitted with.
Source: Mueller H., Bryant, M., Brown, W., and Budinger, A., Hearing aid selection for high-frequency hearing loss. In G. Studebaker, F. Bess, and L. Beck (Eds.), The Vanderbilt Hearing-Aid Report II. Parkton, MD: York Press (1991).

or BTE group at the time of their hearing aid fitting. Six months after the hearing aids were given to the patients, they were asked questions about the *other* style, that is, the style that they were *not* fitted with. As shown in Table 11.2, the responses overwhelmingly favor the ITE style. It appears that people fitted with ITE hearing aids continue to favor this style, whereas people fitted with the BTE style believe that they received an inferior product.

These findings suggest that overall satisfaction with hearing aids will be enhanced if the patient is allowed to choose the hearing aid style. Their choice, of course, will almost always be an ITE rather than a BTE. Fortunately, in most cases the ITE hearing aid fitting will satisfy the patient's amplification needs; digitally programmable circuitry now is available in ITE and *ITC* models, which enhances the flexibility of

these instruments. The patients with more severe hearing loss who need the amplification provided by a BTE instrument will accept this style following counseling and a trial period to demonstrate the advantages.

HEARING AID ARRANGEMENT

Hearing aid arrangement, encompassing options such as monaural versus binaural, or the use of a CROS/BICROS system is an important consideration in determining how to proceed with amplification for a given patient. The fitting arrangement can determine if amplification is successful and accepted by the patient.

Binaural Versus Monaural

Should a patient with a bilateral loss of hearing be fitted with one or two hearing aids? While logic dictates that two hearing aids would be fitted whenever there are two aidable ears, sales statistics reveal that approximately 50% of people are fitted monaurally (Cranmer, 1991). It also has been shown that many patients choose a monaural fitting because an audiologist or other medical professional informed them that they "could get by with only one hearing aid" (Mueller, 1986). It is perhaps helpful, therefore, to review briefly some of the major advantages of binaural hearing aid uses.

Elimination of Head Shadow. Monaural hearing aid fittings may result in attenuation of important high-frequency speech signals by as much as 12 to 16 dB if they originate from the nonaided side of the head. Because these high-frequency speech signals have relatively low intensity (see Fig. 11.1), the head-shadow effect may render them inaudible. With binaural fittings, a talker positioned on either side of the listener is always speaking into a hearing aid microphone, and the head shadow is thereby eliminated (assuming relatively equal hearing loss for each ear).

Loudness Summation. Binaural hearing aids allow for the summing of two signals, resulting in binaural thresholds that are approximately 3 dB better than monaural. The summation effect can be several decibels greater than this for suprathreshold levels. Theoretically, therefore, binaural users require less gain from each hearing aid, reducing the chances of exceeding loudness discomfort level (LDL), and reducing the occurrence of acoustic feedback.

Binaural Squelch. When speech and noise are presented binaurally, an improvement in S/N over a similar monaural presentation occurs. This S/N improvement is approximately 2 to 3 dB (see Mueller & Hawkins, 1990). For listening situations that are either very easy or very difficult, this improvement may not be very noticeable to the hearing aid user. For listening situations where the user is understanding only portions of the speech message (e.g., around the 50% point of the articulation function), a 2 to 3 dB improvement in the S/N can result in a 30 to 40% improvement in speech intelligibility.

Localization. Localization of sound in the horizontal plane is dependent on interaural differences in intensity, time, and phase. A monaural fitting disrupts this relationship and in fact might cause localization to be poorer than if the person were unaided. Binaural hearing aids enhance localization over a monaural fitting.

Wider Dynamic Range. As previously stated, binaural hearing lowers a person's threshold due to binaural summation. The patient's loudness discomfort level (LDL), however, is not significantly different for a binaural signal than for a monaural one (Hawkins 1986). The dynamic range, therefore, becomes larger, which is especially helpful for patients with reduced LDLs.

Other advantages of binaural hearing aid use include improved quality of speech and "spatial balance." Given these numerous advantages, and the fact that most hearing-impaired people are binaural candidates, it is surprising that so many patients are fitted monaurally. It could be argued that the cost of a second hearing aid is the major cause of this discrepancy; however, Mueller (1986) reports that even when hearing aids were provided free of charge (as an entitlement for military service) only 43% of the patients chose a binaural fitting. This suggests that several other factors influence the decision to choose a monaural fitting. Mueller and Reeder (1987) and McCarthy, Montgomery, and Mueller (1990) have reported that patient counseling at the time of hearing aid selection and fitting can have a significant influence on the use of and benefit from binaural hearing aids.

Given the numerous advantages of binaural hearing aids, it is clear that this should be considered the standard fitting for nearly everyone. Moderately asymmetric hearing losses are not a major factor, as reasonable success can be obtained with up to 30 dB of *aided* asymmetry. Financial constraints must be considered, although most individuals will pay the extra money if they believe improved communication will result. Regrettably, many third-party reimbursement agencies are narrow-minded on their views of binaural amplification.

CROS/BICROS

For the individual who has an unaidable hearing loss in one ear, and normal hearing or an aidable hearing loss in the other ear, some type of contralateral routing of signal amplification might be the most appropriate hearing aid arrangement. In general, this arrangement is designed to allow the person to have two-sided hearing, although all signals are channeled into a single ear. This arrangement would be a Contralateral Routing of Signal (CROS) hearing aid for the person with normal or near-normal hearing in one ear and an unaidable hearing loss in the other ear (based on pure-tone sensitivity or disproportionate loss in speech recognition ability). For the person with an aidable hearing loss in one ear and an unaidable loss in the other ear, a Bilateral Contralateral Routing of Signals (BI-CROS) arrangement may be most beneficial. A complete discussion of CROS-type amplification can be found in a review by Pollack (1975).

More recently, a new method of CROS amplification has been discussed (Sullivan, 1988). The concept is "transcranial" amplification, provided by a high-gain ITE hearing instrument fitted to an audiometrically "dead" ear, which provides amplification to the better ear via bone conduction crossover. An intriguing concept, to date, this CROS fitting approach has not been systematically studied on a large number of subjects.

SPECIAL CIRCUITRY

Prior to selecting the gain and output characteristics of the hearing aids, it is necessary to determine if special circuitry is needed. Most commonly, decisions are made regarding the use of compression circuitry or automatic signal processing (ASP). As programmable hearing aids continue to grow in popularity, this feature also must be considered routinely.

Compression

Compression circuitry is a method to automatically lower or limit the gain output of hearing aids. Compression can be single channel or multichannel and can be input or output controlled (for review see Preves, 1991). Walker and Dillon (1982) categorize compression circuitry into three types: compression limiting, whole-range syllabic compression, and slow-acting automatic volume control (AVC). Compression limiting frequently is used in place of peak clipping to limit SSPL90 without producing significant harmonic distortion (Mueller & Hawkins, 1990). Whole-range syllabic compression is used to place the amplified speech signal into the narrowed dynamic range of the hearing aid user. Slow-acting AVC systems, not widely used in hearing aids, will automatically alter the gain of the hearing aid for different listening environments.

Given that nearly all individuals fitted with hearing aids have a nonlinear hearing loss (abnormal loudness growth), it is surprising that the majority of audiologists fit their patients with linear instruments. Compression limiting has distinct advantages over peak clipping as a method to limit SSPL90. The additional cost of compression circuitry is minimal, and this feature should be considered for the majority of hearing aid candidates.

Automatic Signal Processing

Hearing aid circuitry that automatically changes the frequency response of the hearing aid as a function of the input signal is termed automatic signal processing or ASP circuits (see Fabry, 1991; Mueller & Hawkins, 1992). Generally, ASP hearing aids are Level-Dependent Frequency Response circuits (Killion, Stab, & Preves, 1990). In the past, the most commonly used ASP circuits reduced gain in the low-frequency region as the intensity of the input signal increased. This type of circuit is referred to as a BILL (Base Increases at Low Levels, or base decreases at high levels) circuit. An alternative approach in ASP circuits is the TILL (Treble Increases at Low Levels, or treble decreases at high levels) circuit. This type of circuit is exemplified in the K-AMP (Killion, 1988), which provides relatively more high-frequency amplification at low-input levels, with a relative decrease in treble as the input intensity of the signal increases. The third type of ASP circuit, the PILL (Programmable Increases at Low Level), will be discussed in the following section on digitally programmable hearing aids.

There is not a straightforward method to decide which patients should receive ASP hearing aids. Like compression instruments, the additional cost is minimal, and ASP circuitry probably could be used more often than it is. In general, the patients who will benefit the greatest from this circuitry are those who have a moderate hearing loss, are actively involved in communication with others, and experience a variety of listening environments. Importantly, these circuits do not *eliminate* background noise, but they might allow for some improvement in speech understanding, or at least more relaxed listening, for speech-in-noise conditions.

Digitally Programmable Hearing Aids

Digitally programmable hearing aids, currently offered by 10 or more different hearing aid manufacturers (Bentler, 1991), offer a degree of flexibility in the hearing aid fitting process that is not available in conventional hearing aids. Depending on the design of the particular instrument, factors such as adjustable compression knees and ratios, two or three adjustable frequency bands, several memory locations for stored programs, BILL/TILL level-dependent ASP, and several other features are available to the audiologist for manipulation and modification at the time of the hearing aid fitting. This is accomplished via the use of some type of digital programming system (handheld programmer, personal computer, specialized hearing aid software) to set the particular electroacoustic characteristics of the hearing aid. Once the hearing aid is disconnected from the programmer, it functions as an analogue hearing aid. It is important, therefore, to characterize these instruments as "digitally programmable" rather than "digital" hearing aids.

Programmable hearing aids allow the audiologist to control many of the electroacoustic parameters critical to the success of the fitting, something that previously was not possible with custom-made ITE and ITC instruments. By coupling programmable hearing aids with probe-microphone measurements, hearing aids can be fitted with a level of preciseness that previously was not possible. The use of programmable hearing aids is growing rapidly, and in a few years, the question will not be *whether* a patient should be fitted with a programmable instrument but rather *what type* of programmable instrument should be selected.

Selection of Electroacoustic Features

Following the preselection decisions regarding hearing aid style, fitting arrangement, special circuitry, and other factors unique to each patient, it is necessary to make specific electroacoustic decisions pertaining to the instrument to be fitted. In the common case of a nonprogrammable ITE- or ITC-style fitting, these decisions are then related to the manufacturer so that the hearing aids can be constructed accordingly. In general, there are two main areas of hearing aid design that must be considered when the hearing aid is selected: selection of the gain/frequency response and the maximum power output (SSPL90).

SELECTION OF GAIN/FREQUENCY RESPONSE

In the overall hearing aid selection and fitting procedure, the selection and verification of the hearing aid's frequency response usually commands the most time and attention. For more than 50 years, researchers have sought to define and verify methods for selecting the best hearing aid frequency response for a given patient's hearing loss. Unfortunately, even today unanimity has not been attained on such basic issues as what unaided measures best predict gain requirements, how much gain is need relative to the hearing loss, or whether speech audiometry should be used to verify the fitting. There is not even a consensus on whether the frequency response should be selected by the audiologist, the manufacturer, or the patient himself or herself.

In general, audiologists usually select the hearing aid's frequency response either by informally making an estimate of required gain across frequencies based on the patient's pure-tone audiogram or by using some type of a formal prescriptive fitting approach.

Informal Prescriptive Procedures

What is meant by an informal prescriptive procedure? In general, this term is used to describe the selection of a hearing aid's frequency response using unaided measures (usually the audiogram) as a guideline but without actually computing desired gain or output values. For example, it is probable that most audiologists would select a hearing aid with little or no gain at 500 to 1000 Hz for someone with normal hearing at these frequencies. The fact that usually a hearing aid with significant gain in the low frequencies is not even considered for this type of hearing loss suggests that some form of a prescriptive fitting is being used, whether or not it is formally recognized as such.

According to the survey of Martin and Morris (1989), 29% of audiologists do not use a formal prescriptive method for the selection of the frequency response. This could be for a variety of reasons. From a theoretical standpoint, it is reasonable to believe that not everyone with the same hearing loss will derive the same benefit from hearing aids with identical frequency responses. This logic, of course, is one of the underlying reasons for favoring the comparative selection approach. A second contributing factor is that some experienced audiologists believe that their accumulated knowledge on the relationship between frequency response and user acceptance negates the necessity of a formal prescriptive method.

As discussed by Mueller (1992a), perhaps the main factor that prevents audiologists from using formal prescriptive methods is the manner in which custom hearing aids can be ordered. Recall that custom instruments account for approximately 80% of hearing aid sales nationwide. Manufacturers will construct a custom hearing aid based simply on a pure-tone audiogram. Surveys have shown that 85 to 90% of custom instruments are ordered using this method (Bratt & Sammeth, 1991; Valente, Valente, & Vass, 1990). This indirect selection procedure, of course, relieves the audiologist from making any major decisions regarding the hearing aid's frequency response.

Overall, the past 10 to 15 years have shown a gradual shift from the comparative approach to informal prescriptive methods to formal prescription methods. It is probable that the increased use of digital technology, programmable hearing aids, and computerized probe-microphone measurements will stimulate further the move to more formalized prescriptive methods.

Formal Selection Procedures

Most users of a formal prescriptive method ascribe to the belief that the frequency responses that will maximize speech understanding can be predicted from the unaided auditory measures (e.g., pure-tone thresholds, loudness growth functions). The previously mentioned survey of Martin and Morris (1989) revealed that 71% of audiologists are using some type of formalized prescriptive fitting procedure. The most popular method at the time that the survey was conducted (March–June 1988) was POGO (Prescription of Gain/Output) (McCandless & Lyregaard, 1983). The Australian National Acoustic Laboratories (NAL) procedure (Byrne & Dillon, 1986) has become more widely used since the time of the Martin and Morris survey and probably rivals POGO in popularity today. The Desired Sensation Level (DSL) of Seewald (1992) has been used primarily with children but also has direct application to adults; its use also is increasing among audiologists.

Several other well-researched prescriptive fitting procedures, which easily could be argued as equal or superior to POGO, the NAL or the DSL, also are available for clinical use. Hawkins (1992a) reviewed the most commonly used prescriptive fitting methods and provided guidance for conducting the calculations. Humes (1986), Byrne (1987), and Humes and Hackett (1990) also provide a review and evaluation of many of the popular fitting techniques.

The use of formalized prescriptive methods has increased significantly in recent years. At least four factors have contributed to this increase: *(1)* the awareness of the unreliability of comparative aided speech audiometry; *(2)* the greater availability and promotion of prescriptive fitting approaches; *(3)* the increase in custom hearing aid fitting (this type of fitting does not lend itself to the comparative approach, as it is unreasonable to order multiple custom instruments for every patient); and *(4)* the development of computerized probe-microphone measures, which have facilitated the real-ear verification of hearing aid performance.

Table 11.3
Calculation of Desired 2-cm³ Coupler Gain Using the NAL Prescriptive Method

	Frequency (Hz)					
	0.5k	1k	1.5k	2k	3k	4k
Pure-tone thresholds	35	40	45	45	50	50
Prescribed REIG (re: NAL)	9	19	21	19	20	20
Average CORFIG (ITE)	0	0	0	2	6	0
Desired 2-cm³ at use VCW	9	19	21	21	26	20
Reserve gain	10	10	10	10	10	10
Desired full-on cm³ coupler gain	19	29	31	31	36	30

Source: Mueller, H., Individualizing the ordering of custom hearing aids. In H. Mueller, D. Hawkins, and J. Northern (Eds.), Probe Microphone Measurements. San Diego, CA: Singular Publishing Group (1992).

Again, assuming that most patients are fitted with custom ITE hearing aids, prescriptive methods conveniently can be used to select a desired response from the manufacturer's matrix book. Once a prescriptive method has been selected, minor mathematical calculations must be made to determine the desired gain at each frequency. A second step is to add reserve gain—most methods suggest using 10 to 15 dB across frequencies. For patients with unusual ear canal resonance or concha effects, it might be necessary to adjust the desired gain accordingly (see Mueller, 1989, 1992a for a review of these procedures). Finally, desired gain levels are then converted to 2-cm³ coupler values, using either average corrections or direct measurement, to facilitate the selection of a frequency response matrix or the explanation of the requested response to the manufacturer. Table 11.3, from Mueller (1992a), is an example of this procedure using the NAL method and 2-cm³ coupler corrections from Hawkins (1992b).

SELECTION OF SSPL90

It often has been suggested that the leading reason for rejection of hearing aids is that the hearing aid's maximum power exceeds the user's loudness discomfort level. The terms *loudness discomfort level (LDL), uncomfortable loudness level (UCL)* and *threshold of discomfort (TD)* are often used interchangeably and refer to the loudness level at which a patient cannot tolerate sound for more than a brief period. It is a level that is below painfully loud but above comfortably loud. As explained by Bentler (1989), not all sounds become uncomfort-

able at the same intensity. It could be argued, therefore, that when referring to the uncomfortable intensity, "threshold" is a more appropriate term than "level."

It is unfortunate that excessive output contributes significantly to hearing aid rejection, as for the most part this undesired outcome can be avoided when the hearing aid is selected and fitted. Although compression circuitry and automatic signal processing are becoming more common in the routine hearing aid fitting, linear circuits probably will continue to control a large share of the market for several years. Regardless of the type of hearing aid output limiting circuitry, a simple task is to assure that the output delivered in the ear canal when the hearing aid is in saturation (maximum output) does not exceed the LDL for the patient (Mueller & Hawkins, 1990).

Clinical Measurement of the LDL

Several procedural factors must be considered when LDL measures are conducted. For example, the LDL of an individual patient may vary by as much as 20 to 30 dB, depending on whether the instructions to the patient use the term "painfully loud" or a term such as "annoying." Patient instructions, therefore, must be easy to understand, must be consistent, and must accurately describe the loudness rating that is desired. Much of the work concerning clinical LDL measures has been conducted by Hawkins and colleagues, and these authors have provided sample patient instructions for use in LDL measures (Hawkins et al., 1987). These instructions are recommended for use in conjunction with descriptive anchors that relate to the different

---
Levels of Loudness

Painfully Loud
Extremely Uncomfortable
Uncomfortably Loud
Loud, But O.K.
Comfortable, But Slightly Loud
Comfortable
Comfortable, But Slightly Soft
Soft
Very Soft

Figure 11.7 Descriptive anchors used for making loudness judgments when conducting loudness discomfort level measurements. (From Hawkins, D., Reflections on amplification: validation of performance. *J. Acad. Rehab. Audiol.,* 18, 42–54 [1985].)

loudness judgments; Figure 11.7 presents an example of these descriptive anchors. One clinical method of administration is to provide the patient a chart showing these anchors; the patient then only has to point to the term that best describes the loudness of the signal. Figure 11.8 illustrates the use of this test approach for earphone LDL measurements.

In addition to considering the instructions and the use of descriptive anchors, the type of stimulus employed also is an important variable in LDL measures. The most common, but not necessarily the most appropriate, stimulus used for these measurements is a live-voice speech signal. Usually selected because of simplicity and convenience, the use of a speech signal makes the assumption that it is speech, with its maximum energy centered in the lower frequencies, that most frequently causes the hearing aid user loudness discomfort problems. Although this may be true with some patients, environmental sounds, especially those with energy peaks at midfrequencies, also contribute significantly to user complaints of loudness discomfort, and the SSPL90 of the hearing aid must be selected or adjusted accordingly.

For the above reasons, we believe it is necessary to measure unaided LDLs at several frequency regions throughout the range of amplification. A reasonable procedure is to conduct LDL measures using a frequency-specific stimulus (e.g., pulsed pure tones, narrow-band noise), for 500, 1000, 1500, 2000, 3000, and 4000 Hz.

Selection of Desired SSPL90

Following the clinical measurement of LDLs across the frequency range for a given patient, it is then necessary to use these values to select the desired SSPL90 for the hearing aid. If the clinical LDL measurements were conducted using standard earphones, it is necessary to convert from HL/6-cm³ to SPL/2-cm³. Several research studies have addressed the 6-cm³ to 2-cm³ to real-ear differences (e.g., Bentler & Pavlovic, 1988; Cox, 1986; Hawkins, 1992b,c; Sachs & Burkhard, 1972), and correction values have been provided for this purpose. There is considerable variation, however, from patient to patient due to such factors as earphone placement, ear canal resonance, middle ear impedance, hearing aid style, and microphone location. Skinner (1988) reported that average correction values between 750 and 2000 Hz appear to be reasonably reliable, as they are least affected by these variables.

To circumvent the potential errors that occur when average corrections are used, it is best to make direct measurements, which can be accomplished easily with probe-microphone equipment (see Hawkins & Mueller, 1992a, for test protocol). By disabling the loudspeaker of the equipment, the probe-microphone can be used to measure directly the ear canal SPL at the patient's LDL for a given frequency. Then, using a hearing aid with a fixed volume control wheel (VCW) setting, a real-ear to coupler difference (RECD) can be measured for each frequency of interest. The RECD values, added to the real-ear LDL in SPL, will provide the desired 2-cm³ SSPL90. The appropriate circuitry then can be selected from the manufacturer's matrix book. Hawkins (1992c) describes this procedure in detail.

Verification of the Fitting

Following the selection of a hearing aid's frequency response and SSPL90 for a given individual, it is necessary to verify that the individual's performance with the hearing aid meets some predetermined standard of goodness. The need for verification is reduced as a function of the thought and effort

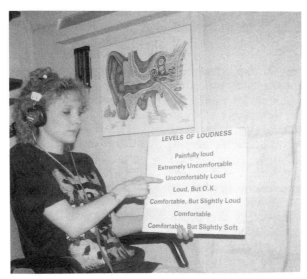

Figure 11.8   Patient using descriptive anchors to rate loudness during unaided loudness discomfort level measurements.

that was expended in the selection procedure. It is somewhat paradoxical, therefore, that in clinical practice, the audiologists who expend the most time on the selection process are also the ones who are the most fastidious regarding the verification of the hearing aid's response characteristics.

While the best verification procedure may be some type of benefit or satisfaction measurement conducted weeks or months after the hearing aid fitting, the discussion in this section will be limited to measures that normally would be conducted at the time that the hearing aid is delivered to the patient. When viewed in this manner, verification procedures can be categorized as either speech based or gain/frequency based.

To a large extent, the verification procedure that is selected is tied to the underlying theoretical model that the audiologist used in the original hearing aid selection process. For example, if the audiologist did not specify desired gain at the time that a custom hearing aid was ordered, then frequency-specific gain measurements at the time of the fitting take on little meaning. At one time, the majority of audiologists professed to use a "comparative hearing aid selection procedure"—that is, hearing aids were selected by performance on a word recognition task (usually monosyllables)

and not by a prescriptive gain-by-frequency procedure. In actuality, this selection procedure really was an informal prescriptive method, as it was not practical, or even possible, to compare all frequency response configurations. Usually, two to four hearing aids were selected for comparison, all having very similar frequency responses. It is not surprising that speech recognition scores rarely differed to a significant degree. Today, while hearing aid selection procedures remain variable, only 17% of audiologists report using a comparative approach for hearing aid selection (Martin & Morris, 1989).

VERIFICATION OF GAIN/FREQUENCY RESPONSE

As discussed earlier in this chapter, we recommend that audiologists use a prescriptive fitting procedure for a first approximation to select the appropriate gain and frequency response of the hearing aid. On the day of the fitting, it is necessary to determine if the desired electroacoustic characteristics have been achieved. Even if the audiologist simply mailed off an audiogram to a custom hearing aid manufacturer, some type of verification procedure is required before the patient is allowed to leave with the hearing aids. The verification process usually involves one or more of the following: speech audiometry, functional gain, or probe-microphone measurements.

Speech-Based Procedures

We cannot question the face validity of using some type of speech-based procedure to verify the choice of a hearing aid's frequency response. At one time (1960s–1970s), nearly 90% of audiologists reported using speech-based procedures for hearing aid selection (Smaldino & Hoene, 1981). The popularity and credibility of speech testing for hearing aid selection/verification has decreased considerably in recent years, however, although surprisingly this procedure remains a common practice for some audiologists (Martin & Morris, 1989). In general, the uses of speech stimuli for verification purposes can be divided into four different areas: *(1)* informal patient judgments; *(2)* measures of speech recognition or understanding; *(3)* patient judgments of quality; and *(4)* patient judgments of intelligibility.

Informal Patient Judgments. "How does that sound?" is often the first phrase spoken to the hearing aid user after the hearing aid is fitted to the ear, and some audiologists might consider the answer to that question an important part of the verification process. In fact, for some people who fit hearing aids, it appears that this might be the extent of the verification process. One survey reported the alarming finding that 23% of dispensers conduct no formal aided testing following the fitting of the hearing aid (Cranmer, 1991). Obviously, for patients fitted by these professionals, the informal speech assessment takes on added importance.

It is possible that an experienced hearing aid user can make reasonably valid judgments regarding the effectiveness of a hearing aid's frequency response simply by listening to conversational speech in one or two familiar listening environments. It is unlikely, however, that new users can make valid judgments of hearing aid performance based on limited exposure to listening to informal conversational speech. Usually, new hearing aid users will prefer the frequency response that sounds the most "natural," which often is a frequency response in opposition to what test results or theoretical models show to be the most bene-

ficial. Given the relative simplicity of conducting formal speech testing (or gain-by-frequency measurements), there would seem to be little reason to rely solely on informal speech measures as the yardstick for the hearing aid's frequency response verification.

Measures of Speech Recognition or Understanding. The measurement of speech understanding, especially the recognition of monosyllabic words, has been a commonly used method for verifying the performance of a hearing aid for over 40 years. In this process, the hearing aid would be judged as satisfactory if the patient scored at a desired level on a standardized speech test. If the desired score is not obtained, the frequency response is altered. The major limitation of this procedure is that the variability inherent in the speech material often equals or exceeds the "true differences" that exist for the different hearing aid frequency response (see reviews by Mueller & Grimes, 1987; Walden et al., 1983). While the likelihood of measuring "true differences" is increased by delivering more speech items (e.g., 250 to 500 words rather than 25 to 50), clinical efficiency or patient endurance usually does not allow for this adjustment. Hence, it is difficult to measure the effects of minor changes in the hearing aid's frequency response using this method.

Alternatives to the traditional monosyllabic word testing are available. For example, Jerger (1987) advocated the use of the Synthetic Sentence Identification (SSI) test. Humes (1988) and Humes and Houghton (1992) suggested using the CUNY nonsense syllable test. Cox et al. (1988) introduced a connected speech test, which they recommended for use in measuring hearing aid benefit. This test has a large number of equivalent forms and reportedly good sensitivity and high content validity.

To some extent, the popularity of the custom ITE hearing aid has made the unreliability of comparative speech measures somewhat of a moot point. Usually there is only one aid to test—the hearing aid that was custom-ordered for the patient. Unless a programmable instrument is used, only minimal changes in the frequency response are possible. Determination of the speech-based pass/fail criteria becomes a challenging task. Does one calculate unaided versus aided improvement or simply make acceptance judgments based on the aided measures? Are these measures made in quiet or in background noise? What performance level necessitates that the hearing aid be returned for alteration of the frequency response? How are the speech recognition scores used to determine what changes are needed in the frequency response?

Judgment of Speech Quality. The popularity of informal measures of speech quality already has been discussed; however, audiologists interested in this type of verification process can adopt more structured and reliable methods. Much of the background work in this area has been done by Gabrielsson and Sjogren (1979), who have provided bipolar adjectives describing sound quality dimensions. An example of these adjectives is shown in Table 11.4, taken from a clinical hearing aid selection/verification procedure recommended by Hawkins (1985).

Two factors are important when conducting these formal speech quality measures. First, the listening environment should be similar (amount of background noise, reverberation) to that normally experienced by the hearing aid user. Research has shown that quality judgments made in a sound suite are very dissimilar to those made in a more typical listening environment (Logan et al., 1984). Second, if the quality judgments are used to compare one hearing aid to another, auditory memory must be considered. Given the time that would elapse to physically remove one hearing aid and insert another, it is not likely that small differences in the hearing aid's frequency response will be detected reliably (Hawkins, 1985). To make reliable speech quality comparisons, therefore, it is necessary to switch rapidly between the different frequency responses, something that can be accomplished easily with most digitally programmable systems (but not too easily using a screwdriver!).

Speech Intelligibility Judgments. Associated with the measurement of speech recognition or understanding is the use of speech intelligibility ratings. Using adaptive methods, intelligibility ratings often can be conducted more efficiently than speech performance measures. Research

Table 11.4
Bipolar Terms That Can Be Used to Rate Hearing Aid Processed Speech Quality

Quality of Speech	
Distinct	Blurred
Mild/Calm	Sharp
Airy/Open	Shut Up/Closed
Bright	Dull
Quiet	Noisy/Hissing
Clear	Hazy
Near	Far
Full	Thin

Source: Hawkins, D., Reflections on amplification: validation of performance. *J. Acad. Rehab. Audiol.*, 18 (1985).

has found the two measures to be highly correlated. Cox and colleagues (e.g., Cox & McDaniel, 1984, 1989) have conducted extensive research on this type of speech assessment procedure, and these authors report good reliability for these measures. Presumably, some predetermined standard determines what rating, or combination of ratings, identifies an inappropriate frequency response. Cox does not recommend using these measures in isolation but rather as part of a complete protocol for hearing aid fitting.

As with quality judgments, it is important to make the intelligibility judgment listening task similar to the environment commonly encountered by the hearing aid user. For example, a task involving continuous discourse, reverberation, background noise, and even visual cues would seem to be the most appropriate. Hawkins and colleagues (1988) reported on a procedure incorporating these variables for speech intelligibility ratings. Although these authors did not specifically advocate this procedure for hearing aid verification, this would seem to be one of the most promising methods to explore for those audiologists who want to continue to use some speech measure in the hearing aid fitting process. If one is concerned with validation of the hearing aid's frequency response, however, the question still remains regarding what speech intelligibility performance is required for the hearing aid to pass the verification procedure and what alteration of the frequency response is made if the hearing aid does not pass the verification procedure.

To summarize, speech audiometry remains a useful measure in the overall hearing aid fitting process. It seems unlikely, however, that a given speech test or procedure will possess the necessary sensitivity to differentiate small variances in the electroacoustic properties of hearing aids or to predict what changes in the electroacoustic response are necessary. We believe the most reasonable approach is to use speech testing to demonstrate the benefits of amplification (aided versus unaided measurements) and to provide a framework for rehabilitation counseling.

Functional Gain

A behavioral method that can be used to verify that the gain of a hearing aid meets some predetermined prescriptive target is the measurement of functional gain. Functional gain simply is the measure of aided versus unaided thresholds for the frequencies of interest. The difference between the two conditions is the functional gain of the hearing aid, and these values can then be compared directly with prescriptive target gain to make a judgment regarding the appropriateness of the fitting.

Compared with rudimentary methods of predicting real-ear gain, such as simply viewing the 2-cm³ coupler response, functional gain offers a significant improvement in validity. No special equipment is required; only a soundfield enclosure for conducting the unaided and aided testing is needed. Because the hearing aid to be fitted is tested on the patient's ear, many of the variables not accounted for in coupler measures now are part of the test condition.

It is important to point out that functional gain is not a method of fitting hearing aids but rather is a method to determine if the audiologist's gold standard has been achieved. Unlike speech audiometry, the functional gain results dictate the frequency-specific alteration to hearing aid gain that is necessary. Without a prescriptive gain target, functional gain findings are of little significance except to assure the audiologist that the hearing aid is providing gain across the frequencies of interest.

The functional gain verification procedure is not without its own limitations (see Haskell, 1987, or Mueller & Grimes, 1987, for review). Prior to probe-microphone measurements, the limitations of functional gain measurement were not as ap-

parent, as there was no other clinical method available. Today, most audiologists use probe-microphone measurements; however, those who continue to use functional gain must consider these issues described by Mueller and Grimes (1987):

Testing at discrete frequencies. Functional gain usually is conducted at octave or half-octave intervals. Although this provides a general estimate of hearing aid gain, important peaks or troughs in the hearing aid's frequency response often can be missed.

Participation of the nontest ear. Unless the patient has a symmetrical hearing loss, masking of the nontest ear is necessary for both the unaided and aided measures. Simply placing an earplug in the nontest ear usually is inadequate.

Noise floor. Due to a combination of the internal circuit noise of the hearing aid and ambient room noise, there is a masking effect when the aided testing is conducted. This will make the aided threshold appear poorer if a patient has hearing thresholds of 25 dB HL or better, and consequently will underestimate functional gain.

Reliability. The test-retest reliability of functional gain precludes the measure of small differences in hearing aid frequency response. Hawkins (1985) shows that critical differences are as large as 10 dB, even at the 0.20 level of confidence. Humes and Kirn (1990) report average test-retest standard deviations of 6 dB for functional gain measures.

If the above limitations are controlled, and functional gain is conducted carefully, this measure can serve reasonably well for hearing aid verification. There are some types of fittings, or comparison of fittings, however, where estimates of gain will continue to be necessary, as it will not be possible to overcome a specific functional gain limitation. For the audiologists who have not yet purchased a probe-microphone system, functional gain testing remains the best method to determine if desired prescription gain has been achieved.

Probe-Microphone Measurements A final method for verification of the hearing aid's frequency response is the use of a probe-microphone system. This equipment has been available for clinical use since the mid-1980s and allows for the direct measure of acoustic output in the patient's ear. There appears to be little reason *not* to use probe-microphone measurements, although Cranmer (1991) reports that only approximately 50% of dispensing audiologists are using this equipment as part of the hearing aid fitting procedure.

While several different types of measurements can be conducted with the probe-microphone equipment for verification of the hearing aid's gain, the most common measurement is the real-ear insertion response (REIR) (Mueller, 1990). This calculation is the electroacoustic equivalent to functional gain; the distinct advantage is that the previously discussed limitations of functional gain have been eliminated. Additionally, no behavioral response is required from the patient, making these measures especially useful for the evaluation of young children and difficult-to-test patients. Because no behavioral response is required, however, probe-microphone measures cannot be used in isolation but must be related to reliable unaided earphone or soundfield behavioral pure-tone thresholds (or reasonable estimates).

To conduct probe-microphone measurements, it is necessary to purchase special equipment for this purpose. This financial outlay ($5000–$14,000) often is viewed by the audiologist or financial administrator as excessive relative to the additional information that can be obtained. This viewpoint is somewhat short-sighted, however, as probe-microphone systems allow for the measure of several important hearing aid parameters in addition to real-ear gain (Mueller, 1992d; Mueller & Hawkins, 1992b).

Since the introduction of clinical probe-microphone measures, there has been some confusion regarding the terminology that is used to describe the various responses. In the past few years there has been some consensus, and the terminology that is presently recommended for use is shown in Table 11.5 (see summary chapter by Mueller, 1992b). As indicated by the definitions in Table 11.4, the probe-microphone measurement that is most directly related to verification of a prescriptive fitting is the REIR, or real-ear insertion gain (REIG), if only one frequency is of interest. As mentioned, logic would suggest that REIG will equal functional gain if both measures are conducted carefully, and this has been supported by research (Humes, Hipskind, & Block, 1987; Popelka & Mason, 1987). In addition to the flexibility and versatility offered by the use of probe-microphone systems, these measures also are reliable (see Hawkins & Mueller, 1992a; Mueller & Sweetow, 1987). Clearly, therefore, this measurement procedure is superior to functional gain for verification of the hearing aid's desired gain and frequency characteristics.

As with speech audiometry or functional gain, following the measurement of the REIR, a decision must be made regarding the accuracy of the hearing aid fit. The general verification rule is that if the REIR is reasonably close to the prescriptive target, then the patient is fitted with the instrument. If the REIR of the hearing aid is not close to target, then the patient presumably is not allowed to use the hearing aid. In the case of an ITE hearing aid, this sometimes means that the instrument is returned to the manufacturer—an outcome that is undesirable for the audiologist, the manufacturer, and the patient.

The preciseness of the probe-microphone gain measurements causes its own set of new problems. Determining a pass/fail criterion is not an easy task, as one must determine what decibel window of acceptance is appropriate. To complicate the issue, this window must be larger at some frequencies than at others and probably needs to vary as a function of the slope and degree of the hearing loss.

Using probe-microphone REIG values, Mueller (1992c) reported on the evaluation of pass/fail criteria for nearly 500 patients with different types of hearing loss configurations fitted with custom ITE hearing aids. Shown in Figure 11.9, from Mueller (1992c), are the REIG results compared to desired prescriptive NAL target gain for five different hearing loss configurations. While examining the target gain-REIG difference, many audiologists prefer to use a fixed decibel difference value to rate the hearing aid as good or bad. Figure 11.9 organizes the target gain-REIG differences so that pass/fail percentages can be observed

Table 11.5
Common Terminology Used for the Real-Ear Measurement of Hearing Aid Performance

Real-ear unaided response	The real-ear unaided response (REUR) is the SPL, as a function of frequency, at a specified point in the unoccluded ear canal for a specified soundfield. This can be expressed either in SPL or a gain in decibels relative to the stimulus level.
Real-ear occluded response	The real-ear occluded response (REOR) is the SPL, as a function of frequency, at a specified point in the ear canal for a specified soundfield, with the hearing aid in place and turned off. This can be expressed either in SPL or as gain in decibels relative to the stimulus level.
Real-ear aided response	The real-ear aided response (REAR) is the SPL, as a function of frequency, at a specified measurement point in the ear canal for a specified soundfield with the hearing aid in place and turned on. This can be expressed either in SPL or as gain in decibels relative to the stimulus level.
Real-ear saturation response	The real-ear saturation response (RESR) is the SPL, as a function of frequency, at a specified measurement point in the ear canal with the hearing aid in place and turned on. The measurement is obtained with the stimulus level sufficiently intense as to operate the hearing aid at its maximum output level.
Real-ear insertion response	The real-ear insertion response (REIR) is the difference, in decibels as a function of frequency, between the REUR and the REAR measurements taken at the same measurement point in the same soundfield.
	The real-ear insertion gain (REIG) is the value, in decibels, of the REIR at a specific frequency.
Real-ear coupler difference	The real-ear coupler difference (RECD) is the difference, in decibels, as a function of frequency, between the outputs of a hearing aid measured in a real-ear versus a 2-cm^3 coupler.

Source: Mueller, H., Terminology and procedures. In H. Mueller, D. Hawkins, and J. Northern (Eds.), *Probe Microphone Measurements*. San Diego, CA: Singular Publishing Group (1992b).

for two different decibel tolerance windows at either 3000 or 4000 Hz. These results show that a rigid cutoff value such as 5 dB would result in an unacceptable number of hearing aid rejections. For 3000 Hz, 10 dB might be considered a reasonable value, but for 4000 Hz, a large number of hearing aids would continue to be rejected even if a 10-dB criterion were used.

By studying the data shown in Figure 11.9, it is possible to generate reasonable pass/fail criteria. Usually, a 90th percentile cutoff will provide a good starting point if the different audiometric configurations and the various degrees of target gain have been separately categorized. The decibel criterion, however, must be reevaluated frequently, as new hearing aid circuitry with improved high-frequency gain and active

tone controls will narrow the tolerance window of acceptance. The use of digitally programmable circuitry will have a similar effect.

VERIFICATION OF SSPL90

As discussed earlier in this chapter, variability exists regarding LDL measures, both in the measurement process itself and in the 2-cm^3 correction calculations used to order or select the hearing aid. It is essential, therefore, that aided LDL measures are conducted after the hearing aid fitting to assure that the output of the hearing aid does not exceed the patient's loudness discomfort level. When possible, it is helpful to use hearing aids that have an output control potentiometer. For ITE instruments (at

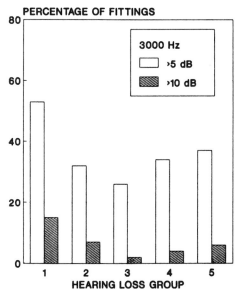

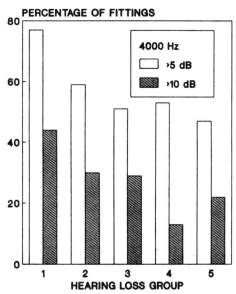

Figure 11.9 Percentage of fittings that exceeded target gain by more than 5 or 10 dB for 3000 Hz and 4000 Hz for five different hearing loss groups. Mean hearing loss at 4000 Hz was equal for all five groups; groups were determined based on the slope of the audiogram, with Group 1 being the most steeply slop-ing and Group 5 having a relatively flat audiometric configuration. (From Mueller, H., Insertion gain measurements. In H. Mueller, D. Hawkins, and J. Northern (Eds.), *Probe Microphone Measurements.* San Diego, CA: Singular Publishing Group [1992c].)

least the larger styles) this trimmer will allow for a 6- to 12-dB adjustment in SSPL90.

In general, the aided LDL measures are conducted in a manner similar to the unaided testing. The goal of the measurements is twofold: The maximum output of the hearing aid should be both *comfortable* and *safe.* The patient uses the same descriptive anchors to make loudness judgments as were used for the unaided testing; these judgments are made when the hearing aid is placed in saturation at each test frequency. If the loudness judgment falls above the "Loud but OK" criterion, then the hearing aid must be adjusted accordingly; the SSPL90 is reduced using the potentiometer. If the judgments are below the "Loud but OK" level (e.g., "Comfortable but slightly loud"), this also is an undesirable outcome, as it may mean that the hearing aid is saturating at an unnecessarily low level (distortion usually is associated with saturation). Again, the output would be adjusted if possible. As a reminder, it is important that the loudspeaker output (in SPL) at each frequency is known prior to aided LDL measures so that an appropriate audiometer dial setting can be selected to saturate the hearing aid.

In addition to the behavioral measurements of LDL, it is also helpful to conduct probe-microphone measurements of the output of the hearing aid. These responses, referred to as the real-ear saturation response (RESR), can provide information regarding the functioning of output limiting circuitry. Most important, these responses clearly detail the unpredictable effects caused by a given patient's external ear. If real-ear LDL measurements were conducted at the time that the hearing aid was ordered, the aided RESR can be matched to these values. With multichannel programmable instruments, with adjustable compression tones and/or ratios, it is possible to shape the SSPL90 function to the patient's LDL in much the same way that the frequency response is shaped to prescriptive target gain. RESR testing also will assure that the output in the ear canal does not exceed the SPL levels considered to be safe for a given patient. There is not a behavioral equivalent for predicting the real-ear output of a hearing aid.

Franks and Beckman (1985) reported on a group of individuals who rejected hearing aid use after a trial period. One of the leading reasons for rejection—reported by 86%

of the respondents—was that the hearing aid "made sounds too loud." The clinical LDL verification procedures described in this section are relatively easy to administer and interpret. The almost-certain enhancement in hearing aid use and acceptance that will result when the SSPL90 is appropriate would seem to make these routine LDL measures well worth the clinical time investment.

Summary

In summary, the focus of this chapter has been to point out the many behavioral and electroacoustic measures that can be used to obtain an optimum hearing aid fitting. Presumably, if all the patient factors and prefitting considerations are taken into account, the verification process will be successful. But, what about the large number of patients who purchase hearing aids and receive no formal testing before or after the fitting other than the pure-tone audiogram that was mailed to the manufacturer to order the instrument? Isn't the fact that most of these individuals do not ask for a refund of their hearing aid purchase a verification method of sorts? After all, it could be argued that if a patient routinely uses his or her hearing aid and reports benefit and satisfaction, then it must be a "good fitting." Although this may be true, it seems that this method of verification usually underestimates the evaluative skills of the audiologist and overestimates the differential judgment capabilities of the patient. Through the careful selection of the hearing aid candidate, consideration of the hearing aid's electroacoustic properties, and use of a reliable validation procedure, we can provide hearing aid fittings that not only will *satisfy* individuals with hearing impairment but also will maximize their speech understanding ability.

References

Bentler, R., Programmable hearing aid review. *Am. J. Audiol.* 1, 25–29 (1991).

Bentler, R., *Output Limitation: Reports in Hearing Instrumentation and Technology.* VI, 4–9 (1989).

Bentler, R., and Pavlovic, C., Transfer functions and correction factors used in hearing aid evaluation and research. *Ear Hear.,* 10, 58–63 (1989).

Bratt, G., and Sammeth, C., Clinical implications of prescriptive formulas for hearing aid selection. In G. Studebaker, F. Bess, and L. Beck (Eds.), The Vanderbilt Hearing-Aid Report II. Parkton, MD: York Press, pp. 35–51 (1991).

Byrne, D., Hearing aid selection formulae: Same or different? *Hear. Instr.,* 38, 5–11 (1987).

Byrne, D., and Dillon, H., The National Acoustic Laboratories' (NAL) new procedure for selecting the gain and frequency response of a hearing aid. *Ear Hear.* 7, 257–265 (1986).

Cavanaugh, W., Farrell, W., Hirtle, P., and Watters, B., Speech privacy in buildings. *J. Acoust. Soc. Am.,* 34(4), 475–483 (1962).

Cokely, C., and Humes, L., Reliability of two measures of speech recognition in elderly people. *J. Speech Hear. Res.,* 35(3), 654–660 (1992).

Cox, R., NBS-9A coupler-to-eardrum transformation: TDH-39 and TDH-49 earphones. *J. Acoust. Soc. Am.,* 79, 120–123 (1986).

Cox, R., Alexander, G., Gilmore, C., and Pusakulich, K., Use of the Connected Speech Test (CST) with hearing impaired listeners. *Ear Hear.,* 9(4), 198–207 (1988).

Cox, R., Alexander, G., Gilmore, C., and Pusakulich, K., The Connected Speech Test Version 3: Audiovisual administration. *Ear Hear.* (10(1), 29–32 (1989).

Cox, R., and McDaniel, M., Intelligibility ratings of continuous discourse: application to hearing aid selection. *J. Acoust. Soc. Am.,* 76, 758–766 (1984).

Cox, R., and McDaniel, D., Development of the Speech Intelligibility Rating (SIR) for hearing aid comparisons. *J. Speech Hear. Res.,* 32, 347–352 (1989).

Cranmer, K., Hearing instrument aid dispensing. *Hear. Instr.,* 42(6), 6–13 (1991).

Davies, J., and Mueller, H., Hearing aid selection. In H. Mueller and V. Geoffrey (Eds.), *Communication Disorders in Aging.* Washington DC: Gallaudet Press, pp. 408–436 (1987).

Fabry, D., Programmable and automatic noise reduction in existing hearing aids. In G. Studebaker, F. Bess, and L. Beck (Eds.), The Vanderbilt Hearing-Aid Report II. Parkton, MD: York Press, pp. 65–78 (1991).

Franks, J., and Beckman, N., Rejection of hearing aids: attitudes of a geriatric sample. *Ear Hear.,* 6(3), 161–166 (1985).

French, N., and Steinberg, J., Factors governing the intelligibility of speech sounds. *J. Acoust. Soc. Am.,* 19, 90–119 (1947).

Gabrielsson, A., and Sjogren, H., Perceived sound quality of sound-reproducing systems. *J. Acoust. Soc. Am.,* 65, 1019–1033 (1978).

Haskell, G., Functional gain. *Ear Hear.,* 8(5), 95S–99S (1987).

Hawkins, D., Reflections on amplification: validation of performance. *J. Acad. Rehab. Audiol.,* 18, 42–54 (1985).

Hawkins, D., Selection of SSPL90 for Binaural Hearing Aid Fittings. *Hear. J.,* 39, 7–10 (1986).

Hawkins, D., Prescriptive approaches to selection of gain and frequency response. In H. Mueller, D. Hawkins, and J. Northern (Eds.), *Probe Microphone Measurements.* San Diego, CA: Singular Publishing Group (1992a).

Hawkins, D., Corrections and transformations relevant to hearing aid selection. In H. Mueller, D.

Hawkins, and J. Northern (Eds.), *Probe Microphone Measurements*. San Diego, CA: Singular Publishing Group (1992a).

Hawkins, D., Corrections and transformations relevant to hearing aid selection. In H. Mueller, D. Hawkins, and J. Northern (Eds.), *Probe Microphone Measurements*. San Diego, CA: Singular Publishing Group (1992b).

Hawkins, D., Selecting SSPL90 using probe-microphone measurements. In H. Mueller, D. Hawkins, and J. Northern (Eds.), *Probe Microphone Measurements*. San Diego, CA: Singular Publishing Group (1992c).

Hawkins, D., and Mueller, H., Test protocols for probe-microphone measurements. In H. Mueller, D. Hawkins, and J. Northern (Eds.), *Probe Microphone Measurements*. San Diego, CA: Singular Publishing Group (1992a).

Hawkins, D., and Mueller, H., Procedural considerations in probe microphone measurements. In H. Mueller, D. Hawkins, and J. Northern (Eds.), *Probe Microphone Measurements*. San Diego, CA: Singular Publishing Group (1992b).

Hawkins, D., Walden, B., Montgomery, A., and Prosek, R., Description and validation of an LDL procedure designed to select SSPL90. *Ear Hear.*, 8, 162–169 (1987).

Hayes, D., and Jerger, J., Aging and the use of hearing aids. *Scand. Audiol.*, 8, 33–40 (1979).

Humes, L., An evaluation of several rationales for selecting hearing aid gain. *J. Speech Hear. Dis.*, 51, 272–281 (1986).

Humes, L., Selecting hearing aids for patients effectively [SHAPE]. *Hear. J.*, 41(1), 15–18 (1988).

Humes, L., Understanding the speech understanding problems of the hearing impaired. *J. Am. Acad. Audiol.*, 2, 59–69 (1991).

Humes, L., and Hackett, T., Comparison of frequency response and aided speech-recognition performance for hearing aids selected by three different prescriptive methods. *J. Am. Acad. Audiol.*, 1, 101–108 (1990).

Humes, L., Hipskind, N., and Block, M., Insertion gain measured with three probe tube systems. *Ear Hear.*, 9, 108–112 (1988).

Humes, L., and Houghton, R., Beyond insertion gain. *Hear. Instr.*, 43(3), 32–35 (1992).

Humes, L., and Kirn, E., The reliability of functional gain. *J. Speech Hear. Dis.*, 55, 193–197 (1990).

Jerger, J., On the evaluation of hearing aid performance. *Asha*, 29, 49–51 (1987).

Killion, M., An "acoustically invisible" hearing aid. *Hear. Instr.*, 39(10), 39–44 (1988).

Killion, M., Staab, W., and Preves, D., Classifying automatic signal processors. *Hear. Instr.*, 41(8), 24–26 (1990).

Kirkwood, D., 1991 U.S. hearing aid sales summary. *Hear. J.*, 44(12), 9–15 (1991).

Logan, S., Schwartz, D., Ahlstrom, J., and Ahlstrom, C., Effects of the acoustic environment on hearing aid quality/intelligibility judgments. Annual convention of the American Speech-Language-Hearing Association, San Francisco, CA (1984).

Martin, F., and Morris, L., Current audiologic practices in the United States. *Hear. J.*, 4, 25–44 (1989).

McCandless, G., and Lyregaard, P., Prescription of gain/output (POGO) for hearing aids. *Hear. Instr.*, 34(1), 16–21 (1983).

McCarthy, P., Montgomery, A., and Mueller, H., Decision making in rehabilitative audiology. *J. Am. Acad. Audiol.*, 1(1), 23–30 (1990).

Mueller, H., Binaural amplification: attitudinal factors. *Hear. J.*, 39, 7–10 (1986).

Mueller, H., Individualizing the ordering of custom hearing instruments. *Hear. Instr.*, 40, 18–22 (1989).

Mueller, H., Probe tube microphone measures: some opinions on terminology and procedures. *Hear. J.*, 42(1), 1–5 (1990).

Mueller, H., Individualizing the ordering of custom hearing aids. In H. Mueller, D. Hawkins, and J. Northern (Eds.), *Probe Microphone Measurements*. San Diego, CA: Singular Publishing Group (1992a).

Mueller, H., Terminology and procedures. In H. Mueller, D. Hawkins, and J. Northern (Eds.), *Probe Microphone Measurements*. San Diego, CA: Singular Publishing Group (1992b).

Mueller, H., Insertion gain measurements. In H. Mueller, D. Hawkins, and J. Northern (Eds.), *Probe Microphone Measurements*. San Diego, CA: Singular Publishing Group (1992c).

Mueller, H., and Bender, D., Reasons for obtaining hearing aids: Do they relate to subsequent benefit? *Corti's Organ*, 11 (Abstract) (1988).

Mueller, H., Bryant, M., Brown, W., and Budinger, A., Hearing aid selection for high-frequency hearing loss. In G. Studebaker, F. Bess, and L. Beck (Eds.), The Vanderbilt Hearing-Aid Report II. Parkton, MD: York Press, pp. 35–51 (1991).

Mueller, H., and Budinger, A., Selection of hearing aid style. *Reports Hear. Instrument. Technol.*, 2, 5–10 (1990).

Mueller, H., and Calkins, A., Dichotic speech measures for predicting hearing aid benefit. *Asha*, 30(10), 104 (Abstract) (1988).

Mueller, H., and Grimes, A., Amplification systems for the hearing impaired. In J. Alpiner and P. McCarthy (Eds.), *Rehabilitative Audiology: Children and Adults*. Baltimore: Williams & Wilkins (1987).

Mueller, H., and Hawkins, D., Considerations in hearing aid selection. In R. Sandlin (Ed.), *Handbook of Hearing Aid Amplification, II: Clinical Considerations and Fitting Practices*. San Diego: College Hill Press, pp. 31–60 (1990).

Mueller, H., and Hawkins, D., Assessment of fitting arrangements, special circuitry and features. In H. Mueller, D. Hawkins, and J. Northern (Eds.), *Probe Microphone Measurements*. San Diego, CA: Singular Publishing Group (1992).

Mueller, H., and Killion, M., An easy method for calculating the articulation index. *Hear. J.*, 43, 14–17 (1990).

Mueller, H., and Sweetow, R., A Clinical comparison of probe microphone systems. *Hear. Instr.*, 38, 20–21, 57 (1987).

Olsen, W., Hawkins, D., and Van Tasell, D., Representations of the long-term spectra of speech. *Ear Hear.*, 8(5), 1003–1085 (1987).

Pascoe, D., Clinical implications of nonverbal methods of hearing aid selection and fitting. *Sem. Hear.*, 1, 217–229 (1980).

Pavlovic, C., Articulation index predictions of speech intelligibility in hearing aid selection. *Asha*, 30(6), 63–65 (1988).

Pavlovic, C., Speech recognition and five articulation indexes. *Hear. Instr.*, 42, 20–24 (1991).

Pearsons, K., Bennett, R., and Fidell, S., Speech levels in various noise environments. Project Report on

Contract 68 01-2466. Washington DC, Office of Health and Ecological Effects, U.S. Environmental Protection Agency (1977).

Pollack, M., Special applications of amplification. In M. Pollack (Ed.), *Amplification for the Hearing-Impaired.* New York: Grune & Stratton (1975).

Popelka, G., and Mason, D., Factors which affect measures of speech audibility with hearing aids. *Ear Hear.,* 8(5), 109(s)–118(s) (1987).

Preves, D., Output limiting and speech enhancement. In G. Studebaker, F. Bess, and L. Beck (Eds.), The Vanderbilt Hearing-Aid Report II. Parkton, MD: York Press, pp. 35–51 (1991).

Sachs, R., and Burkhard, M., Zwislocki coupler evaluation with insert earphones. Report 20022-1. Franklin Park, IL: Knowles Electronics (1972).

Seewald, R., The desired sensation level approach for children: selection and verification. *Hear. Instr.,* 39, 18–22 (1992).

Skinner, M., *Hearing Aid Evaluation.* Englewood Cliffs, NJ: Prentice-Hall (1988).

Smaldino, J., and Hoene, D., A view of the state of hearing aid fitting practices: Part I. *Hear. Instr.,* 32, 1–15, 38 (1981).

Stach, B., Hearing aid amplification and central processing disorders. In R. Sandlin (Ed.), *Handbook of Hearing Aid Amplification, II: Clinical Considera-*

tions and Fitting Practices. Boston: College-Hill Press, pp. 87–111 (1990).

Stach, B., Spretnjak, M., and Jerger, J., The prevalence of central presbycusis in a clinical population. *J. Am. Acad. Audiol.,* 1(2), 109–115 (1990).

Sullivan, R., Transcranial ITE CROS. *Hear. Instr.,* 39(1), 11–13 (1988).

Tyler, R., Measuring hearing loss in the future. *Br. J. Audiol.,* 2, (Suppl.), 29–40 (1979).

Valente, M., Valente, M., and Vass, W., Selecting an appropriate matrix for ITE/ITC hearing instruments. *Hear. Instr.,* 41, 20–24 (1990).

Walden, B., Schwartz, D., Williams, D., Holum-Hardigan, L., and Crowley, J., Test of the assumptions underlying comparative hearing aid evaluations. *J. Speech Hear. Dis.,* 48, 264–273 (1983).

Walker, G., and Dillion, H., *Compression in Hearing Aids: An Analysis, a Review and Some Recommendations.* National Acoustic Laboratories Report #90. Canberra: Australian Government Publishing Service (1982).

Ventry, I., and Weinstein, B., Identification of elderly people with hearing problems. *Asha,* 25(7), 37–42 (1983).

12

Management of the Hearing-Impaired Adult

ALLEN A. MONTGOMERY, Ph.D.

In the practice of aural rehabilitation for the adult, a hearing-impaired individual seeks help from a specialized professional for the communication breakdowns and emotional reactions caused by a loss of normal hearing function. Typical clients range in age from 20 to 70 years (older clients are discussed in Chapter 13) and have acquired their sensorineural hearing losses over a period of years. Losses may range from mild to severe. Many individuals wear hearing aids and may have been fitted just prior to enrolling in rehabilitation. The chapter focuses primarily on the rehabilitation of these representative clients.

Clinical Truths

A few obvious but sometimes neglected principles have accumulated in the collective experience of audiologists in the past several years.

1. Amplification does not provide complete remediation of a hearing loss.
2. The hearing aid is the beginning of rehabilitation, not the end.
3. Recognition of speech is the most important auditory activity that people engage in.
4. Listening in noise is much more difficult than listening in quiet. It is difficult to learn to listen in noise.
5. Speech, except over the telephone, is a bisensory event involving the integration of audition and vision (lipreading).

6. Bisensory speech perception is superior to audition or vision alone.
7. People learn by doing and practicing, not by being told to do or practice.
8. People learn information well in a one-to-one situation with a teacher; they change behavior and attitudes only in the presence of a group.

These assumptions and the implications they generate lead to the principles and practices of adult aural rehabilitation discussed below. First, a brief picture of the nature of adult aural rehabilitation and its practice in the last decade of the 20th century is presented.

The Nature of Aural Rehabilitation

Traditionally, aural rehabilitation arose in medical settings such as rehabilitation hospitals following World War II. It continues today in rehabilitation centers, in VA hospitals, in community and university clinics, and, increasingly, in private audiological practices where some enterprising audiologists are conducting hearing aid orientations, comprehensive follow-ups, and group meetings of hearing aid users. (See Chapter 3 for more information on aural rehabilitation and private practice.)

From its early beginnings in the lipreading classes promoted at the turn of the century, aural rehabilitation has always reflected the culture and conditions under which it is practiced. At no time in its 90-year history has this been more true than today. In this chapter we consider aural rehabilitation in the context of the 1990s and offer not only a description of the many facets of a successful aural rehabilitation program but also a projection of the changes and challenges that clinicians will face in the remaining years of the 20th century. It is alternately an exciting and a frightening prospect to consider the practice of aural rehabilitation at this time.

Three major developments are likely to have a heavy impact on the conduct of adult aural rehabilitation in the 1990s. These are the social-economic-demographic trends so evident in our society. The social component refers to the rapid development of a multicultural society in which nonwhite minority members and women will soon be the majority workers and black, Hispanic, and Asian populations have established roles. Minority groups almost invariably have a higher prevalence of handicapping conditions, and the need for adult aural rehabilitation services is undoubtedly large and growing. Some minority-oriented programs have emerged, such as the Spanish language HOLA program of Serrano-Navaro, Arana, and Cram (1991). The economic reality of the 1990s is the increasing likelihood of a major health care crisis. This crisis may bring potential for benefit as well as harm to adult aural rehabilitation. Finally, the demographic forces produced by the aging population—36 million over age 65 by 2000 A.D. (Asha, 1990)—will put tremendous strain on all rehabilitative services, including aural rehabilitation.

It is interesting to note that in direct contrast to the education of deaf children, adult aural rehabilitation has suffered from almost a *lack* of controversy and direction and "schools" and "methods." In the coming health care crisis, when we (as a society) are forced to choose between care for the elderly, transplants, prolonged neonatal care, drug rehabilitation, and other expensive procedures, we (as audiologists) will be forced to develop brief, effective, accountable, *billable* activities if aural rehabilitation is to be conducted anywhere outside of subsidized university clinics on a wide-spread basis. In some ways this pressure to produce efficient therapeutic techniques and ways to measure progress (or lack of deterioration) is good. It forces us to examine our clinical procedures critically and come up not only with improved rehabilitative methods but also with more sensitive and specific diagnostic and prognostic tests. These new procedures will draw heavily on high technology but also on rehabilitative psychology and cognitive science. On the other hand, it is probably true that such time-honored traditions as the specific lipreading group and isolated auditory training will give way to counseling, assertive situation control, spouse training, and audiovisual instruction.

We think that aural rehabilitation is at a crossroads that could lead to growth and new directions such as that seen after World War II or to a diminution and trivializing effect wherein aural rehabilitation is considered only in the aftermath of hearing aid fitting and available only to financially secure retirees. The growth will come from the high-tech revolution and the elevation of rehabilitation in general accompanying the resolution of the health care crisis. The stagnation would occur if demographics and economic conditions interact in ways that produce financial disincentives for prolonged treatment of any sort. In the long run, however, it is hard to believe that the tremendous general need for rehabilitative services associated with the increasingly older population will not spin off benefits to aural rehabilitation. These benefits, presumably in the form of public awareness, third-party payments, and rehabilitative teams and centers, would be available to us only if we are prepared with *(1)* accurate, quantitative assessment procedures; *(2)* efficient treatment methods; and *(3)* a supply of well-trained personnel.

The remainder of the chapter is devoted to introducing rehabilitative principles and techniques that are in clinical use today or are under development.

WHAT CAN AURAL REHABILITATION DO?

In this section we present a series of examples of what aural rehabilitation for the adult can accomplish. The list is somewhat extended but is necessary to demonstrate the diversity of ways in which the goals of adult aural rehabilitation may be realized. Some of the situations described involved immediate and dramatic improvements, whereas others yielded substantial long-term benefits. We hope that the reader will sense some of the excitement and rewarding nature inherent in the modern practice of aural rehabilitation.

Some clinical examples follow:

1. An older woman is clinging to her independence by doing food shopping and other things for herself. As her hearing deteriorates, it becomes difficult, and she begins thinking about a nursing home. We provide her with the lipreading skills and strategies (and confidence!) to extend her independence for several years.
2. An old man moves in with his daughter and son-in-law, and they cannot agree on how loud to play the television set. An infrared system transmitting to a personal headset solves the problem.
3. Our adult rehabilitation group helps a couple to stop yelling at each other when the husband does not understand and to adopt effective strategies for coping with his difficulties.
4. The owners of a small business raised questions about their need to conform to the ADA91 guidelines and were advised on the definition of small business and given some options to consider in making their workplace more accessible to their deaf and hard-of-hearing workers and customers.
5. A personal FM system allows a young professional woman to attend and participate in the frequent small meetings necessary for her work.
6. Some assertive behavior, rehearsed in our group, helps a shy woman speak to her minister about acoustic conditions in her church. The minister agrees to modernize the public address system and the woman is able to hear the sermon better.
7. A man with a progressive hereditary loss comes to us for counseling and advice. We provide information on deafness, sign language and lipreading, and cochlear implants. He becomes informed and

is more prepared to face the future. Afterward, we follow up. On our advice, he joins Self-Help for the Hard of Hearing (SHHH) and meets another person with similar problems.
8. An old man in a nursing home communicates very little because of excessive shyness and because of his withdrawal and refusal to try. We are able to talk to the staff, reduce some of the noise, and boost his confidence and willingness to guess. He is now able and willing to entertain visitors and neighbors in his room.

These eight examples were drawn from our clinical practice of adult aural rehabilitation to illustrate the wide variety of circumstances where aural rehabilitation may be necessary. Several observations can be made on the basis of the examples. First, there is obviously a positive impact on human happiness in all of the examples, but especially in numbers 1, 2, 3, and 7. However, there are also specific occupational and financial benefits in cases 1 and 5. Furthermore, these examples demonstrate larger, less tangible benefits to society as well. The impact of keeping young and middle-aged people working and working more productively for a lifetime is certainly substantial. Also the effect of allowing older citizens to remain independent and active for additional years is clearly cost-effective and humane compared to extended nursing home care and the steady deterioration that comes with loss of self-sufficiency.

Finally, note that some of the cases involved the use of special amplifiers and transmitters, known collectively as assistive listening devices (ALDs), which provide specific technical solutions to communication problems. An important part of aural rehabilitation is the ALD interview, where hardware and needs are matched up. In addition, several of the situations called for assertive behavior on the part of the individual to resolve the difficulties. It will become obvious that hardware and "skinware" (the client) cannot passively solve the problems of communicating in a noisy, busy society. It is often necessary for the client to speak up and act on his or her own behalf to improve listening conditions and prevent future problems. These topics are considered in more detail below.

OVERALL GOAL OF ADULT AURAL REHABILITATION

The general overall goal of aural rehabilitation is to increase the *probability* that communication will occur between a hearing-impaired person and his or her verbal environment. This is stated in probabilistic terms because conditions and circumstances change so much from moment to moment and day to day that there is no guarantee our client will be successful in a given situation, despite the best amplification, lipreading, and assertive listening skills. We strive to increase the "odds" that communication will take place without difficulty. We seek better communication *on the average* throughout the client's life. This definition acknowledges that there are many aspects of the situation that are out of anyone's control—that have a statistical rather than a definite predictable basis. Approached in this way, the successes and failures that the hearing-impaired person experiences are viewed realistically. The hearing-impaired person cannot understand everything, but on the average he or she can increase the percentage of "hits" while reducing the frustration and isolation previously experienced. Hence we use buzzwords like "maximize" and "optimize" in the sections that follow.

This overall goal translates into addressing several factors that are emphasized or deemphasized, depending on the client's particular needs, strengths, and weaknesses. Major factors that contribute to increasing the likelihood of communication are:

1. Reducing negative emotional reactions such as anger, frustration, fear, and withdrawal related to communication difficulties
2. Making cognitive processes and attitudes toward hearing impairment more realistic
3. Increasing knowledge of the context of the communication, including the language/dialect used, current news, the talkers, the topic, the history of the participants, and so on
4. Maximizing auditory input through professionally fitted hearing aids and through assistive listening devices for specific problems/situations
5. Improving the listening and viewing (i.e., lipreading) conditions by increasing the auditory and visual signal-to-noise ratio (S/N) through assertive and educational behavior
6. Optimizing audiovisual input through speechreading and improved viewing habits combined with the amplified auditory signal.
7. Minimizing communication breakdown through preventive action and, when breakdown occurs, using effective repair strategies

These factors can be viewed in terms of the time frame in which they operate: 1 and 2 (emotion and cognition) are long-term, slowly responding changes that continue through life; 3 and 4 (contextual knowledge and amplification) occur before and while rehabilitation is conducted; 5 (assertive listening) should happen before or immediately on entering a difficult situation; 6 (audiovisual integration) occurs during the situation; 7 (conversion repair) comes into play only after something is missed or misunderstood. In this chapter we concentration on factors 3 through 7.

The successful aural rehabilitation client accomplishes several things. He or she works on long-term goals of emotional and cognitive health, obtains hearing aids and assistive listening devices, works actively to prevent difficult situations before they occur/recur, reacts promptly to improve the overall S/N ratio when entering difficult situations, makes optimal use of audiovisual input during a difficult situation, and repairs misunderstandings immediately after they have occurred. Thus there is *always* something that the hearing-impaired person can do when anticipating, encountering, or repairing communication difficulties. This knowledge and the skills that accompany it provide the hearing-impaired client with the confidence and ability to succeed or improve in almost any communication situation.

HEARING LOSS AS A SOURCE OF AMBIGUITY

Note that all of the seven factors mentioned above increase the likelihood of communication directly or indirectly by reducing the number of alternatives that must be considered in resolving an ambiguous message. If successfully resolved, the message is said to be disambiguated.

The way in which the seven factors come into play can be illustrated by an example. Consider the sentence that occurred while two men were watching television: "I_in__e mi_ have _ good year i_ hi_ ba_or_ _om_ _ough." Factors 1 and 2 prevent the listener from trying to figure out what was said: "If I miss it the first time, I never get it" (cognitive discord). If he is wearing a hearing aid, the "s" (z sound) in his . . . _omes will become audible as will the unstressed "a" (factor 4). Also, if he can integrate lipreading with the amplified auditory signal (factor 6), he will get the "th" in thin_ and through. The sentence now looks like this: "I thin_ _e mi_ have a good year if his ba_or_ _omes through." Of course, if he had been assertive and asked that the volume on the TV set be turned off during the commercial, he would have heard enough to understand it correctly (factor 5). As it is, he must depend on his knowledge of the context (they are discussing the basketball coach of the local team—factor 3), to supply the key phrase "back court" (lipreading had already ruled out backboard as an option) and decide on "I think he might have a good year if his back court comes through."

The point is that the hearing-impaired person must call on several sources of information and assistance in his search for understanding. If all else had failed, he could have repaired the breakdown by asking a specific question (not just "What?") like "If his what comes through?" (factor 7), which reduces the possibilities very quickly to the correct one. Obviously, all seven factors must be addressed in the rehabilitation of hearing-impaired adults, with different emphasis on each factor depending on the client's needs.

MODELS OF AGING

Given the fact that hearing deteriorates over age, even in the absence of active pathology (unless you are considering aging itself to be pathological!), it is not surprising that many adult aural rehabilitation clients are middle-aged or older. It is therefore important that our approach to adult aural rehabilitation consider the aging process and models of aging. Until recently, aging was almost uniformly considered to be characterized by a gradual constant decline in physical, sensory, and mental capabilities, starting as early as age 40. Many studies show exactly such a trend, based on groups of people at each age, tested on various characteristics, such as strength, alpha rhythm, memory, and reaction time. This is a decidedly negative model. It implies that one can expect aural rehabilitation clients to steadily degenerate on all fronts despite our efforts. One is fighting a brief holding action at best. This is especially discouraging because sometimes the degenerative physical and mental problems are more serious impediments to rehabilitation than the hearing loss itself.

Recently, however, a much more positive and perhaps more representative model has appeared. It is called the terminal drop model (Smith, 1989). Essentially, it says that many people retain performance levels near those of their middle age long into their 70s and 80s or older. At some point, they then experience a terminal drop—a more rapid decline in capability, often leading to death. In other words, they are relatively healthy until they "drop." Smith believes that the gradual decline data show a misleadingly steep straight-line decline. The steepness in this view is due to the likelihood that the sample of people at each age group included a mix of healthy people and those already in their terminal drop stage. The decline is due primarily to simply having more subjects who have "dropped" in each successive age group. The implications of this are quite profound. It says that many people will lead long, healthy lives until late in life. Individuals will experience only minor loss of function until some major catastrophe hits, such as dementing disease, stroke, cancer, or heart attack. We have all known people who fit the terminal drop model.

At this point the critical reader will ask, "If the terminal drop model holds so well, why are there so many people who gradually lose their hearing over time? " The answer seems to be that the terminal drop model best describes physical and mental capabilities but not sensory capacity, especially hearing, which does seem to share the gradual loss predicted by the steady decline model. So, in a sense we can have the best of both models in a particular client—a sensory loss whose consequences clinicians can relieve to a considerable extent and a capable mind and body that allow the client not only to succeed in rehabilitation but to enjoy the benefits.

Along these lines, it is also encouraging to note that some forms of senility and loss of mobility, which would seem to be the terminal drop itself, are actually reversible in the elderly with a modest, steady program of physical exercise.

The Process of Communication

Verbal communication is an interactive process where two or more talker-listeners exchange information using a common language and a shared set of rules concerning the manner in which the exchange is conducted. (Note that we do not designate a distinct talker and listener because talking and listening occur simultaneously and roles change very rapidly.). The process includes, among other components, a message to be conveyed, a purpose and intent to convey it, and a medium through which the message is transmitted. The form of the message is spoken sentences and sentence fragments accompanied by verbal and nonverbal pragmatic mechanisms that follow the rules of exchange and streamline the interactive aspects of the communication process. These mechanisms include pauses filled with "uh" or "um" to signal the talker's intent to continue talking, facial expressions indicating understanding or disagreement with the message, and ways to repair the conversation when a misunderstanding or communication breakdown has occurred. The message is thus conveyed between talker-listeners through two channels: the auditory channel, which receives the speech and audible markers, and the visual channel, which receives the dynamic image of the talker's lips (i.e., lipreading) and the visible pragmatic markers, such as facial expression and the information as to who (among three or more participants) is speaking.

UNIMPAIRED COMMUNICATION IS NOT SMOOTH

It is often naively assumed that the process of verbal communication proceeds smoothly in the absence of sensory impairment, but that is far from the truth! A typical communication exchange among two or three people is a constant stream of interruptions, rephrasings, two (or more) people talking at once, corrections, topic shifts, and unclear references to people and things not present. The messages are constantly being checked or verified with facial expressions and phrases like "right?" It is a useful and eye-opening experience for students to transcribe a typical audio recording of a conversation among three people. This exercise illustrates several points: *(1)* It is sometimes difficult to tell who is speaking without the visual information. *(2)* Similarly, the visible pragmatic markers are lost, especially head nodding and facial expressions that signal the talker to proceed or back up. *(3)* If it is a monophonic recording it is hard to separate the speech from the background noise because the important binaural advantage in separating signal from noise spatially is lost. *(4)* Much of the speech is in the form of sentence fragments and rephrasings, many of which are redundant. *(5)* The transcript contains only the words spoken and fails to convey the emotions, spirit, and even the meanings of the conversation itself. That is, a conversation is much more than the words spoken. *(6)* The talkers share a common knowledge base, whereas the transcribers have no way of knowing such contextual references as to whom "you" or "they" refer to or what "my problem" is. *(7)* Further, if the recording is "impaired" at all (noisy or low fidelity), some of the words are transcribed incorrectly. Errors occur involving speech sounds that are acoustically similar (like "b" or "v"), low intensity ("f," "th," or unstressed "th") or have high-frequency energy ("s," "t," "k"). Many of these errors were not made by the actual conversants because they had better acoustic conditions and also could lipread the talker, thereby eliminating the b/v and f/th errors, for example. The transcribers, of course, had the further disadvantage that they could not interact with the talkers and request clarification or repetition. They could not *repair* the conversation.

IMPLICATIONS FOR AURAL REHABILITATION

From this exercise we can draw several conclusions and implications for aural rehabilitation where one of the talker-listener's auditory channels is impaired. First, the visual channel is very important—it provides lipreading, contextual clues, pragmatic markers, facial expressions, and eye-gaze direction. The hearing-impaired client must learn to use vision to the greatest extent possible. Therefore, we would expect telephone conversations where visual cues are absent to be especially difficult for some clients.

Second, the loss of binaural or "stereo" listening has a serious effect on listening in noise. Our clients must be fit with two hearing aids if at all possible (Chapter 11 has more on the advantages of binaural hearing aids). Third, the communication process involves, indeed is dependent on, interaction among the participants. The aural rehabilitation client must acquire considerable skill in directing—even manipulating—the conversation and in repairing it when it breaks down. The transcribers couldn't ask for a clarification of an indistinct passage, whereas the client can. Furthermore, much of the transcription difficulty arose from the background noise, which would also severely limit the ability of the client to understand speech. However, if the client has learned assertive listening skills, he or she can act to reduce or eliminate the noise ("Can we move out of the hallway? I'm having trouble hearing you" or "I'm going to turn the radio down for a minute while we are talking"). Assertive noise control can provide as much benefit to an impaired adult as the hearing aids and lipreading combined. The successfully rehabilitated adult interacts in an effective, focused way to improve the chances for clear communication. On the other hand, if the aural rehabilitation client is so frustrated or discouraged by the difficulty in hearing that he or she withdraws (physically or mentally) from the conversation, or acts inappropriately, then all possibility of constructive interaction, assertive intervention, or repair is lost. In some clients, emotional reactions, fears, and attitudes are the primary obstacles to rehabilitation and must be addressed.

Fourth, much of the meaning is conveyed with tone of voice, manner and rate of speaking, and facial expression. These characteristics are usually available to the hearing-impaired adult and can be used to great advantage.

Fifth, knowledge of the topic and the background and attitude of the talker is a great help in filling in words and phrases that a client might miss. The more the hearing-impaired individual knows about current events, sports, local news, agendas of meetings, and the topic of conversation, the better off he or she is.

A more complete view of the verbal communication environment for the typical hearing-impaired adult thus involves at least six elements: a talker-listener with normal hearing; a message; two-way auditory and visual channels with varying amounts of noise or competing messages; a talker-listener with acquired sensorineural hearing loss; a common language and pragmatic system; and a shared intent to communicate.

The Nature of the Hearing Loss

For prognostic purposes, the hearing loss should be broken down further into three components whose relative rehabilitative impact varies considerably among individuals: hearing threshold, loss of frequency selectivity, and effects of noise.

FIRST COMPONENT: HEARING THRESHOLD

The first component defines the presence of hearing loss and is shown in the audiogram as the sensitivity curve—that is, the threshold of audibility across frequency. Obviously, a person who cannot hear the high-frequency energy in speech will have reduced speech recognition ability. If a hearing aid is used, the reduction is to the extent that the aid fails to restore normal thresholds in the soundfield. There is also some modest effect of distorted loudness relationships among acoustic speech cues due to recruitment. On the whole, it is approximately as if the speech had been filtered (usually low-pass filtered) by the hearing loss. When the filtering is counteracted by frequency-selective amplification, speech recognition is restored to near-normal levels. Threshold filtering by itself is an excellent prognostic factor.

Unfortunately, two other components prevent many hearing-impaired adults from receiving anywhere near that amount of benefit from amplification. For example, a recent aural rehabilitation client in our adult group had a relatively flat bilateral loss averaging around 75 dB HL, yet we could find no level or type of amplification that would produce monosyllabic speech recognition performance above 35% correct. The more availability of amplified speech energy in his region of audibility was not sufficient to make the speech intelligible. Obviously, other distortions are present in his auditory system beyond any threshold filtering that might be present.

SECOND COMPONENT: LOSS OF
FREQUENCY SELECTIVITY

The second component involves the loss of frequency selectivity and can be thought of as internal distortion of the signal. Here, the client has less than normal ability to discriminate between similar speech sounds, such as "s" and "sh" or "t" and "k," even though the sounds are audible and presented at a comfortable loudness level. The loss of frequency selectivity was clearly demonstrated by Walden et al. (1981), who experimentally removed the effects of filtering and found that perhaps a third of the patients still had significant loss of speech recognition in addition to that attributable to the filtering. The second component probably involves a loss of temporal resolution as well, where the rapid changes in the speech waveform may be distorted or go undetected by the impaired auditory system (Humes, 1982). The loss of spectral and temporal resolving power is present under quiet, ideal amplification conditions and probably is due to cochlear pathology in most cases. More information

on this phenomenon can be found in Pickles (1988, Chapter 10) and Sachs, Winslow, and Blackburn (1988). Clients who have significant amounts of internal distortion are not likely to receive great benefit from hearing aids and will need aural rehabilitation to reach their full communication potential.

THIRD COMPONENT: EFFECTS OF
NOISE

The third component reflects the difficulty experienced by many hearing-impaired adults (and surprisingly, some people with normal-thresholds as well) in separating speech from background noise. This component is often characterized as the signal-to-noise ratio (S/N) problem because the client's speech recognition ability is affected much more seriously by moderate levels of noise than is a normal-hearing individual. Whether the S/N component is truly independent of the loss of frequency resolution ability is debatable. The S/N difficulty may simply reflect the ear's broadened internal "filters" inability to reject the noise. Plomp quantifies some aspects of this question in two important papers (1978, 1986). However, the well-documented existence of clients whose speech recognition ability in quiet is near-normal but deteriorates badly in noise argues strongly for the presence of a specific S/N component to the individual's hearing loss. Further, many clients report difficulty only in noisy conditions and for rehabilitation purposes are most effectively treated as a distinct category of client with emphasis on assertive listening, binaural amplification, and lipreading. The prognosis for a pure S/N client depends largely on his or her ability to employ these three remedial techniques.

Four Stages in Speech Recognition

In designing an aural rehabilitation program for an individual, it is useful to break down the process of speech recognition into four stages. To the extent that the stages are distinct and have unique behavioral manifestations, they will be valuable in assessing a client's perceptual strengths and weaknesses and focusing on problem areas. It is possible to delineate four stages of speech understanding in a conversational situation.

PREPOSITIONING

The purpose of the prepositioning stage is to prepare for maximum sensory input and linguistic disambiguation. As the hearing-impaired adult enters into a conversation, he or she ideally experiences several things, which include becoming aroused to start the brain and body working optimally; performing orientation in space to occupy the location best for lipreading; using binaural input and paying mental attention to the talker to cut down on background interference; focusing eye gaze on the talkers' lips; and pulling up to consciousness old knowledge of the talker and likely topics. If possible, some assertive listening activities may be undertaken prior to the conversation to eliminate noise, learn the topic, adjust the lighting, and so on.

SENSORY PROCESSING

The sensory stage results in the visual information and the degraded auditory signal being transduced in the eye and ear and subjected to preliminary decoding, sharpening, and extraction from noise. The signals are integrated to some extent (see Massaro, 1987) and processed through the primary sensory projection areas in the cortex to some other "association" areas for cognitive processing.

COGNITIVE PROCESSING

The ideal result of cognitive processing is lexical access and sentence comprehension, where incoming sensory images and words stored in memory are matched to provide meaning. With degraded auditory signals, the auditory and visual input must be combined and then used with knowledge of the language and situation to reduce the number of ambiguous word candidates and select the most likely one (or decide to wait for additional input). Such personality factors as attitude, willingness to guess, and

ability to tolerate uncertainty enter in at this stage.

INTERACTIVE PROCESSING

Finally, because of difficulty with any or all of the preceding stages, the impaired individual must be prepared to interact positively in the conversation by verifying hunches, asking specific questions, supplying information, interrupting, and repairing breakdowns as they occur.

The Practice of Adult Aural Rehabilitation

THE ADULT AURAL REHABILITATION GROUP

Throughout the chapter we have referred to experiences and benefits gained by client participation in an adult aural rehabilitation (AR) group. In this section we describe the AR group as an important, almost essential, part of adult rehabilitation. The information is based largely on the group that is conducted at the University of South Carolina, although many clinics conduct their own version of the adult AR group. (See Binnie and Hession, 1990, for a good description of a similar group.). Our group reflects years of experimenting and refining procedures and content, with David Hawkins, Terry New and the author contributing to the continually evolving product. An outline of the current group, which meets 2 hours a week for 6 weeks, is included in Appendix 12.1.

Group Structure The ideal group involves four or five couples or families with one or both spouses having a hearing loss. (One group had a grandmother with a hearing loss, her daughter, and her teenage grandson!). The clinician acts as group leader and facilitator, with two graduate students participating and eventually leading the group as part of their training. The AR group meetings are designed to include three types of experiences. First, the members share feelings, experiences, successes, and failures related to coping with their hearing loss and their spouse's hearing loss. Members actively help each other to identify and solve specific communication problems. Second, some structured thera-peutic activities are conducted, such as lip-reading, assertive listening practice and role playing, learning to speak clearly to the hearing-impaired spouse, conversation re-pair, and situation analysis. Finally, each class has some time devoted to didactic in-formation on various topics such as care of hearing aids, ALDs, and other consumer-related issues. (See Appendices 12.1 and 12.2).

Four Essential Components of Rehabilitation

Throughout the six classes it is stressed that there are four essential components to the members' rehabilitation. These primary components of Efficient Aural Rehabilita-tion (we refuse to use the acronym EAR!) are:

1. Effective amplification. This includes a properly fitted hearing aid and appro-priate ALDs, with orientation and fol-low-up.
2. Auditory-visual integration. Here we stress the use of speechreading in com-bination with available auditory infor-mation through a variety of exercises. A handout (available in Appendix 12.3) is discussed and practiced.
3. Assertive listening. Assertive listening is also called situation control or asser-tiveness for the hearing impaired. It in-volves the use of assertive control of the communication environment and inter-active communication strategies.
4. Consumer awareness. Here, the client is guided through the acquisition of knowl-edge about hearing loss and the accept-ance of responsibility for his or her own rehabilitation and growth.

Benefits of Group Experience

The group situation allows several ben-eficial things to be experienced by the par-ticipating group members:

1. It produces the rapid gains in spee-chreading and auditory-visual (A-V) speech recognition that occur in the in-itial three or four sessions of practice. (See section ''Can Lipreading Be Taught?'' for a list of reasons why this improvement occurs.)

2. It allows the group members (hearing impaired and spouses) to benefit from "the group experience." These benefits include *(a)* sharing feelings of frustra-tion, anger, disappointment, and so on; *(b)* receiving support and encourage-ment; *(c)* gaining perspective on one's situation: "My loss isn't as serious as I thought it was" or "I'm glad I don't have *that* spouse's problem"; and *(d)* being ex-posed to healthy, even inspirational, role models in the group who demonstrate strong, positive approaches to assertive listening and problem solving in general.
3. It provides an emotionally safe situation where people can admit their hearing losses and practice communication strategies and assertive behaviors before attempting them in the outside world.
4. It provides ongoing contact with an au-diologist during the initial hearing aid adjustment period. Anecdotal evidence suggests that one primary reason people reject hearing aids is the cumulative ef-fect of several small malfunctions and irritations coupled with unmet (and per-haps unrealistic) expectations for hear-ing aid benefit. Both of these reasons are addressed effectively in the weekly group meetings.

A list of these benefits phrased as goals is used as a handout and discussion guide for the group and is available in Appendix 12.2.

In summary, it is clear that the group experience involves a great deal more than lipreading practice, although some of the members refer to it as their "lipreading class." Finally, we are convinced that group participation is the most effective form of insurance that a new hearing aid user will continue to use the aid after it is purchased (Montgomery, 1991). It is foolish and un-professional to limit contact with the client after hearing aid fitting and to cease reha-bilitation with only one of the four primary components completed.

CONVERSATION REPAIR

The topic of conversation repair has been mentioned several times previously. It represents an important skill that many hearing-impaired adults seem to lack, and it is an ideal activity for the aural rehabilitation group as well as for individual therapy. "Conversation repair" is a modern term for the interactive process that, ideally, follows a conversation breakdown of the type commonly experienced by hearing-impaired individuals. Three interesting studies have recently appeared that attest to the growing interest in this topic. Gagne (1989) showed that in lipreading, receiving a paraphrase or synonym after an error was more helpful than a repetition. In a similar study, Tye-Murray et al. (1990) indicated that each of five different strategies improved performance but that no one strategy was superior to the other. Asking for a simple repetition, however, remains a popular strategy (Tye-Murray et al., 1991), although it is not necessarily effective. This is not surprising because as long ago as 1951, Miller, Heise, and Lichten showed that simply repeating the controlled presentation of words that had been misunderstood in a list increased overall intelligibility by only a few percent. There must be some additional information to supplement the incomplete impression of the word created by the hearing loss. A pure repetition adds nothing to assist the client in the laboratory. However, repetition helps to the extent it does in real life because it buys the client time to think about the context and come up with a better guess, and because the talker often produces the repetition more slowly and loudly in isolation. That is, the repeated word or phrase is said in a different, more intelligible manner.

One of the most effective ways for the impaired listener to take advantage of the improved repetition of isolated words is to ask as specific a question as possible, rather than just saying, "What?" This latter approach elicits the whole rapidly produced sentence rather than only the single word, which may be all that was missed. Better, "You're going *where* on vacation?" or simply "Where?" than 'Huh?" Or better still, verify a hunch, "Did you say *George* was there or *Joe*?" These skills can be practiced very effectively in the aural rehabilitation group by having the leader distort a word or phrase in a sentence, and the group members try to come up with the shortest, most specific question possible to elicit only the distorted part. This strategy does much to streamline the dialogue between hearing

and hearing-impaired people. Other strategies such as asking for a synonym or a paraphrase produce much less predictable behavior from the talker and are not generally advisable. Actually, if the talker were willing to paraphrase for a hearing-impaired listener, he or she might be willing to speak in a controlled, clear manner that would eliminate much of the need for repair! (See Erber, 1988, Chapter 5 for information on training the talker.). Conversation repair, like all other interpersonal rehabilitative techniques, works best if the hearing person knows the listener has a hearing loss.

SIMPLE SOLUTIONS

The clinician's role in the group and in individual therapy and counseling is much like a detective, seeking to discover those elements that contribute to the client's communication difficulty. In many cases, the assistive listening device interview and information revealed in the group and in individual/family counseling will indicate specific problems that can be reduced or eliminated with the clinician's knowledge and attention. Sometimes the client's life can be significantly improved (and the spouse's life as well) with simple changes in behavior or through an inexpensive assistive listening device. For example, many couples, where one or both members are hearing impaired, have fallen into an angry, confrontational reaction style when communication breakdown occurs. Because this may happen several times a day, major improvements in the quality of life can be achieved if better reactions to frustration can be found. It may be as simple as establishing rules for handling the common problem when one person is in another room and the other person calls to him or her: the "I can't hear you when I'm in the bathroom" problem. (The two-room situation is almost always doomed to failure because of *(1)* lack of lipreading, *(2)* weak or distorted acoustic signal, *(3)* interfering noise and resulting poor S/N, *(4)* poor room acoustics, and *(5)* lack of a common context or topic.) In the group, we lead the couples to analyze these (and other) reasons for difficulty and help them to come up with an agreed-on set of rules to handle the "bathroom" problem. A typical set might be as follows: Step 1—Establish the communication channel: "Can you hear me, Mary?" If yes, proceed with the room-to-room communication; if no, say "I can't hear you, Fred." Step 2—the *initiator* of the conversation must move to the room where the recipient is. We have found that if the group members come up with the rules themselves, with our guidance, they are much more likely to adopt them than if the group leader simply tells them how to handle the situation. Obviously, it is necessary for both spouses to be involved in the process of setting the rules or it doesn't become "their" solution.

Another example comes out of the assistive listening device interview. A frequent problem involves setting the loudness on the TV audio signal when hearing-impaired and nonimpaired adults watch TV. "Grandma wants the volume up so loud it drives me out of the room!" This is again an important problem because it occurs daily, and it is easily solved with the appropriate assistive listening device. Grandma must be involved in the decision, however, and must help arrive at the solution or she will reject a heavy-handed imposition of the "newfangled headset."

These examples illustrate several principles: *(1)* It is most effective to attack the problems that occur often; *(2)* many communication problems are solved with changes in behavior or attitude, and this is best accomplished in the adult group with the spouses present; and *(3)* a surprising number of communication difficulties can be resolved quickly and easily once the situation has been analyzed and dialogue between the participants has been opened.

A CASE STUDY

The principles and practices discussed above are probably best illustrated in a case study of a typical adult hearing-impaired client.

During a problem-sharing session in the adult group a 57-year-old man with a moderate high-frequency hearing loss, "Mr. Jones," indicated that he had a recurring, frustrating situation that he was sure had no solution, but he would share it anyway. The problem involved a group of six to eight businessmen who met once every 3 or 4 weeks as a dinner club for social conversation at a local restaurant. Mr. Jones reported having considerable difficulty hearing and following the various conversations. The men were all longtime friends, and some were in their 70s. After some questioning, the aural rehabilitation group came up with the following suggestions: *(1)* Start eating earlier or later to avoid the most crowded time in the restaurant; *(2)* have all the men learn sign language; *(3)* encourage Mr. Jones to improve his lipreading skills; *(4)* get the men to agree to give a verbal signal when a new person starts talking ("Well, . . . "); *(5)* purchase a personal FM system so that Mr. Jones can pass the microphone around as needed; *(6)* have Mr. Jones bring up the topic of his hearing loss for discussion among the men; *(7)* teach the men to announce changes of topics as they occur; *(8)* have the club ask for a better table (round, not long and rectangular, and away from the kitchen door); and *(9)* get the men to decide on the likely topics for the evening beforehand.

Obviously, many of the suggestions are impractical (the men aren't going to become proficient in sign language), but all suggestions were written on the board for the aural rehabilitation group to consider. The group encouraged Mr. Jones to at least bring up the topic with the men in the dining club and to analyze exactly which factors seem to cause the most difficulty. Mr. Jones reported 2 weeks later than he had brought up the fact of his hearing loss with the men and found, to his surprise, that two other members were also experiencing some difficulty. The club decided to start one-half hour earlier and requested a better table, which the restaurant owner was happy to provide for his long-term customers. Mr. Jones also seated himself in a better position to lipread and hear the one man he had the most difficulty understanding. Most important, Mr. Jones felt much freer than before to ask for clarification, now that the club members knew he had a hearing loss. Finally, by the time of the second club meeting, Mr. Jones had improved his viewing and attending strategies considerably and was able to accommodate more audiovisual integration than previously. He reported having an enjoyable, relaxing experience for the first time, and the aural rehabilitation group applauded him.

Mr. Jones's success illustrates several things: the power of peer pressure in the group to change behavior; the value of assertive listening, starting with admitting that the hearing loss exists; the generally accommodating nature of talkers once they are aware of the listener's difficulty; and the value of analyzing the situation to determine the specific factors that are interfering with communication.

THE NONHEARING AID WEARER

In our opinion, one of the least appreciated and most tragic (and undoubtedly largest) groups of hearing-impaired adults is the *non*hearing aid wearer. Least appreciated, because they are clinically invisible—they rarely appear in an audiologist's practice. This is unfortunate because they frequently can benefit from a hearing aid, almost always can use specific assistive listening devices, and invariably profit from aural rehabilitation. We define this person as an adult who has consciously rejected wearing a hearing aid, either by refusing to try one or by having worn one for a period of time and then discarding it. Of course, by rejecting or avoiding audiological services they miss the opportunities for assistive listening devices and aural rehabilitation as well. Unfortunately, among some audiologists there is a tendency to reject these people in return or dismiss them as unreachable. Typically, the nonhearing aid users have been told a hearing aid can't help them, or they have tried an aid sometime in the past and rejected it for various reasons. Many are poor or financially very conservative and will not invest the money needed for a modern hearing aid. In these cases (and in general in a professional hearing aid practice) the use of loaner aids and trial periods, including rehabilitation, is very valuable. It is important to note that generally the nonhearing aid wearer is in *greater need* of rehabilitation services than the aided individual because he or she is denied the obvious benefits of amplification. Today, with digital fitting procedures, advanced compression circuits, noise suppression capability, and in-the-canal aids, there are very few people in the men-

tally competent mild-to-severe "typical" group we have targeted who cannot be fitted beneficially. However, the cardinal rule in rehabilitating the nonhearing aid wearer is, *do not try to talk him or her into a hearing aid!* They will simply vanish again and perhaps confirm whatever beliefs led to the original antiaid attitude! The correct approach is to accept the individual's reasons for not wanting an aid and get on with the rehabilitation. Of course, he or she may decide to try an aid at some point in the rehabilitation process, but the decision must be the individual's, based on new information and attitudes acquired, not on your salesmanship. Rehabilitation should include three components: *(1)* the adult aural rehabilitation group, *(2)* the assistive listening device interview, and *(3)* individual audiovisual integration training and assertive listening as needed.

The rationale for these three components is as follows: The adult group is a very important experience for the nonhearing aid wearer because in it he or she sees people who are in the process of adjusting to their new (or not so new) hearing aids and using them successfully. Also, the other group members will undoubtedly ask why the nonhearing aid wearer doesn't have an aid, and this leads to a useful sharing of feelings and attitudes.

The assistive listening device interview is important because often the nonhearing aid wearer has specific difficult listening situations and actually may not need an aid for general use if these situations can be handled with assistive listening devices and speechreading. Three assistive listening devices (TV audio transmitter, telephone amplifier, FM system) are especially useful in these cases.

Finally, the need for individual audiovisual training and assertive listening training as seen in the group interaction or rehabilitation evaluation is often necessary because, without amplification, the nonhearing aid wearer with a significant loss is quite dependent on lipreading in combination with residual hearing. In addition, any improvement in signal level or S/N that can be attained through assertive listening is of great benefit to the nonhearing aid wearer. Given that these people are likely to have more serious problems than the hearing aid wearer, and that they may come to accept amplification and/or assistive listening devices, working with a nonhearing aid wearer would seem to be a very efficient form of rehabilitation. The potential exists for large benefits from a small amount of rehabilitation effort.

Once one accepts the value of rehabilitating nonhearing aid wearers, the question arises of how to reach or find them. Various forms of follow-up and advertising may be employed. This varies greatly depending on the type of rehabilitative audiology practice involved. One of the most effective ways is to enroll them in the aural rehabilitation group program. Because the group is promoted as an educational as well as therapeutic experience and does not depend on having a hearing aid, and because it focuses on speechreading (in audiovisual contexts) and assertive listening and problem solving, it may appeal to the nonhearing aid wearer as an alternative to hearing aids. The USC adult group has attracted several nonhearing aid users through its promotion as a continuing or adult education class (along with macramé, Spanish, and Tai Chi!). Also, the large population of adults who receive hearing evaluations but who reject (or fail to return for) the hearing aid evaluation must be made aware of the possibility of rehabilitation with *or without* a hearing aid and encouraged to attend some form of rehabilitation. We contend that it is impossible to reach the nonhearing aid wearer without rehabilitation and assistive listening devices.

INDIVIDUAL AURAL REHABILITATION

Traditionally, aural rehabilitation has focused on lipreading (or speechreading—a more comprehensive term), auditory training, and hearing aid orientation. Much of the therapeutic activity was conducted in individual training sessions, which sometimes extended over a period of weeks or months.

Although the long-term individual-session paradigm may not be cost-effective in the 1990s, many of the techniques can be adapted to a short-term or self-administered therapy format. In this section, unisensory lipreading and auditory training are considered, and circumstances when unisensory training may be helpful are discussed. A variety of other clinical activities are then considered briefly and placed in a framework of five areas where the client may work to make maximum achievement either individually or in a group setting.

Individual aural rehabilitation takes place under several circumstances. First, much of a rehabilitory nature occurs naturally between audiologist and hearing aid client during the selection and follow-up stages, especially if a formal hearing aid orientation is included. The orientation typically includes information on how the aid works and how to troubleshoot and maintain it. Much time is spent encouraging the client to have realistically low expectations for performance in real-world conditions, and the client may be exposed to noise or taken outside to the street. Also, lipreading and the existence of self-help groups like SHHH may be mentioned. Second, a client may be scheduled for one-on-one therapy sessions at a university clinic or rehabilitation facility to allow more intensive or long-term exposure to auditory or visual stimuli or for counseling on personal adjustment problems. Finally, a variety of audiovisual materials such as videocassettes or disks are available from libraries or other agencies for self-paced practice in lipreading at home or in the clinic (Tye-Murray, 1992).

LIPREADING

There is no doubt that lipreading is of vital importance to almost every hearing-impaired person. The crucial questions, however, are whether lipreading can be taught and what the best way is to do it.

Can Lipreading Be Taught?

Several studies indicate that lipreading can be improved with individual, concentrated training (Walden et al., 1981; Walden et al., 1977) and that most of the improvement comes during the first few hours of therapy. On the other hand, there is a general feeling that adults with acquired hearing losses do not show much improvement beyond some predetermined individual limit (De Filippo, 1990). These seemingly contradictory observations can be easily reconciled, however.

It seems likely that there are indeed limits to the sensory process—at least in the visual system, although their nature is not clear (Samar & Sims, 1983; Shepherd et al., 1977)—and thus a limit to performance. Recall the four stages of speech recognition: prepositioning, sensory processing, cognitive processing, and interactive processing. The gains in lipreading performance with short-term training, then, come from pre-processing (learning to attend and watch effectively) and cognitive skills (willingness to guess [Lyxel & Ronnberg, 1987; Van Tasell & Hawkins, 1981], increased confidence, learning the test procedures). If this explanation is correct, it has clinical implications. It means that the improvement is based on important skills (apart from learning the test procedures) that provide more and better visual speech input and a higher probability that the correct word will be included in the ambiguous set of alternatives. These skills could well translate into better lipreading in the real world, although that is difficult to evaluate, and thus these skills are well worth pursuing. For prognostic purposes, a client with poor viewing habits and restricted guessing should be able to improve considerably in lipreading performance, whereas a person who attends well and guesses well probably has low potential for progress.

Lipreading is in no way a substitute for audition. Unfortunately, it is impossible to lipread a conversation without some sound included. This is because many of the phonemes (speech sounds) have little or no visible manifestation. They simply do not appear in the anterior part of the talker's mouth. It is sometimes said that another reason lipreading is so difficult is that the phonemes appear so rapidly that the eye cannot follow the movements. This explanation is incorrect. It is a very "eye-opening" educational experience to watch a videotape or disk of conversational speech in slow motion and count the number of actual visible movements. As few as one or two per second may be seen for some talkers. The problem is that there are too few visible aspects of speech, not too many! Another difficulty is that many of the movements look alike. Thus the "s" in "I knew Sue" looks very similar to the "sh" in "a new shoe." The rounded vowel context obscures any natural differences that might exist between "s" and "sh." It is often pointed out that phonemes like "p," "b," and "m" look alike and thus constitute a single visible element, a viseme. This concept unfortunately is confined to sounds occurring in isolation or with open vowels, like "ba," and does not relate well to sounds in more complex contexts like the "s"/"sh" example above (Montgomery, Walden, & Prosek, 1987). The viseme concept is of limited value in clinical practice where the emphasis is properly on words and sentences. Incidentally, the ideal clinical material, in our experience, is the prepositional phrase. A list of 300 prepositional phrases generated over the years is good for several graded lipreading lessons.

Analytic and Synthetic Approaches

The use of simple materials like isolated sounds, consonant-vowel (CV) syllables ("da" or "sa," and so on), or single words may be necessary for some lipreaders who need to gain experience with short-duration clear stimuli. The goal is to move to longer, more realistic stimuli as the client's skill and attention span permit. This approach is called the analytic method because the speech is analyzed into its component parts. This method has been used frequently because it is simple and highly structured. The alternative is the synthetic method, which uses phrases, sentences, and real-life situations as therapeutic material to encourage the client to bring together (synthesize) speech elements into larger units of meaning. Jeffers and Barley (1971) have produced lipreading materials and teaching methods of both types. Many people now believe that lipreading is best taught with some voice added so that the difficulty of the task can be controlled. That is, the client's performance level can be varied from near zero (no voice) to good understanding (strong voice) to suit the client's needs for success and challenge (De Filippo, 1990).

AUDITORY TRAINING

Much of what has been presented above on lipreading has a direct analogue in auditory training. Analytic approaches are often used to help the client make finer auditory discriminations such as comparing "ba" with "va" (without lipreading, of course) or "sa" and "fa." More severely impaired individuals may benefit from even grosser distinctions, including presence or absence of sound, long or short words, and one or two syllables. Sometimes noise is added to make the task more difficult or more realistic. (A friend of ours says that is like a baseball player practicing hitting foul balls—not a very positive thing to do!)

It is our experience that the more severely impaired clients benefit from pure auditory training, especially when experiencing amplification for the first time, but that listening to noise is rarely indicated. The trend seems to be toward doing combined auditory-visual (A-V) training rather than either sensory channel in isolation.

THE FIVE MAX'S

Aural rehabilitation, however, is now seen as consisting of much more than lipreading and auditory training. To illustrate this, Appendix 12.4 shows clinical activities organized under five categories, with each category representing one level or type of activity. The first level is concerned with "maximizing" auditory and visual input—simply making sure that as much sensory information as possible is available to the client's brain. Note the recommendation of a *vision* test at this stage.

The activities at Level II are aimed at improving discrimination, A-V integration, and memory. These are largely analytic in nature and may be skipped for most people with mild-to-moderate losses.

Level III is designed to focus the client's attention on the linguistic aspects of speech, including vocabulary, topic awareness, and conversational context awareness. An excellent source of ideas and materials at this level is Erber (1988).

Level IV is directed at interactive communication strategies, including assertive listening (and situation analysis) and conversation repair. Note the presence of the tracking task (De Filippo, 1988) in which a clinician reads textual material to the client for perfect repetition. If the client misses any word the two conversants engage in a highly structured repair process until it is correct. Performance is scored as words correctly repeated per minute. This procedure has been recommended as a rehabilitative technique as well as a possible test of performance (Levitt et al., 1986; Owens & Telleen, 1981; but see Tye-Murray and Tyler, 1988). The tracking task is an intensive and invigorating experience that may be of benefit to the more severely impaired client or to the client who needs carefully controlled auditory, visual, or auditory-visual speech stimuli.

The fifth level is directed specifically at improving the client's ability to interact effectively with his or her family. It assumes a motivated client and spouse. Activities are tailored to specific problems and may include helping the spouse to speak more clearly (an excellent group demonstration, incidentally) and designing and practicing conversational teamwork where the spouse will signal a new topic or indicate who in a group is speaking.

Obviously, no one client would receive all these activities either in individual or group form. The clinician's role is to get to know the client well enough to help the client select the exercises and experiences that will produce the most benefit in the time available.

Summary

In this chapter we have presented a variety of clinical aspects of the practice of aural rehabilitation. It can be seen that the goal of aural rehabilitation for the adult is ambitious—to increase the likelihood, the level, of successful communication over the client's lifetime. This is accomplished through giving him or her the skills and the hardware to understand and control the process of communication. All elements of verbal communication are shown to be in the client's domain of influence—the talker, the message, the auditory and visual channels, and the impaired listener whose emotional reactions, cognitive processes, and interactive strategies are tailored to prevent, minimize, and repair communication breakdown.

Because of its potential to help individuals and society, aural rehabilitation offers an excellent opportunity for audiologists and speech pathologists who choose to practice this exciting specialty.

Acknowledgments. The author's interest in adult aural rehabilitation was developed through stimulating friendships with six dedicated scientists and clinicians: Brian Walden, Carl Binnie, Marilyn Demorest, Lynne Bernstein, Charlene Scherr, and Sue Erdman. Their contributions, although perhaps unrecognizable here, are gratefully acknowledged.

References

Binnie, C.A., and Hession, C.M., A four-week communication training program. *Acad. Dispensing Audiol., ADA Feedback*, winter issue, 37–41 (1990).

De Filippo, C.L., Tracking for speechreading training. In C. De Filippo and D. Sims (Eds.), *New Reflections on Speechreading, Volta Rev.*, 90 (September 1988).

De Filippo, C.L., Speechreading training: believe it or not! *Asha*, 32, 46–48 (1990).

Erber, N.P., *Communication Therapy for Hearing-Impaired Adults*. Abbotsford, Victoria, Australia: Clavis Press (1988).

Gagne, J.P., and Wyllie, K.A., Relative effectiveness of three repair strategies on the visual-identification of misperceived words. *Ear Hear.*, 10, 368–374 (1989).

Garstecki, D.C., Audio-visual training paradigm for hearing impaired adults. *J. Acad. Rehabil. Audiol.*, 14, 223–228 (1981).

Herer, G.R., Inventing our future. *Asha*, 31, 35–37 (1989).

Humes, L.E., Spectral and temporal resolution by the hearing impaired. In G. Studebaker and F. Bess (Eds.), *The Vanderbilt Hearing Aid Report*, Upper Darby, PA: Monographs in Contemporary Audiology (1982).

Jeffers, J., and Barley, M., *Speechreading (Lipreading)*. Springfield, IL: C.C. Thomas (1971).

Levitt, H., Waltzman, S.B., Shapiro, W.H., and Cohen, N.L. Evaluation of a cochlear prosthesis using connected discourse tracking. *J. Rehabil. Res. Develop.*, 23, 147–154 (1986).

Lyxell, B., and Ronnberg, J., Guessing and speechreading. *Br. J. Audiol.*, 21, 13–20 (1987).

Massaro, D.W., *Speech Perception by Ear and Eye: A Paradigm for Psychological Inquiry*. Hillsdale, NJ: Lawrence Erlbaum (1987).

Miller, G.A., Heise, G.A., and Lichten, W., The intelligibility of speech as a function of the contrast of the test materials. *J. Experiment. Psychol.*, 41, 329–375 (1951).

Montgomery, A.A., Aural rehabilitation: review and preview. In G. Studebaker, F. Bess, and L. Beck (Eds.), *The Vanderbilt Hearing Aid Report II*. Parkton, MD: York Press (1991).

Montgomery, A.A., Walden, B.E., and Prosek, R.A., Effects of consonantal context on vowel lipreading. *J. Speech Hear. Res.*, 30, 50–59 (1987).

Owens, E., and Telleen, C., Tracking as an aural rehabilitation process. *J. Acad. Rehabil. Audiol.*, 14, 259–273 (1981).

Pickles, J. O., *An Introduction to the Physiology of Hearing*, 2nd edition. London: Academic Press (1988).

Palmer, C.V., Assistive devices in the audiology practice. *Am. J. Audiol.*, 1, 37–57 (1992).

Plomp, R., A signal-to-noise ratio model for the speech reception threshold of the hearing impaired. *J. Speech Hear. Res.*, 29, 146–154 (1986).

Plomp, R., Auditory handicap of hearing impairment and the limited benefit of hearing aids. *J. Acoust. Soc. Am.*, 63, 533–549 (1978).

Sachs, M.B., Winslow, R.L., and Blackburn, C.C., Representation of speech in the auditory periphery. In G. Edelman, E. Gall, and M. Cowan (Eds.), *Auditory Function: Neurobiological Bases of Hearing*. New York: John Wiley & Sons (1988).

Samar, V., and Sims, D., Visual evoked-response correlates of speechreading performance in normal-hearing adults: a replication and factor analytic extension. *J. Speech Hear. Res.*, 26, 2–9 (1983).

Serrano-Navaro, M., Arana, M., and Cram, J.E., HOLA: a new trend in aural rehabilitation. Paper presented at Academy of Rehabilitative Audiology, Summer Institute, Breckenridge, CO (June 1991).

Shepherd, D., DeLavergne, R. Frueh, F., and Clobridge, C., Visual-neural correlate of speechreading ability in normal-hearing adults. *J. Speech Hear. Res.*, 20, 752–765.

Smith, M.C., Neurophysiology of aging. *Sem. Neurol.*, 9, 64–77 (1989).

Tye-Murray, N., Repair strategy usage by hearing-impaired adults and changes following communication therapy. *J. Speech Hear. Res.*, 34, 921–928 (1991).

Tye-Murray, N., Laser videodisc technology in the aural rehabilitation setting: good news for people with severe and profound impairments. *Am. J. Audiol.*, 1, 33–36 (1992).

Tye-Murray, N., and Tyler, R.S., A critique of continuous discourse tracking as a test procedure. *J. Speech Hear. Disord.*, 53, 226–231 (1988).

Tye-Murray, N., Purdy, S., Woodworth, G., and Tyler, R.S., The effect of repair strategies on the visual identification of sentences. *J. Speech Hear. Dis.*, 55, 621–627 (1990).

Van Tassel, D.J., and Hawkins, D.B., Effects of guessing strategy on speechreading test scores. *Am. Ann. Deaf*, 126, 840–844 (1981).

Walden, B.E., Prosek, R.A., Montgomery, A.A., Scherr, C.K., and Jones, C.J., Effects of training on the visual recognition of consonants. *J. Speech Hear. Res.*, 20, 130–145 (1977).

Walden, B.E., Schwartz, D.M., Montgomery, A.A., and Prosek, R.A., A comparison of the effects of hearing impairment and acoustic filtering. *J. Speech Hear. Res.*, 24, 32–43 (1981).

Walden, B.E., Erdman, S.A., Montgomery, A.A., Schwartz, D.M., and Prosek, R.A., Some effects of training on speech recognition by hearing-impaired adults. *J. Speech Hear. Res.*, 24, 207–216 (1981).

APPENDIX 12.1 *Adult Aural Rehabilitation Group Outline**

Session one

1. Introductions, orientation
2. Discussion of what to expect from the group, what situations are difficult. Development of list of individual problem areas
3. Presentation of information on hearing and causes of hearing loss

HANDOUTS: notebooks
diagrams of the ear
list of purposes of the group

OUTSIDE WORK: Begin list of difficult situations

Session two

1. Discussion of difficult situations, introduction of CPHI
2. Presentation of information on the audiogram
3. Performance of brief lipreading test, discussion of lipreading

OUTSIDE WORK: Start on CPHI, lipreading assignment

Session three

1. Discussion of CPHI, discussion of lipreading assignment
2. Demonstration, pep talk on maximizing the chances for lipreading
3. Presentation of information on hearing aids

OUTSIDE WORK: Assertive lipreading assignment

Session four

1. CPHI inventory due
2. Discussion of lipreading assignment, situation analysis
3. Videotape demo
4. More information on hearing aids

OUTSIDE WORK: Analyze two situations that you encounter in everyday living

Session five

1. Conversation repair, demo and practice
2. Discussion of CPHI inventory results, individual counseling
3. Presentation of information and demonstration of assistive listening devices

HANDOUT: List of assistive listening devices and addresses

SUGGESTION: Attend a concert at Koger Center; use their excellent infrared listening system

Session six

1. Review of specific strategies for difficult listening situations
2. Lipreading practice, situation management
3. Course evaluation: "Y'all tell us what YOU think."
4. Wrap-up!

---

*Outline handed out to members of adult aural rehabilitation group. This groups meets for 2 hours each week for 6 weeks.

APPENDIX 12.2 *Specific Goals and Purposes for the Class**

1. To get together and share and discuss problems with other hearing-impaired individuals and couples.
2. To provide a place to practice new communication skills before trying them in the "real world."
3. To gain information and understanding about hearing loss and to have the opportunity to ask questions about your specific situation.
4. To provide a place where you don't have to hide your hearing loss.
5. To give you the opportunity to analyze and practice the art of conversation and conversation "repair."
6. To provide a chance for your spouse/friend/caregiver to gain understanding of your hearing difficulties and learn how to communicate more effectively with you (and you with them!).
7. To gain knowledge about new technology in hearing aids and assistive listening devices.

APPENDIX 12.3 *Ways to Maximize Your Chances of Lipreading in Combination with Your Hearing Aid***

1. Indicate to the talker in some way that you are hearing impaired.
2. Adjust the communication situation so that noise sources are nearer the talker than to you (all's fair in lipreading!). Reduce noise as much as possible.
3. Look around and become familiar with the situation so that you will know what the talkers are referring to.
4. Watch the talker's lips, not his or her eyes. Look around only during pauses (there are *plenty* of them) and changes of talkers. You can see facial expressions and eye movements without leaving the lips.
5. Adjust the situation so that the light is on the talker's face and not yours. Avoid glare and backlighting that obscure the talker's face or cause you to squint or strain to see.
6. Arrive early for situations that are more formal or structured, such as meetings, church, classes, or any place where people will be seated, so that you can stake out the best spot. Don't be afraid to move if you made a mistake or if the structure of the group changes. If there is one primary talker, sit so that you can see him or her without strain. Talk to the organizers beforehand about seating, amplifiers, and so on.
7. Learn to relax, even in tough listening situations. Avoid tension—keep your shoulders down, don't wrinkle your forehead, and so on. (One version of this list said, "Work hard at relaxing"; that's *not* what we mean!)
8. Concentrate on phrases and ideas rather than trying to pick out single words.
9. Make an effort to stay current on recent events, news, sports, and so on. The more you know about likely topics of conversation, the better off you are.

---

*Handout for members of adult aural rehabilitation group.
**Handout for members of adult aural rehabilitation group.

10. Interact with the talker or group to clarify or verify the message when you miss something. Don't wait until you're lost and three sentences behind.

APPENDIX 12.4 *Goals and Methods in Adult Aural Rehabilitation**

I. **Maximize Sensory Input**
   AUDITORY (A)
   1. Hearing aid(s)
   2. Assistive listening devices
   3. Improve S/N
      a. reduce noise
   4. Improve talker intelligibility
   5. Improve listener attention

   VISUAL (V)
   1. Vision check, glasses
   2. Improve visual S/N
      a. larger, taller image
      b. better lighting
   3. Improve talker intelligibility
   4. Improve viewer attention: focus on lips

II. **Maximize Sensory Processing**
   1. Analytic auditory or visual training
      a. same/different drill (A or V)
      b. contrasts, easy—difficult
   2. Memory training (A or V)
   3. Auditory training in noise
   4. Relaxation practice
   5. A-V training (e.g., Garstecki [1981] hierarchy)

III. **Maximize Cognitive Processing**
   1. V, A, and A-V depending on client's needs
   2. Develop and work on specialized vocabulary
   3. Topic cueing—sentences, paragraphs
   4. Context awareness
      a. filling in missing words
      b. predicting the next word
   5. Erber's syntactic practice (Erber, 1988, p. 106)
   6. Erber's semantic practice (Erber, 1988, pp. 107–108)
   7. Awareness of current events

IV. **Maximize Interactive Communication**
   1. Assertive listening situation control
   2. Conversation repair strategies
   3. Tracking procedure
   4. Handling changes of topic: cues and strategies

V. **Maximize Family Communication**
   1. Spouse training—talker improvement
   2. Solving specific problems
   3. Signals, cues, signs, and teamwork

---

*Activities useful in implementing the five "Max's"

13

Rehabilitative Considerations with the Geriatric Population

PATRICIA A. McCARTHY, Ph.D., JULIE VESPER SAPP, M.S.

The 1980s saw the reemergence of a "new ageism" in this country, centered on the belief that there are too many social, financial, and health care benefits for the elderly. Myths contributing to this ageism abound. Some even have claimed that the condition of children as a group has deteriorated because of the inordinate cost of the elderly. Yet in reality the older group receives more federal expenditures than the young, while children's education is supported on a community basis by state and local property taxes. Therefore, it is highly unlikely that the welfare of children will improve by stripping the elderly. Furthermore, already less than half (44%) of health care costs for the elderly are covered through Medicare (Zones, Estes, & Binney, 1987). Another popular myth is that the elderly in this country are affluent and have a large disposable income. Yet only 6% of people over the age of 65 years have incomes greater than $50,000, and older women endure the highest poverty rates (Zones et al., 1987). And the fact that almost 74% of the elderly live either alone or with a spouse (Coward, Cutler, & Schmidt, 1989) belies the image of the frail nursing home resident surviving on government largesse.

Negative stereotyping of both aging and hearing loss has produced a challenging dilemma for rehabilitative audiologists. Indeed, the negative image of aging held in this country is pervasive. Because hearing loss is often associated with aging, it is not surprising that older individuals often feel that admitting to a hearing loss is admitting to growing old. In fact, hearing aids are viewed as such overt, negative signs of aging that until recently the American Association of Retired Persons (AARP) did not allow them to be advertised in its publication, *Modern Maturity*. Unfortunately, the logic of "avoiding hearing loss avoids aging" may prevent older hearing-impaired adults from taking advantage of rehabilitative services. Consequently, successful rehabilitation of the older hearing-impaired adult can occur only if these deeply rooted psychological and social barriers are overcome.

The overwhelming demographic projections of the growth of the older population in the United States suggest that these attitudes need to change. There are almost 30 million people in the United States over the age of 65 years (U.S. Bureau of the Census, 1986), and an estimated 9.4 million of these have hearing problems (Williams, 1989). Furthermore, it is estimated that by the year 2010, there will be 39 million people ≥ 65 years (U.S. Census Bureau, 1986). Selker (1987) estimates that between the years 2020 and 2030, 75% of allied health care workers' time will be spent with the geriatric population. It can be expected that audiologists' caseloads will continue to grow commensurately, and older persons will ac-

Table 13.1
Sensory Changes with Aging

Visual	Auditory	Body Sensations
Structural	**Structural**	**Structural**
Depigmentation and atrophy of iris	Loss of elasticity in cartilaginous portion of outer ear	Loss of elasticity in skin and muscles
Yellowing of sclera	Reduced elasticity and atrophy of middle ear muscles	Decreased collagen in connective tissue
Decreased size of pupil		
Functional	Arthritic middle ear joints	**Functional**
Decreased acuity	Atrophy and degeneration of hair cells in basal coil of cochlea	Decreased sensitivity to touch
Decreased accommodation		Lessened sensitivity to pain
Decreased darkness adaptation	Alteration of motion mechanics of cochlea	Slower healing of wounds due to loss of collagen
Increased sensitivity to glare	Loss of auditory neurons	
Decreased ability to discriminate colors	**Functional**	
	Bilaterally symmetrical high-frequency sensorineural hearing loss	
	Inordinate reduction in speech recognition	

count for 59% of our services by 2050 (Fein, 1983, 1894).

Intolerance for ageism can begin with health care professionals. One way to eliminate this ageism is for health care professionals, including audiologists and speech-language pathologists, to prepare for the "graying" of their caseloads (Raiford & Shadden, 1985). Indeed, Oyer (1984) has suggested that audiologists and speech-language pathologists must have not only a knowledge of communication disorders but also a thorough understanding of the normal aging process. Unfortunately, Raiford and Shadden (1985) found in their survey of university training programs that only limited progress has been made in incorporating gerontology into communication disorders coursework. As such, audiologists and speech-language pathologists may feel unprepared to work with this population. Consequently, the potential for ageism may be intensified by feelings of ill-preparedness to work with the older hearing-impaired adult (Weinstein, 1987).

Knowledge of aging of the hearing mechanism must go beyond just the anatomic and physiologic changes. Senescent changes in the auditory system may produce dramatic effects on the overall functioning of the older individual. For example, social isolation, frustration, embarrassment, and anxiety have all been reported as by-products of hearing loss. Indeed, Herbst and Humphrey (1980) found a twofold greater incidence of depression in elderly persons with hearing losses. These are among the factors that contribute to the complexity of rehabilitation of the older hearing-impaired adult. The purpose of this chapter, therefore, is to present many of the facets of aging that can affect this rehabilitation process. It is hoped that as audiologists become more knowledgeable about aging and less prone to rely on misperceptions, service delivery to the older population will be more successful and older adults will be more likely to participate in their own hearing rehabilitation.

Normal Aging Processes

CHANGES IN SENSORY PROCESSES WITH AGING

Audition

No part of the auditory system is impervious to age-related changes (Table

13.1). And while the traditional view of *presbycusis* has centered on the inner ear, the term represents a variety of pathologic processes in the auditory system that result from aging.

Although no hearing loss results, even the outer ear experiences age-related structural changes. Visual inspection of the auricle often reveals a physical enlargement due to a loss of skin elasticity and muscle tonicity. Loss of elasticity in the cartilaginous portion of the external auditory meatus, however, may introduce audiologic testing problems. The pressure exerted by earphone placement can result in collapsed ear canals, thereby causing an artifactual conductive hearing loss. Audiologists have developed a variety of solutions to this problem, including using insert earphones, canal-retaining earmolds, or soundfield audiometry, or simply pulling the auricle upward and backward prior to earphone placement (Maurer & Rupp, 1979). Loss of elasticity of the skin and cartilage also can interfere with the proper fit of an in-the-ear hearing aid or earmold because of the difficulty of getting a tight fit. Improper fit may produce an auditory feedback problem that can lead ultimately to rejection of amplification.

Histologic studies suggest the presence of senescent changes throughout the middle ear, including reduced elasticity and atrophy of middle ear muscles (Schuknecht, 1955). Ethol and Belal (1974) reported arthritic middle ear joints with increasing age but with apparently no associated conductive hearing loss. Interestingly, audiologic testing has shown no significant changes in the transmission characteristics of the middle ear despite these structural changes with age (Jerger, Jerger, & Mauldin, 1972; Sataloff, Vassalo, & Menduke, 1965).

Degeneration of the structures of the inner ear appear to most markedly interfere with hearing function. The classic histologic studies of Schuknecht (1955) have contributed greatly to our understanding of the age effects on the inner ear and central auditory structures. Schuknecht observed that atrophic changes involving the membranous labyrinth, including afferent and efferent fibers along the organ of Corti, spread from the base to the apex of the cochlea. The slow progression of this process is consistent with the gradual high-frequency hearing loss seen in presbycusic patients. Schuknecht further described degenerative changes and a decrease in the number of auditory neurons of the eighth cranial nerve and central auditory pathway.

Later study by Schuknecht (1974) classified four general types of presbycusis: *(1) Sensory* presbycusis involves atrophy and degeneration of the hair cells and support cells in the basal coil of the cochlea; *(2) metabolic* presbycusis is characterized by atrophy of the stria vascularis with disruption of the nutritive supply necessary for cellular function; *(3) mechanical* presbycusis involves alterations in the motion mechanics of the cochlear duct probably implicating the tectorial membrane and basilar membrane; and *(4) neural* presbycusis includes degeneration and loss of auditory neurons. Corso (1977) cautions that despite the categorization of these different types of presbycusis, these various types rarely will occur separately.

The diffuse effects of the aging process on the auditory structures contribute to the unique differences seen in the auditory functioning of aging individuals. A discussion of the classic manifestations of aging on audiometric results follows.

Hearing Sensitivity. The physical changes in auditory structure with aging are accompanied by changes in hearing. In general, the hearing loss associated with aging, termed presbycusis, is bilateral, sloping, and sensorineural. Both longitudinal and cross-sectional studies with older subjects have demonstrated that the degree of hearing loss progresses throughout age (Gates et al., 1990; Milne, 1977). In other words, individuals in their 80s suffer even more hearing loss than individuals in their 60s. Another consistent finding is that hearing loss is greater among elderly men than among elderly women. These values, of course, are averages, and great individual variability in hearing levels is present within the elderly population, making age alone a poor predictor of hearing thresholds.

Aging itself is not the sole cause of hearing loss among the elderly. The longer one lives the more likely one has been exposed to high noise levels and personal and environmental factors, such as ototoxic drugs and vascular insufficiencies, which can contribute to hearing loss. These factors interact with the aging process in bringing about changes in hearing sensitivity. For example, in a study examining the interaction between aging and noise exposure on hearing levels, Rosenhall, Pederson, and Svanborg (1990) found that for elderly men aged 70 years, hearing levels were worse for those with a history of noise exposure than for those who had no history of noise exposure. By age 79 these differences had disappeared. The 79-year-old men with no noise exposure had now lost enough hearing to have thresholds not significantly different from men the same age with a history of noise exposure.

Speech Understanding. Clinical audiologists are accustomed to hearing the report from elderly clients that even when they can "hear," they often cannot "understand what is being said." Much research has investigated this phenomenon, yielding a better understanding of the factors that influence speech understanding ability for the elderly. Schum, Matthews, and Lee (1991) have demonstrated that in quiet, word recognition scores for groups of elderly subjects can be predicted from pure-tone thresholds using the articulation index. It appears from this that group differences between older and younger listeners on word recognition scores in quiet are caused primarily by differences in hearing thresholds. The greater hearing loss among elderly listeners accounts for their greater difficulty understanding speech in quiet. Of course, these are group findings and do not account for the individuals who do not conform to group averages. Bess and Townsend (1977) found that for older individuals with hearing thresholds worse than 60 dB HL, word recognition scores were worse than for younger listeners with similar thresholds. For most elderly listeners, however, reduction in word recognition in quiet can be explained based on peripheral hearing loss as demonstrated on the pure-tone audiogram.

The difficulties elderly listeners experience understanding speech in degraded listening conditions is not so easily explained based on peripheral hearing loss alone. Numerous studies have demonstrated a further decline in speech understanding ability in the presence of competing noise for elderly listeners compared to younger listeners. Schum et al. found that in the presence of a competing babble, the Articulation Index overestimated word recognition scores. So, as a group, the scores for the elderly subjects were 25% worse than predicted from the Articulation Index based on their hearing thresholds and the masking effect of the noise. Consequently, peripheral hearing loss alone could not account for the differences between young and elderly listeners on speech understanding in noise.

The presence of background noise is not the only degraded speech condition in which the elderly exhibit greater difficulty understanding speech. Blumberg et al. (1976) found that older listeners performed less well than younger listeners when the rate of the speaker increased, when the speech signal was filtered, or in a reverberant listening environment. Nabelek and Robinson (1982) found that across reverberation times, older listeners were more adversely affected than younger listeners. Because most listening in the real world takes place in situations with less than optimal conditions, these findings are very important in understanding the communication problems of the hearing-impaired elderly patient.

Much research has been performed in an attempt to determine the cause or causes of the discrepancy between young and elderly listeners on speech understanding tasks when peripheral hearing sensitivity has been controlled. Currently, the most frequently cited possible contributors to speech understanding problems for the elderly are central auditory processing problems, cognitive deficits, and attentional changes with age. Willott (1991) suggests that an interactive model including peripheral, central, and cognitive-linguistic factors is most appropriate. As he points out, if the peripheral system is impaired, additional stress is placed on central and cognitive functions, and if cognitive function is reduced, the ability to process sounds is affected. The specific ways in which these factors interact are not yet clear.

Once it has been determined that an elderly patient is experiencing speech understanding problems, particularly in background noise, rehabilitative intervention is important. Aside from selecting hearing aids to address the peripheral components of the speech perception deficit, the rehabilitative audiologist can counsel the elderly patient regarding environmental management techniques for controlling or avoiding noise, emphasize the importance of using visual cues, and make recommendations for appropriate assistive listening devices.

Central Auditory Processing. Changes in the function of auditory structures within the central nervous system, termed central auditory processing disorder (CAPD), are frequently held to be a significant contributing factor to the speech understanding problems of elderly listeners (Humes & Christopherson, 1991; Marshall, 1981). Tests for central auditory dysfunction include dichotic listening tasks, degraded speech tasks, and comparisons of PB-Max to SSI-Max.

Estimates of the prevalence of central auditory processing disorder among the elderly vary depending on how the sample was selected and what measures and criteria were used to identify CAPD. Prevalence of central auditory processing disorder among the elderly has been estimated to be as low as 22.6% for those 65 years of age and older (Cooper & Gates, 1991). These data were collected from a large sample, the famed Framingham cohort from cardiovascular research. As such they were not selected based on any communicative complaints. Prevalence estimates as high as 70% for listeners over 60 years of age have also been reported (Stach, Spretnjak, & Jerger, 1990). A clinical population was used in the second study. Prevalence of central auditory processing disorder was lower in the same study for a nonclinical volunteer group but still much higher than that reported by Cooper and Gates. Both of these studies showed higher prevalence of CAPD for those over 80 than for those in their 60s, and no significant differences were found between men and women. In the Stach et al. study, the prevalence among the clinical population for those over 80 was 95%, and for the nonclinical population of the same age the prevalence was 72%.

The impact of identified central auditory processing disorder in elderly patients on the aural rehabilitation process is a growing area of study. Jerger, Oliver, and Pirozzolo (1990) found that subjects who were identified with a central auditory processing disorder reported greater hearing handicap on the Hearing Handicap Inventory for the Elderly (HHIE) than did non-CAPD subjects. This findings was consistent across subjects with normal hearing, as well as those with mild and moderate hearing losses. The implications of this study were that the presence of a central auditory processing disorder was communicatively handicapping for the elderly in and of itself and added to the handicapping effect of any peripheral hearing loss.

When a peripheral hearing loss is present, the likelihood of benefit from amplification appears to be the same for elderly patients with CAPD as for those without. Using the Hearing Aid Performance Inventory (HAPI), Kricos et al. (1987) found similar scores of hearing aid benefit comparing a CAPD group to a non-CAPD group. The ranges of HAPI scores were also similar between the two groups. Both groups experienced the greatest benefit in quiet environments and the least benefit in noisy environments. This finding is encouraging in its implication that hearing aids are of benefit to elderly patients with CAPD and concomitant peripheral hearing loss. However, it is discouraging that hearing aids for both CAPD and non-CAPD individuals may be of limited benefit in the noisy listening environments that cause the greatest difficulty for older listeners. Indeed, using the HAPI, Schum (1992) found that elderly respondents reported less perceived hearing aid benefit than did the generally younger subjects from the original HAPI normative study of Walden et al. (1984).

Vision

The decrease in visual acuity after age 40 is a well-accepted aging phenomenon commonly referred to as presbyopia. In fact, after age 60, normal vision even with corrective lenses is rare. Dramatic changes in visual acuity occur with age. However, acuity is not the only aspect of vision that changes with age. Like the ear, almost every structure experiences age-related changes. As a result, many of these structural changes effect functional changes that have implications for rehabilitation of the hearing-impaired geriatric individual. In the following discussion, a brief review of the anatomy of the eye is provided to facilitate understanding of these structural/functional changes.

The iris, which is situated between the cornea and the lens, is responsible for controlling the amount of light that enters the eye. The lens controls the quality of light by changing its shape, while the size of the pupil (controlled by the iris) dictates the amount of light that will be focused on the retina. The rods and cones of the retina encode the spatial, spectral, and temporal aspects of the visual stimulus. This information is then transmitted from the retina over the optic nerves through the lateral geniculate nuclei to the visual cortex, where integration occurs.

Depigmentation and atrophy of the iris together with a decrease in pupil diameter contribute to the diminished amount of light that enters the aging eye. It has been estimated that the eye of the average 60-year-old allows only about one-third as much light to enter the eye as that of the average 20-year-old (Atchely, 1988). Consequently, older individuals may need three to four times brighter illumination than their younger counterparts. Interestingly, the retina itself is relatively free of age-related changes (Leopold, 1965).

Yellowing of the lens with age results in a decreased ability to discriminate colors. This yellowing causes the lens to filter out violets, blues, and greens, whereas reds, yellows, and oranges are easier to see (Corso, 1971). Visual adaptation to darkness also changes with age. Botwinick (1978) has suggested that older people adapt as fast as the young, but their adaptation is not nearly as good. A reduced ability of the eye to discriminate detail, called accommodation, has been reported to decrease with age (Bruckner, 1967). Furthermore, the ability to visualize distant objects has been reported to decline in the fifth and sixth decades (Riffle, 1979). Finally, sensitivity to glare reportedly increases with age (Wolf, 1960).

Clearly, these structural and functional changes can undermine the success of rehabilitation of the older hearing-impaired individual. As such, these changes should be considered in any rehabilitative planning. Most older individuals will need glasses in addition to large-print reading materials. This includes information given by the audiologist regarding hearing aids and communication strategies. Attention also should be given to levels of illumination in therapy rooms, audiometric test suites, waiting rooms, and offices. Levels of illumination need to be significantly higher for the aged individual to receive the same visual effect as a younger person.

Color discrimination should be taken into account when dealing with the older population. When possible, use of red or orange print for signs and therapy materials will facilitate visualization. Decreases in accommodation with age present a particularly difficult problem during the hearing aid orientation. The older patient's ability to distinguish the external components of the hearing aid may be severely limited. (This represents a challenge for some younger eyes as well!) Some audiologists have enhanced the visualization of these hearing aid components by highlighting them with a red marking pen or nail polish. This technique capitalizes on the older person's ability to easily visualize the color red. Increased glare sensitivity can also interfere with battery insertion in a hearing aid, since the "+" sign indicating the correct insertion side may be difficult to see. With some patients, the use of tactile cues to differentiate the positive side of the battery from the negative side may work. For others, marking the "upside" with red, orange, or yellow may be helpful.

Many of the methods, procedures, and strategies used with younger adults in the rehabilitative process are undermined by the visual changes that occur with aging. As such, knowledge of these changes in visual structures and functions with age allows audiologists to be creative in rehabilitative planning. The suggestions offered above are but a few of the practical suggestions that can enhance the success of rehabilitation of the older hearing-impaired adult.

Body Sensations

Touch and pain, two of the so-called body sensations (Atchely, 1988), undergo aging changes that can have an impact on the success of rehabilitation. Interestingly, the sense of touch starts to become somewhat dulled after about 45 to 50 years of age. In a study by Axelrod and Cohen

(1961), sensitivity to light touch on the palm and thumb was significantly less in older subjects (63 to 78 years) than in younger subjects (20 to 36 years). Concomitantly, sensitivity to pain appears to decrease with aging. Although these changes may appear to have little relationship to impaired hearing, they have implications for successful rehabilitation of the older hearing-impaired individual.

Decreased manual touch sensitivity may have an immense impact on the older individual's ability to manipulate a hearing aid. Hearing aid controls are so small that only minimal movement is needed to effect large changes in the hearing aid response. As such, the older person with decreased touch sensitivity may not be able to make the fine adjustments necessary to set the hearing aid at the most comfortable loudness level. Ultimately, this may lead to rejection of the hearing aid. Hearing aid manufacturers have responded to this situation somewhat by adding optional features such as enlarged and stacked volume control wheels, finger grips, and removable handles. These features coupled with the relative ease of inserting a custom in-the-ear hearing aid should overcome the problem of decreased touch sensitivity in most older patients. However, a mild gain body aid, albeit cosmetically unappealing, may be recommended for some older patients because of the size of the controls and the ability to manipulate the instrument at chest level.

Changes in pain sensitivity with age are difficult to quantify because pain is more than a sensory phenomenon. Responses to pain can be influenced by individual personality and cultural factors (Schwartz, Snyder, & Peterson, 1984). Although it is difficult to generalize about pain sensitivity with age, the clinical impression of gerontologists is that a decrease in pain sensitivity occurs with aging.

If decreased pain sensitivity does occur, then there is an increased likelihood of an older individual ignoring a pathologic condition caused by an improperly fit earmold or ITE hearing aid. It is not uncommon to find this auricular irritation among geriatric hearing aid wearers because elasticity changes in the cartilage of the outer ear may preclude a proper fit of the aid or earmold.

If the older patient ignores the condition, it can become chronic, which may preclude wearing the hearing aid until the irritation has healed. The seriousness of this situation is compounded by the fact that collagen, one of the compounds of connective tissue found throughout the body, decreases with age. Collagen aging causes wounds to heal more slowly (Kimmel, 1974). Consequently, the older patient may be prevented from wearing his or her hearing aid for a long period of time as the result of a slow healing process. This situation occurred with a 79-year-old severely hearing-impaired man seen by one of the authors. Unfortunately, the healing process was so slow that this man was without one of his hearing aids for 6 weeks.

The situation described above can be avoided by doing a careful inspection of the initial fit of the aid or earmold and by conducting frequent checks for auricular irritation during the first several weeks of hearing aid wear and on a regular basis thereafter.

CHANGES IN PSYCHOLOGICAL PROCESSES WITH AGING

Memory

To engage successfully in the aural rehabilitation process, the elderly patient must learn and recall information that will facilitate improved communication. It is important to understand the changes in memory that can occur with age and the variability seen among elderly individuals that can present challenges to the rehabilitative audiologist. Basic models of memory have attempted to define stages in the memory process, including encoding, storage, and retrieval of information. Much of the research on memory and aging has focused on which components of the process are most likely to be affected as we grow older, and on what variables related to the environment or the assigned task affect memory for older individuals.

Craik (1977) proposed a three-stage model that includes an information storage stage, a transfer to short-term memory, and a transfer to long-term memory. Current thought on memory includes further distinctions within memory processes. One important distinction is that of automatic versus effortful encoding (Kausler, 1990). Automaticity refers to the encoding of information without the conscious attempt to encode it. In other words, it refers to the way in which individuals "pick up" information without concentrating on trying to remember it. Effortful encoding, on the other hand, requires attention and concentration. The unconscious (automatic) process appears to be little affected by aging, while the active, conscious process (effortful) is affected more severely. This effortful encoding process is limited by working memory capacity. Working memory is another important concept in current research and theory related to memory. According to Hultsch and Dixon (1990), working memory is a limited capacity system that involves the simultaneous storage of recent information and processing of additional information. Working memory capacity apparently decreases with age. Hasher and Zacks (1988) have suggested that younger subjects use inhibitory attentional mechanisms to exclude irrelevant information from working memory. According to their theory, aging is associated with a reduction in these inhibitory attentional mechanisms. As a result, older subjects experience a reduced ability to exclude extraneous information from the task at hand and focus their attention on the storage and processing of the desired information.

Another important distinction is between implicit and explicit memory (Hultsch & Dixon, 1990). Implicit memory refers to the effect of prior exposure on later performance of a task that is not a direct request for recall of material. Explicit memory, on the other hand, involves the conscious attempt to remember. Elderly individuals tend to have greater difficulty than younger individuals on tasks involving explicit memory. Little difference has been noted between the young and the elderly for implicit memory. Retrieval of previously stored information is also affected by aging. Interference from extraneous distractors once again appears to have a greater effect on elders' ability to retrieve information (Gerard et al., 1991). Additionally, older people may require more time to retrieve information once they have stored it. This has been demonstrated by improved performance on memory tasks when response time has been increased (Canestri, 1964). Younger subjects' scores also improved with increased response time, but the older subjects benefited more from the slower pace.

These changes in encoding and retrieval of information with advancing age do not imply that older individuals cannot learn. Rather, they suggest that some older people may require more time to learn and to retrieve what they have learned. Audiologists working with elderly clients must be sensitive to the time their clients require to master new information. Additionally, attention should be paid to reducing distractions, to providing information clearly, and to focusing the elderly individual's attention to the task at hand. It should be kept in mind that great variability in memory skills exists within the elderly population. Therefore, the rehabilitative program and the time allotted to it must be tailored to the needs of the individual elderly hearing-impaired patient.

Slowing and Cautiousness

An often observed phenomenon among older people is a slowness of behavior. Simple reaction time, meaning the simple response to the onset of a stimulus, becomes longer as we age. Older individuals are particularly slow to respond if the stimulus is unexpected (Botwinick & Brinley, 1962). Reaction time can, however, improve with practice (Botwinick & Thompson, 1967). Slowness in response behavior has also been observed for more complex cognitive tasks. In general, the more complex and demanding the task, the slower the response. However, variability is high (Botwinick, 1984). This variability makes age alone a poor predictor of speed of response.

An issue related to slowness of response behavior is cautiousness. Botwinick (1984) describes the elderly as being willing to sacrifice speed for the sake of accuracy. Additionally, the elderly may fail to respond at all rather than risk making a mistake. In audiology, cautiousness by the elderly has been well documented on pure-tone threshold tasks (Rees & Botwinick, 1971). This caution can yield elevated thresholds on standard pure-tone audiometric tasks. However, elderly listeners do not appear to respond more cautiously than younger listeners on tests of word recognition (Gordon-Salant, 1986; Vesper & McCarthy, 1990). Vesper and McCarthy (1990) examined this issue by studying the frequency of occurrence of the omission error. Omission of a response during a behavioral task is regarded as a product of cautiousness. In this study an adaptive procedure was employed to set the level of a competing babble to equalize task difficulty and to create the need for guessing. Using a word recognition task, elderly normal-hearing listeners showed no greater rate of omission errors than did younger listeners. However, while greater cautiousness in the elderly group was not observed in this study, further research is needed to determine if hearing-impaired elderly perform similarly.

In the aural rehabilitation process, the tendency to respond slowly or not at all can affect an elderly patient's progress. During hearing aid orientation, for example, the elderly patient may require more rehearsal and encouragement to effectively and confidently manipulate and maintain a hearing aid independently. Once again, this highlights the importance of providing the elderly client with sufficient time to master a skill or task. This may require more patience on the part of the audiologist, but the greater rehabilitative success gained with the elderly client is ample reward.

Motivation

Implicit in the aural rehabilitation of individuals of any age is the factor of motivation. Elias and Elias (1977) suggest that the age differences in a variety of human activities may be related to motivation rather than intellectual or physiologic competence

Included in the definition of motivation are the factors of drive and incentive. Theorists suggest behavior is *pushed* through the action of motivating drives and *pulled* through the perception of a goal or valuable object (Bolles, 1967). Drive then appears to be internally generated as from a biologic or psychological need. Incentives are provided externally by the reinforcement of achieving a goal or an object.

Motivation for successful aural rehabilitation can be viewed from both a *push* and *pull* perspective. While the hearing-impaired individual provides the *push* or

drive, the audiologist can provide the *pull* or incentive. With hearing loss, a biologic need for better communication is produced. Theoretically, increased hearing deprivation should result in increased drive to improve communication. In practice, however, this is not always the case. Older hearing-impaired individuals often appear to lack the push or drive necessary for improved communication. To compensate for the lack of drive, the audiologist can provide the pull or incentive. The incentive can be the goal of successful use of amplification, improved use of visual cues, or development of better listening skills and communication.

The audiologist has the responsibility to ensure that the goals for the hearing-impaired individual truly are viewed as valuable. For this reason, goals for aural rehabilitation should be mutually established with the hearing-impaired individual. If input is not obtained from the older client, the value of the goals may be insufficient to provide the incentive necessary to achieve them. Unfortunately, the input of the client often is not considered in treatment planning. Perhaps this is why so many older clients appear to be lacking motivation. The audiologist can increase the older person's motivational level by ensuring that the end goal of treatment is of value to the individual.

HEALTH CARE ISSUES IN AGING

Physical Health of the Elderly

Sociologists believe that health is of major importance to aging individuals because it determines their ability to perform those tasks that enable them to participate in family, community, jobs, and leisure activities (Shanas & Maddox, 1976). Moreover, health can be a major determinant of the geriatric individual's ability to participate in his or her own rehabilitation. Therefore, a discussion of the general health status of the elderly follows.

Unfortunately, there is a strong association between advancing chronological age and an increased incidence of disease and disability. However, it is interesting to note that on the average, older people are afflicted with *acute* disease comparatively less often than younger people. In fact, Ries

(1979) reported an average of 1.1 acute conditions per year in the 65+-year-old population, which represents the lowest occurrence across age groups. However, when this older group experiences an acute condition, they experience more days of restricted activity than younger individuals do. From these data it appears that there is no reason to suspect a higher rate of absenteeism among geriatric patients in an audiology practice. However, when absenteeism is due to an acute illness, it may be more long term than expected.

The incidence of *chronic* conditions increases with age, and it is estimated that only a small percentage of persons over 65 years have *no* chronic conditions. However, Atchley (1988) cautions that a chronic condition is seldom disabling. Therefore, any generalizations about the frequency of occurrence of a chronic condition or the percentage of the geriatric population with chronic conditions must be interpreted in that light. Atchley reports that the number of older individuals with no limitations on activity has increased substantially in recent years.

While health is not a seriously limiting factor for most older hearing-impaired patients, general health status should be considered when developing a rehabilitative plan for a geriatric individual. Rehabilitative goals should be made with respect to the individual's general health status.

Use of Medication by the Elderly

Given the incidence of chronic diseases and disorders, it is not surprising that use of medication by the elderly is higher than among younger patients (Vestal, 1984). And as the geriatric population grows, so will the expenditures for drugs and medications. In 1976, the elderly population spent about 25% of the national total for drugs and drug sundries, and it has been estimated that by the year 2030, expenditures for drugs by the elderly in the United States will reach 30 to 40% of the national total (Vestal, 1978). Furthermore, multiple drug use by elderly individuals is the rule rather than the exception. Consequently, the potential for medication errors among the elderly is great. Complicating the situation is the fact that older adults are prone to increased drug sensitivity (Braithwaite, 1982; Schumaker,

1980). These factors contribute to the higher incidence of adverse drug reactions in the elderly than in the young (Vestal, 1978).

Medication compliance in the elderly has been the subject of several investigations. In a review of over 50 studies, Blackwell (1972) found that complete failure to take medication occurred in 25 to 50% of all outpatients. Schwartz et al. (1962) studied 178 chronically ill elderly patients and found that 59% made one or more medication errors, with 26% making potentially serious mistakes. Furthermore, Schwartz et al. found that error-prone patients were likely to make multiple mistakes more than single mistakes. The most frequent mistake was omission of medication, followed by lack of knowledge about the medications, use of medications not prescribed by the physician, and errors of dosage, timing, or sequence. A study by Parkin et al. (1976) found that a lack of understanding of the drug regimen was the greatest problem in medication compliance.

Another possible issue in medication compliance is the complexity of the language used in the directions found on the labels of the bottles and containers. Tymchuk (1990) investigated the readability of over-the-counter medications using a standard readability formula. His results showed that elderly persons using some common over-the-counter medications would have to have a reading ability anywhere between grade 6 and college level to comprehend the information. Previous studies in medical decision making found that the average reading comprehension levels of competent elderly people were between fourth and fifth grade (Tymchuk, Ouslander, & Rader, 1986; Tymchuk et al., 1988). In addition, Tymchuk (1990) reported that the obtained grade levels found on the labels actually masked the complexity of some of the medical, technical, and scientific language used. As such, only a very well-informed layperson, pharmacist, or physician would understand most of the language. Tymchuk suggests that this lack of understanding may contribute to misuse of medication among the elderly.

In addition to misuse, older adults have a higher incidence of adverse drug reactions (Vestal, 1978). The combination of multiple

Table 13.2
Possible Adverse Effects of Prescription Drugs

Drug Class	Adverse Effects
Antihypertensives Reserpine Methyldopa Propranolol Clinidine Hydralazine	Sedation, fatigue, depression, constipation, confusion, weakness
Analgesics Narcotics Morphine Codeine Meperidine Pentazocine Propoxyphene	Sedation, hallucinations, confusion, withdrawal, constipation
Non-Narcotic Indomethacin	Headache, dizziness, confusion, depression
Antiparkinsonian L-Dopa Carbidopa Bromocriptine Trihexyphenidyl	Confusion, hallucinations, depression
Antihistamines Dipheniramine Hydroxyzine	Sedation, anxiety, confusion
Antimicrobials Gentamicin Isoniazid	Psychosis, depression, agitation, hallucination, memory disturbance
Cardiovascular Digitalis Lidocaine Atropine	Fatigue, psychosis, irritability, confusion
Hypoglycemics Insulin Sulfonylureas	Anxiety, irritability, confusion, lethargy
Laxatives	Habituation, withdrawal, irritability, insomnia, confusion

Reprinted with permission. From Illness and Psychopathology in the Elderly by J.G. Ouslander, L.F. Jarvik, and G.W. Small (eds.), *Psychiatric Clinics of North America* (vol. 5), Harcourt, Brace, Jovanovich, Orlando, FL [46, p. 155], 1982.

health problems combined with a decline in physiologic functioning of the elderly may predispose elderly adults to adverse drug reactions (Cherry & Morton, 1989). Physiological changes with aging can have dramatic effects on the absorption and distribution of drugs in the body. Often dosages of medications have to be adjusted up or down to achieve desirable levels in the body.

Misuse of medications, adverse drug reactions, and aging changes related to drug sensitivity all can have negative effects on the elderly person both physiologically and behaviorally. Table 13.2 displays many of the commonly observed side effects associated with several classes of drugs. Although these side effects can occur with any age group, the factors discussed in the preceding section suggest that the elderly may be particularly at risk.

Clearly, communication can be severely compromised if the elderly patient is experiencing any of the adverse effects shown in Table 13.2. Furthermore, elderly patients experiencing these adverse effects may have a great amount of difficulty participating in their own hearing rehabilitation. Unfortunately, audiologists may be tempted to consider such behaviors as confusion, irritability, memory loss, or depression as normal albeit negative aspects of aging. As a consequence, the elderly person's "rehabilitation potential" may appear limited, and recommendations for amplification and communication therapy may not be made. As such, the elderly person in this situation experiences "double jeopardy." Not only has this older person experienced serious side effects from prescribed medication, but he or she may have appropriate rehabilitative recommendations withheld by the audiologist.

Audiologists working with elderly patients must be aware of the potentially serious side effects that older patients may experience from medications. Furthermore, they must be knowledgeable of the medications that their own patients are taking and look for signs of these behavioral side effects. While attributing irritability and confusion to aging may be the easy answer, it may lead to inappropriate rehabilitative decision making by the audiologist.

Health Care Providers' Relationships with the Elderly

The continuing growth of the geriatric population suggests a great need for health care providers who are knowledgeable about care of the elderly. It has been estimated that even with minimum use, more than 24,000 primary care physicians knowledgeable about geriatric medicine will be needed by the year 2010, when there will be as many as 35 million people in the United States 65 years of age and older (Belgrave et al., 1982). This projection implies more than the demand for a large number of physicians; it suggests these physicians must be knowledgeable of and sensitive to the special medical needs of the geriatric population. Furthermore, the importance of physicians' attitudes toward the elderly is underscored by the critical role physicians play in the lives of older persons. Indeed, the elderly use about three times the health care resources of the rest of the population (U.S. Department of Health and Human Services, 1983).

Unfortunately, studies that have examined the attitudes and practices of medical students and physicians suggest that ageism and stereotyping may influence treatment received by older patients. Several studies have shown that first-year medical students reveal little interest in geriatric medicine (Geiger, 1978; Perotta et al., 1981). Furthermore, Cicchetti et al. (1973) reported little change in the attitudes of medical students as a function of exposure to a social medicine course focusing on the elderly. Medical students typically characterized the elderly as lacking ambition, resisting change, and representing less of a loss to society than younger individuals. More recently, a study of six successive entering classes at a medical school found students' general attitudes toward the elderly were not negative (Wilderom et al., 1990). However, only 3% of the students expressed an interest in specializing in geriatric medicine.

Interestingly, attitudes toward the elderly have been found to differ by medical specialty. Ford et al. (1967) found that physicians in specialties where a relatively large number of the patients were elderly were less likely to express a dislike of them. Belgrave et al. (1982) observed less stereotyping of the elderly among medical students who had selected primary care specialties (family practice and internal medicine) than those who had selected surgery and other specialties (pediatric, obstetrics, psychiatry).

Unfortunately, even when stereotypes appear not to be pervasive, the quality of care provided to the elderly may be suboptimal. One indicator of quality of care is the time spent with elderly patients. In an examination of national surveys of physicians' professional practices, it was found that physicians spent less time with their older patients in the 65- to 75-year age range than they did with younger patients (Radecki et al, 1988a). Internists and cardiologists spent substantially more time with older patients than did general and family practitioners. In a follow-up study of the quality of care provided to the elderly, Radecki et al. (1988b) found that diagnostic testing falls off significantly for patients 75 years of age or older. However, internists used substantially more tests for each age group than did family practice and general practitioners and generally were better at recognizing changes associated with aging than were other specialists. Unfortunately, even among internists some signs of ageism were evident. For example, internists were less likely to perform routine cancer screenings on older women. From these studies, the authors conclude that the elderly may indeed need *more* time rather than less time for giving and receiving information than do younger patients. Furthermore, primary care physicians need more training in health care of the elderly to offset signs of ageism.

One way that physicians and health care professionals have attempted to improve the state of geriatric medicine is through the establishment of Geriatric Education Centers (GECs). The GEC's have been developed to expand education and training in geriatric health care so that health care professionals can work together to improve the nature and quality of care provided to elderly persons (Hubbard & Kowal, 1988). The U.S. Department of Health and Human Services has funded this nationwide network of GECs to improve the interdisciplinary approach to health care for the elderly. This is done by providing educational and clinical opportunities for health care professionals to learn from one another (Weinstein, 1987). All GECs provide training for physicians and nurses, and many include dentistry, social work, occupational therapy, physical therapy, and pharmacy. A few centers also involve audiology and speech-language pathology (Weinstein & Clark, 1989). The mission and efforts of the GECs represent a step forward in meeting the challenge of providing quality health care to the burgeoning geriatric population.

An interdisciplinary approach to learning about aging and health represents the most hopeful approach for the future of geriatric health care. This approach will provide reciprocal benefit to both participating professionals and geriatric patients. To that end, all allied health care professionals need to be resolute in *(1)* eliminating stereotypes about the elderly as patients; *(2)* improving the educational preparation of health care professionals by expanding curricula to include interdisciplinary training in geriatric health care; and *(3)* improving the quality

of health care service delivery to the burgeoning geriatric population.

Hearing Health Care Knowledge: Professionals and Consumers

Because physicians and health care workers are often the first to see the elderly person with presbycusis, it is of utmost importance that they be knowledgeable about hearing loss and the effects of aging. If myths and stereotypes about aging and hearing loss persist among primary care physicians and other health care workers, then these patients may never be referred to the audiologist. As such, the geriatric patient is the loser.

Unfortunately, a review of some investigations of the hearing health care knowledge of health care professionals is disconcerting. Taylor (1991) reported the results of a survey administered to 585 family practitioners and internal medicine specialists who responded that at least 25% of their practice was dedicated to elderly patients. A large majority of these physicians (77.8%) described amplification or amplification followed by aural rehabilitation as the preferred treatment for older hearing-impaired patients. However, only about half of these physicians said that amplification is "always" or "frequently" effective in treating hearing loss in the elderly. Moreover, only 47.1% responded that they refer elderly patients suspected of hearing loss for audiologic services. And nearly 20% indicated that they "always" or "frequently" advise *against* amplification for elderly hearing-impaired patients. From these results, it would appear that a significant number of hearing-impaired elderly individuals are not being referred by their physicians for audiologic services perhaps in large part because these physicians were unaware of the benefits of audiologic remediation.

Olinger, Dancer, and Patterson (1991) surveyed students in four health professions to determine their knowledge of hearing loss in the elderly. Two hundred thirty-two students in speech-language pathology, nursing, physical therapy, and occupational therapy were administered a questionnaire that included 30 statements about hearing loss, hearing aids, and aging. Although the speech-language pathology students presented the highest mean score, all four groups performed similarly and answered most of the items correctly. However, Olinger et al. found that all the occupational groups were misinformed in seven areas. Five of these items related to misinformation about hearing aids, and the other two items related to hearing loss and aging. The authors suggest that a questionnaire of this type can be used to help plan teaching strategies for programs educating health care professionals about hearing health care.

Because few health care workers have received formal training in the identification, treatment, management, and needs of patients with communication disorders, Sarvela, Odulana, and Sarvela (1990) developed a questionnaire to use as a staff training tool in a geriatric care setting. The Communication Disorders Questionnaire (CDQ) was pilot-tested with long-term care facility workers including therapists, physicians, administrators, and support staff. The final form of the CDQ consists of 23 items that test general knowledge in these categories: identification of commonly occurring hearing disorders, identification of commonly occurring speech disorders, and knowledge about communication disorders therapy. The authors report the CDQ is reliable and valid as measured through content and construct validity procedures. They recommend that the CDQ be used for three major purposes: *(1)* as a needs assessment instrument to determine the need for employee education in communication disorders in geriatric care settings; *(2)* as a teaching tool to be used by audiologists, speech-language pathologists, health educators, nurses, and/or physicians during inservice training programs; and *(3)* as a posttest on completion of training for quality assurance purposes.

The CDQ represents a viable tool for use with health care workers in a geriatric care setting. The scope of it goes beyond hearing loss to include other communication disorders. However, Sarvela et al. report that researchers and practitioners may add, delete, or modify certain items to meet the needs of their own target group of health care workers.

In the 1990s, consumer education has become one of the major goals of health care providers. Certainly, patients who are knowledgeable about their disorder will be more effective in participating in their own rehabilitation. However, until recently little has been known about the aging adult's knowledge of hearing impairment and rehabilitation. In an ongoing study of hearing health knowledge of aging adults, Garstecki (1990) investigated older adults' knowledge about hearing assessment, impact of hearing loss, factors known to contribute to hearing loss, and approaches to treatment of hearing loss. Subjects in this study displayed age-normal hearing, less than maximal self-assessed hearing handicap, good to fair physical health, average or above educational accomplishment, and income sufficient to meet hearing health care needs. Subjects completed Part II of the Hearing Health Inventory (Singer & Brownell, 1981), which consists of 35 correct and incorrect statements relating to hearing and hearing health. Respondents indicated agree, disagree, or undecided for each item. Results showed that subjects were uninformed of the relationship between hearing loss and other sensory functions, common medications, and ear disease. Furthermore, these respondents were not well-informed of the benefits of binaural amplification and speechreading. Garstecki (1990) concludes that greater emphasis must be directed toward educating the general aging population regarding the impact of hearing loss; the influence of drugs, diseases, and chemical agents; and the benefits of binaural amplification and speechreading.

It is an underlying tenet of rehabilitative audiology that patient education in part can ameliorate the handicapping effects of hearing loss. Yet in a large survey of Self-Help for Hard of Hearing (SHHH) members, consumers reported that information that should have come from professionals typically has not been provided. Furthermore, consumers in this survey thought that neither physicians nor audiologists do a very good job at helping people adjust to a newly diagnosed hearing loss. And although the respondents reported that audiologists were usually more helpful than physicians, few were rated very highly (Glass & Elliott, 1992).

The results of both of these studies underscore the need for hearing health care professionals to provide more and better patient education. Furthermore, audiologists have a dual responsibility. We must not only be more diligent about educating consumers about hearing health care, we must also educate physicians and other allied health professionals of the importance of our rehabilitative services.

Relationship of Health to Rehabilitative Audiology

The goal of virtually every older person with a disabling condition is restoration of his or her independence and autonomy (Williams, 1989). Concomitantly, a major goal of medical practice is to assist elderly patients in achieving independence (Cluff, 1981). However, a prerequisite to independence and autonomy for the elderly appears to be maintenance of good general health. While such disabilities as cardiac problems and arthritis present known, quantifiable limitations on one's functioning, less is known about the influence of hearing impairment on overall health status and functioning. Nonetheless, given the ubiquitous presence of hearing impairment among the elderly, this is clearly an issue of interest to all health care professionals working with this population.

Studies of the impact of hearing impairment on the overall health status of the elderly have garnered conflicting results. Herbst (1983) found that hearing loss in the elderly was associated with poor health, increased depressive symptoms, and a reduction in mobility, activities, interpersonal relations, and enjoyment of life. Yet, Salomon (1986) found no direct relationship between hearing level in the elderly and life satisfaction, self-perception, and general activity level. Neither of these studies, however, adjusted for confounding variables (Bess et al., 1989).

Given these conflicting results, Bess et al. (1989) conducted a study to clarify whether hearing loss imposes adverse functional and psychosocial consequences on elderly patients. The impact of hearing impairment was analyzed on 153 patients over the age of 65 years. Pure-tone audiometry was conducted to determine hearing levels, and functional health status was assessed using the Sickness Impact Profile. The SIP, a 136-time standardized questionnaire that assesses physical and psychosocial function, has 12 subscales: ambulation, mobility, body care/movement, social interaction, communication, alertness, sleep/rest, eating, work, home management, and recreation/pastimes. Three main scales are formed by combining subscales: physical (ambulation, mobility, body care/movement), psychosocial (social interaction, communication, alertness, emotional), and overall (combining all 12 subscales). The higher the SIP score, the higher the level of functional impairment (Bess et al., 1989).

Results of this study demonstrate that poor hearing was associated with higher SIP scores and increased overall dysfunction. Furthermore, progressive hearing impairment in elderly patients was associated with progressive physical and psychosocial dysfunction. The authors conclude that hearing loss appears to be an important determinant of function in elderly persons.

If hearing impairment is such a strong determinant of physical and psychosocial function, then all health care professionals working with the elderly should have a vested interest in the assessment and rehabilitation of hearing impairment in their elderly patients. This can happen only if audiologists educate other health care professionals about the possible deleterious effects of hearing loss on the overall functioning of the hearing-impaired elderly. Clearly, the impact of ignoring a hearing impairment in the elderly person may extend beyond the simple inability to hear. Indeed, the neglected hearing loss may contribute to a diminished overall quality of life for the elderly person.

Given the findings of Bess et al., it is conceivable that efforts to rehabilitate hearing function could result in a significant improvement in the overall quality of life of the older person. These kinds of results were found by Harless and McConnell (1982) in their study of self-concept and hearing aid use in older individuals. Older hearing aid wearers were found to have a better self-concept and higher self-esteem than their unaided hearing-impaired counterparts. These findings suggest improved psychosocial functioning may be a beneficial by-product of amplification and the rehabilitation process. However, although these results are encouraging, further study of the effects of aural rehabilitation on improved physical and psychosocial functioning in the hearing-impaired elderly is needed.

Alternative Hearing Health Care Delivery

With the changing face of health care practice in the United States, there has been an increase in alternative sites for delivering services to the elderly (Weinstein & Clark, 1989). Consequently, service delivery in the home as well as in long-term care facilities has become more prevalent for speech-language pathology and audiology.

Speech-language pathologists have developed a successful delivery model for provision of in-home services to patients with neurogenic speech and language disorders due to strokes and traumatic brain injury. In fact, the American Speech-Language-Hearing Association Task Force on Home Care (1986) characterized home health care as the most dynamic segment in health care in the 1980s. They provided four reasons for the growth of home care. First, it is a response to the rapidly expanding elderly population. Second, there is pressure on hospitals to decrease costs by reducing length of stay and limiting bed growth. Third, there is a strong consumer need or preference for receiving services within the home. And fourth, government agencies and private businesses are stressing cost containment in health care. This task force stressed that given the unique characteristics of the home, speech-language pathologists and audiologists need to work with the family as well as other professionals to ensure continuity of patient care. Indeed, Selker (1987) states that home care requires home adaptation of treatment regimens and training of caregivers/family members to ensure proper care.

Although home health care in general is not new, its growth in the past 10 years has been phenomenal. Waldo, Levit, and Lazenby (1986) estimate that the average annual growth rate of the home care industry in recent years has been 20 to 25%. For example, in 1961 there were only 208 agencies in the United States providing home care, while in 1990 there were an estimated 12,000 to 14,000 providers (Applebaum & Phillips, 1990). Furthermore, total spending for home care services and products was estimated to be at $16 billion (Sabatino, 1989).

Although audiologists may think there is a negative stigma associated with the provision of audiologic services in the home, it may be an excellent alternative for the hearing-impaired older individual with mobility problems. The accuracy of diagnostic and hearing aid evaluations done in the home may be questionable. However, hearing aid fittings and orientations as well as aural rehabilitation could be conducted ideally in the patient's home. Indeed, the face validity of these procedures might increase greatly if rehabilitative decisions and planning were done in the patient's own communication environment. As the home health care industry grows, audiologists must overcome resistance to offering services in the patient's home and develop appropriate models for effective delivery of a full range of aural rehabilitation services in that environment.

The proliferation of long-term care facilities in the past decade presents another alternative site for service provision by audiologists. However, Bebout (1991) reports that while there were 15,607 nursing homes in this country, only 33.3% offered audiology services. This is in stark contrast to the 76% of these facilities that offered speech-language therapy.

Bebout (1991) suggests that the expanding population of senior residential facilities offers both challenges and opportunities. This potential is enhanced by the revisions in federal laws that regulate nursing homes certified for Medicare funds. The Omnibus Budget Reconciliation Act (OBRA) of 1987 requires that as of October 1, 1990, nursing homes certified for Medicare coverage must complete a comprehensive assessment, including hearing screening, of all residents (*Federal Register*, February 2, 1989, p. 5364). Specialized rehabilitation services requirements state that a facility must provide or obtain rehabilitation services. Furthermore, facilities have to ensure that residents receive proper treatment and assistive devices to maintain hearing abilities. The facility must also assist the resident in making appointments and arranging transportation to and from the medical practitioner "specializing in the treatment of hearing impairment" (White, 1989).

At present, the new regulations do not specify who is to conduct the assessments, but in practice it is typically a nurse or social worker (Bebout, 1991). Clearly, provision of hearing screenings by nonaudiologists may produce a wide margin of error. As such, appropriate referrals as mandated by law may never be made. One reason that audiologists may not be involved with this population is that currently hearing screening is not reimbursable by Medicare. However, audiologists can charge Medicare for full audiological assessments. Given the incidence of hearing loss in the elderly population, the number of patients ultimately referred for audiological assessments and rehabilitation would appear to justify the provision of "free" hearing screenings by the audiologist.

The case for development of a systematic audiometric screening of all nursing home residents has been made by Voeks et al. (1990) in their study of hearing assessment practices in nursing homes. To determine whether audiometric screening duplicated the observations of other medical personnel, audiometric results for each resident were compared to the nursing and physician assessments. Nurses' observations of hearing status were either "good" or "impaired," while physicians' observations were either "within normal limits" or "impaired." Results indicated that 16% of nursing home residents with significant hearing loss (PTA > 40 dB HL) were not identified using either the nursing or physician assessments. Furthermore, 76% of the nursing home admissions were at risk or significantly hearing impaired, and 60% complained of hearing difficulties during daily activities. The authors conclude that since standard practice fails to identify many individuals in need of hearing health care, a systematic audiometric screening program should be instituted. Moreover, the authors contend that when over three-fourths of the individuals in an institution share the same disability, institutional policy should be directed toward accommodating the disability in question.

It is unlikely that nursing home administrators will change their standard practices in dealing with hearing-impaired nursing home residents without the input of audiologists. Unquestionably, there is a legislative mandate that opens the door to re-habilitation of the hearing-impaired nursing home resident. Audiologists have the opportunity and the responsibility to be proactive in better meeting the hearing health care needs of older individuals, whether the individuals live in their own homes or in long-term care facilities.

Successful Rehabilitation Strategies

SCREENING

Traditionally, hearing screenings have consisted of pass/fail pure-tone audiometric tasks. A criterion level is determined, and the patient who responds at this level passes, while the patient who does not respond fails and is referred for further testing. For the screening to be effective, the criterion level must be chosen so that those who pass are not experiencing communication problems due to hearing loss. Those who fail, on the other hand, should be those who will benefit from follow-up testing and rehabilitative services.

The selection of an effective criterion level for use with the elderly is difficult. Unlike young children, all of whom have intense communicative demands placed on them by the need for language acquisition and successful education, hearing handicap for the elderly is not easily predictable from pure-tone thresholds alone. An elderly individual may be working or retired; may be socially active or not; or may live with family, in a retirement community, in a nursing home, or alone. These life-style factors will affect the degree of hearing loss that the individual will be able to cope with before the loss affects the ability to communicate successfully. In reviewing literature related to the issue of selecting a criterion level, Schow (1991) suggests that a 40-dB HL screening level at 1000 and 2000 Hz may be appropriate for elderly living in an institutional setting. While these criteria also are recommended frequently and used for screenings with noninstitutionalized elderly individuals, Schow points out that 25% of noninstitutionalized elderly hearing aid users would pass such a screening. Lowering the criterion level to 25 dB HL, as is commonly used when younger adults are screened, causes concern for overreferral. A single criterion level for pure-tone screening cannot take into account the variability within the elderly population, which has an impact on determining the communicative needs of the elderly individual.

An alternative or adjunct to pure-tone screening with the elderly is the screening self-assessment inventory. These screening scales are designed to separate those who perceive themselves as having communication problems resulting from their hearing loss from those who do not. The Hearing Handicap Inventory for the Elderly—Screening Version (HHIE-S) (Ventry & Weinstein, 1982, 1983) and the Self-Assessment of Communication (SAC) (Schow & Nerbonne, 1982) (Appendix 10.1) were recommended in proposed ASHA Guidelines (1989) as tools for screening hearing handicap in the elderly population. The proposed ASHA Guidelines state that the choice of the instrument to be used should be based on the population to be screened. However, the SAC purportedly can be used with individuals from 20 to 80 years of age, while the HHIE-S was standardized on individuals age 65 years or greater. Consequently, a choice between the HHIE-S and SAC must be made when screening the elderly population. Lee and McCarthy (1991) investigated whether differences exist between these two inventories in their ability to screen hearing handicap in individuals age 65 years or older. Results of this study showed no significant differences between the HHIE-S and the SAC. Schow, Smedley, and Longhurst (1990) compared these two inventories using large groups of young and elderly adults. Test predictive measures such as sensitivity, specificity, positive predictive value (PPV), and negative predictive value (NPV) were examined when pure-tone findings were used as a criterion measure. Results of this study suggested that the overall efficiency of the SAC was slightly higher than that of the HHIE-S. However, Schow et al. (1990) concluded that the SAC and the HHIE-S perform very similarly even though the SAC was standardized on a broad age range and the HHIE-S was standardized on the elderly. Furthermore, Frank, Bennett, and Blood (1989) reported a high correlation (.918) between the HHIE-S and the SAC.

Although there are no significant differences between these two inventories in screening hearing handicap, qualitative differences may exist. For example, the response format of the HHIE-S may be more suitable for the elderly population. The yes/no/sometimes format of the HHIE-S may be easier and less time consuming than the five-point multiple-choice format of the SAC for some older individuals. This may be particularly true if the inventory is administered face to face rather than as a paper-and-pencil screening tool.

Lichtenstein, Bess, and Logan (1988) evaluated the utility of the HHIE-S as a tool for screening hearing loss. They compared HHIE-S results from 178 elderly subjects with audiometric results obtained during the same visit. The diagnostic performance of the HHIE-S was compared against five different definitions of hearing loss. They found that the HHIE-S is a valid, robust screening tool for identifying hearing-impaired elderly irrespective of the audiometric definition used.

Jupiter (1989) used both a pure-tone task and a self-assessment scale (HHIE-S) in a screening protocol. She found that based on the HHIE-S, 36.2% of the elderly screened fell into referral priority categories, while 66% failed a pure-tone screening. When comparing a group screened using both the pure-tone task and HHIE-S to a group screened using only a pure-tone task, equal percentages were referred for follow-up. Interestingly, of those referred for follow-up from either group, most who chose to proceed (approximately 30% of those who failed) went to physicians for follow-up. Few of these were seen for further testing or obtained a hearing aid. Use of other rehabilitative services was not surveyed. These findings suggest the need for greater education for older patients failing a hearing screening. Patients should be informed of audiologic services and the potential benefits of amplification. Clearly, a hearing screening program for the elderly can be considered successful only if it ultimately leads to appropriate rehabilitation for the elderly hearing-impaired individual.

THE USE OF HEARING HANDICAP INVENTORIES WITH ELDERLY LISTENERS

Evaluating the impact of hearing loss on communicative and psychosocial function is imperative before planning and instituting a rehabilitative program. This is no less true for older listeners than for younger listeners, but the instrument selected should be appropriate for the individual being served. Hearing handicap scales have been specifically designed for use with elderly patients, and others have been developed through modification of existing questionnaires. In general, inventories for the elderly tend to use fewer items, most notably omitting vocational questions. Fewer response choices are used for each item to simplify administration. Face-to-face presentation is often recommended rather than the more traditional paper-and-pencil format (Weinstein, Spitzer, & Ventry, 1986). A review of these scales highlights the unique qualities of each of these instruments for the elderly.

One of the first scales designed specifically for the older population was the Denver Scale of Communication Function for Senior Citizens Living in Retirement Centers (Appendix 13.1). Zarnoch and Alpiner (1977) modified the original Denver Scale of Communication Function for use with older individuals. It was designed for presentation through an individual interview, since self-scoring scales often are not feasible with older persons. This scale consists of seven major questions covering the topics of family, emotions, other persons, general communication, self-concept, group situations, and rehabilitation. These are scored by a plus (yes) or minus (no). Under each main question is a "Probe Effect" and an "Exploration Effect." The Probe Effect attempts to specify the problem areas related to the general question. The Exploration Effect determines how applicable the general question is to the individual. This aspect of the scale helps to eliminate questions that are irrelevant to the individual and consequently unnecessary in establishing goals for aural rehabilitation. A scoring form is included to help in interpretation of the responses. This scale does not provide norms or group comparisons. Rather it allows the individual to provide his or her communication performance prior to and following any rehabilitative procedures.

The Denver Scale of Communication Function (DSSC) was also modified for use with older individuals by Kaplan, Feeley, and Brown (1978). To make the DSSC more

usable for older people living in retirement settings or with their families, several basic modifications were made. First, the interview technique was adopted. Second, the seven-point scale was reduced to five points with each point defined for the patient. Third, all items concerned with vocation were eliminated, since most older persons are not employed. Fourth, the "family" category was changed to "peer and family attitudes," since many older people do not live with their families. Fifth, the "self" and "socialization" categories were combined into one category aimed at probing degrees and feelings of participation in social activities. Finally, a new category, "specific difficult listening situations," was added. While the DSSC-Modified (Appendix 13.2) was found to be reliable when using group data, individual test-retest reliability was variable. Therefore, the authors caution against using the scale as a pre- or postmanagement evaluation tool.

The unique problems of the elderly living in nursing homes are the focus of the Nursing Home Hearing Handicap Index (NHHHI) developed by Schow and Nerbonne (1977) (Appendix 13.3). The 20-item scale is divided into two sections named "Self" and "Staff." The premise of the NHHHI is that input from both of these sources is superior to either one alone. Both sections can be administered as a paper-and-pencil test. A five-point rating scale for each item is used. In evaluating the scale, the authors found that the staff members' ratings of hearing handicap correlated much better with the pure-tone average than did the residents' self-perception scores. They concluded that staff members were probably more objective observers of residents' hearing difficulties. However, the fact that there was a discrepancy between the ratings may be of rehabilitative value. As such, this scale may provide information for treatment planning that includes nursing home staff in-service education.

Alpiner and Baker (1981) developed the Communication Assessment Procedure for Seniors (CAPS) (Appendix 13.4). It attempts to evaluate communication status in terms of both attitudes and specific communication situations. CAPS enables the clinician to evaluate subjectively how a person living in an extended care facility reacts to his or her hearing loss. Questions are included for five communication areas: general communication, group situations, other persons, self-concept, and family. A final section is included to determine if an individual is interested in and could benefit from remediation. CAPS is also an interview-type scale and is interpreted subjectively.

One of the best designed and most widely researched assessment instruments is the Hearing Handicap Inventory for the Elderly (HHIE) by Ventry and Weinstein (1982) (Appendix 13.5). This scale was developed to assess the social and emotional effects of hearing impairment in the non-institutionalized older person. The HHIE is composed of an emotional and a social/situational subscale. It was standardized on 100 noninstitutionalized individuals over the age of 65 years. It was found to be highly reliable and contains a high degree of content validity. Scoring involves "yes" (4 points), "sometimes" (2 points), and "no" or "not applicable" (0 points). The total score can range from 0 to 100, wherein the higher the score, the greater the self-assessed hearing handicap. This scale can be administered in either a face-to-face or a paper-and-pencil format (Newman & Weinstein, 1989). The HHIE-S is the screening version of the scale and consists of five emotional items and five social/situational items (Appendix 13.6). Statistical analysis suggests this short form is of comparable reliability and validity to the long form.

One of the most exciting uses for the HHIE and HHIE-S is in the area of assessing hearing aid benefit. Weinstein, Spitzer, and Ventry (1986) determined that the 95% confidence interval for change on the HHIE is 18%. In a pre/postintervention comparison, a change of 18% can therefore be considered significant clinically. In group studies, Newman and Weinstein (1988) and Malinoff and Weinstein (1989) assessed hearing handicap among elderly clients prior to hearing aid fitting and again following hearing aid fitting. Newman and Weinstein found that after a year of hearing aid use, the perception of hearing handicap as measured by the HHIE was significantly reduced. Malinoff and Weinstein assessed benefit following 3 weeks, 3 months, and 1 year of hearing aid use. They found that after 3 weeks of hearing aid use, a sharp reduction in hearing handicap occurred. Perception of handicap increased between 3 weeks and 3 months but still represented a significant improvement over the prefit scores. The perception of handicap remained stable between 3 months and 1 year. These findings suggest that the typical return visit by the new hearing aid user after 2 to 3 weeks of hearing aid use may not be sufficient to monitor the elderly client's long-term adjustment to and success with amplification. Additional follow-up at longer intervals may allow the audiologist to provide the elderly client with further rehabilitation once the perceived benefit from the hearing aid has stabilized.

The HHIE-S, being a shorter scale, requires less time for the audiologist to administer and for the elderly patient to complete. To determine whether the HHIE-S also could be used to assess hearing aid benefit, Newman et al. (1991) administered this scale to new hearing aid users prior to hearing aid fitting and 3 weeks following hearing aid fitting. They established a 95% confidence interval of 9.3 points on the HHIE-S as indicating true change from the prefit to postfit scores. They found significant reductions in perceived handicap on both the emotional and social/situational subscales of the HHIE-S after 3 weeks of hearing aid use.

These studies suggest that self-assessment inventories are viable tools to be used to measure hearing aid outcome. Because providing amplification is the cornerstone of effective aural rehabilitation, it is important that success with hearing aids be measured and documented (McCarthy, 1990). As such, use of self-assessment inventories in measuring hearing aid benefit is recommended for use with the geriatric population.

HEARING AIDS

Advances in hearing aid technology and hearing aid fitting practices have revolutionized our ability to select amplification for hearing-impaired patients. In spite of these advances, however, hearing aids continue to be underused by the hearing-impaired elderly. Fino et al. (1992) looked at audiometric data, hearing aid status, and follow-up from 178 elderly individuals who had been screened in primary care facilities. Eighty-three, or 47%, of these individuals were considered candidates for amplification. Of the 83 hearing aid candidates, 58 simply opted not to obtain amplification. Of the remaining 25 elderly hearing-impaired patients, 14 already owned a hearing aid and only 11 purchased a hearing aid as a result of audiologic recommendations. In all, 67% of the elderly hearing-impaired patients who were considered candidates for amplification chose not to obtain a hearing aid. Commonly reported reasons that elderly individuals will choose not to obtain a hearing aid include concerns regarding cost, amplification of background noise, fear of drawing attention to a hearing handicap, deceptive dealer practices, and where to obtain a hearing aid (Fino et al., 1992; Franks & Beckman, 1985).

Another factor in the underuse of amplification by the elderly is nonuse of hearing aids after they have been purchased. Surr, Schuchman, and Montgomery (1978) found that overall postfit hearing aid use decreased as age increased. Using an open-ended question to elicit comments about amplification from elderly hearing aid users, Smedley and Schow (1990) judged that 63 to 66% of the responses were negative, while only 10 to 19% were positive. The authors categorized most of the negative comments into four problem areas: *(1)* the effects of background noise/groups; *(2)* fitting, comfort, and mechanical problems; *(3)* too little benefit from the hearing aids; and *(4)* the cost of the hearing aids, repairs, and batteries. This suggests that for many of the elderly hearing aid owners who use their hearing aids, serious concerns affecting user satisfaction still remain.

The data on hearing aid use and satisfaction raise important issues for the rehabilitative audiologist who works with the geriatric population. How can we predict which elderly patients will use a hearing aid and which will not? How can we improve the rate of success and the level of satisfaction for elderly hearing aid users? In general, those with a greater degree of hearing loss are more likely to follow recommendations and obtain a hearing aid. Within any particular degree of hearing loss category, the individuals who report the most handicap are most likely to obtain a hearing

aid (Fino et al., 1992). For the elderly individual with a mild to moderate hearing loss, the level of perceived hearing handicap is a factor in determining candidacy, once again highlighting the usefulness of hearing handicap scales with the elderly population. In looking at elderly individuals after they had obtained amplification, Nabelek, Tucker, and Letowski (1991) identified three groups: full-time hearing aid users, part-time hearing aid users, and nonusers. They compared them to each other and to an elderly normal hearing group and a young normal hearing group. Unaided, under headphones, the subjects listened to a story and were asked to set the highest intensity of various background noises that they could "put up with." The full-time users tolerated a lower signal-to-noise ratio with music as the background noise than any other group. With speech-spectrum noise, the full-time users tolerated more noise than the part-time users and nonusers. Overall, the full-time hearing aid users were more tolerant of relatively high noise levels. Because these measures were made postfitting, the predictive ability of these measures cannot be addressed. Additionally, the HHIE was given to the hearing-impaired subjects. No significant differences were found between the full-time, part-time, and nonusers on hearing handicap without a hearing aid as measured by the HHIE. Comparing perceptions of hearing handicap without amplification and with amplification using the HHIE, only the full-time users demonstrated a significant reduction of handicap with the hearing aid. These data suggest that there may be a relationship between the ability to tolerate background noise and hearing aid benefit.

Hearing Aid Selection Issues

When amplification for elderly patients is selected, the standard hearing aid selection questions arise regarding the style of the aids, monaural versus binaural fitting, gain and output characteristics, and special hearing aid circuits and features. The audiologist must keep in mind how age-related changes in function may affect the elderly patient's hearing aid use. The choice of the style of hearing aid may be affected not only by gain limitations and the cosmetic preferences of the patient but also by changes in manual dexterity, changes in touch sensitivity, and changes in the texture of the pinna. The patient with impaired dexterity and/or reduced sensitivity at the fingertips may not be a good candidate for an in-the-canal (ITC) hearing aid because of the smaller controls and batteries. For some, even a full concha in-the-ear (ITE) hearing aid may not be easily manipulated and used. Modifications, such as stacked volume control wheels and removal notches should also be considered when an ITE fitting is recommended. For clients with very soft pinnae, difficulties controlling feedback may make a behind-the-ear (BTE) hearing aid fitting preferable because of the greater distance to the microphone.

The VA/Vanderbilt Hearing Aid Conference Consensus Statement (1990) recommends that binaural hearing aid fittings are preferred "unless clear contraindications exist." As a group, the elderly experience the same binaural advantages as do younger listeners, including improved speech understanding in noisy and reverberant listening environments, binaural summation, and sound localization. However, additional factors must again be considered. A monaural fitting could result in more successful training in the manipulation and use of a hearing aid in instances where dexterity, learning, and/or memory are limited. Additionally, elderly people living on fixed incomes simply may be unable to afford to purchase two hearing aids and to keep them in good repair.

The common complaint of reduced speech perception in the presence of background noise has led the hearing aid industry to create circuitry designed to reduce the effects of noise. Circuitry such as automatic signal processors (ASP), which automatically adjust low-frequency gain, the K-amp, which automatically adjusts high-frequency gain, and the Zeta, which is also an adaptive filter, are commonly available and frequently recommended. Group studies assessing the success of such circuitry in improving speech understanding in noise has been equivocal (Schum, 1990; Tyler & Kuk, 1989; VanTasell, Larsen, & Fabry, 1988). It is possible that such circuitry is beneficial for some subjects but not for others. Because each elderly patient will be affected to a different extent by the changes that can characterize aging, the unique array of skills and needs for each patient must be considered. This need to recognize the variability among aging patients and respond to each patient individually represents both the challenge and the reward for the rehabilitative audiologist working with the geriatric population.

Hearing Aid Counseling and Follow-Up

Ultimately, orientation and counseling are the keys to successful hearing aid use by the older individual. Without adequate orientation and follow-up, a hearing aid is much more likely to be rejected. As with all hearing aid counseling, time must be spent discussing hearing aid parts and function; rehearsing hearing aid insertion and removal, battery changing procedures, and manipulation of the controls; and emphasizing realistic expectations for the benefits and limitations of the hearing aid. The client who expects more than the hearing aid alone can achieve will be a dissatisfied hearing aid owner. Additional counseling regarding adjustment to amplification should be stressed. The counseling should be tailored to the unique listening needs, skills, and strategies of the individual.

The greatest difference in counseling and follow-up between older and younger hearing aid purchasers is in the time that will need to be allotted to the task. Smedley and Schow (1990) recommend a minimum of three follow-up visits within the first month after fitting an elderly patient with a hearing aid. This schedule will allow the audiologist to repeat vital information and will allow the new hearing aid owner to rehearse hearing aid care skills with needed supervision and reinforcement. The goal for the elderly hearing-impaired user is to master the skills necessary to use the hearing aid and to develop a thorough understanding of how to use and what to expect from the aid. Almost all elderly individuals will be able to learn to use a hearing aid independently, but many will require a longer time to master the necessary skills and information.

In the cases where the hearing aid user will require assistance, a significant other must also be trained. The individual chosen must be someone who is regularly available to assist the patient. This may be the spouse or other family member. In a nursing home these tasks will fall within the duties of staff members. Because of high turnover rates in institutional settings and reassignments within a nursing home, frequent, periodic in-services may be necessary to ensure that the hearing-impaired patient will be able to use his or her hearing aid consistently. The need for these follow-up services within the nursing home is clear. Thibodeau and Schmitt (1988) found that 72% of hearing aids in a sample of nursing homes and retirement centers were malfunctioning, with dead/weak batteries and clogged vents and sound openings composing the majority of the problems. Clearly, the importance of in-service education of nursing home personnel cannot be overemphasized. The use of the CDQ discussed earlier in this chapter or some other tool may represent a good starting point for educating other health care professionals as to the importance of hearing and communication.

Computer-Assisted Therapy

In Chapter 17, computer applications to rehabilitative audiology are discussed in depth. In the elderly, however, questions about "computer phobia" linger. Can older individuals who are experiencing so many aging changes use a computer to assist in their own rehabilitation?

The answer to this question was answered in a study by Hurvitz and Goldojarb (1988) in which two methods of providing aural rehabilitation to nursing home residents were compared. Elderly residents of a Veterans Administration nursing home were assigned to one of three groups. The first group received a six-lesson aural rehabilitation program presented on an Apple IIC computer with a color display monitor. Lessons were designed to be user friendly, and only a few key strokes were required. Topics included mechanisms of the ear, audiograms, management of hearing problems, speechreading, hearing aids, and communication skills training. Group Two also had a six-lesson program covering the same material, but it was led by an instructor. A third group served as a control and received no therapy. The effectiveness of the methods was measured by administer-

ing a 25-question pre/posttest to each subject. Questions required remembering specific information and giving problem-solving answers to situational questions. Results showed that both Groups I and II achieved significantly higher performance after instruction than did Group III. No significant difference was found between Groups I and II in performance.

The authors of this study concluded that each method of offering aural rehabilitation was valuable and offered unique advantages. While the class offered greater opportunity for support and socialization, the computer-assisted method allowed each subject to proceed through the material at his or her own pace. In addition, an audiologist was not required to be present while subjects were working on the computer.

Perhaps an even more important finding of this study relates to the fact that elderly nursing home residents were successful with user-friendly software. Moreover, they were able to learn via this method. These encouraging results suggest that audiologists should not make presumptions about their older patients' facility with technology. With the right software, use of the computer in educating the older population about hearing health care may be a viable option. Further study of this is needed.

Summary

Ageism can take the form of misperceptions about or a lack of knowledge of the aging process. In either case, ageism can contribute to a denial of services or provision of inadequate services to elderly persons. The underlying premise of this chapter has been that hearing health care delivery can be improved if the effects of aging are known, understood, and incorporated into the rehabilitation process. As the geriatric population continues to expand, indeed as we all become part of it, quality services that meet the unique needs of the elderly will be demanded. Survival of audiology as a profession may, in large part, be dependent on how we respond to meeting the needs of the growing elderly hearing-impaired population.

References

Alpiner, J.G., and Baker, B., Communication assessment procedures in the aural rehabilitation process. *Sem. Speech, Lang. Hear.*, 2, 189–204 (1981).

American Speech-Language-Hearing Association, The delivery of speech-language and audiology services in home care. *Asha*, 28, 49–52 (1986).

American Speech-Language-Hearing Association, Guidelines for the identification of hearing impairment/handicap in adult/elderly persons. (Draft for peer review.) *Asha*, 31, 59–60 (1989).

Applebaum, R., and Phillips, P., Assuring the quality of in-home care: the "other" challenge for long-term care. *Gerontologist*, 30(4), 444–450 (1990).

ASHA, Guidelines for the identification of hearing impairment/handicap in adult/elderly persons. (Draft for peer review.) *Asha*, 31, 59–63 (1989).

Atchley, R., *Social Forces and Aging.* Belmont, CA: Wadsworth (1988).

Axelrod, S., and Cohen, L.D. Senescence and embedded-figure performance in vision and touch. *Percept. Psychphysiol.,* 12, 283–288 (1961).

Bebout, M., A new window of opportunity opens for hearing health care services. *Hear. J.*, 44(11), 11–17 (1991).

Belgrave, L., Lavin, B., Breslau, N., and Haug, M., Stereotyping of the aged by medical students. *Gerontol. Geriatr. Ed.*, 3(1), 37–44 (1982).

Bergman, M., Blumenfeld, V., Cascardo, D., Dash, B., Levitt, H., and Margulies, M., Age-related decrement in hearing for speech: sampling and longitudinal studies. *J. Gerontol.* 31, 533–538 (1976).

Bess, F., and Townsend, T., Word discrimination for listeners with flat sensorineural hearing losses. *J. Speech Hear. Disord.*, 42, 232–237 (1977).

Bess, F., Lichtenstein, J., Logan, S., Burger, J., and Nelson, E., Hearing impairment as a determinant of function in the elderly. *J. Am. Geriatr. Soc.*, 37, 123–128 (1989).

Blackwell, B., The drug defaulter. *Clin. Pharmacol. Therap.*, 13, 841 (1972).

Bolles, R.C., *Theory of Motivation.* New York: Harper & Row (1967).

Botwinick, J., *Aging and Behavior.* New York: Springer (1978).

Botwinick, J., *Aging and Behavior: A Comprehensive Integration of Research Findings (3rd ed.).* New York: Springer (1984).

Botwinick, J., and Brinley, J., Aspects of RT set during brief intervals in relation to age, sex and set. *J. Gerontol.*, 17, 295–301 (1962).

Botwinick, J., and Thompson, J., Practice of speeded response in relation to age, sex, and set. *J. Gerontol.*, 22, 72–76 (1967).

Braithwaite, R., The pharmacokinetics of psychotropic drugs in the elderly. In D. Wheatley (Ed.), *Psychopharmacology of Old Age.* New York: Oxford University Press (1982).

Bruckner, R. Longitudinal research on the eye. *Gerontol. Clin.*, 9, 87–95 (1967).

Canestri, R., Paced and self-paced learning in young and elderly adults. *J. Gerontol.*, 18, 165–168 (1963).

Cherry, K., and Morton, M., Drug sensitivity in older adults: the role of physiologic and pharmacokinetic factors. *Intl. J. Aging Human Develop.*, 28(3), 159–174 (1989).

Cicchitti, D., Fletcher, C., Lerner, E., and Coleman, J., Effects of a social medicine course on the attitudes of medical students toward the elderly. *J. Gerontol.*, 28(3), 370–373 (1973).

Cluff, L., Chronic disease, function and quality care. *J. Chronic Dis.*, 34, 299 (1981).

Cooper, J.C., and Gates, G.A., Hearing in the elderly—the Framingham cohort, 1983–1985: Part II. Prevalence of central auditory processing disorder. *Ear Hear.* 12(5), 304–311 (1991).

Corso, J.F. Sensory processes and age effects in normal adults. *J. Gerontol.*, 26(1), 90–105 (1971).

Coward, R., Cutler, S., and Schmidt, I., Differences in the household composition of elders by age, gender and area of residence. *Gerontologist*, 29(6), 814–821 (1989).

Craik, F.I.M., Age difference in human memory. In J.E. Birren and K.W. Schaie (Eds.), *Handbook of the Psychology of Aging.* New York: Van Nostrand Reinhold (1977).

Dubno, J.R., Dirks, D.D., and Morgan D.E., Effects of age and mild hearing loss on speech recognition in noise. *J. Acoust. Soc. Am.*, 76(1), 87–96 (1984).

Elias, M.F., and Elias, P.K., Motivation and activity. In J. Birren and K. Schaie (Eds.), *Handbook of the Psychology of Aging.* New York: Van Nostrand Reinhold (1977).

Ethol, B., and Belai, A. Senile changes in the middle ear joints. *Ann Otol.*, 83, 49–54 (1974).

Federal Register, p. 5364 (February 2, 1989).

Fein, D., Projection of speech and hearing impairments to 2050. *Asha*, 25(11), 25 (1983).

Fein, D., On aging. *Asha*, 26(8), 25 (1984).

Fino, M.S., Bess, F.H., Lichtenstein, J.J., and Logan, S.A., Factors differentiating elderly hearing aid wearers and non-wearers. *Hear. Instru.*, 43(2), 6–10 (1992).

Ford, A., Liske, R., Ort, R., and Denton, J., *The Doctor's Perspective: Physicians View Their Patients and Practice.* Cleveland, OH: Case Western Reserve University (1967).

Frank, T., Bennett, S., and Blood, I., Relations between hearing handicap and impairment. Paper presented to annual convention of the American Speech-Language-Hearing Association, St. Louis (1989).

Franks, J., and Beckman, N., Rejection of hearing aids: attitudes of a geriatric sample. *Ear Hear.* 6, 161–166 (1985).

Garstecki, D., Hearing health knowledge of aging adults. *J. Acad. Rehabil. Audiol.*, 23, 79–88 (1990).

Gates, G., Cooper, J., Kannell, W., and Miller, N., Hearing in the elderly: the Framingham Cohort, 1983–1985. *Ear Hear.*, 11(4), 247–256 (1990).

Geiger, D., Note: How future professionals view the elderly. *Gerontologist*, 18, 591–594 (1978).

Gerard, L., Zacks, R., Hasher, L., and Radvansky, G., Age deficits in retrieval: the fan effect. *J. Gerontol.*, 46(4), 131–136 (1991).

Glass, L., and Elliott, H., The professionals told me what it was, but that's not enough. *SHHH J.*, 26–28 (January/February 1992).

Gordon-Salant, S., Effects of aging on response criteria in speech-recognition tasks. *J. Speech Hear. Res.*, 29, 155–162 (1986).

Harless, E.L., and McConnell, F., Effects of hearing aid use on self-concept in older persons. *J. Speech Hear. Dis.*, 47(3), 305–309 (1982).

Hasher, L., and Zacks, R., Working memory, comprehension, and aging: a review and new view. In G.H. Bower (Ed.), *The Psychology of Learning and Motivation*, Vol. 22, New York: Academic Press (1988).

Herbst, K., and Humphrey, C., Hearing impairment and mental state in the elderly living at home. *Br. Med. J.*, 281, 903 (1980).

Hubbard, R., and Kowal, J., Guest editorial: from the guest editors. An issue devoted to the Geriatric Education Centers. *Gerontol. Geriatr. Ed.*, 8, 1–5 (1988).

Hultsch, D., and Dixon, R., Learning and memory in aging. In J.E. Birren and K.W. Schaie (Eds.), *Handbook of the Psychology of Aging*. San Diego: Academic Pres (1990).

Humes, L., and Christopherson, L., Speech identification difficulties of hearing-impaired elderly persons: the contributions of auditory processing deficits. *J. Speech Hear. Res.*, 34, 686–693 (1991).

Hurvitz, H., and Goldojarb, M., Comparison of two aural rehabilitation methods in a nursing home. Paper presented to the annual convention of the American Speech-Language-Hearing Association, Boston (1988).

Jerger, J., Jerger, S., and Mauldin, L., Studies in impedance audiometry: I. Normal and sensorineural ears. *Arch. Otolaryngol.*, 96, 513–523 (1972).

Jerger, J., Jerger, S., Oliver, T., and Pirozzola, F., Speech understanding in the elderly. *Ear Hear.*, 10(2), 79–89 (1989).

Jerger, J., Oliver, T., and Pirozzolo, F., Impact of central auditory processing disorder and cognitive deficit on the self-assessment of hearing handicap in the elderly. *J. Am. Acad. Audiol.*, 1, 75–80 (1990).

Jupiter, T., A community hearing screening program for the elderly. *Hear. J.*, 42(1), 14–17 (1989).

Kaplan, H., Feely, J., and Brown, J., A modified Denver scale: test-retest reliability. *J. Acad. Rehabil. Audiol.*, 11, 15–32 (1978).

Kausler, D.H., Automaticity of encoding and episodic memory processes. In E.A. Lovelace (Ed.), *Aging and Cognition: Mental Processes, Self-Awareness and Interventions*. North-Holland: Elsevier Science (1990).

Kimmell, D.C., *Adulthood and Aging*. New York: John Wiley & Sons (1974).

Kricos, P.B., Lesner, S.A., Sandridge, S.A., and Yanke, R.B., Perceived benefits of amplification as a function of central auditory status in the elderly. *Ear Hear.*, 8(6), 337–342 (1987).

Lee, J., and McCarthy, P., A comparison of self-reported handicap in two hearing handicap inventories. Paper presented to annual convention of the American Speech-Language-Hearing Association, Atlanta (1991).

Leopold, I., The eye. In J.T. Freeman (Ed.), *Clinical Features of the Older Patient*. Springfield, IL: Charles C. Thomas (1965).

Lichtenstein, M., Bess, F., and Logan, S., Diagnostic performance of the HHIE-S against differing definitions of hearing loss. *Ear Hear.*, 9, 208–211 (1988).

Malinoff, R.L, and Weinstein, B.E., Changes in self-assessment of hearing handicap over the first year of hearing aid use by older adults. *J. Acad. Rehabil. Audiol.*, 22, 54–60 (1989a).

Malinoff, R.L., and Weinstein, B.E., Measurement of hearing aid benefit in the elder. *Ear Hear.*, 10(6), 354–356 (1989b).

Marshall, L., Auditory processing in aging listeners. *J. Speech Hear. Disord.*, 46(3), 226–240 (1981).

Mauer, F.J., and Rupp, R.R., *Hearing and Aging: Tactics for Intervention*. New York: Grune & Stratton (1979).

McCarthy, P., Self-assessment inventories as quality assurance tools. *Rocky Mountain J. Communication Disord.*, 6, 17–21 (1990).

Milne, J.S., A longitudinal study of hearing loss in older people. *Br. J. Audiol.*, 11(4), 7–14 (1977).

Nabelek, A.K., and Robinson, P.K., Monaural and binaural speech perception in reverberation for listeners of various ages. *J. Acoust. Soc. Am.*, 71, 1242–1248 (1982).

Nabelek, A.K., Tucker, F.M., and Letowski, T.R., Toleration of background noises: relationship with patterns of hearing aid use by elderly persons. *J. Speech Hear. Res.*, 34, 679–685 (1991).

Newman, C.W., Jacobson, G.P., Hug, G.A., Weinstein, B.E., and Malinoff, R.L., Practical method for quantifying hearing aid benefit in older adults. *J. Am. Acad. Audiol.*, 2, 70–75 (1991).

Newman, C.W., and Weinstein, B.E., The hearing handicap inventory for the elderly as a measure of hearing aid benefit. *Ear Hear.*, 9(2), 81–85 (1988).

Newman, C.W., and Weinstein, B.E., Test-retest reliability of the hearing handicap inventory for the elderly using two administration approaches. *Ear Hear.*, 10(3), 190–191 (1989).

Olinger, B., Dancer, J., and Patterson, K., Misconceptions of health professionals regarding hearing loss in the elderly. *Ed. Gerontol.*, 17, 33–40 (1991).

Ouslander, J., Jarvick, L., and Small, G., Illness and psychopathology in the elderly. *Psychiatric Clin. North Am.*, 5(46), 155 (1982).

Owens, E., and Raggio, M., the UCSF tracking procedure for evaluating and training of speech reception by hearing-impaired adults. *J. Speech Hear. Disord.*, 52, 120–128 (1987).

Oyer, H., Preface. In L. Jacobs-Codit (Ed.), *Gerontology and Communication Disorders*. Rockville, MD: American Speech-Language-Hearing Association (1984).

Palmore, E., Facts on aging: a short quiz. *Gerontologist*, 17, 315–320 (1977).

Parking, D., Henney, C., Quirk, J., and Crooks, J., Deviation from prescribed drug treatment after discharge from hospital. *Br. Med. J.*, 2, 686–688 (1976).

Perotta, P., Perkins, D., Schimpfhauser, F., and Calkins, E., Medical student attitudes toward geriatric medicine and patients. *J. Med. Ed.*, 56, 478–483 (1981).

Radecki, S., Kane, R., Solomon, D., Mendenhall, R., and Beck, J., Do physicians spend less time with older patients? *J. Am. Geriatr. Soc.*, 36, 713–718 (1988a).

Radecki, S., Kane, R., Solomon, D., Mendenhall, R., and Beck, J., Are physicians sensitive to the special problems of older patients? *J. Am. Geriatr. Soc.*, 36, 719–725 (1988b).

Raiford, C, and Shadden, B., Graduate education in gerontology. *Asha*, 27, 37–43 (1985).

Rees, J.N., and Botwinick, J., Detection and decision factors in auditory behavior of the elderly. *J. Gerontol.*, 26(2), 133–136 (1971).

Ries, P.W., Acute conditions: incidence and associated disability: U.S., 1977–1978. Vital and Health Statistics, Series 10, Number 132, Washington, DC: U.S. Government Printing Office (1979).

Riffle, K.L., Physiological changes in aging and nursing assessment. In A.J. Reinhardt and M.D. Guinn (Eds.), *Current Practice in Gerontological Nursing*, St. Louis, MO: C.V. Mosby (1979).

Rosen, S., Bergman, M., and Plester, D., Presbycusis study of relatively noise free population in the Sudan. *Ann. Otol. Rhinol. Laryngol.*, 71, 727 (1962).

Rosenhall, U., Pedersen, J., and Svanborg, A., Presbycusis and noise-induced hearing loss. *Ear Hear.*, 11, 257–263 (1990).

Salomon, G. Hearing problems in the elderly. Special Supplement Series, 3, *Danish Medical Bulletin,* 1 (1986).

Sarvela, P., Odulana J., and Sarvela, J., The communication disorders questionnaire: a staff training tool for the geriatric care setting. *Ed. Gerontol.*, 16, 73–86 (1990).

Sataloff, J., Vassalo, L., and Menduke, H., Presbycusis: air and bone conduction thresholds. *Laryngoscope*, 75, 889–901 (1965).

Schow, R.L., Considerations in selecting and validating an adult/elderly hearing screening protocol. *Ear Hear.*, 12(5), 337–347 (1991).

Schow, R., and Nerbonne, M.A., Assessment of hearing handicap by nursing home residents and staff. *J. Acad. Rehabil. Audiol.*, 10, 10–12 (1977).

Schow, R., Smedley, T., and Longhurst, T., Self-assessment and impairment in adult/elderly screening: recent data and new perspectives. *Ear Hear.*, 11, 17s–27s (1990).

Schuknecht, H., Presbycusis. *Laryngoscope*, 65, 419–420 (1955).

Schuknecht, H., *Pathology of the Ear.* Cambridge, MA: Harvard University Press (1974).

Schum, D.J., Noise reduction strategies for elderly hearing-impaired listeners. *J. Am. Acad. Audiol.*, 1, 31–36 (1990).

Schum, D.J., Responses of elderly hearing aid users on the Hearing Aid Performance Inventory. *J. Am. Acad. Audiol.*, 3, 308–314 (1992).

Schum, D.J., Matthess, L.J., and Lee, F.S., Actual and predicted word-recognition performance of elderly hearing-impaired listeners. *J. Speech Hear. Res.*, 34, 636–642 (1991).

Schumacher, G., Using pharmacokinetics in drug therapy. VII. Pharmacokinetics factors influencing drug therapy in the aged. *Am. J. Hosp. Pharmacol.*, 33, 559–562 (1980).

Schwartz, A.N., Snyder, C.L., and Peterson, J., *Aging and Life: An Introduction to Gerontology.* New York: Holt, Rinehart and Winston (1984).

Schwartz, D., Wang, M., Feitz, L., and Goss, M., Medication errors made by elderly, chronically ill patients. *Am. J. Public Health*, 52, 2018–2029 (1962).

Selker, L., Special Issue: an aging society. Implications for health case needs impacts on allied health practice and education. *J. Allied Health*, 16 (1987).

Shanas, E., and Maddox, G.L., Aging, health and organization of health resources. In R. Binstock and E. Shanas (Eds.), *Handbook of Aging and the Social Sciences.* New York: Van Nostrand Reinhold (1976).

Shock, N., System integration. In C. Finch and L. Hayflick (Eds.), *Handbook of the Biology of Aging.* New York: Van Nostrand Reinhold (1977).

Singer, W., and Brownell, J., Assessment of knowledge about hearing and hearing loss. Paper presented at the Northeastern Gerontological Society meeting, Newport, RI (1984).

Smedley, T.C., and Schow, R.L., Frustrations with hearing aid use: candid observations from the elderly. *Hear. J.*, 41(6), 21–27 (1990).

Stach, B.A., Spretnjak, M.L., and Jerger, J., The prevalence of central presbycusis in a clinical population. *J. Am. Acad. Audiol.*, 1, 109–115 (1990).

Surr, R.K., Schuchman, G.I., and Montgomery, A.A., Factors Influencing hearing aid use. *Arch. Otolaryngol.*, 104, 732–736 (1978).

Taylor, S., Survey finds physicians often fail to refer hearing impaired elderly. *Hear. J.*, 44(11), 36–39 (1991).

Thibodeau, L.M., and Schmitt, J., A report on condition of hearing aids in nursing homes and retirement centers. *J. Am. Acad. Audiol.*, 21, 99–112 (1988).

Tyler, R.S., and Kuk, F.K., The effects of noise suppression hearing aids on consonant recognition in speech-babble and low-frequency noise. *Ear Hear.*, 10, 243–249 (1989).

Tymchuk, A., Ouslander, J., and Rader, N., Informing the elderly: a comparison of four methods. *J. Am. Geriatr. Soc.*, 34, 818–822 (1986).

Tymchuk, A., Ouslander, J., Rahbar, B., and Fitten, J., Medical decision making among elderly people in long term care. *Gerontologist*, 28 (Suppl.) 59–63 (1988).

U.S. Department of Commerce Bureau of the Census, Statistical abstract of the U.S. (1986) (106th ed.). Washington, DC: U.S. Government Printing Office (1986).

U.S. Department of Health and Human Services, *Health, United States 1983.* Washington, DC: U.S. Government Printing Office (1983).

VA/Vanderbilt Hearing Aid Conference 1990 Consensus Statement, Recommended components of a hearing aid selection procedure for adults. In G.A. Studebaker, F.H. Bess, and L.B. Beck (Eds.), *The Vanderbilt Hearing-Aid Report II.* Parkton, MD: York Press (1990).

VanTasell, D.J., Larsen, S.Y., and Fabry, D.A., Effects of an adaptive filter hearing aid on speech recognition in noise by hearing-impaired subjects. *Ear Hear.*, 9, 15–21 (1988).

Ventry, I., and Weinstein, B., The hearing handicap inventory for the elderly: a new tool. *Ear Hear.*, 3, 128–134 (1982).

Ventry, I., and Weinstein, B., Identification of elderly people with hearing problems. *Asha*, 25, 37–42 (1983).

Vesper, J.A., and McCarthy, P.A. Omission errors in word recognition by elderly listeners. Annual convention of American Speech Language Hearing Association, 1990.

Vestal, R., Drug use in the elderly. A review of problems and special considerations. *Drugs*, 16, 358–382 (1978).

Vestal, R., Geriatric clinical pharmacology: an overview. In R. Vestal, *Drug Treatment in the Elderly.* Sydney, Australia: ADIS Health Science Press (1984).

Voek, S., Gallagher, C., Langer, E. and Drinka, P. Hearing loss in the nursing home. *J. Am. Gerontol. Soc.,* 38, 141–145 (1990).

Walden, B.E., Demorest, M.E., and Hepler, E.L., Self-report approach to assessing benefit derived from amplification. *J. Speech Hear. Res.,* 27, 49–56 (1984).

Waldo, D., Levit, K., and Lazenby, H., National Health Care. *Health Care Financing Rev.,* 8(1), 1–21 (1985).

Weinstein, B., Audiology and the geriatric education centers. *J. Acad. Rehab. Aud.,* 20, 83–87 (1987).

Weinstein, B., and Clark, L., An aging society. *Asha,* 4, 67–69 (1989).

Weinstein, B., Spritzer, J., and Ventry, I., Test-retest reliability of the hearing handicap for the elderly. *Ear Hear.,* 7, 295–299 (1986).

White, S., Medicare and nursing home services. *Asha,* 31, 75 (1989).

Wilderom, C., Press, E., Perkins, D., et al., Correlates of entering medical students' attitudes toward geriatrics. *Ed. Gerontol.,* 16, 429–446 (1990).

Williams, T.F., Teamwork for the problems of aging. *Asha,* 31, 77–78 (1989).

Willott, J.D., *Aging and the Auditory System: Anatomy, Physiology and Psychophysics.* San Diego: Singular (1991).

Wolf, E., Glare and age. *Arch. Ophthalmol.,* 64, 514–520 (1960).

Zarnoch, J.M., and Alpiner, J.G., The Denver scale of communication function for senior citizens living in retirement centers. Unpublished study.

Zones, J., Estes, C., and Binney, E., Gender, public policy and the oldest old. *Aging Soc.,* 7, 275–302 (1987).

APPENDIX 13.1   The Denver Scale of Communication Function for Senior Citizens Living in Retirement Centers

NAME: _____   DATE OF PRE-TEST: _____
ADDRESS: _____   DATE OF POST-TEST: _____
AGE: _____   EXAMINER: _____
SEX: _____

1. Do you have trouble communicating with your family because of your hearing problem?
   Yes _____ No _____

   Probe Effect I
   a. Does your family make decisions for you because of your hearing problem?
      Yes _____ No _____
   b. Does your family leave you out of discussions because of your hearing problem?
      Yes _____ No _____
   c. Does your family get angry or annoyed with you because of your hearing problem?
      Yes _____ No _____

   Exploration Effect
   a. Do you have a family? Yes _____ No _____
   b. How often does your family visit you?
   c. How far away does your family live? In a city _____ Other _____
   d. How often do you visit your family?

2. Do you get upset when you cannot hear or understand what is being said?
   Yes _____ No _____

   Probe Effect I (to be used only if person responds yes)
   a. Do your friends know you get upset? Yes _____ No _____
   b. Does your family know you get upset? Yes _____ No _____
   c. Does the staff know you get upset? Yes _____ No _____

   Probe Effect II (to be used only if person responds no)
   a. Do your friends realize you are not upset? Yes _____ No _____
   b. Does your family realize you are not upset? Yes _____ No _____
   c. Does the staff realize you are not upset? Yes _____ No _____

   Exploration Effect (to be used only if person responds yes)
   a. How does your behavior change when you become upset?

3. Do you think your family, your friends, and the staff understand what it is like to have a hearing problem? Yes _____ No _____

   Probe Effect
   a. Do they avoid you because of your hearing problem? Yes _____ No _____
   b. Do they leave you out of discussions? Yes _____ No _____
   c. Do they hesitate to ask you to socialize with them? Yes _____ No _____

Exploration Effect
a. Family   Yes _____   No _____
b. Friends   Yes _____   No _____
c. Staff   Yes _____   No _____

4. Do you avoid communicating with other people because of your hearing problem?
   Yes _____   No _____

   Probe Effect
   a. Do you communicate with people during meal times?   Yes _____   No _____
   b. Do you communicate with your roommate(s)?   Yes _____   No _____
   c. Do you communicate during the social activities in the home?
      Yes _____   No _____
   d. Do you communicate with visiting family or friends?   Yes _____   No _____
   e. Do you communicate with the staff?   Yes _____   No _____

   Exploration Effect
   a. Is your roommate capable of communication?   Yes _____   No _____
   b. What are the social activities of the home? _____
   c. Which ones do you attend? _____

5. Do you feel that you are a relaxed person?   Yes _____   No _____

   Probe Effect
   a. Do you think you are an irritable person because of your hearing problem?
      Yes _____   No _____
   b. Do you think you are an irritable person because of your age?
      Yes _____   No _____
   c. Do you think you are an irritable person because you live in this home?   Yes _____
      No _____

   Exploration Effect

   Do you have to live in this home?   Yes _____   No _____

6. Do you feel relaxed in group communicative situations?   Yes _____   No _____

   Probe Effect
   a. Do you get nervous when you have to ask people to repeat what they have said if
      you have not understood them?   Yes _____   No _____
   b. Do you feel nervous if you have to tell a person that you have a hearing
      problem?
      Yes _____   No _____

   Exploration Effect
   a. Do you watch facial expression?   Yes _____   No _____
   b. Do you watch gestures?   Yes _____   No _____
   c. Do you think you are a good listener?   Yes _____   No _____   Why? _____
   d. Do you have a hearing aid?   Yes _____   No _____
   e. Do you wear your aid?   Yes _____   No _____

7. Do you think you need help in overcoming your hearing problem?
   Yes _____   No _____

   Exploration Effect I
   a. A person can improve his communication ability by using lipreading (or
      speechreading) which means watching the speaker's lips, facial expressions, and
      gestures when he's speaking to you.

b. Do you agree with that definition of lipreading?

Probe Effect

a. If lipreading training was available, would you attend?   Yes _____   No _____
b. Do you think this home provides adequate activities to make you want to communicate?
Yes _____   No _____

Exploration Effect II

a. Is your vision adequate?   Yes _____   No _____
b. Are you able to get around unassisted?   Yes _____   No _____

Reprinted by permission from Zarnock, J.M., and Alpiner, J.G., The Denver Scale of Communication Function for Senior Citizens Living in Retirement Centers. Unpublished study, 1977.

THE DENVER SCALE OF COMMUNICATION FUNCTION FOR SENIOR CITIZENS LIVING IN RETIREMENT CENTERS

_____ Initial Evaluation

_____ Final Evaluation

by
Janet M. Zarnoch, M.A. and Jerome G. Alpiner, Ph.D.

NAME: _____   DATE OF PRE-TEST: _____

ADDRESS: _____   DATE OF POST-TEST: _____

AGE: _____ SEX: _____   EXAMINER: _____

CATEGORY	MAIN QUESTION	PROBE EFFECTS	EXPLORATION EFFECTS	PROBLEM	NO PROBLEM
Family	1 + ☐ − ☐	a ☐ b ☐ c ☐	a. _____ b. _____ c. _____ d. _____		
Emotional	2 + ☐ − ☐	I a ☐ b ☐ c ☐ II a ☐ b ☐ c ☐	a. _____ _____		
Other Persons	3 + ☐ − ☐	a ☐ b ☐ c ☐	a. _____ _____ b. _____ c. _____		
General Communication	4 + ☐ − ☐	a ☐ b ☐ c ☐ d ☐ e ☐	a. _____ _____ b. _____ _____ c. _____		
Self Concept	5 + ☐ − ☐	a ☐ b ☐ c ☐	a. _____ _____		
Group Situations	6 + ☐ − ☐	a ☐ b ☐ c ☐	a. _____ b. _____ c. _____ d. _____ e. _____		
Rehabilitation	7 + ☐ − ☐	a ☐ b ☐	Ia. _____ b. _____ IIa. _____ b. _____		

Key + = person responded yes to question
    − = person responded no to question

Additional Client Comments:

1. _____
2. _____
3. _____
4. _____
5. _____
6. _____

APPENDIX 13.2 *The Denver Scale of Communication Function—Modified*

PRE-THERAPY _____ POST-THERAPY _____

DATE _____

NAME _____ AGE _____ SEX _____

ADDRESS _____
_____

AUDIOGRAM (Examination Date) _____

Pure tone	250	500	1000	2000	4000	8000	Hz
RE	_____	_____	_____	_____	_____	_____	db (re:
LE	_____	_____	_____	_____	_____	_____	(ANSI)

Discrimination Score (%)

Speech _____

SRT		Quiet	Noise (S/N=)
RE _____ dB		RE _____	_____
LE _____ dB		LE _____	_____

Hearing Aid Information:

Aided _____ For How Long _____ Aid Type _____

Ear _____ Satisfaction _____

Examiner _____

INSTRUCTIONS

I am going to say some statements relating to hearing loss. For each statement, I want you to tell me if you: (1) definitely agree, (2) slightly agree, (3) irrelevant, (4) slightly disagree, or (5) definitely disagree. If you consider the statement to be irrelevant or unassociated to your communication problem, please tell me.

Scoring

(1) Definitely agree   (2) Slightly agree   (3) Irrelevant
(4) Slightly disagree   (5) Definitely disagree

Attitude Toward Peers

1. The people I live with are annoyed by my loss of hearing. Comments:

   _____ 1. Definitely agree
   _____ 2. Slightly agree
   _____ 3. Irrelevant
   _____ 4. Slightly disagree
   _____ 5. Definitely disagree

2. The people I live with sometimes leave me out of conversations or discussions. Comments:

   _____ 1. Definitely agree
   _____ 2. Slightly agree
   _____ 3. Irrelevant
   _____ 4. Slightly disagree
   _____ 5. Definitely disagree

3. Sometimes people I live with make decisions for me because I have a hard time following discussions. Comments:

_____ 1. Definitely agree
_____ 2. Slightly agree
_____ 3. Irrelevant
_____ 4. Slightly disagree
_____ 5. Definitely disagree

4. People I live with become annoyed when I ask them to repeat what was said because I did not hear them. Comments:

_____ 1. Definitely agree
_____ 2. Slightly agree
_____ 3. Irrelevant
_____ 4. Slightly disagree
_____ 5. Definitely disagree

5. Other people do not realize how frustrated I get when I cannot hear or understand. Comments:

_____ 1. Definitely agree
_____ 2. Slightly agree
_____ 3. Irrelevant
_____ 4. Slightly disagree
_____ 5. Definitely disagree

6. People sometimes avoid me because of my hearing loss. Comments:

_____ 1. Definitely agree
_____ 2. Slightly agree
_____ 3. Irrelevant
_____ 4. Slightly disagree
_____ 5. Definitely disagree

Socialization

7. I am not an "outgoing" person because I have a hearing loss. Comments:

_____ 1. Definitely agree
_____ 2. Slightly agree
_____ 3. Irrelevant
_____ 4. Slightly disagree
_____ 5. Definitely disagree

8. I now take less of an interest in many things as compared to when I did not have a hearing problem. Comments:

_____ 1. Definitely agree
_____ 2. Slightly agree
_____ 3. Irrelevant
_____ 4. Slightly disagree
_____ 5. Definitely disagree

9. I am not a calm person because of my hearing loss. Comments:

_____ 1. Definitely agree
_____ 2. Slightly agree
_____ 3. Irrelevant
_____ 4. Slightly disagree
_____ 5. Definitely disagree

10. I tend to be negative about life in general because of my hearing loss. Comments:

_____ 1. Definitely agree
_____ 2. Slightly agree
_____ 3. Irrelevant
_____ 4. Slightly disagree
_____ 5. Definitely disagree

11. I do not socialize as much as I did before I began to lose my hearing. Comments:

_____ 1. Definitely agree
_____ 2. Slightly agree
_____ 3. Irrelevant
_____ 4. Slightly disagree
_____ 5. Definitely disagree

12. Since I have trouble hearing, I do not like to participate in activities. Comments:

_____ 1. Definitely agree
_____ 2. Slightly agree
_____ 3. Irrelevant
_____ 4. Slightly disagree
_____ 5. Definitely disagree

13. Since I have trouble hearing I hesitate to meet new people. Comments:

_____ 1. Definitely agree
_____ 2. Slightly agree
_____ 3. Irrelevant
_____ 4. Slightly disagree
_____ 5. Definitely disagree

14. Other people do not understand what it is like to have a hearing loss. Comments:

_____ 1. Definitely agree
_____ 2. Slightly agree
_____ 3. Irrelevant
_____ 4. Slightly disagree
_____ 5. Definitely disagree

15. I do not feel relaxed or comfortable in a communicative situation. Comments:

_____ 1. Definitely agree
_____ 2. Slightly agree
_____ 3. Irrelevant
_____ 4. Slightly disagree
_____ 5. Definitely disagree

Communication

16. Because I have difficulty understanding what is said to me I sometimes answer questions wrong. Comments:

_____ 1. Definitely agree
_____ 2. Slightly agree
_____ 3. Irrelevant
_____ 4. Slightly disagree
_____ 5. Definitely disagree

17. Conversations in a noisy room prevent me from attempting to communicate with others. Comments:

_____ 1. Definitely agree
_____ 2. Slightly agree
_____ 3. Irrelevant
_____ 4. Slightly disagree
_____ 5. Definitely disagree

18. I am not comfortable having to communicate in a group situation. Comments:

_____ 1. Definitely agree
_____ 2. Slightly agree
_____ 3. Irrelevant
_____ 4. Slightly disagree
_____ 5. Definitely disagree

19. I seldom watch other people's facial expressions when talking to them. Comments:

_____ 1. Definitely agree
_____ 2. Slightly agree
_____ 3. Irrelevant
_____ 4. Slightly disagree
_____ 5. Definitely disagree

20. Most people do not know how to talk to a hearing-impaired person. Comments:

_____ 1. Definitely agree
_____ 2. Slightly agree
_____ 3. Irrelevant
_____ 4. Slightly disagree
_____ 5. Definitely disagree

21. I hesitate to ask people to repeat if I do not understand them the first time they speak. Comments:

_____ 1. Definitely agree
_____ 2. Slightly agree
_____ 3. Irrelevant
_____ 4. Slightly disagree
_____ 5. Definitely disagree

22. Because I have difficulty understanding what is said to me, I sometimes make comments that do not fit the conversation. Comments:

_____ 1. Definitely agree
_____ 2. Slightly agree
_____ 3. Irrelevant
_____ 4. Slightly disagree
_____ 5. Definitely disagree

23. I do not like to admit that I have a hearing problem. Comments:

_____ 1. Definitely agree
_____ 2. Slightly agree
_____ 3. Irrelevant
_____ 4. Slightly disagree
_____ 5. Definitely disagree

Specific Difficulty Listening Situations

24. I have trouble hearing the radio or the television unless I turn the volume on very loud. Comments:

_____ 1. Definitely agree
_____ 2. Slightly agree
_____ 3. Irrelevant
_____ 4. Slightly disagree
_____ 5. Definitely disagree

25. If someone calls me when my back is turned, I do not always hear him. Comments:

_____ 1. Definitely agree
_____ 2. Slightly agree
_____ 3. Irrelevant
_____ 4. Slightly disagree
_____ 5. Definitely disagree

26. If someone calls me from another room, I have much trouble hearing. Comments:

_____ 1. Definitely agree
_____ 2. Slightly agree
_____ 3. Irrelevant
_____ 4. Slightly disagree
_____ 5. Definitely disagree

27. When I sit talking with friends in a quite room, I have a great deal of difficulty hearing. Comments:

_____ 1. Definitely agree
_____ 2. Slightly agree
_____ 3. Irrelevant
_____ 4. Slightly disagree
_____ 5. Definitely disagree

28. When I use the phone, I have much difficulty hearing. Comments:

_____ 1. Definitely agree
_____ 2. Slightly agree
_____ 3. Irrelevant
_____ 4. Slightly disagree
_____ 5. Definitely disagree

29. When I play cards, understanding my partner gives me much difficulty. Comments:

_____ 1. Definitely agree
_____ 2. Slightly agree
_____ 3. Irrelevant
_____ 4. Slightly disagree
_____ 5. Definitely disagree

30. At lectures or discussions I have much difficulty hearing the speaker. Comments:

_____ 1. Definitely agree
_____ 2. Slightly agree
_____ 3. Irrelevant
_____ 4. Slightly disagree
_____ 5. Definitely disagree

31. In church, when the minister gives the sermon, I have much difficulty. Comments:

_____ 1. Definitely agree
_____ 2. Slightly agree
_____ 3. Irrelevant
_____ 4. Slightly disagree
_____ 5. Definitely disagree

32. When a movie is shown, I have much difficulty hearing what is said. Comments:

_____ 1. Definitely agree
_____ 2. Slightly agree
_____ 3. Irrelevant
_____ 4. Slightly disagree
_____ 5. Definitely disagree

33 I have difficulty understanding announcements sent through the loudspeaker even when the speaker is in the same room. Comments:

_____ 1. Definitely agree
_____ 2. Slightly agree
_____ 3. Irrelevant
_____ 4. Slightly disagree
_____ 5. Definitely disagree

34. I have trouble understanding messages sent over the intercom. Comments:

_____ 1. Definitely agree
_____ 2. Slightly agree
_____ 3. Irrelevant
_____ 4. Slightly disagree
_____ 5. Definitely disagree

Reprinted by permission from Kaplan, H., Feeley, J., and Brown, J., A modified Denver Scale: Test-Retest Reliability. *J. Acad. Rehab. Audiol.*, **11**, 15–32 (1978).

APPENDIX 13.3 *Nursing Home Hearing Handicap Index (NHHI): Self Version for Resident*

	Very Often				Almost Never
1. When you are with other people do you wish you could hear better?	5	4	3	2	1
2. Do other people feel you have a hearing problem (when they try to talk to you)?	5	4	3	2	1
3. Do you have trouble hearing another person if there is a radio or TV playing (in the same room)?	5	4	3	2	1
4. Do you have trouble hearing the radio or TV?	5	4	3	2	1

5. (How often) do you feel life would be better if you could hear better?   5 4 3 2 1

6. How often are you embarrassed because you don't hear well?   5 4 3 2 1

7. When you are alone do you wish you could hear better?   5 4 3 2 1

8. Do people (tend to) leave you out of conversations because you don't hear well?   5 4 3 2 1

9. (How often) do you withdraw from social activities (in which you ought to participate) because you don't hear well?   5 4 3 2 1

10. Do you say "what" or "pardon me" when people first speak to you?   5 4 3 2 1

Total _____ × 2 = _____
$$\frac{}{-20}$$
_____ × 1.25 = _____ %

Reprinted by permission from Schow, K.L., and Nerbonne, M.A., Assessment of hearing handicaps by nursing home residents and staff. *J. Acad. Rehabil. Audiol.*, 10, 2–12 (1977).

Nursing Home Hearing Handicap Index (NHHI): Staff Version

		Very Often				Almost Never
1.	When this person is with other people does he/she need to hear better?	5	4	3	2	1
2.	Do members of the staff, family and friends make negative comments about this person's hearing problems?	5	4	3	2	1
3.	Do they have trouble hearing another person if there is a radio or TV playing in the same room?	5	4	3	2	1
4.	When this person is listening to radio or TV do they have trouble hearing?	5	4	3	2	1
5.	How often do you feel life would be better for this person if they could hear better?	5	4	3	2	1
6.	How often are they embarrassed because they don't hear well?	5	4	3	2	1
7.	When they are alone do they need to hear the everyday sounds of life better?	5	4	3	2	1

8. Do people tend to leave them out of conversations because they don't hear well?   5   4 3 2   1

9. How often do they withdraw from social activities in which they ought to participate because they don't hear well?   5   4 3 2   1

10. Do they say "what" or "pardon me" when people first speak to them?   5   4 3 2   1

Total _____ × 2 = _____
                   −20
                   _____ × 1.25 = _____ %

Reprinted by permission from Schow, K.L., and Nerbonne, M.A., Assessment of hearing handicaps by nursing home residents and staff. *J. Acad. Rehabil. Audiol.*, 10, 2–12 (1977).

APPENDIX 13.4 Communications Assessment Procedure for Seniors (CAPS)

Name: _____ Date: _____ Birthdate: _____ Sex: _____
Address: _____
Telephone: _____ Pre-Service: _____ Post-Service: _____

A. General Communication

1. Do you avoid talking to other people because of your hearing problem?
   Always _____   Never _____
   Sometimes _____   Not applicable _____

2. Do you talk with your roommate?
   Always _____   Never _____
   Sometimes _____   Not applicable _____

3. Do you talk with people during the social activities of this home?
   Always _____   Never _____
   Sometimes _____   Not applicable _____

4. Do you talk with people during your meals?
   Always _____   Never _____
   Sometimes _____   Not applicable _____

5. Do you talk to the staff here?
   Always _____   Never _____
   Sometimes _____   Not applicable _____

6. Do you have trouble hearing in certain situations? (Example: watching television, listening to the radio, etc.)
   Always _____   Never _____
   Sometimes _____   Not applicable _____

B. Group Situations

1. Do you feel relaxed in group situations?
   Always _____   Never _____
   Sometimes _____   Not applicable _____

2. Do you ask a person to repeat if you don't understand what he says?
   Always _____   Never _____
   Sometimes _____   Not applicable _____

3. Does it make you nervous to ask a person to repeat what he said?
   Always _____   Never _____
   Sometimes _____   Not applicable _____

4. Does it make you nervous to tell a person you have a hearing problem?
   Always _____   Never _____
   Sometimes _____   Not applicable _____

5. Do you think your hearing problem annoys other people?
   Always _____   Never _____
   Sometimes _____   Not applicable _____

6. Do you get annoyed when people don't speak loudly enough for you to hear?
   Always _____   Never _____
   Sometimes _____   Not applicable _____

7. Do you feel isolated from group discussions because of your hearing loss?
   Always _____   Never _____
   Sometimes _____   Not applicable _____

C. Other Persons: Family, Friends, and Staff

1. Do you think other people understand what it's like to have a hearing problem?
   Always _____   Never _____
   Sometimes _____   Not applicable _____

2. Do others avoid you because of your hearing loss?
   Always _____   Never _____
   Sometimes _____   Not applicable _____

3. Does anyone ever leave you out of conversations because of your hearing problem?
   Always _____   Never _____
   Sometimes _____   Not applicable _____

4. Do you mind telling people that you have a hearing loss?
   Always _____   Never _____
   Sometimes _____   Not applicable _____

5. Do other people understand how frustrated you get when you can't hear them?
   Always _____   Never _____
   Sometimes _____   Not applicable _____

Comments: Tell me how other people, like your friends, your family, and the staff here, react to your hearing loss.

D. Self-Concept

1. Would you describe yourself as a relaxed person?
   Always _____   Never _____
   Sometimes _____   Not applicable _____

2. Does your hearing loss make you irritable?
   Always _____   Never _____
   Sometimes _____   Not applicable _____

3. Do you like living here?
   Always _____   Never _____
   Sometimes _____   Not applicable _____

4. Are you an interesting person?
   Always _____   Never _____
   Sometimes _____   Not applicable _____

5. Are you a happy person?
   Always _____   Never _____
   Sometimes _____   Not applicable _____

6. Do you keep busy with hobbies and other activities?
   Always _____   Never _____
   Sometimes _____   Not applicable _____

Comments: Is there anything else you'd like to tell me about yourself or about living here?

E. Family

Do you have a family? How much do you see your family? Where do they live? (If the person does not have family, do not use this section.)

1. Does your family get annoyed with you when you can't hear them?
   Always _____   Never _____
   Sometimes _____   Not applicable _____

2. Do they make decisions for you because of your hearing loss?
   Always _____   Never _____
   Sometimes _____   Not applicable _____

3. Does your family leave you out of discussions because of your hearing loss?
   Always _____   Never _____
   Sometimes _____   Not applicable _____

4. Do members of your family speak loudly enough for you to hear them?
   Always _____   Never _____
   Sometimes _____   Not applicable _____

5. Does your family understand what it's like to have a hearing problem?
   Always _____   Never _____
   Sometimes _____   Not applicable _____

Comments: How does your family feel about your hearing loss?

F. Rehabilitation

1. Do you think you need help in overcoming your hearing problem?
   Always _____   Never _____
   Sometimes _____   Not applicable _____

2. Are you a good listener?
   Always _____   Never _____
   Sometimes _____   Not applicable _____

3. Do you watch facial expressions when someone is speaking to you?
   Always _____   Never _____
   Sometimes _____   Not applicable _____

4. Do you watch gestures or "body language" when someone is talking to you?
   Always _____   Never _____
   Sometimes _____   Not applicable _____

5. Do you have a hearing aid? (If person responds yes, proceed.)
   Always _____   Never _____
   Sometimes _____   Not applicable _____

6. Do you wear your hearing aid?
   Always _____   Never _____
   Sometimes _____   Not applicable _____

Comments: If lipreading training were available, would you be interested in attending?

Reprinted by permission from Alpiner, J.G., and Baker, B., Communication assessment procedures in aural rehabilitation process. *Semin. Speech, Lang. Hear.*, 2(3), 189–204 (1981).

APPENDIX 13.5 *The Hearing Handicap Inventory for the Elderly*

Instructions:

The purpose of this scale is to identify the problems your hearing loss may be causing you. Answer *YES, SOMETIMES*, or *NO* for each question. *Do not skip a question if you avoid a situation because of your hearing problem.* If you use a hearing aid, please answer the way you hear *without* the aid.

		Yes (4)	Some-times (2)	No (0)
S-1.	Does a hearing problem cause you to use the phone less often than you would like?	____	____	____
E-2.	Does a hearing problem cause you to feel embarrassed when meeting new people?	____	____	____
S-3.	Does a hearing problem cause you to avoid groups of people?	____	____	____
E-4.	Does a hearing problem make you irritable?	____	____	____
E-5.	Does a hearing problem cause you to feel frustrated when talking to members of your family?	____	____	____
S-6.	Does a hearing problem cause you difficulty when attending a party?	____	____	____
E-7.	Does a hearing problem cause you to feel "stupid" or "dumb"?	____	____	____
S-8.	Do you have difficulty hearing when someone speaks in a whisper?	____	____	____

E-9.   Do you feel handicapped by a hearing problem? _____ _____ _____

S-10.   Does a hearing problem cause you difficulty when visiting friends, relatives, or neighbors? _____ _____ _____

S-11.   Does a hearing problem cause you to attend religious services less often than you would like? _____ _____ _____

E-12.   Does a hearing problem cause you to be nervous? _____ _____ _____

S-13.   Does a hearing problem cause you to visit friends, relatives, or neighbors less often than you would like? _____ _____ _____

E-14.   Does a hearing problem cause you to have arguments with family members? _____ _____ _____

S-15.   Does a hearing problem cause you difficulty when listening to TV or radio? _____ _____ _____

S-16.   Does a hearing problem cause you to go shopping less often than you would like? _____ _____ _____

E-17.   Does any problem or difficulty with your hearing upset you at all? _____ _____ _____

E-18.   Does a hearing problem cause you to want to be by yourself? _____ _____ _____

S-19.   Does a hearing problem cause you to talk to family members less often than you would like? _____ _____ _____

E-20.   Do you feel that any difficulty with your hearing limits or hampers your personal or social life? _____ _____ _____

S-21.   Does a hearing problem cause you difficulty when in a restaurant with relatives or friends? _____ _____ _____

E-22.   Does a hearing problem cause you to feel depressed? _____ _____ _____

S-23.   Does a hearing problem cause you to listen to TV or radio less often than you would like? _____ _____ _____

E-24.   Does a hearing problem cause you to feel uncomfortable when talking to friends? _____ _____ _____

E-25.   Does a hearing problem cause you to feel left out when you are with a group of people? _____ _____ _____

FOR CLINICIAN'S USE ONLY: Total Score: _____

Subtotal E: _____

Subtotal S: _____

Reprinted by permission from Ventry, I., and Weinstein, B., The hearing handicap inventory for the elderly: a new tool. *Ear Hear.*, 3, 128–134 (1982).

APPENDIX 13.6 *Hearing Handicap Inventory for the Elderly—Screening Version (HHIE-S)*

Please answer "yes," "no," or "sometimes" to each of the following items. Do not skip a question if you avoid a situation because of a hearing problem. If you use a hearing aid, please answer the way you hear without the aid.

		Yes	No	Some-times
E-1.	Does a hearing problem cause you to feel embarrassed when you meet new people?	___	___	___
E-2.	Does a hearing problem cause you to feel frustrated when talking to members of your family?	___	___	___
S-3.	Do you have difficulty hearing when someone speaks in a whisper?	___	___	___
E-4.	Do you feel handicapped by a hearing problem?	___	___	___
S-5.	Does a hearing problem cause you difficulty when visiting friends, relatives, or neighbors?	___	___	___
S-6.	Does a hearing problem cause you to attend religious services less often than you would like?	___	___	___
E-7.	Does a hearing problem cause you to have arguments with family members?	___	___	___
S-8.	Does a hearing problem cause you difficulty when listening to TV or radio?	___	___	___
E-9.	Do you feel that any difficulty with your hearing limits or hampers your personal or social life?	___	___	___
S-10.	Does a hearing problem cause you difficulty when in a restaurant with relatives or friends?	___	___	___

Reprinted by permission from Ventry, I., and Weinstein, B., Identification of elderly people with hearing problems. *Ear Hear.*, 3, 128–134 (1982).

14

Counseling Hearing-Impaired Adults

SUE ANN ERDMAN, M.A.

· ·

The effectiveness of audiologists' counseling influences many aspects of patients' adjustment to hearing impairment. This may range from acceptance of the hearing impairment, to compliance with recommended rehabilitation measures, to resolution of communication problems. As technological advances increasingly depersonalize many of the diagnostic and rehabilitative procedures employed in audiology, establishing rapport and credibility with one's clientele becomes both more important and more difficult. Consequently, it is imperative that renewed emphasis be placed on the importance and actual nature of effective counseling in clinical practice. The ultimate goal of rehabilitative audiology is to facilitate adjustment to the auditory and nonauditory consequences of hearing impairment. By definition, counseling is the process wherein clinicians facilitate clients' adjustment. In this chapter, counseling is presented not merely as an essential clinical skill but as the essence of successful rehabilitative intervention. Successful rehabilitation entails the following: (1) establishing the requisite therapeutic conditions to facilitate change, (2) actively engaging patients in the rehabilitation process, (3) identifying pertinent communication and concomitant adjustment problems, (4) implementing appropriate intervention strategies, and (5) monitoring patients' benefit from and compliance with treatment regimens. These aspects of the counseling process in rehabilitative audiology are discussed from philosophical, the-

oretical, and practical perspectives to illustrate the need to focus on hearing disability and handicap as opposed to hearing impairment in rehabilitative intervention.

The rationale for counseling, the characteristics of the counselor-client relationship, and the specific approaches reviewed in this chapter are relevant for counseling most hearing-impaired patients. Inasmuch as other sections of this book specifically address the geriatric population, this chapter emphasizes the counseling needs of adults with postlingually acquired hearing impairments who rely on oral communication. Corsini (1989) refers to individuals he counsels in a private office as *clients* and those he counsels in a hospital setting as *patients*. Inasmuch as audiologists practice in both of these clinical settings and use the terms interchangeably, both terms are used throughout this chapter.

Defining the Role of Counseling in Rehabilitative Audiology

Counseling has been slow to evolve into a systematic, well-defined process in rehabilitative audiology. This is not to say that counseling is not a constant aspect of audiologists' practice. Nonetheless, in spite of growing awareness of the psychosocial consequences of hearing impairment and related communication dysfunction, an organized approach to counseling individuals with hearing impairment has not been developed. Audiologists are more uneasy about being "counselors" than with counseling per se. Many are reluctant to recommend "counseling" and cite reservations about patients' perceptions of needing counseling. There is also concern that payment for rehabilitation counseling may not be available through a third-party source. As with any diagnostic or treatment regimen previously unknown or unproven, this is not surprising. Historically, as a need for intervention is demonstrated, and its benefits and effectiveness are documented, change occurs in this regard. Meanwhile, given the communication and adjustment difficulties associated with hearing loss, there is no justifiable reason for counseling not to be readily available.

Audiologists' reluctance to accept the counselor's role may have other roots as well. The extent to which training emphasizes and provides experience in counseling affects how comfortable clinicians are assuming the role of counselor. In a survey of ESB-accredited programs in communication disorders McCarthy, Culpepper, and Lucks (1986) found considerable variability in availability of counseling courses, in course content, and in requirements for such coursework. Three-quarters of the programs surveyed offered counseling courses through their own or another department; however, the courses were required only 45% of the time.

The American Speech-Language-Hearing Association (ASHA, 1974, 1984) cites counseling as a minimal competency for those providing aural rehabilitation services. Given that counseling occurs in most interactions with clients, it is safe to assume that students gain insight into the counseling process through clinical observations and their practicum experience. There is evidence that training per se is not always essential for counseling to be successful (Thomas, Butler, & Parker, 1987). Nonetheless, the professional responsibility for counseling hearing-impaired individuals about hearing loss and subsequent communication and adjustment problems lies clearly with the audiologist. Audiologists' understanding of hearing impairment and the problems it creates exceeds that of any other group of professionals. Hence, audiologists are ideally suited to counsel hearing-impaired persons and family members regarding the problems they experience. Failure to accept this responsibility undermines audiologists' credibility among consumers and other professionals. By questioning audiologists' qualifications to counsel hearing-impaired patients relative to the effects of hearing impairment, the profession's role in management of hearing disorders is questioned.

Audiologists' ambivalence regarding their role in counseling hearing-impaired patients warrants a systematic delineation of the counseling process in rehabilitative audiology. This entails defining communicative difficulties and adjustment problems experienced secondary to hearing impairment; defining rehabilitative strategies; monitoring and defining outcome through quality assurance, program evaluation, and clinical follow-up studies; and documenting and disseminating this information. By doing so, the requisite knowledge base to enhance clinician training and services for hearing-impaired populations can be developed. There is much to be said for clinical data that is "there for the taking." Those who despair of ever finding time to conduct research in a busy practice are referred to Barlow, Hayes, and Nelson (1984) for an enlightening perspective on conducting clinical research within the confines of clinical practice. As demands increase for program evaluation and quality assurance to justify one's existence, expansion, and/or expenditures, the need to define the scope and nature of services becomes more critical. The information gathered for such purposes identifies client needs, effective methodologies, and areas in need of expansion. Documentation of the counseling needs of hearing-impaired patients, the nature of counseling services, and the outcome of intervention has been woefully neglected.

What Is Counseling?

The term *counseling* conjures up different notions for different people and in different contexts. For some, counseling connotes psychotherapy. Indeed, counseling and psychotherapy textbooks (Corsini &

Wedding, 1989; Patterson, 1986) acknowledge that definitions of one serve equally well as definitions of the other, the same theories and methods apply in each, and hence, the terms are used interchangeably. Often, a difference in severity is inferred; psychotherapy tends to imply intervention for more serious problems, such as personality disorders, whereas counseling denotes help in adjusting to specific or situational problems. Counseling has also been equated with interpersonal communication effectiveness (Gerrard, Boniface, & Love, 1980; King, Novik, & Citrenbaum, 1983), and problem solving (Golightly, 1981; Patterson, 1986; Thomas et al., 1987). Even the term *patient education* is applied to the counseling process (Falvo, 1985).

Sanders (1975, 1980) describes two types of counseling in rehabilitative audiology: informational counseling and personal-adjustment counseling. Although this breakdown simplifies categorization of many activities in which audiologists are involved, it suggests a dichotomy, as Wylde (1987) has pointed out, that is inconsistent with the adjustment process. Counseling, as most definitions hold, is designed to facilitate resolution of problems by enabling individuals to find appropriate solutions for their difficulties. The provision of information specific to hearing problems, in many instances, facilitates personal adjustment. Patterson (1986) maintains that counseling includes the affective realm, that is, attitudes, feelings, and emotions, and that when these are not involved, the process does not constitute counseling but rather "teaching, information giving, or an intellectual discussion." Few individuals report an absence of emotional reactions to the myriad of difficulties posed by hearing impairment. Thomas's findings (1984, 1988) indicate that adjustment to hearing loss is a psychological process consisting of numerous affective factors for which counseling is indeed warranted. Further, he places the counseling responsibility on providers of audiological services, stressing that rehabilitation success is not likely if the social and psychological factors relevant to each individual are not considered.

The distinction between informational and personal adjustment counseling is even less apparent when the process is viewed from a problem-solving perspective, remembering of course, that counseling is a process wherein the resolution of problems is facilitated. An initial step in problem solving is problem identification. The ease with which this first step is completed varies depending on how cognizant one is of the specific difficulties experienced secondary to hearing loss. As an example, husbands with high-frequency hearing loss often do not recognize the relationship between that diagnosis and their wives' seeming inability to speak clearly anymore. Inherent in accepting an identified problem is understanding the problem. The extent to which individuals accept their hearing impairment is facilitated by increased understanding of the nature of the loss. The husbands described above make statements like, "I hear just fine! I hear her talking, I just can't understand her because she mumbles all the time." Many people do not have a clear understanding of the relationship between low and high frequencies and speech loudness and clarity. They equate hearing loss with decreased "volume" or audibility, not a lack of clarity. Understandably, individuals with that notion find it hard to believe they have a real hearing problem. Hence, understanding must precede true acceptance of a problem. Acceptance, in turn, precedes assuming responsibility to effect change or to try and resolve the problem. Problem-solving approaches to counseling are designed to facilitate personal adjustment, yet they rely heavily on the dissemination or sharing of information. The emphasis in problem-solving approaches to counseling, as Thomas et al. (1987) explain, is on systematic resolution of pertinent problems using any and all available resources. The versatility and goal-orientedness of these approaches are ideal for rehabilitation counseling. Rather than being a separate entity or distinctly different function, informational counseling in rehabilitative audiology is an essential and integral aspect of the overall counseling process that is intended to facilitate personal adjustment. Categorizing or labeling specific facets of the overall process limits, rather than enhances, awareness of the scope and nature of counseling.

Counseling is also communication behavior; effective counseling constitutes effective communication. Insofar as behavior is learned, it is possible to become more effective as a communicator and counselor. Ironically, the communication disorders professions have yet to explore the role of communication effectiveness in treatment outcome. There is a wealth of information regarding effective communication in the health/helping professions applicable to counseling hearing-impaired patients (Barrett & Wright, 1984; Egan, 1986; Falvo, 1985; Gerrard et al., 1980; Golightly, 1981; King et al., 1983; Maguire, 1984; Purtilo, 1978). Information regarding variables that affect counseling effectiveness and compliance with treatment regimens can be borrowed from other health/helping professions. Existing patient-education models, counseling techniques, and counselor training methods can be adapted for rehabilitative audiology. In so doing, the role of counseling in rehabilitative audiology can be defined, providing it with identifiable objectives, methods, and results.

Review of Counseling Approaches

When counseling is integral to rehabilitation, clinicians often find that a combination of specific aspects of different counseling approaches is desirable. This is in contrast to adhering to a specific theory or model regardless of the patient's particular adjustment problems or the counselor's philosophy and skills. The eclectic approach to counseling has gained wider recognition in recent years (Bohart & Todd, 1988; Brearley & Birchley, 1986; Corsini, 1989; Meier, 1989; Patterson, 1986; Thomas et al., 1987). Patterson (1986) cautions against approaches that are atheoretical and unsystematic, noting that a true eclectic model has yet to be developed. The recent convergence among many counseling approaches in terms of theory and practice, however, suggests that foundations for an integrative approach to counseling now exist. To appreciate fully these converging trends and commonalities in counseling, a basic understanding of existing methodologies is indicated. This review is included to stimulate interest in counseling theory

and to introduce theories and methods that have potential applications in rehabilitative audiology.

Estimates of the different approaches to counseling range up to 400 (Karasu, 1986). Hence, it is difficult to categorize the various approaches with any degree of ease. It can be argued that counseling always encompasses learning, albeit via different modalities and mechanisms. Indeed, adjustment is facilitated by helping people *learn* to think, feel, or behave differently. It is possible, therefore, to review counseling methods within an arbitrary framework as follows: *cognitive* or *rational* approaches, *affective* or *humanistic* approaches, and *behavioral* approaches. Cognitive approaches focus primarily on thought processes and logic to enable individuals to think differently. Humanistic approaches are aimed at modifying feelings and emotions. Behavioral approaches, in turn, emphasize the body and physical actions as opposed to the mind, intellect, or affective realm. This somewhat simplistic framework serves to outline the methods shown in Table 14.1. Naturally, there are limitations to arbitrary categorizations such as this one. Meichenbaum's (1974, 1977) cognitive behavioral modification can be considered a cognitive approach. Adler (1963), a cognitive psychologist, has been referred to as a humanist whose ideas mirror existential psychologists. Also, many humanistic and cognitive approaches could be categorized as phenomenological or perceptual-phenomenological approaches instead. Approaches differ relative to the theories on which they are based (e.g., learning theory, behavior theory, personality theory, psychoanalytic theory, cognitive theory of emotion), the specific techniques employed, and the mechanisms involved in the therapeutic process. How an approach is labeled may be a function of its underlying theory, the orientation of those who first developed or described it, the techniques employed, or the learning modality involved. Or, it can be based on an interpretation of any or all of those variables by authors or editors attempting to organize the approaches for purposes of comparison. A cursory review of counseling textbooks provides testimony to that fact. Because counseling in rehabilitation is approached

Table 14.1
Cognitive, Behavioral, and Humanistic Approaches to Counseling

Approach	Originator	Landmark Publications
Cognitive Approaches		
Individual psychology	Alfred Adler	Adler (1963) Ansbacher & Ansbacher (1964)
Cognitive therapy	Aaron T. Beck	Beck (1976) Beck & Emery (1985) Beck, Rush, Shaw, & Emery (1979)
Rational-emotive therapy	Albert Ellis	Ellis (1962) Ellis & Grieger (1977)
Transactional analysis	Eric Berne	Berne (1961, 1964, 1966)
Behavioral Approaches		
Behavior therapy	Joseph Wolpe	Wolpe (1958, 1982)
Social learning methods	Albert Bandura	Bandura (1969, 1977, 1986)
Multimodel therapy	Arnold Lazarus	Lazarus (1976, 1981)
Cognitive behavior modification	Donald Meichenbaum	Meichenbaum (1974, 1977)
Humanistic Approaches		
Person-centered therapy	Carl Rogers	Rogers (1942, 1951, 1961, 1980)
Gestalt therapy	Friedrich Perls	Perls, Hefferline, & Goodman (1951) Perls (1969, 1973)
Existential psychotherapy	Rollo May	May (1961, 1977)

from a problem-solving perspective, the counseling methods outlined here are loosely categorized on the basis of *how* the adjustment process is primarily facilitated: by modifying behaviors, thoughts, or feelings. It is generally believed that psychoanalysis is not appropriate for counseling that is specifically rehabilitative in nature. Hence, classical Freudian analysis is not included in Table 14.1. Cognitive, behavioral, and humanistic approaches to counseling, however, can all be said to have roots in some aspect of psychoanalytic theory; some (e.g., Adler's individual psychology) are referred to as "neopsychoanalytic" therapies. Despite widespread influence, psychoanalysis is often not a viable or appropriate option for intervention. Among its limitations are cost, length of therapy, and the level of cooperation required from the patient. Psychoanalysis is typically not recommended in rehabilitation counseling because it is too time consuming to be applied efficiently, and requires education and training atypical of most professionals in rehabilitation

settings. Familiarity with psychoanalytic theory, particularly in terms of personality structure, defense mechanisms, and the unconscious, is relevant to an understanding of personality and behavior and the counseling process in general. Freudian ego defenses, including repression, projection, reaction formation, and regression, are often discussed in treatises on adjustment to disability, although research findings in support of Freudian explanations of adjustment to disability are equivocal at best (Cook, 1987; English, 1977). The influence of psychoanalytic theory and methods on other approaches to counseling has been widespread; the limitations of psychoanalysis, however, have given rise to a wide body of different approaches.

COGNITIVE APPROACHES

Cognitive methods in counseling emphasize intellectual or logical means of resolving problems. Cognitions include thoughts, ideas, beliefs, opinions, interpretations, values, and perceptions, which may or may not be conscious. From the cognitive perspective, abnormal behavior and emotional disturbance are caused or mediated by cognition. Cognitions can be modified by active means such as self-analysis or by passive means in which the counselor assumes an essentially didactic role. Beck's cognitive therapies (1976) and Ellis's (1962) rational-emotive therapy (RET) employ active, directive methods to address patients' assumptions and beliefs that are viewed as irrational or dysfunctional. Both therapies are present oriented and employ a reality testing approach to problem solving. In Beck's cognitive therapies and RET the counselor assumes an accepting yet confrontational role in which persuasion and argument are used to help explore the inappropriateness of clients' perceptions. This confrontational role is somewhat more didactic in RET than in Beck's approach, where a collaborative relationship between counselor and client is encouraged. In both approaches the patient is aided in identifying, confronting, and modifying inappropriate underlying assumptions that have triggered emotional distress or behavior problems. Ellis acknowledges Adler's individual psychology (1963) as a precursor to rational-emotive therapy. Both view emotions as a product of thought processes; inasmuch as people are capable of reason, they can control their feelings by controlling their thoughts. Adler's ideas on self-worth, including the view that inferiority feelings result when differences exist between concepts of ideal self and actual self, are clinically relevant in counseling individuals who have not accepted their disability. Adlerian theory is viewed as a cooperative educational enterprise with specific goals including reducing inferiority feelings, overcoming discouragement, helping individuals to recognize and use their resources, encouraging individuals to recognize equality among people, and helping individuals become contributing human beings (Mosak, 1989). Adler's individual psychology addresses modifications of motivation through changing goals and concepts; hence, it is cognitively oriented. RET is specifically intended to minimize irrational consequences, that is, emotional disturbances, such as anxiety (self-blame) and hostility (blaming others or cir-

cumstances), which result from impossible "shoulds," "oughts," and "musts" that people inflict on themselves. The positive effects of alleviating, if not eliminating, these emotional tolls may include recognition of the rights of others, self-direction, independence and responsibility, flexibility and openness to change, scientific thinking, commitment to something outside oneself, willingness to try things, and self-acceptance (Patterson, 1986). Here, too, the emphasis is on modification of cognitive patterns.

The appeal of cognitive approaches is their logical, indeed common sense, approach to what people think, say, and do. This is illustrated in Ellis's A-B-C model of adjustment difficulties. When a highly charged emotional consequence (C) follows a significant activating event (A), A may seem to, but actually does not, cause C. Emotional consequences, in fact, are caused by the person's belief system (B). Undesirable emotional consequences can be eliminated or alleviated by effectively disputing the irrational beliefs via rational or behavioral challenges. The cognitive skills required in RET might preclude using this approach with some people. Its appropriateness for individuals with low self-esteem or for those having difficulties adjusting to specific situations or problems (e.g., a disability) makes it useful in rehabilitative counseling.

Berne's (1961, 1964) transactional analysis (TA) is considerably more complex than the RET A-B-C paradigm, but it also is intended to facilitate clients' understanding of adjustment and the counseling process. TA is described as a psychology of human relationships that emphasizes increasing understanding of interactive/communication behavior to facilitate adjustment. An outgrowth of the human potential movement, TA has been strongly influenced by Gestalt psychology, Satir's family dynamics concepts, and Berne's training and early career in psychoanalysis. The TA framework of behavior is also based on three ego states: parent, adult, and child. Unlike psychoanalysis however, in which the id, ego, and superego are hypothetical constructs, the ego states in TA are considered to be dynamic, observable phenomena. Symbols and diagrams, including the egogram, a bar graph depicting the function and energy of the ego states (Dusay, 1977, 1978), are used to facilitate both communication between the counselor and client and the mechanisms involved in promoting adjustment or learning: understanding and insight. The terms adapted to describe TA concepts, such as transactions (units of human communication), games (series of ulterior transactions), scripts (life plans based on existential decisions that constitute belief systems), and strokes (human contact and recognition, either positive or negative), are sometimes viewed as colloquialisms. Nonetheless, their use is rigidly adhered to by those who use this approach. The rationale is that this demystifies the counselor and the counseling process and enables clients to understand, label, analyze, and interpret their behavior and relationships, directly supporting the TA goal of enhancing personal responsibility. The simple language eliminates the need to clarify and redefine concepts, goals, and techniques. Proponents of TA stress that the terms are easily learned and have been successfully taught to and used with those who are intellectually disabled. The potential disadvantage is that the "new language" can become a substitute for ideas and concepts. TA's "trendy" popularity, a function of its easily adopted terminology and Berne's best-selling books, has had a rather negative effect on professionals unfamiliar with the actual complexity and scope of Berne's original ideas and theory. Pollack (1978) has applied TA concepts to explain adjustment to hearing loss. The role of communication theory in the development of TA concepts and the success of TA in group settings are relevant when considering this approach for use in rehabilitative audiology.

These contributors to cognitive approaches to psychotherapy and counseling—Adler, Beck, Berne, and Ellis—departed from their original psychoanalytic orientation to enhance the therapeutic process. The constructs of cognitive approaches are more easily explained than those of psychoanalytic or humanistic methods. Cognitive methods are expedient and effective, and although systematic and structured, they are more flexible than many of the behavioral approaches.

BEHAVIORAL APPROACHES

Behavioral counseling is based on learning theory to an even greater extent than the cognitive methods are. Behavior therapies employ learning principles to change inappropriate behaviors and to teach adaptive behavior. Although approaches differ widely, behavioral counseling is typically described as having roots in experimental and social psychology and as being analytic and empirical in nature. The focus of intervention is on the observable and measurable. Familiarity with the work of Pavlov (1927, 1928) and Skinner (1938, 1953, 1971) is warranted to appreciate behavioral counseling methods. A Russian biologist with interests in nutrition and digestion, Pavlov contributed to the conceptualization of classical conditioning and extinction following his observations of salivation responses in dogs. Skinner's instrumental or operant conditioning, exemplified in experiments with key-pecking pigeons and bar-pressing rats, is fundamental to an understanding of token economies and other behavior modification programs. The work of these renowned behaviorists is basic to introductory psychology courses.

Joseph Wolpe, yet another psychoanalyst, first introduced behavioral concepts into the clinical arena. A South African who became interested in Pavlov's theories, Wolpe developed what is now known as systematic desensitization, originally termed reciprocal inhibition (Wolpe, 1958). This method is used to treat phobias and anxiety by introducing an incompatible response such as relaxation paired with a hierarchy of stimuli that evoke the undesirable emotional response. Wolpe's original model involved having clients imagine feared stimuli progressing through hierarchies from the least to the most anxiety-provoking stimulus conditions. In vivo desensitization, often used to assess the successfulness of intervention, involves exposure to the actual stimulus rather than an imagined one. Other behavioral strategies employed by Wolpe (1982) that have been used to treat a wide range of problems include aversion therapy and assertiveness training. The latter has been applied with hearing-impaired populations in a number of settings (DiMichael, 1985; Erdman, 1980). Wolpe has been criticized for not acknowledging the probable impact of cognitive and relational variables inherent in his or any behavioral approach. Indeed, behavior therapy often includes cognitive and affective variables, such as correction of misconceptions, teaching, acceptance, expressions of concern and of interest, reassurance, suggestions, persuasion, and a desire to help (Patterson, 1986), which are known to influence counseling outcome.

During the 1970s, emphasis on the cognitive processes increased among the behavioral approaches. Bandura's social learning theory (1969, 1977), Lazarus's multimodal therapy (1976, 1981), and Meichenbaum's cognitive behavior modification (1974, 1977) were developed in response to limitations inherent in strictly behavioral explanations of emotional disturbances and other aspects of human functioning. Bandura (1986) believes learning is cognitively mediated rather than an automatic association of a stimulus with a response. His theory of social learning includes learning through observation, imitation, and modeling, and acknowledges the role of expectations and environmental considerations in understanding behavior. Social learning models promote performance and observational approaches to learning over verbal (didactic or persuasive) methods. Meichenbaum's (1974, 1977) cognitive behavioral modification approach is based on self-instructional procedures. Clients engage in self-observation to monitor thoughts, feelings and behaviors. In therapy, internal communication, or "self-speech" is modified, thus enabling the person to adapt a flexible rather than fixed set of coping strategies. The versatility of this approach is evidenced by its use with clients ranging from hyperactive children to chronic pain patients (Meichenbaum, 1974; Turk, Meichenbaum, & Genest, 1983).

The overlapping of behaviorism with the cognitive perspective is evident in social learning theory, Meichenbaum's methods, Ellis's rational-emotive therapy, and Beck's cognitive therapy. Lazarus, a behaviorist, considers his multimodal approach to therapy (1976, 1981) to be responsive to the multitude of problems with which patients often present. To address the range of prob-

lems adequately, a multimodal assessment is conducted to determine the individual's "BASIC I.D." (Behavior, Affect, Sensation, Imagery, Cognition, Interpersonal relationships, Drugs/biology). The BASIC I.D. is an assessment and intervention model as well as Lazarus's view of personality dimensions. Lazarus (1989) contends that the assessment provides an operational means of determining what works, for whom, and under what conditions. In that respect, the multimodal approach is touted as being flexible and versatile, if not eclectic. Because it is based on observations, testing of hypotheses, and empirically derived data, Lazarus maintains that multimodal therapy is a behavioral approach. The original label, "multimodal behavior therapy," has been dropped, however, in favor of stressing customized treatment based on each patient's needs.

Behavioral approaches to counseling have made shorter cost-effective treatment a possibility in many instances. Specific treatment methods spawned by behavioral approaches have been particularly beneficial in clinical settings. Among these are many aspects of behavioral medicine including biofeedback. Behavioral therapy has also led to a resurgence of interest in the use of hypnosis in treatment. Behavioral therapists respond to criticism that they are "social control agents" by pointing out that clients determine their own therapy goals. Although this would not always apply to children, or some mentally handicapped and institutionalized individuals, Bohart and Todd (1988) acknowledge the egalitarian nature of behavior therapy and cite evidence that behavior therapists are rated as highly as other therapists in warmth, empathy, and genuineness. As in any counseling relationship, this may be one of the most salient ingredients of the therapeutic process. Some believe behavioral therapy is passé; others believe its potential is only now beginning to be realized.

AFFECTIVE APPROACHES

Affective or humanistic approaches to counseling focus on emotion or feelings to facilitate adjustment rather than on behavior or thought processes. An inherent problem in affective approaches is that emotions can only be dealt with indirectly. The premise underlying affective counseling methods is that clients can redirect their lives given an empathic, therapeutic climate conducive to self-exploration. The client is viewed as the agent of change in humanistic counseling models.

Carl Rogers's client-centered therapy, now frequently referred to as person-centered therapy, is based on extensive theories of personality and development (1942, 1951). Rogerian theory is another distinct departure from psychoanalysis; individuals are viewed as innately good, basically realistic or rational, constructive, and growth oriented. Also considered to be a phenomenological approach (i.e., one that holds that although a real world may exist, its existence is inferred on the basis of perceptions), the intent of person-centered therapy is to change the way the client perceives his or her phenomenal field. Rogers's approach differs markedly from cognitive counseling approaches in terms of the counselor's role. The client-centered counselor is characteristically *nondirective*. This is entirely consistent with the overall goal of enhancing the self-directed growth process, *self-actualization*. Concepts central to Rogers's client-centered therapy include congruence, unconditional positive regard, and empathy—critical factors in the therapist's role that are essential to the therapeutic process. Self-concept, locus of evaluation, and experiencing are concepts that apply to the client. These constructs have been carefully investigated with respect to outcome of the counseling process. Outcome is enhanced when clients receive congruence, unconditional positive regard, and empathy for the counselor, as this enables them to become more positive, realistic, self-expressive, self-directed, and open in their experiencing. Rogers's methods have been used with a wide range of patients and in a variety of settings. Because personal attributes rather than extensive training in psychotherapy are considered to be essential counselor ingredients, this approach is within the purview of counselors in rehabilitation settings (Thomas et al., 1987). The impact of Rogers's theories on rehabilitation counseling has been enormous. Rogers's concepts regarding ideal-self versus real-self discrepancies (i.e., differences in how people view themselves and how they wish to view themselves) are central to understanding why people react differently to physical disabilities; it is not the disability but the significance one attaches to it that determines acceptance and adjustment. Rehabilitation is impeded when the realities of disability are unacceptably inconsistent, or incongruent, with the ideal self (Cook, 1987). Self-acceptance (wherein the real self, even if not consistent with the ideal self, is satisfactory or acceptable) is instrumental in adjustment to disabilities, including hearing impairment. Erdman and Demorest (1986b) found strong relationships between self-acceptance and overall psychological adjustment to hearing impairment, maladaptive compensatory strategies, and perceptions of others' attitudes and behavior. Among the potential benefits of person-centered therapy are greater self-acceptance and effectiveness in problem solving, more realistic and objective perceptions, less defensiveness, maturity, a greater capacity for dealing with stress, and a sense of self-control (Raskin & Rogers, 1989; Rogers, 1986). Corsini (1989) contends that those considering careers in counseling, regardless of their philosophical orientation, would do well to begin with Rogers's *Counseling and Psychotherapy* (1942).

Gestalt therapy (Perls, 1969, 1973; Perls, Hefferline, & Goodman, 1951), a phenomenological-existential approach, is similar to person-centered therapy inasmuch as the goal of this holistic approach is to integrate the individual to the point that he or she is self-directive. The counselor's role and the therapeutic process are, however, distinctly different. Gestalt therapy focuses on the here and now to increase the person's ability to remain in contact with the current situation. This includes an awareness of all the elements that configure one's *gestalt* or whole field. The exercises employed in Gestalt therapy, including enactment, exaggeration, and guided fantasy, are experiential and are designed to enhance awareness. Bohart and Todd (1988) dub this "behavioral existentialism." Counselors are confrontative, probing, and authoritative to the point of actively frustrating patients so that they can find the support and resources they seek within themselves. Extensive training and personal therapy are requirements to be a Gestalt therapist. This, in and of itself, limits its application in rehabilitation settings. The process is neither easy nor pleasant; many who begin treatment reportedly do not continue. Unlike person-centered counseling, Gestalt therapy has not been the subject of systematic investigations. Nonetheless, this approach has also made its contributions. Expressions that have become idiomatic, such as "getting in touch with" and "consciousness raising" have roots in Gestalt techniques. Experiential exercises used in Gestalt therapy have been adapted for a wide variety of purposes in workshops. The Gestalt focus on nonverbal communication has been influential in many arenas. There is evidence of a softening of many hitherto rigid stances in Gestalt methods, particularly with respect to "frustrating" the patient (Patterson, 1986; Yontef & Simkin, 1989). The popularity of Gestalt therapy has grown over the last couple decades despite early perceptions that the approach was appropriate for individuals stereotypically viewed as rigid, inhibited, or perfectionistic.

Although Rogers's and Perls's approaches can be considered existential in nature, there are those who espouse a more distinctly existential approach. In the United States, the most influential of these has been Rollo May (1961 1977), whose writings reflect the existential philosophy of Husserl, Kierkegaard, and Nietzsche. May and Yalom (1989) predict existential therapy will be absorbed into other approaches inasmuch as it deals with presuppositions underlying counseling of any kind. One might say the approach constitutes a philosophy of therapy that understands "man as being." Because existential therapy is meant to transcend the therapy process, there are no specific methods. The significance of its philosophical underpinnings are such, however, that the writings of Rollo May are strongly recommended to those who will consider adapting converging trends in counseling to their own practice.

The contributions of humanistic, phenomenological, existential counseling are many. The critical nature of counselor characteristics and their importance to the counselor-client relationship are especially noteworthy. Rogers's influence in this domain may well be unsurpassed. Similarly, his theory of self, and the rigorous study to which the concepts embodied in this have been subjected, are now cornerstones in the understanding of personality. Role playing and the "empty chair" technique have proved to be effective therapy tools that have been adapted from Gestalt therapy by counselors of various orientations.

Commonalities and Converging Trends: Implications for Counseling in Rehabilitative Audiology

In recent years counselors have increasingly admitted to an eclectic approach to clinical practice. From the preceding descriptions it is apparent that few, if any, approaches adhere rigidly to just one theory, one method, or one modality. In each approach, behavioral, cognitive, and affective influences are apparent. Patterson (1986), Brohart and Todd (1988), and Corsini (1989) acknowledge and identify converging trends in counseling. Corsini believes successful counselors adopt or develop theories and methods best suited to their personality. He condones this practice when the approach is based on sound knowledge of existing theories and methods and entails doing the right thing with a client in light of that body of knowledge. Patterson (1986) claims eclectic approaches increase the potential for haphazard use of techniques and methods without a theoretical rationale for doing so. He optimistically observes the convergence of concepts and methods in counseling, however, as an indication that "true eclectic counseling" may be a possibility.

The convergence in counseling approaches can best be understood in the context of how much is actually common to the counseling experience as well as a historical review of what has proved to be successful. The proclivity for coining new terms or adding a new twist to create yet another innovative counseling approach notwithstanding, there are common threads among those approaches documented in the literature. Self-acceptance and self-growth are goals common to humanistic, psychoanalytic, and cognitive approaches. Each of these perspectives also views adjustment problems as the result of rigid, maladaptive, or similarly inadequate, inappropriate perceptions of reality (Brohart & Todd, 1988). Cognitive and behavioral approaches have many similarities; they tend to be present centered, problem oriented, systematic, structured, efficient, empirical, and less esoteric than other approaches.

Patterson (1986) cites seven implicit commonalities among counseling approaches:

1. The counseling approaches agree that humans can change or be changed.
2. The approaches agree that some behaviors are undesirable, inadequate, or harmful, or result in dissatisfaction, unhappiness, or limitations that warrant change.
3. Counselors expect patients to change as a result of their particular techniques and intervention.
4. Individuals who seek counseling experience a need for help.
5. Clients believe change can and will occur.
6. Counselors expect clients to be active participants.
7. Intervention characteristically includes persuasion, encouragement, advice, support, and instruction.

The implications for counseling in rehabilitative audiology are readily apparent in each of the above. Certainly the effects of hearing impairment can be minimized (changed). Communicative behavior, subsequent to hearing impairment, may be undesirable, inadequate, or harmful, or result in dissatisfaction, unhappiness, or limitations that warrant change. Audiologists expect patients to change as a result of intervention. Those individuals who benefit from the process seek help and believe change can occur. Similarly, clients are expected to participate actively in the rehabilitative process in terms of accepting and adjusting to the use of amplification, learning to watch speakers' faces, exploring their communication difficulties and the ramifications of those problems, and adhering to the rehabilitative regimen presented via persuasion, encouragement, advice, support, and instruction.

Corsini and Rosenberg (1955), in an extensive literature review, identified nine mechanisms of change in therapy. Corsini (1989) maintains that these are equally applicable today despite four decades of intervening innovations in counseling. He describes the mechanisms as cognitive, affective, and behavioral factors. The cognitive factors include *universalization, insight,* and *modeling.* Universalization is the recognition that human suffering is universal; one benefits from realizing "I'm not alone." Insight relates to the benefits incurred through increased understanding of one's self and others. Modeling facilitates change because people learn and benefit from watching others.

Affective factors that facilitate adjustment include *acceptance, altruism,* and *transference.* Acceptance pertains to a sense of being part of a group (in group counseling) and receiving unconditional positive regard from others, notably from the counselor. Change is engendered altruistically by the awareness that one is loved and cared for and that one loves and cares for others. Transference, a global recognition of the significance attached to the counselor by the client (not limited here to strict psychoanalytic connotations), is another factor to which change is frequently attributed.

The behavioral mechanisms identified as effecting change in counseling include *reality testing, ventilation,* and *interaction.* Reality testing facilitates change when new behaviors and concepts can be experimented within the safety of the counseling session and are subsequently reinforced or modified as a result of success, feedback, and support. Ventilation refers to benefits derived from the opportunity to express pent-up emotions or previously unvoiced fears and preoccupations. Lastly, interactions with a counselor or group members, in which clients essentially admit to a problem, facilitate adjustment.

Clinicians who have conducted groups sessions with hearing-impaired patients will immediately recognize the above mechanisms of change as cogent factors in adjustment to hearing loss. Hearing-impaired clients benefit from the realization that others experience similar difficulties as a result of hearing loss (universalization) and from increased awareness and understanding of the effects of hearing loss (insight). They also learn from observing how others with hearing impairment cope with their difficulties and how situational coping strategies can be employed (modeling). Individuals engage in reality testing by experimenting with amplification to verify and explore its potential benefits and comparing unaided/aided performance, by practicing lipreading, and by evaluating other verbal and nonverbal communication strategies. Hearing-impaired patients also benefit from verbalizing the stress and frustration caused by hearing difficulties (ventilation) to one another or to the audiologist (interaction). The camaraderie engendered within the group by the cognitive and behavioral mechanisms, in turn, promotes the affective conditions that further facilitate—and perhaps ultimately ensure—adjustment: trust in and respect for the audiologist (transference), whose recommendations are now more likely to be followed, and a sense of rapport, of once again belonging (acceptance) and of being cared for (altruism), in spite of one's hearing problems. Although these mechanisms of change are more readily apparent in group counseling, each also contributes to change in individual counseling. The mechanisms are highly interdependent; the effectiveness of one is likely to enhance the presence and effectiveness of another. Recognition of these factors is of paramount importance in developing, implementing, and evaluating counseling programs. They are also relevant in understanding the process of adjustment to hearing loss.

The most frequently cited and discussed variables in counseling involve the *nature of the counselor-client relationship,* which, many believe, defines and determines the counseling process. Patterson (1986) claims that those who debate evidence supporting the counseling relationship as the most powerful, effective variable in the counseling process are simply threatened by the implications of this incontrovertible fact. These implications suggest that warmth, empathy, trust, respect, and unconditional positive regard—personal attributes that the effective counselor presents to the client and that thereby define the counseling pro-

cess—are more salient than any other variables in the treatment process. For those whose theories and methodologies are trivialized by what Patterson believes is perhaps the most well-documented and supported conclusion in the psychology of human behavior, some resistance is largely understandable. Although the evidence does not confirm that these relational conditions are sufficient for therapeutic change, it also does not confirm that they are not. More important, there is no evidence of the effectiveness of other treatment variables in the absence of these relational conditions. The findings, replicated in varied settings, with varied populations, in varied contexts, and in varied languages, simply and categorically demonstrate that those who communicate warmth, genuineness, and accurate empathy are more effective in interpersonal relationships regardless of their role or the purpose of the interaction (Rogers, 1957; Truax & Carkhuff, 1967; Truax & Mitchell, 1971).

The features common to the counseling experience discussed above are clearly relevant to intervention with hearing-impaired patients. Yet the process wherein they become operative has yet to be implemented systematically into audiologists' practice. Why? The answer may lie in whether audiologists function from a medical model (Illich, 1976) or from a rehabilitation/helping process model (Anderson, 1977; Brammer, 1985) perspective of health care delivery. The clinical implications of the disparities inherent in these perspectives merit consideration.

Professionals functioning within a medical model of treatment react differently to the adjustment problems experienced by a patient secondary to illness or disability than do professionals in a rehabilitation model. Those trained in the behavioral sciences tend to be supportive in their efforts to help individuals adapt coping strategies to minimize or alleviate the debilitating effects of disease or disability. Hence, in a rehabilitative model, health care reflects a cooperative, collaborative helping process (Brammer, 1985; Egan, 1986); patients participate actively in the identification and resolution of pertinent problems. In the medical model, patients are passive recipients of diagnostic and treatment procedures; the patient is poked, probed, and prodded by the practitioner, who subsequently identifies the problem and proceeds to give instructions to resolve the problem. The patient may not agree with, understand, or accept the professional's diagnosis (identification of the problem) or regimen (solution to the problem), which results in noncompliance with recommended treatment. The professional's role in compliance is of paramount importance (Falvo, 1985; Garrity, 1981; Squier, 1990). Research findings suggest that the more authoritative the professional is, the less compliant the client is likely to be (Anderson, 1977). The traditional medical model essentially contributes to noncompliance inasmuch as patients are not actively engaged in the decision-making process relative to their treatment. Recent focus on the role of behavior in disease emphasizes the importance of compliance in prevention and treatment of health problems. Compliance problems abound in audiology, although they have yet to be investigated as such. Among the problems constituting noncompliance are hearing aid recommendations that patients fail to pursue, hearing aids that end up in dresser drawers, and failure to use hearing protection in noise hazardous areas. The role audiologists play in patients' noncompliance has also not been addressed. Nonuse of hearing aids has been attributed to cosmetic concerns, to denial, to limitations posed by certain hearing impairments, and to limitations in amplification technology. Rarely, if ever, has the effectiveness of counseling/patient-education/interpersonal communication skills (call it what you will!) been evaluated as a factor in patients' acceptance of and adjustment to hearing impairment or the use of amplification. Inasmuch as counselor characteristics are among the most powerful variables in facilitating adjustment and change, the parameters of clinical demeanor that determine outcome must be acknowledged. Adherence to treatment programs is enhanced when patients are engaged in the management (i.e., identification and resolution) of their problems. Counselor characteristics are the key to engaging patients in this process. The essential relational conditions of empathy, warmth, understanding, and respect provide a basis of trust that patients need to accept, assimilate, and act on the information given them. This complex interaction exemplifies the rehabilitation model and helping process; when clinicians engage patients in their own treatment, outcome is more likely to be successful. This is the essence of the counseling process. Paradoxically, if patients are not engaged in their own adjustment they fail, and the clinician fails. Hence, counseling is an integral aspect of successful rehabilitative intervention.

Implications of Hearing Impairment

Recognizing the applicability of varied counseling approaches to practice in rehabilitative audiology is the first step in appreciating the wealth of information available on facilitating adjustment. The literature pertaining to psychosocial reactions to disability and to rehabilitation counseling is replete with information applicable to rehabilitative audiology. The psychosocial implications of hearing impairment, in many respects, are similar to those stemming from other disabling conditions. Ergo, the conceptual and methodological underpinnings of rehabilitation counseling are also relevant.

Implementing effective counseling methods in rehabilitative audiology has been stymied by the fact that the course of adjustment to hearing impairment cannot be predicted. It is possible to generalize and describe problems *typically* experienced by hearing-impaired individuals; however, no one adjustment pattern can be determined from a given audiometric configuration. Individuals with a particular type and/or degree of hearing impairment may tend to report similar communication problems and adjustment difficulties. It is not uncommon for individuals with identical audiograms, however, to experience dissimilar communication difficulties and adjustment patterns. The unpredictable nature of adjustment to hearing loss is not atypical; there is considerable evidence that adjustment to disability is universally unpredictable (Cook, 1987; English, 1977; Geis, 1977; Falvo, 1985; Schontz, 1977). Importantly, however, these results also reveal that disability affects individual behavior and can have a profound psychosocial impact. Factors that impinge on adjustment to disability are related to (*1*) negative reactions from others (stigma), (*2*) dependency on others, (*3*) changes in interpersonal relationships, (*4*) isolation or lack of accessibility to the environment, (*5*) acceptance of the disability, and (*6*) low self-esteem or difficulty reintegrating the self-concept (Scadden, 1987; Thomas et al., 1987). It is noteworthy that these variables are associated with the individual and his or her environment and not with characteristics of the disability per se. Knutson and Lansing (1990) found that specific communication strategies and accommodations to hearing impairment, rather than the hearing impairment, contribute to individuals' psychological adjustment among those with profound acquired hearing impairment.

Notwithstanding this multidisciplinary evidence, many studies have been conducted to examine the relationship between hearing impairment and its resultant communication and adjustment difficulties. Correlations between audiometric variables and self-report measures, obtained to explore the predictive capability of audiometric data or the validity of self-assessment tools, albeit significant, have typically not been strong (Brainerd & Frankel, 1985; Erdman & Demorest, 1990; Kielinen & Nerbonne, 1990; Hawes & Niswander, 1985; Rowland, J. P. et al., 1985; Speaks, Jerger, & Trammell, 1970; Weinstein & Ventry, 1983a, 1983b). One can infer from this that there is a relationship between hearing loss and its concomitant communication and adjustment problems; the relationship, however, is not one that permits prediction of adjustment problems for a given individual.

Nonetheless, audiologists seem compelled to attempt to quantify the handicapping effects of hearing loss. Perhaps this can be attributed to the fact that audiology's foundation is steeped in measurement. There are, of course, intrinsic advantages to quantifying hearing handicap for compensation purposes and to monitor progress. The tendency to equate something as complex as communicative behavior and personal adjustment with a handful of au-

diometric variables, however, is unwise. Regardless of how much more expedient it might be to do so, *for rehabilitative purposes, degree or nature of handicap cannot be determined from audiometric data alone.* Information regarding auditory factors, as Thomas (1988) stresses, does not suffice when it comes to explaining the psychological stress that results from hearing loss.

The terminology employed to describe the consequences of hearing impairment has stimulated considerable discussion. Diverse definitions of *disability* and *handicap* (AMA/AAO, 1979; ASHA, 1981; PL 101-336, 1990; Susser & Watson, 1970; WHO, 1980), as shown in Table 14.2, have prompted concern about subsequent problems in discussing and studying these phenomena (Giolas, 1990; Noble, 1988; Schow & Gatehouse, 1990; Stephens & Hétu, 1991; Ward, 1983, 1988). The World Health Organization (1980) definitions closely follow those proffered by Susser and Watson (1970), which delineate three facets of handicapping conditions: organic, functional, and social. The organic component of the disease process constitutes impairment; disability is composed of the functional limitations imposed by an impairment; and handicap consists of the manner and extent to which impairment and disability impinge on an individual's roles and relationships.

The AMA and ASHA definitions relate disability to compensation. The ASHA (1981) definitions were developed by a task force appointed specifically to consider the issue of when hearing impairment constitutes a handicap and to recommend a definition of hearing handicap. The members focused their efforts specifically on the formulation of a definition that could be used as a basis for determining hearing disability for workers' compensation. Although the ASHA definitions are frequently cited, the task force report clearly states that it does not constitute ASHA policy; the report is not a position paper. Inasmuch as the stated purpose was to define handicap specifically for compensation purposes, broader definitions can certainly be applied as a basis for understanding the sequelae of hearing loss.

The AMA and ASHA definitions do not distinguish between auditory and nonau-

Table 14.2
Classifications of Auditory Dysfunction Domains as Defined by the American Academy of Otolaryngology (AAO, 1979), American Speech-Language-Hearing Association (ASHA, 1981), the Americans with Disabilities Act of 1990 (PL 101-336, 1990), Susser and Watson (1970), and the World Health Organization (WHO, 1980)[a]

AAO, 1979

Permanent Impairment. A change for the worse in either structure or function, outside the range of normal, is permanent impairment. The term is used here in a medical rather than a legal sense. Permanent impairment is due to any anatomic or functional abnormality that produces hearing loss. This loss should be evaluated after maximum rehabilitation has been achieved and when the impairment is nonprogressive at the time of evaluation. The determination of impairment is basic to the evaluation of permanent handicap and disability.

Permanent Handicap. The disadvantage imposed by an impairment sufficient to affect a person's efficiency in the activities of daily living is permanent handicap. Handicap implies a material impairment.

Permanent Disability. An actual or presumed inability to remain employed at full wages is a permanent disability. A person is permanently disabled or under permanent disability when the actual or presumed ability to engage in gainful activity is reduced because of handicap and when no appreciable improvement can be expected.

ASHA, 1981

Hearing impairment is used to mean a deviation or change for the worse in either auditory structure or auditory function, usually outside the range of normal.

Hearing handicap means the disadvantage imposed by a hearing impairment on a person's communicative performance in the activities of daily living.

Hearing disability means the determination of a financial award for the loss of function caused by any hearing impairment that results in significant hearing handicap.

PL 101-336, 1990

Disability The term "disability" means, with respect to an individual:
(A) a physical or mental impairment that substantially limits one or more of the major life activities of such individual;
(B) a record of such an impairment; or
(C) being regarded as having such an impairment.

Susser and Watson, 1970

Impairment is the organic component, a static condition of the process of disease.

Disability is the functional component, or the limitation of function imposed by the impairment and the individual's psychologic reaction to it.

Handicap is the social component, the manner and degree in which the primary impairment and functional disability limit the performance of social roles and relations with others.

WHO, 1980

Disorder occurs as a result of some type of disease process or malformation of the auditory system.

Impairment is any loss or abnormality of psychological, physiological, or anatomical structure or function.

Disability is any restriction or lack (resulting from an impairment) of ability to perform an activity in the manner or within the range considered normal for a human being.

Handicap is a disadvantage for a given individual, resulting from an impairment or a disability, that limits or prevents the fulfillment of a role that is normal (depending on age, sex, and social and cultural factors for that individual).

[a] Adapted from Schow, R.L., and Gatehouse, S., Fundamental issues in self-assessment of hearing. *Ear Hear.*, 11(5), 6S–16S (1990).

ditory effects of hearing impairment as do WHO-based classifications. Hence, they do not facilitate delineation of specific cause/ effect relationships for assessment, intervention, or research purposes. As others have also indicated (Schow & Gatehouse, 1990; Stephens & Hétu, 1991), a consensus regarding terminology would facilitate discussion and understanding among rehabilitative audiologists. Public Law 101-336 (1990), the Americans with Disabilities Act of 1990 (ADA-1990), protects the rights of those with disabilities, including communication disorders. The regulatory definition of disability introduced in ADA-1990 makes no reference to compensation; moreover, the definition approximates the WHO definition of disability. As guidelines for enacting PL 101-336 and references to the implications of the law continue to appear, future interpretations of "disability" are likely to be more consistent.

References to impairment, disability, and handicap in this chapter reflect applications of the WHO (1980) definitions presented by others who have investigated aspects of adjustment to hearing impairment (Davis, 1983; Stephens & Hétu, 1991; Swan & Gatehouse, 1990; Thomas, 1984, 1988). In large part, this is because *psychosocial implications* of hearing impairment are integral aspects of the conceptual basis of these classifications, consistent with literature relating to other physical disabilities and rehabilitation counseling. There are also relevant clinical and academic advantages to differentiating between the auditory and nonauditory effects of hearing impairment in this straightforward, logical fashion. Additionally, adhering to this paradigm acknowledges the significant contributions of those who have employed this schema in addressing psychosocial consequences of hearing impairment.

Classifications of auditory dysfunction based on WHO nomenclature have been the basis of numerous proposals for counseling-based aural rehabilitation (Davis, 1983; Hétu et al., 1988; Stephens & Hétu, 1991; Thomas, 1984, 1988). The four-domain schema of auditory dysfunction

Disorder > Impairment
> Disability > Handicap

is a sequential framework that distinguishes between site of lesion, specific auditory symptoms, effects on abilities or performance, and psychosocial consequences. *Disorder* refers to the specific diagnosis in anatomical, physiological, and diagnostic terms, for example, otosclerosis. Appropriate remedial intervention for a disorder is most likely to entail medical or surgical treatment. *Impairment* refers to the resulting abnormal function of the auditory system. This may be manifested as reduced hearing sensitivity or discrimination, localization difficulties, or tinnitus. The extent of auditory impairments can be measured. Medical intervention may be indicated; however, remediation could also be rehabilitative in nature, for example, a hearing aid. The extent to which an impairment affects performance or ability to use hearing in everyday activities, be it in speech perception or environmental awareness, constitutes the *disability*. Disability may vary as a function of communication need, environmental conditions, and other situational variables. Hearing disabilities are the auditory consequences of the individual's hearing impairment. The negative impact on well-being and quality of life, the nonauditory effects of hearing impairment and hearing disability, constitute hearing *handicap*. This may include repercussions on interpersonal relationships, on emotional health, and on educational, social, or occupational interactions and aspirations. In short, handicap amounts to the psychosocial consequences of the dysfunction. This interpretation is consonant with the rehabilitation counseling view of handicap as the cumulative negative fallout of psychological and sociological barriers.

In many ways, disability and handicap are inextricably interwoven. Adjustment is predicated on the person's capacity to cope with a disability. Lazarus and Folkman (1984) define coping as "constantly changing cognitive and behavioral efforts to manage specific external and/or internal demands that are appraised as taxing or exceeding the resources of the person" (p. 141), an appropriate working definition for what is involved in contending with hearing impairment. The ability to cope effectively can be affected by the very psychological and sociological variables one endeavors to control (Lazarus & Folkman, 1984; Menaghan, 1983; Turner, 1983). For example, depression, not an uncommon reaction to long-standing stress, loneliness, or isolation, can result in apathy. Apathy and lethargy inhibit the effort and energy needed to compensate effectively for hearing difficulties and thereby lead to further failure, isolation, and depression. In short, handicap can exacerbate disability, which, in turn, further exacerbates handicap. Rehabilitation counseling attempts to prevent or minimize handicap by focusing on the elimination or alleviation of these psychosocial problems so as to facilitate adjustment (Thomas & Parker, 1984).

Thomas (1988) maintains that involvement or intervention within any one domain of auditory dysfunction can be expected to influence that domain and those to the right of it. One can argue, however, that if intervention in the handicap domain engenders the insight and motivation necessary to develop and adapt effective compensatory behaviors, disability can be ameliorated. Grappling with the interrelatedness of the auditory and nonauditory consequences of hearing impairment exemplifies the inadequacy of equating hearing handicap with a combination or permutation of variables reflective of the impairment alone: Myriad variables are involved in individuals' personal backgrounds and environments that contribute to disability and handicap. The four-domain framework is extremely useful in treatment design. Systematic identification of relevant auditory and nonauditory involvement facilitates selection of appropriate cognitive, affective, and/or behavioral approaches in counseling a particular client.

Identifying Communication and Adjustment Difficulties

The importance of viewing rehabilitative needs as a function of patients' idiosyncratic characteristics and circumstances has been acknowledged more readily in recent years. The philosophical and practical underpinnings of clinical services in audiology, however, have been slow to reflect this. Focus remains primarily on diagnosis of hearing impairment. In light of evidence that patients seek assistance because of the disability and handicap experienced, which may not correspond to their hearing impairment (Swan & Gatehouse, 1990), the clinical focus in audiology must be expanded. Evaluations of the disabling and handicapping effects of hearing impairment, when conducted, are often intended to assess hearing aid candidacy. The scope and nature of hearing problems are relevant inasmuch as they provide a rationale for the clinician to present to the client when recommending amplification. For this purpose, short "screening" tools, which can be administered routinely in an expedient fashion, are employed. Among the instruments that can be used for this purpose are the Hearing Handicap Scale (High, Fairbanks, & Glorig, 1964), the Hearing Measurement Scale (Noble & Atherley, 1970), the Social Hearing Handicap Index (Ewertsen & Birk-Nielsen, 1973), the Hearing Handicap Inventory for the Elderly (HHIE) (Newman & Weinstein, 1989; Ventry & Weinstein, 1982; Weinstein, Spitzer, & Ventry, 1986; Weinstein & Ventry, 1983a, 1983b), the Hearing Handicap Inventory for Adults (HHIA) (Newman et al., 1990), and the Feasibility Scale for Predicting Hearing Aid Use (FSPHAU) (Rupp, Higgins, & Maurer, 1977).

Insofar as it goes, screening for handicap to establish hearing aid candidacy is a reasonable clinical practice. If hearing aids, in fact, resolved the auditory and nonauditory effects of hearing loss, this would also probably be adequate clinical practice. But hearing aids are of limited and varying benefit. There is overwhelming evidence that the majority of those who have worn amplification for a number of years still have "residual" disability and handicap (Alberti et al., 1984; Thomas, 1984; Thomas & Gilhome-Herbst, 1980). Even if perfect hearing aids and perfect fitting protocols were a reality, people would accept and adjust to amplification differently. Additionally, some effects of hearing impairment and disability are not immediately or automatically resolved even with an optimal hearing aid fitting. Learned responses to adverse listening conditions or to repeated communication failure must often be "unlearned" for adjustment to occur. A person with long-standing hearing impairment may have an aversion to social gatherings due to the cumulative effect of frustration experienced in such settings over time. Smiling and nodding, while not understanding the majority of what is being said, ceases to be enjoyable very quickly. Why bother to go if the experience ranges from boredom to torture? Not all individuals with hearing impairment attribute such negative reactions and subsequent avoidance to hearing problems. Some may attribute it to age, others to a preference to staying home. Many do not bother to analyze their feelings at all. Even the most successful hearing aid fittings do not resolve learned stress and avoidance patterns automatically. And, if the person is comfortable at home, so be it. But social isolation has implications over time, if not for the hearing-impaired person then for family members whose social activities and outings have also been curtailed.

In short, hearing aids are not perfect substitutes for normal hearing; people benefit differently from amplification; and many learned responses to communication difficulties, even with an optimal hearing aid fitting, do not resolve automatically. Stated differently, *the auditory and nonauditory effects of hearing impairment warrant rehabilitative intervention beyond the recommended use of amplification.*

If hearing impairment is a handicapping condition and audiologists are the appropriate professionals to manage this condition, how is this responsibility to be shouldered? First and foremost, *audiologists must view each hearing-impaired patient as a unique individual with idiosyncratic needs.* This entails a commitment to ascertain, rather than assume, the extent and nature of the auditory and nonauditory consequences of each individual's hearing impairment. To facilitate adjustment to hearing impairment, the adjustment problems must be identified. As demonstrated by a host of studies conducted to examine the relationship between perceived handicap and audiometric variables, the audiogram does not provide the necessary information. In addition to documenting the degree of hearing impairment, the auditory and nonauditory effects of that impairment must be documented and interpreted in

light of the psychological, interpersonal, environmental, and social variables relevant to each individual. A variety of comprehensive self-assessment tools including the Communication Profile for the Hearing Impaired (CPHI) (Demorest & Erdman, 1986, 1987, 1988, 1989a, 1989b), the Denver Scale of Communication Function (Alpiner, 1982; Alpiner et al., 1974), and the Hearing Performance Inventory (Giolas et al., 1979; Lamb, Owens, & Schubert, 1983) are available to aid in the identification of auditory and nonauditory consequences of hearing impairment. Skinner (1988) and Schow and Gatehouse (1990) outline many of the wide-ranging self-assessment tools that have been developed for use with varied populations and in varied settings. Clinicians should select standardized instruments appropriate for their clinical population's characteristics and needs. Self-assessment inventories constitute "psychological tests" (Demorest & Erdman, 1984b). Hence, there are ethical considerations relative to the administration and interpretation of these instruments. Inherent in the clinical use of psychometric instruments are certain responsibilities. Among these are a thorough knowledge of the instrument's content, scope, applications, psychometric properties, and administration and scoring procedures to ensure valid measurement and interpretation (Demorest & Walden, 1984).

Routine use of a specific assessment tool with a particular clinical population benefits the clinician in a variety of ways. In addition to quantifying and documenting the pertinent adjustment difficulties of each client, the cumulative results yield normative data that describe the characteristic needs and problems of one's clientele. In addition to providing a basis for determining appropriate goals and procedures, this information serves as a reference for interpreting individuals' scores, and a baseline for monitoring program effectiveness (Erdman & Demorest, 1990). An awareness of the type and extent of problems characteristically experienced also has value when focusing on prevention of handicap, a continuing aspect of rehabilitation counseling (Gellman, 1977).

One concern relative to using specific criteria to designate disability or handicap is the subsequent use of these criteria to determine who is eligible for rehabilitative services. This is a legitimate concern. Even those with minimal hearing impairment should be viewed as having a *potentially handicapping condition* that could manifest itself insidiously, gradually, or suddenly as personal circumstances or environmental conditions change. Patients often report a sudden marked decrease in hearing ability that is not evident in an audiological reassessment. A multitude of factors may precipitate sudden difficulties. Something as innocuous as installing an air conditioner can lead to sudden, significant hearing difficulties with a rash of new frustrations and emotional strain for the entire family. Prevention of handicap involves familiarizing clients with the typical auditory and nonauditory effects of hearing impairment, the variables that facilitate or exacerbate adjustment to hearing impairment, and the skills necessary to minimize the difficulties that may develop as communication needs or personal circumstances change.

Case history and anecdotal information obtained during interviews should also be included in assessment of rehabilitative needs. Automated (computerized) data repositories for personal information, audiometric results, and self-assessment inventories provide a viable mechanism for immediate feedback relative to each patient and to one's clientele in general (Demorest & Erdman, 1984a; Demorest et al., 1988). Clinical databases can be customized to include relevant information needed to establish counseling goals and monitor progress. The very technology that many fear distances audiologists from patients can be used to gain insight into hearing handicap. Over time, the database becomes a valuable source of information about trends in the clinical population and can be explored to answer a multitude of questions. The scope of questions is limited only by the nature and number of variables in the database and the extent of one's clinical and investigative curiosity. As databases increase in size, patients return for follow-up visits, and one learns to query data, a wealth of information with implications for managing hearing-impaired patients becomes available. The vast potential of such databases has yet to be exploited for purposes of rehabilitative audiological care. But, assorted means to create and explore them exist. Consequently, so does the opportunity to address many unanswered questions about the need for—and benefits of—counseling hearing-impaired clients.

Whether records are maintained in traditional "hard-copy" folders or in computer-age, automated databases, the information to be included in clients' records must be determined a priori. Uniformity and consistency in record keeping facilitates documentation and record reviews. There are clinical, administrative, and research implications in ensuring that records contain the information that has been deemed relevant and essential. Inconsistency precludes meaningful quality assurance reviews, program evaluations, or accurate descriptions of the characteristics, needs, or progress of one's clientele. The scope of clinical services is dictated by the characteristics and needs of the populations served. To identify and document patients' counseling needs, it is of paramount importance that accurate and complete records be maintained.

Hearing Impairment, Disability, and Handicap: Counseling Implications

Thomas's (1984) investigation of National Health Service hearing aid owners constitutes a major contribution to the understanding of psychological and psychosocial implications of acquired hearing loss. On the basis of his results and a thorough review of the literature, Thomas concludes that basic personality structure is *not* affected by hearing loss. He refutes the notion that suspiciousness and paranoid psychoses are more prevalent in the hearing-impaired population. Meadow-Orlans (1985) also concludes that the alleged higher incidence of paranoia among hearing-impaired individuals is a "persistent myth." Thomas's and Meadow-Orlans's conclusions are consistent with observations that type and degree of disabilities in general are not associated with type or degree of personality traits or with adjustment (Cook, 1987; Shontz, 1977; Wright, 1983). These findings, however, also unequivocally reveal that many people are profoundly affected by their disabilities. Thomas's (1984) results indicate that a significant number of hearing-impaired people—*irrespective of the type or degree of loss*—experience a high level of psychological disturbance. Hence, rehabilitative audiologists must be prepared to address hearing impairment as an experience that is likely to be very stressful and psychologically disturbing. The audiologist who is fully prepared to address these consequences recognizes the central and indispensable role counseling will play in doing so.

Counseling, the facilitative process employed to resolve problems experienced secondary to hearing impairment, is the cornerstone of rehabilitative audiology. The effectiveness of counseling determines the extent to which *all* other rehabilitative measures—from hearing aid use to speechreading—succeed or fail. Counseling enables individuals to cope effectively with the communicative difficulties (disability) they have experienced and the extent to which they can resolve subsequent adjustment problems (handicap). In short, counseling effectiveness determines the outcome of one's clinical services.

The full implications of counseling's essential role in the rehabilitative process have not yet been assimilated into training and practice in audiology. There is, however, greater awareness among rehabilitative audiologists of the need for counseling. As in rehabilitation counseling, counseling in rehabilitative audiology can effectively be conducted using an eclectic, problem-solving approach. Intervention is designed to resolve or minimize communication and adjustment problems experienced secondary to hearing loss. Counselors proceed on the assumption that patients' problems, behavior, and adjustment are products of their idiosyncratic psychological makeup, life histories, and environments. This "somatopsychological" perspective, which employs a *person by situation* paradigm to analyze adjustment to disability, stresses the personal meaning of the disability (Cook, 1987). The empathic counselor must deter-

mine the personal meaning of disability to facilitate adjustment.

THE EMPATHIC CLINICIAN-CLIENT RELATIONSHIP

The role of the counseling audiologist should be facilitative, directive, and supportive. Counselor variables including warmth, empathy, genuineness, and unconditional positive regard are critical factors in treatment. These requisite elements and the implications for audiologist-patient relationships have been stressed (Caccavo & Geist, 1986; Erdman, Crowley, & Gillespie, 1984; Roberts & Bouchard, 1989; Skinner, 1988; Wylde, 1987); however, the effects of relational variables have not been explored in audiology. Moreover, development of effective interpersonal skills in clinician-client relationships typically receives little systematic attention in audiologists' clinical training. Without such training, health care professionals may not recognize which aspects of their relationships with patients are therapeutically beneficial or may simply lack confidence in how to foster such relationships (Squier, 1990). Consequently, patients may receive appropriate technical care physically but inadequate psychological care on a personal level. This results in overall dissatisfaction with treatment. Swan and Gatehouse (1990) conclude that hearing-impaired patients seek audiological assistance because of disability and handicap but are managed on the basis of puretone thresholds. The appropriateness of "treating the audiogram" is severely compromised by its inadequacy. Inasmuch as this is analogous to providing technical care for a physical problem while ignoring the psychosocial factors that prompted the individual to seek assistance, the probability that individuals will not be satisfied with overall treatment warrants consideration.

Interestingly, younger, less experienced practitioners tend to exhibit more empathy than do those who are older and more experienced (Hall & Dornan, 1988). Novice and experienced counselors alike can assess their counseling style by monitoring their interactions with clients. Listening attentively, a prerequisite to determining the scope of adjustment difficulties, communicates care and concern, critical elements of empathic rapport. Time constraints are often cited as an excuse for not listening to a patient's "litany of complaints" and may account for a clinician's harried, distracted affect, which the patient interprets as a lack of interest, concern, or understanding. In short, the clinician is perceived as lacking empathy.

Squier (1990) describes two facets of empathy that have implications for the counseling relationship. *Perspective taking,* a cognitive skill, is the ability to take another's point of view. *Emotional reactivity* is the capacity to respond affectively to another's emotional state. Squier's (1990) model of empathic understanding and adherence to treatment regimens in practitioner-patient relationships is based on well-documented findings concerning relational variables and treatment outcome. This model has been adapted to illustrate the treatment process in rehabilitative audiology as shown in Figure 14.1. Cognitive and affective aspects of empathy, as presented by the clinician, facilitate patients' awareness and understanding of the consequences of hearing impairment while facilitating motivation to resolve them as well. This enhances patients' comprehension of problems and their confidence that they will be able to cope. Greater understanding of problems, on the part of both clinician and client, serves to clarify problems further and facilitates discussions relative to how they can be managed. By virtue of feeling that clinicians care and understand, patients are more relaxed and optimistic about treatment outcome. The interaction between increased knowledge and motivation can be expected to result in increased adherence to treatment programs. Empathic understanding is particularly critical in cases of chronic, long-term illness and handicapping conditions (Falvo, 1985; Squier, 1990; Thomas et al., 1987). The empathic understanding model lends itself to monitoring the effects of cognitive problem solving and changes in patients' affective states as intervention continues. This, in addition to the importance of empathic understanding in treating those with handicapping conditions, underscores the potential clinical, research, and training applications of an empathic understanding model in rehabilitative audiology. Evalua-

tions of clinician empathy have been conducted using the Empathy Scale (Hogan, 1969) and the Questionnaire Measure of Emotional Empathy (Mehrabian & Epstein, 1972), which related empathy to other personality characteristics. The Accurate Empathy Scale (Truax, 1967) and the Relationship Questionnaire (Truax and Carkhuff, 1967) have been employed to study empathy specifically within the context of the counselor-client relationship as espoused by Rogers (1957, 1975). Hence, they have potential in audiology training programs and in clinical investigations of treatment effectiveness.

Some patients elicit more empathy from clinicians than others. Little research has been conducted, however, to examine patient communication style. The results of one study (Pettegrew & Turkat, 1986) suggest three patient typologies: assertive, ideal, and stoic. Assertive patients see health care providers more frequently, receive more medication, apply for more disability payments, and are perceived by raters to be contentious, if not manipulative. Ideal patients are described as such because they are attentive, are precise in delivering and requesting information, and do not exaggerate their health problems. (If actual assertion training terminology were being applied here, the assertive patients would be labeled aggressive and the ideal patients assertive.) The stoic typology is characteristically relaxed, exhibits passive communication in the health care relationship, and is viewed as easily controlled. These preliminary findings support the notion that although therapeutic empathy is generated primarily by the clinician, patients' communication style may have a mitigating effect on this critical variable.

Managing patients who are seemingly uncooperative or otherwise difficult is a challenge best met by striving even more to see things from their perspective. Barriers erected by patients, more often than not, are indicative of efforts to cope with a situation that they perceive (on some level) to be unmanageable or overwhelmingly stressful. Falvo (1985) discusses a multitude of patient reactions to infirmity with which practitioners must deal to ensure adherence to treatment regimens. Among these are denial, forgetting, detrimental or overcom-

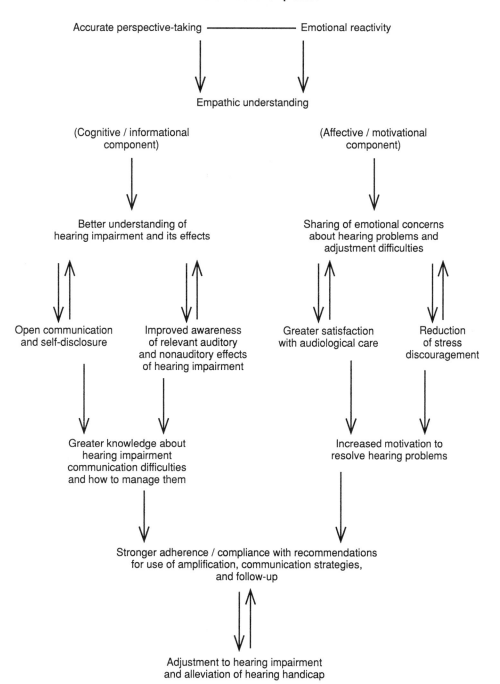

Counselor Relationship Skills

Accurate perspective-taking —————————— Emotional reactivity

Empathic understanding

(Cognitive / informational component)   (Affective / motivational component)

Better understanding of hearing impairment and its effects

Sharing of emotional concerns about hearing problems and adjustment difficulties

Open communication and self-disclosure

Improved awareness of relevant auditory and nonauditory effects of hearing impairment

Greater satisfaction with audiological care

Reduction of stress discouragement

Greater knowledge about hearing impairment communication difficulties and how to manage them

Increased motivation to resolve hearing problems

Stronger adherence / compliance with recommendations for use of amplification, communication strategies, and follow-up

Adjustment to hearing impairment and alleviation of hearing handicap

Figure 14.1   Squier's (1990) model of empathic understanding and adherence to treatment regimens in practitioner-patient relationships adapted for use in rehabilitative audiology.

pensation, retreating or withdrawing, regression, ascribing blame, self-blame, rationalization, hiding feelings, projection, and hyperactivity. Counselors must be alert to the implications of these behaviors. Denial of significant communication difficulties and/or related adjustment problems, for instance, should not be taken at face value. There may be manifold difficulties the individual is reluctant to reveal. The disinclination to discuss them may reflect concerns relative to the implications of the diagnosis or may be an attempt to downplay the significance of the problem by refusing to focus on the negative. Even when faced with incontrovertible evidence (e.g., frequent misunderstandings or requests for repetition), rather than refute a patient's stance, efforts should be made to focus on issues he or she is willing to discuss. This facilitates an understanding that is anchored in a realistic assessment of the problem. Missed appointments are a frequent problem in clinical settings. Patients attribute this to their forgetfulness. Given that people tend to forget what they do not want to remember, chronic missed appointments should alert clinicians to probable difficulties in accepting a diagnosis or a lack of motivation relative to the specific treatment regimen.

Although often viewed as innate characteristics or abilities, in fact, many skills exemplified by those who are rated highly empathic are learned. Reflection of feeling and restatement of content, two methods of pacing (i.e., following the client's expressed thoughts and feelings) that promote empathic understanding, are skills in which counselors receive training. Reflection of feeling and restatement of content exemplify the emotional reactivity and accurate perspective-taking facets of empathy essential to the counselor-client relationship portrayed in the empathic understanding model in Figure 14.1. Also, termed active or reflective listening, these counseling skills can be modeled, practiced through role playing, and evaluated by peers or supervisors.

Many variables that affect communication between clinician and patient are environmental variables that can be controlled. Messages communicated in a quiet, private area such as an office or test suite will be heard more easily and will be taken more seriously than messages delivered in noisy, public areas such as lobbies or waiting areas. Above and beyond the fact that effectiveness is precluded, *in view of patients' absolute right to privacy and confidentiality, counseling—regardless of its purpose or nature—should not be conducted in a public area.*

Clinicians must also be aware of nonverbal cues that influence counseling/communication effectiveness. Facial expression, eye contact, gestures, body posture, proximity, speaking rate, and tone of voice influence perceptions of clinician empathy, genuineness, and unconditional positive regard. To provide optimal care, counselors' interpersonal skills must be inextricably interwoven with technical skills. The quality of audiologists' relationships with patients tempers the impersonal isolation of the audiometric test suite, the intimidating effects of electronic and computerized technology, and the apprehension patients experience when faced with the diagnosis of hearing impairment and the prospect of hearing aid use.

Limitations of Traditional Hearing Aid Orientation

Audiologists' counseling skills are critical in facilitating acceptance of and adjustment to hearing impairment and hearing aid use. Allaying patients' concerns relative to diagnosis and instilling an optimistic yet realistic awareness that the personal experience of hearing disability and handicap can be managed effectively requires empathic understanding. Unfortunately, the vehicle for this essential counseling all too often consists of a brief, didactic hearing aid orientation that minimizes interactive exchanges fundamental to empathic counselor-client relationships and effective counseling.

The traditional hearing aid orientation class focuses primarily on technical aspects of hearing aid use. The new hearing aid user has a multitude of questions about the instrument when first becoming familiar with it. The initial preoccupation with technical matters precludes focusing on identification or remediation of communication difficulties and adjustment problems within the confines of the hearing aid orientation. Albeit inadequate from a truly rehabilitative perspective, the traditional hearing aid orientation is far more appropriate than the mere dissemination of information via pamphlets, brochures, or video recordings to familiarize patients with their new hearing aids.

The *assumption* underlying the continued perception of hearing aid orientations as adequate rehabilitative intervention is that hearing aids resolve the disabling, handicapping consequences of hearing impairment for the majority of hearing-impaired clients. This assumption is false. First, hearing aids may alleviate the communicative disabilities experienced secondary to hearing impairment, but they do not eliminate them. Second, hearing aid use cannot, in and of itself, resolve the psychosocial handicap experienced secondary to hearing impairment and hearing disability. Hence, at best, some hearing-impaired clients benefit from a reduction of some hearing disabilities and subsequent handicapping experiences. If hearing aid use *did* adequately resolve the disabling and handicapping consequences of hearing impairment, hearing aids would not end up in dresser drawers, fewer hearing aids would be returned to manufacturers, more than only 15 to 20% of hearing-impaired people would want hearing aids, and hearing aid orientations might be adequate intervention for the majority of hearing-impaired people.

The major problem in addressing the rehabilitative needs of hearing-impaired patients is that current service delivery models do not provide for doing so; audiology is practiced from the perspective of a medical model rather than a rehabilitative model. By adhering to a medical model, genuine rehabilitative counseling in audiology practice is tacitly and systematically precluded. Some claim that a need for rehabilitation is an exception to the rule. Data do not support this. Thomas (1984) found that the vast majority of those who have worn amplification for a number of years manifest residual disability and handicap. Alberti et al. (1984), in a follow-up survey of 1000 hearing aid users, found that

continued hearing aid use was not a reliable indicator of treatment success. In recent surveys of hearing aid consumers, approximately two-thirds of those fitted by dispensers (66%) and by dispensing audiologists (63%) volunteered negative comments about their benefit from and adjustment to amplification (Smedley & Schow, 1990). The rate of hearing aids returned to manufacturers (although influenced by a multitude of factors) is so high many manufacturers would like to see the traditional 30-day trial period abolished (Gallagher, 1990). Conversely, those who receive thorough counseling report greater short-term and long-term satisfaction with hearing aid use (Brooks, 1989). Despite improved technology and fitting procedures, most hearing aid users cite continuing problems in background noise or other difficult listening conditions that detract from their overall satisfaction with hearing aid use and from their satisfaction with overall audiological care. Patients naively expect the disabling and handicapping effects of hearing impairment to be resolved by a hearing aid fitting. Indeed, the provision of new hearing aids with a brief instructional period minus a meaningful discussion of relevant communication and adjustment difficulties perpetuates the myth that simply wearing the hearing aid will resolve whatever problems have been experienced. When this does not occur, the patient's trust in the process, the clinician, and the hearing aid is severely compromised. Moreover, these patients are not satisfied consumers who purchase future hearing aids, and they do not refer other hearing-impaired individuals for services. In other words, the myth that hearing aids are not beneficial is also perpetuated.

Audiologists' direct involvement in the dispensing of hearing aids has enormous potential for enhancing rehabilitation of hearing-impaired clients inasmuch as it streamlines the hearing health care process. Dispensing audiologists who are committed to resolving the disability and handicap experienced secondary to hearing impairment are in an ideal position to evaluate the appropriateness of hearing aid fittings and monitor clients' progress and problems. By assuming responsibility for comprehensive audiological management of hearing-impaired patients, audiologists can assert their role—not just as hearing aid dispensers but as experts in what Jerger (1991) describes as audiology's mission—the evaluation and treatment of auditory communication disorders. There are, nevertheless, inherent disadvantages to audiologists' direct involvement in the sale of hearing aids. Hearing-impaired consumers reportedly have more confidence in recommendations for hearing aid use that come from those not directly involved in selling the instruments (Libby, 1990). This stems from a concern that those who dispense do not act in the client's best interest. Consumer confidence in audiologists' recommendations was found to be related to whether the audiologist did or did not dispense hearing aids. Clinicians who establish empathic understanding with clients and base recommendations for hearing aid use on patients' admitted difficulties can dispel concerns that recommendations are not based on patients' best interests.

The hearing aid fitting plus hearing aid orientation model of service provision constitutes, as Swan and Gatehouse (1990) contend, management of patients on the basis of pure-tone thresholds. Elevated pure-tone thresholds are not why patients seek audiological assistance; hearing disability and hearing handicap prompt them to do so. The rationale for recommended hearing aid use must be based on the clinician's and client's assessment of the specific communication and adjustment difficulties experienced. The resolution of these problems must be directly and adequately addressed throughout the hearing aid fitting process. Investigations have consistently demonstrated that continued hearing aid use and satisfaction with amplification are related to the pre- and postfitting counseling patients receive (Alberti et al., 1984; Brooks, 1979, 1985; Brooks & Johnson, 1981; Surr, Schuchman, & Montgomery, 1978). The audiologist's counseling must facilitate a realistic understanding of the scope and nature of the hearing impairment, its auditory and nonauditory consequences, and the benefits and limitations of hearing aid use. Moreover, to facilitate adjustment to hearing impairment, the adequacy and appropriateness of specific compensatory skills and coping behavior must be determined.

Interviews, clinical observations, and formal and informal assessment procedures are indispensable when formulating an initial impression of a client's perception of his or her hearing difficulties. The high incidence of hearing impairment in the general population coupled with clinicians' daily exposure to those with hearing impairment must not result in a nonchalant or complacent attitude regarding the implications of the diagnosis for the client. Discounting patients' personal reactions to the diagnosis of hearing impairment by inadvertently implying that hearing loss is just an ordinary, everyday problem is the antithesis of empathic understanding. For the hearing-impaired individual, the diagnosis and its implications are intensely personal. Although the person may have been aware of hearing-related difficulties for some time, the formal diagnosis of a clinically significant hearing loss may cause distress. In all probability, the individual would much rather learn there is no problem or that it is an insignificant one. The manner in which the clinician deals with a patient's overt and covert concerns is vitally important in enhancing the likelihood that hearing aid use will be viewed as a positive and plausible option. Timing is an extremely critical variable at this juncture. All too often clinicians forge ahead and schedule another appointment for a hearing aid evaluation or proceed to make an ear impression without establishing patients' readiness to accept the diagnosis and the responsibility for doing something about it. Readiness is a prerequisite to accepting the option of amplification with enthusiasm, optimism, and motivation. The clinician can alleviate patients' concerns by suggesting that the actual significance of hearing impairment be viewed in terms of the specific communication problems that have arisen and the implications of those problems for patients and their families, coworkers, and friends. This encourages patients to assume an active role in decision making and problem solving and dispels any sense of their not having a choice relative to the treatment options. By actively engaging patients in this process, it is more likely that the decisions made will be acceptable to them.

Self-assessment inventories are invaluable in facilitating the identification of pertinent communication difficulties and the variables that contribute to those problems. The audiogram, as an explanation of hearing impairment, is not particularly meaningful to most clients. Descriptions of the types of communication difficulties and frustrations they have experienced, as found in various self-assessment inventories, provide meaning and relevance to the diagnosis. Indeed, completion of a self-assessment questionnaire can be of benefit in focusing patients on the extent to which hearing difficulties have actually progressed. It also assists them in verbalizing vague complaints that they have downplayed and tried to ignore in order to cope with their hearing difficulties. Scores from instruments such as the Hearing Performance Inventory (HPI) (Giolas et al., 1979; Lamb et al., 1983) and the Communication Profile for the Hearing Impaired (CPHI) (Demorest & Erdman, 1986, 1987) can be used as a baseline to assess the extent and nature of hearing disability and handicap, to outline counseling goals, and to monitor progress. In most instances, patients can complete these questionnaires in approximately 20 minutes with little or no supervision. They may do so in the clinic or, alternatively, at home. Automated scoring procedures typically take less than 2 minutes per patient. Hence, with a minimal amount of time and effort, clinicians can obtain a wealth of information relative to an individual's specific communication difficulties, coping behaviors, and adjustment problems. This information is of fundamental importance in facilitating emotional reactivity and perspective taking, the key ingredients of empathic understanding. A comprehensive assessment of hearing disability and handicap is a prerequisite to treatment of the communicative consequences of hearing impairment and resultant adjustment problems.

Problem-solving exercises are another method of enabling patients to address their hearing difficulties and resultant adjustment problems in a cognitive manner. The exercises shown in Table 14.3 have been used with hearing-impaired clients in a variety of clinical settings. Reviewing assignments with clients engages them in the problem-solving process while enhancing clinicians' awareness of maladaptive coping strategies and adjustment problems (Erdman et al., 1984).

Identifying and analyzing difficulties experienced secondary to hearing impairment can be therapeutic in and of itself. Rehabilitative counseling, however, must also include mechanisms to ensure resolution of the problems that have been identified. A variety of techniques that can be used in individual, group, or family counseling have been successfully applied by rehabilitative audiologists to address hearing disability and handicap.

Specific Counseling Applications: Assertiveness Training, Stress Management, and Problem Solving

Assertiveness training (AT) is well-suited to addressing communication difficulties related to hearing impairment (DiMichael, 1985; Erdman 1980) because it focuses on communication effectiveness; moreover, it emphasizes situational behavior. In AT, clients learn to distinguish aggressive, passive, and assertive behavior in terms of verbal and nonverbal communication variables, reactions of others, and the consequences of communication interactions. Aggressive, passive, and assertive behavior patterns are described in Table 14.4. Passive communication is often ineffective because the individual fails to convey needs or feelings adequately or directly. Although passive behavior may initially elicit sympathy from others, over time they may become exasperated and angry if the individuals they care about fail to stand up for themselves. Aggressive communication often alienates others. Aggression may elicit a passive response from others; conversely it may trigger a hostile reaction. In either case, effective communication is precluded. By communicating assertively individuals are able to start, maintain, and terminate conversations; to stand up for themselves; to express disagreement or annoyance; to give and re-

Table 14.3
Sample Problem-Solving Exercises

Exercise 1—Problem Identification

Describe a situation in which your hearing loss has affected your ability to communicate.

1. Describe as completely as you can the environment in which this problem typically occurs including your immediate surroundings, the adjacent areas, and the ambient noise.
2. What is the nature or purpose of your communication in this situation (e.g., negotiations, learning, social conversation)?
3. Describe your typical reaction to the communication difficulty.
   a. What do you usually do and say when this occurs?
   b. What are your thoughts when this occurs?
   c. How do you feel when this happens?
4. Given that communication is a two-way process, it is likely that someone else is involved. As best you can, describe the other person's reaction to the communication problem.
   a. What does the other person do or say when this happens?
   b. What does it seem like they are thinking?
   c. How do you think they feel?

Exercise 2—Exploring Potential Solutions

1. Many of the situations that have been problems in the past may continue to be somewhat difficult because hearing aids are not substitutes for normal hearing. It is hoped that these situations will be less difficult and will not occur as frequently. But, when they do occur there are other things you and others can do to lessen the communication difficulty and frustration. Examine each aspect of the communication difficulties you have already described. What possibilities exist for resolving these problems?
   a. What aspects of the environment can be modified?
   b. What alternatives exist for making such modifications?
   c. How might these changes minimize your hearing problems?
2. In view of the nature of the communication, what alternatives exist for conducting this exchange in some other way (e.g., in person, in writing, in private, via recording)?
3. There are effective and ineffective ways to cope with hearing problems. If how you reacted in the past contributed to the problem:
   a. What might you do or say differently?
   b. How might this change things for you?
   c. What do you think and feel about these alternative ways of handling your hearing problems?
4. The only thing more difficult than changing your own behavior is trying to change someone else's. If you are now beginning to understand your hearing loss better, imagine what it is like for someone who has never experienced it before. Even though others may know you have a hearing problem, they probably don't know what they should do to help you hear better. They are confused by the fact that often you seem to hear just fine. They don't understand the effects background noise, fatigue, or listening to something else can have on your ability to hear them. How can you help them understand so that they can help you minimize the effects of your hearing loss?

ceive compliments and criticism; and to make requests in an effective manner. In situations that are demanding or stressful, being assertive is most difficult and most necessary. Inasmuch as hearing problems are demanding, stressful experiences, AT concepts are applicable in facilitating communication effectiveness and adjustment. Assertive communication skills are essential when asking others to speak up or repeat, when requesting clarification or verification, and when soliciting help in modifying the listening environment. Common examples of passive, aggressive, and assertive reactions to hearing difficulties are shown in Table 14.5. AT's emphasis on the reactions one's behavior elicits from others enhances hearing-impaired patients' aware-

Table 14.4
Definitions and Characteristics of Aggressive, Passive, and Assertive Behavior

Aggressive behavior is that type of behavior in which a person stands up for his or her rights in such a way that the rights of others are violated. The goal of aggressive behavior is to get one's way without regard for the other person. When communicating in an aggressive manner individuals may be perceived as:

Condescending	Manipulative	Domineering
Boisterous	Obnoxious	Insincere
Intimidating	Rude	Pompous
Inconsiderate	Threatening	Explosive

Passive behavior is that type of behavior exhibited when anxiety prevents an individual from standing up for his or her own rights and expressing honest emotions in an effective way. When behavior is passive one may be perceived as:

Shy	Inhibited	Afraid
Powerless	Submissive	Pathetic
Helpless	Nervous	Indecisive
Defensive	Apologetic	Guilty

Assertive behavior is reflected in the spontaneous, honest, and direct expression of one's feelings, beliefs, opinions, and needs stated in an appropriate manner. Within such behavior there is a high regard for one's personal rights and the rights of others. When behavior is assertive in nature one may be perceived as:

Confident	Honest	Calm
Affectionate/caring	Friendly	Optimistic
Respectful	Good-natured	Considerate
Open	Understanding	Sincere

Table 14.5
Assertive, Passive, and Aggressive Reactions to Communication Difficulties Experienced by Those with Hearing Impairment

Assertive Reactions

Request repetition or clarification appropriately
Admit hearing problem to others
Explain difficulty and suggest solution
Modify listening conditions
Use amplification devices as needed

Passive Reactions

Withdraw from family and friends
Pretend to understand
Pretend not to hear
Avoid social situations
Fail to seek assistance
Fail to ask for repetitions or clarification as needed

Aggressive Reactions

Accuse others of mumbling or not speaking up
Deny hearing problem when others suggest it
Dominate conversation to avoid listening
Interrupt conversation to avoid listening
Blame others when unable to hear

ness of the effects their hearing difficulties have on those with whom they communicate. Role playing and script writing are effective rehearsal strategies in assertiveness training. Rehearsing is of benefit in reducing anxiety related to specific problems (Wolpe, 1958) and in formulating alternative ways of managing the problems.

Assertiveness is characteristically viewed as an effective way to cope with stressful situations. Hallberg and Carlsson (1991a, 1991b) describe two coping styles exhibited by hearing-impaired persons: controlling the social scene and avoiding the social scene. The former is characterized by actively managing situations, planning one's activities, and preventing difficulties within the environment. Hallberg and Carlsson's data suggest that individuals coping in this manner assume responsibility for outcome, assign responsibility appropriately to environmental factors, inform others as needed, and ask for repetition or clarification. This controlling pattern is similar to the "reaction" pattern revealed in factor analysis of the CPHI (Demorest & Erdman, 1989b), which is characterized by a frequent need to communicate, a poor communication environment, strong problem awareness, and frequent use of verbal and nonverbal communication strategies. The CPHI "reaction" factor and the "controlling of the social scene" pattern illustrate assertive management of hearing difficulties.

Hallberg and Carlsson (1991a) characterize avoidance of the social scene as attempting to avoid situations that are demanding or threatening, thereby controlling which situations one is willing to face. There is also evidence of minimizing the disability and using nonverbal strategies to avoid attracting attention to one's disability. The combination of withdrawal and avoidance behaviors is similar to patterns exhibited by those with low scale scores for "Withdrawal and Maladaptive Behavior" and a low factor score for "Interaction" on the CPHI. Such manifestations are characteristic of passive behavior patterns. Although Hallberg and Carlsson have not defined an aggressive pattern of coping, they report incidents of irritation and aggressive behavior in the home environment. This is consistent with findings (Erdman et al., 1984) that reveal anger and irritation as the most frequently reported reactions to hearing problems at home. Aggressive behavior is often manifested by angry outbursts.

Stress management techniques are closely related to AT; Wolpe's (1958) desensitization concepts are fundamental to both. Successful stress management entails giving individuals a sense of control over variables that contribute to their stressful condition. Actually exerting control in a situation is not as important as the perception of being able to do so if one wishes (Blechman & Dannemiller, 1976; Glass & Singer, 1972). Stress is perhaps the most universal reaction to hearing loss, a problem over which patients often feel they have no control. Indeed, beyond gains achieved with amplification, one's hearing levels are essentially fixed. Even individuals with severe hearing impairments, however, can describe ideal situations in which they hear well (e.g., a quiet listening environment, one-to-one conversation, ability to see the speaker's face) and can understand what is being said. While these situations are not stressful, others are. But, when difficulties

are experienced, individuals attribute the subsequent stress to their hearing impairment. Identifying variables in stressful situations that are different from ideal situations enables clients to recognize that variables other than hearing loss preclude hearing in these situations and that those variables are responsible for the stress. Moreover, these variables, in all probability, can be controlled. Cognitive awareness of one's ideal listening environment is often, in and of itself, stress reducing because it demonstrates that hearing loss isn't always impossible to manage. Additionally, however, it introduces the notion that control is possible because, if and when it's important enough, ideal listening conditions can be re-created. When deemed necessary or worthwhile, options exist to move to another room, to eliminate background noise, or to meet later face to face. The essential element for stress management is not controlling stress-related variables as much as it is recognizing that one can do so. The combined effect of reducing stress by exerting that control from time to time and recognizing that one has that option mitigates the residual stress that occurs when options for control truly do not exist.

Heppner (1978), employing D'Zurilla and Goldfried's (1971) five-stage model for facilitating behavior modification training, describes counseling as a problem-solving process. The process consists of five definable stages: general orientation or mind set, problem definition and formulation, generating alternatives, decision making, and verification. Orientation refers to an inferred predisposition to behave in a certain way. The optimal orientation for problem solving includes (1) the awareness that problems are normal and are something with which it is possible to cope, (2) an ability to identify and label problematic situations, and (3) behavior that is not impulsive or avoiding. Counselors help clients define problems by increasing their awareness of information and by specifically delineating variables, events, and relationships among events or variables that are associated with the problem. Homework assignments are recommended to monitor behaviors, feelings, and consequences. Generating alternatives can be complicated by past failures or emotional reactions that inhibit the formulation of alternative solutions. Perceptual restructuring and brainstorming are techniques employed to help clients generate alternative solutions. The decision-making stage involves selecting appropriate alternatives in such a way that clients will be comfortable and satisfied with their decisions. Clients' ability to assess probabilities, preferences, and consequences of the various alternatives are relevant issues at this stage. The final stage, evaluating the selected alternative and verifying its appropriateness, entails determining whether the outcome and consequences are satisfactory or not. This behavioral execution of the selected solution is analogous to reality testing. Success is reinforcing; dissatisfaction or failure necessitates continued problem solving. Heppner and Petersen (1982) identify dimensions of real-life problem solving that apply to all phases of the problem-solving process. These include confidence in one's problem-solving ability, an approach-avoidance style (consistent with generating alternatives as needed), and personal control.

The problem-solving approach to counseling, as mentioned earlier in this chapter, is well-suited to rehabilitation counseling because the emphasis is on systematic resolution of the specific problems with which clients present. Problem-solving approaches have been used in counseling hearing-impaired patients in a variety of settings including teaching hospitals (Alberti et al., 1984), military hospitals (Erdman et al., 1984), programs for those with occupational hearing loss (Lalande, Riverin, & Lambert, 1988), elderhostel programs (Bally & Kaplan, 1988; Kaplan, 1983), hospital hearing clinics in Sweden (Eriksson-Mangold et al., 1990), and private practices (Caccavo & Geist, 1986).

Although the specific problems experienced by hearing-impaired clients vary, the ultimate goals in counseling hearing-impaired patients are similar:

1. Acceptance of and adjustment to hearing impairment
2. Acceptance of and adjustment to amplification
3. Effective communication ability

Audiologists are responsible for ensuring that hearing-impaired clients attain these goals. Empathic understanding in clinician-client relations and a problem-solving approach to facilitating adjustment to hearing impairment constitute an appropriate framework for intervention designed to achieve goals.

To achieve the ultimate or long-term goals that define successful rehabilitative intervention in audiology, it is necessary to establish concrete short-term goals. For example, the following goals and strategies might be set:

1. An understanding of hearing impairment (explain auditory system and audiogram)
2. Awareness of effects of hearing impairment (explain audibility and clarity of speech in terms of vowel and consonant energy, effects of background noise)
3. An understanding of communication variables (explain importance of visual input, audiovisual integration, environmental conditions, listening behavior)
4. Identification of pertinent difficulties (problem-solving exercises and self-assessment inventories completed and discussed)
5. Awareness of adaptive/maladaptive compensatory behaviors and consequences (explore present strategies and alternatives)

The specific techniques employed in counseling will necessarily vary by virtue of patients' orientation, audiologists' expertise and comfort level with various concepts and methods, the nature of the difficulties identified, the structure of the counseling sessions, and what does or does not seem to be working. A problem-solving framework is flexible and compatible with an assortment of methods including assertiveness training, stress management, traditional "aural rehabilitation" techniques including speechreading and auditory training, and behavioral training as in communication repair strategies (Tye-Murray, 1991). Traynor (1987) suggests that many traditional aural rehabilitation procedures are not necessary for all hearing-impaired persons who acquire hearing aids but stresses the importance of pre- and postfitting counseling to ensure adjustment to hearing aid use.

The precise course counseling takes is determined by patient needs and by constraints posed by available resources. The latter, however, does not negate the necessity for effective counseling nor should it preclude routine provision of adequate, appropriate counseling for each patient. Successful outcome results in satisfied clients who return and who refer others. Dispensing hearing aids in a cursory fashion to clients arbitrarily designated as "routine" is incompatible with a rehabilitative model of health care. Dissatisfied clients do not refer; they may also influence potential new clients to go elsewhere. Hence, even viewed from a shrewd business perspective, hearing aid dispensing devoid of appropriate rehabilitative intervention is imprudent. Counseling is a necessary and integral aspect of rehabilitation; how (not if) it is provided is dictated by the needs of the patient and the constraints of the delivery system.

Communication Needs of Hearing-Impaired Adults

Emphasis on pediatric and geriatric populations sometimes undermines the significance of hearing impairment among young and middle-aged adults. The fact that hearing impairment may not be as prevalent or as severe among younger adults belies the significance of the disability and handicap posed by hearing impairment of individuals in their 20s, 30s, 40s, and 50s. The communicative demands on young and middle-aged adults warrant increased efforts to identify and remediate hearing impairment in this population. Findings relative to the effects of age on adjustment to hearing impairment have, at times, seemed contradictory. Reports of better adjustment among "older" hearing-impaired active-duty soldiers and better adjustment among "younger" hearing-impaired veterans, for example, appear to be inconsistent (Erdman et al., 1990). In fact, however, the different findings can be attributed to the different age ranges of subjects in these studies. Adjustment may vary as a function of self-acceptance and communication demands, which, in turn, may vary as a func-

tion of age. This remains to be demonstrated. For a variety of reasons, however, young adults appear less likely to accept and pursue assistance for their hearing problems (Hétu et al., 1990; Kochkin, 1990). In view of the potential consequences to family harmony, job performance, and career progression, this is particularly worrisome. Hearing impairment has been implicated in underemployment (Markides et al., 1979; Thomas, Lamont, & Harris, 1982), criminality (Belenchia & Crowe, 1983; Crowe & Jackson, 1990; Jacobson, Jacobson, & Crowe, 1989), and marital stress (Thomas, 1984).

Between the ages of 18 and 65 adults experience peak communication demands in relation to education, occupation, marriage, and childrearing. Hearing impairment can thwart any or all of these major life endeavors either directly or indirectly. Ineffective communication may preclude career progression or marital happiness. Stress, withdrawal, or anger related to continued communication difficulties can ruin relationships, result in dismissal from a job, or suppress the motivation necessary to succeed in any aspect of life.

EMPLOYMENT ISSUES

Thomas et al. (1982) found that although hearing impairment may not result in unemployment, it does contribute to work-related problems. Their results suggest that individuals with hearing impairment are often underemployed. They were unable to discern whether underemployment was specifically related to hearing difficulties, to performance issues unrelated to hearing, or to discrimination on the basis of hearing impairment. The consequences of hearing impairment on job performance and career progression have not been systematically investigated. The listening demands associated with the average workday, however, result in complaints of fatigue, irritability, and stress from individuals with even mild hearing impairments. Active-duty service members with mild-to-moderate hearing impairments frequently report feeling stressed, frustrated, incompetent, angry, embarrassed, and discouraged as a result of work-related hearing problems (Erdman et al., 1984).

Hearing conservation efforts in noise hazardous work environments focus on identifying and monitoring individuals who are at risk for noise-induced hearing impairment and who have already sustained hearing damage. This complicates workers' ability to hide hearing impairment, a tendency related to the stigma attached to hearing impairment and to workers' need to protect their self-image (Hétu et al., 1988; Hétu et al., 1990). In these studies, individuals working in mines, lumbermills, and wood and metal products factories were particularly preoccupied with the demeaning attitudes and comments of coworkers. Beaudry and Hétu (1990) reviewed the literature related to attitudes of those with normal hearing toward the hearing impaired. Their findings suggest that attitudes toward people with hearing impairment are generally positive. Additional research is being conducted to investigate the inconsistent trend exhibited among industrial workers. Kyle, Jones, and Wood (1985) report that manual laborers are less likely to acquire hearing aids than are nonmanual workers. The latter engage in more verbal activities, recognize the effects of their hearing impairment, and are, therefore, more apt to acquire hearing aids. This pattern is evident among military personnel; officers are more likely to obtain hearing aids provided gratis through the military than are enlisted personnel (Erdman & Demorest, 1990). Kyle et al. (1985) postulate that adjustment to hearing impairment is a function of the control individuals exert over "access features" of information they receive (i.e., speed, intensity, and density of information). Hearing impairment necessitates the exertion of additional control over access features to maximize information reception. As the additional control becomes unacceptable to others, the awareness of hearing impairment increases. At this juncture, individuals can increase the level of control at all costs, accept reduced control and information, or avoid situations in which the level of control is threatened. Adjustment is predicated on the extent to which the reduced and varying access to information can be tolerated. Consistent with this model, management-level employees might exert more control and

may engage in denial; conversely overt acceptance is also a plausible option.

The reluctance to reveal hearing impairment in some work settings is clearly associated with fears relative to career advancement. Denial, one aspect of individuals' reluctance to acknowledge hearing difficulties, may be adaptive or maladaptive. If the perspective is one in which negative aspects of a situation are merely downplayed to maintain optimism and adjustment, it may be an adaptive coping mechanism. If, however, denial precludes addressing conditions that have a negative impact on health, job performance, or interpersonal relationships, it adversely affects adjustment and is, therefore, maladaptive. Self-reports, whether in an interview or questionnaire format, may underestimate difficulties as a function of patients' efforts to protect their self-image. Although, there is a relationship between self-acceptance, acceptance of loss, and denial (Erdman & Demorest, 1986b), Hétu et al. (1990) quite correctly point out that denial is not necessarily related to response to rehabilitation. Indeed, participation in group counseling enables individuals to admit to problems they have heretofore been reluctant to acknowledge. Audiologists should anticipate denial of adjustment-related problems and minimization of communication difficulties. *Denial should not be interpreted to mean that the individual does not experience these problems.* The gradual onset of hearing impairment and the insidious way in which concomitant communication problems develop cause many individuals to attribute difficulties to something other than hearing ability. By exerting extra effort and energy, these individuals compensate when necessary, believe they are hearing what they need to hear, and are often oblivious to how much they are missing. They are slow to recognize others' reactions to their apparent inattentiveness, forgetfulness, or aloofness. They fail to realize that others may view them as "slow" or uninformed when they don't understand what is said. Albeit needlessly, such reactions can adversely affect career progression. From the standpoint of preventing handicap, it is the audiologist's responsibility to counsel patients about the limitations hearing impairment can impose in order to prevent these insidious disadvantages. Hearing-impaired adults who are reluctant to admit to hearing-related problems can effectively be counseled by focusing on the documented hearing impairment and on the prevention of problems hearing impairment is likely to create. This approach, particularly when applied in group counseling, permits individuals to gain insight into hearing problems, become cognizant of the limitations hearing impairment may actually be imposing on them, and develop alternative coping strategies in the safety of a supportive environment.

It is all too easy to take patients' declaration that they have no difficulties at face value. This is a problem faced by all health care practitioners. Stoic patients who maintain an "everything's just fine" attitude are a significant part of the reason practitioners end up treating the pathology rather than the patient; conflicting messages from the diagnostic report on the one hand, and the patient's smiling countenance on the other, do not facilitate selection of appropriate treatment regimens. Patients may inadvertently belittle the significance of their problems by trying to appear cheerful and nonproblematic so that health care providers will like them and, subsequently, take good care of them. Individuals with hearing impairment behave no differently. Clinicians must focus on covert messages from patients and help them explore the impact hearing impairment has had on job performance, social life, relationships, energy level, and motivation to meet new challenges. Comprehensive self-assessment inventories such as the CPHI (Demorest & Erdman, 1986, 1987) and the HPI (Giolas et al., 1979) can be administered to determine the extent of communication difficulties experience in work-related settings as well as the use of adaptive and/or maladaptive coping strategies. The CPHI's Denial and Problem Awareness scales provide clinicians with additional insight into patients' willingness to acknowledge specific communication difficulties typical of hearing impairment and related adjustment problems. This information is useful in interpreting other scale scores and in recognizing a priori patients' reluctance to admit to hearing problems, thereby facilitating counselors' perspective taking and emotional reactivity.

Lalande et al. (1988) emphasize the importance of meeting the unique needs of those with high-frequency sensorineural hearing impairment incurred as a result of occupational noise exposure. Specifically, they recommend (*1*) information and counseling to promote understanding of the nature of the problem and greater acceptance and adjustment to the hearing handicap, (*2*) development of skills and strategies to reduce communication breakdown, and (*3*) stress management. These components are similar to those included in military rehabilitation programs for service members who also have primarily noise-induced hearing impairments (Erdman, 1983; Gaeth, 1979; Sedge, 1979; Sedge & Walden, 1979).

In addition to increasing employer and employee awareness of the hazards of noise exposure, industrial audiologists have an important role in increasing awareness of the consequences of hearing impairment and the implications for productivity. Individuals who have attended rehabilitation programs after acquiring noise-induced hearing impairment not only become strong proponents of hearing conservation efforts but also enhance participation in rehabilitation efforts (Lalande et al., 1988). Counseling is a critical element of hearing conservation efforts. The success of hearing conservation programs is directly related to compliance with the recommended use of hearing protection in the workplace and other noise hazardous areas. Improving adherence to hearing protection guidelines is a critical aspect of the industrial audiologists' counseling activities.

MARITAL AND FAMILY ISSUES

The effects of hearing impairment on family life have been largely ignored in the literature. One person's hearing impairment affects all family members. Communication difficulties occur as a direct result of hearing impairment and because of misconceptions about hearing problems. The marital relationship probably represents the most intensely interactive communication dyad in society. The successful growth and development of this relationship depends on the quality of partners' communication with one another. Although couples may be expected to understand each other's weaknesses and limitations, it is also quite likely that they take certain things about one another for granted. When one partner is hearing impaired, the quality of their communication is affected by that impairment, as well as by the couple's overall understanding of and adjustment to the limitations it imposes. Spouses' perceptions of the handicapping effects of hearing impairment are often inconsistent with those of their hearing-impaired partners (Erdman & Demorest, 1986a, 1990; Hétu, Lalonde, & Getty, 1987; McCarthy & Alpiner, 1983; Newman & Weinstein, 1986). There is a tendency for spouses to underestimate the degree of difficulty their hearing-impaired partners report. Spouses characteristically respond in contradictory ways to their partner's hearing difficulties. They may complain about the extent of the hearing problem and a spouse's refusal or reluctance to do anything about it. At the same time, they may claim that the spouse (*1*) hears just fine when he or she wants to, (*2*) just doesn't pay attention, (*3*) doesn't care enough to listen, or (*4*) all of the preceding. These same spouses refuse to repeat or speak up, fail to get the hearing-impaired person's attention before they speak, talk from other rooms, and say "forget it" or "never mind" when the hearing-impaired partner asks them what they said. The hearing-impaired individual's ability to hear well at times essentially negates the significance of a diagnosed hearing problem. In view of not sharing the same perceptions, it is not surprising that hearing-impaired patients and their partners fail to resolve satisfactorily their shared communication problems. Hétu et al. (1987) report that couples do not spontaneously attempt to find mutually acceptable solutions. Consequently, it is essential that family members be included in at least some phases of the counseling process.

To facilitate counseling of hearing-impaired patients and their spouses (or other family members), all parties' perceptions of the related difficulties must be considered. To do so, self-assessment inventories can be administered to the patient as well as to the significant other. This approach has been advocated by many clinicians. Erdman and Demorest (1986a, 1990) have documented spouses' and offsprings' perceptions of communication performance, environmental variables, use of coping strategies, and personal adjustment, and have counseled couples and families using the CPHI. McCarthy and Alpiner (1983) developed a scale specifically for use in family counseling. The disparity in hearing-impaired patients' and their partners' perceptions, as assessed by both the CPHI and the McCarthy-Alpiner Scale, exemplifies the difficulties couple and families experience in adjusting to hearing impairment. The hearing-impaired person may be more or less aware of hearing difficulties than family members are, differences may exist relative to their perceptions of the nature of the problems, or family members may differ in their views of how to cope with hearing difficulties. Screening instruments including Schow and Nerbonne's (1982) Self-Assessment of Communication and the Hearing Handicap Inventory for the Elderly (Newman & Weinstein, 1986) have also been employed to assess discrepancies in couples' perceptions of hearing handicap.

Audiologists' role in counseling couples who are dealing with hearing impairment is a delicate one; both parties live with the effects of the hearing impairment but view the problems from different perspectives. In addition to providing an empathic, supportive atmosphere, clinicians can furnish objective information about hearing impairment, evaluate the disparate views of hearing problems, identify common ground, and offer potential explanations for the disparities as well. Counseling sessions provide neutral time and territory in which alternative solutions can be generated with guidance from an informed mediator who can empathize with each person, and with the couple as a unit, to facilitate adjustment. Scores from self-assessment inventories help identify disparities in couples' perceptions of their communication difficulties. They are also invaluable in describing each party's perception of his or her partner in an objective manner. Once the partners are aware of the difference in their perceptions, they can begin to focus on the problems these differences have caused. For example, a hearing-impaired person who has worked all day in a busy office, straining to listen in meetings or on the phone to irate customers and a demanding boss, arrives home in dire need of time out, during which listening is the last thing he or she wants to do. Meanwhile, spouse and children are anxiously waiting to share news, to ask for help with homework, to discuss family crises, to interact—in short, to be heard. Unfortunately, family members' need to be heard coincides with the hearing-impaired person's need to "tune out." Inasmuch as not listening to someone communicates a disinterested, uncaring attitude, the family's solidarity can be severely shaken. Family members are insensitive to the fatigue, often specifically related to listening, and unknowingly place unreasonable demands on the hearing-impaired person. The family's failure to recognize and address the necessity for time out results in communication problems far more significant than the degree of hearing impairment. These issues and similar ones are common in families with a hearing-impaired member. Ironically, the milder the impairment, the less likely everyone in the family is to attribute the problems to hearing loss.

Group counseling affords couples an opportunity to learn that other families grapple with the same frustrations and difficulties as a result of hearing impairment. This arrangement facilitates adjustment for individual partners as well as couples as they discover that other hearing-impaired people, other spouses, and other couples can identify with the individual and shared problems experienced in a marriage. In a couples' group, clinicians must attend to individual reactions, couples' interactions, and of course, interactions among all group members. The therapeutic advantages of shared insights, problem solving, and commiseration are particularly effective and efficient when counseling groups of couples and outweigh any potential disadvantages posed by the complexities of the group's member composition.

Other Auditory Disabilities and Handicaps: Counseling Considerations

Hearing disabilities and handicaps are commonly associated with communication difficulties and subsequent adjustment problems; however, there are other aspects of auditory dysfunction that warrant counseling intervention. Thomas (1984) and Hétu et al. (1988) categorize difficulties in environmental awareness as hearing disability. This may include hearing warning signals or other environmental sounds ranging from a turn signal clicking to a bird chirping. The significance of one's ability to hear nonspeech sounds is readily appreciated when considered in the context of safety and job performance. Hearing-impaired health care workers often need amplified stethoscopes to enhance their ability to monitor cardiac and pulmonary function. Law enforcement officials, military personnel, guards, assembly line workers, miners, and loggers find the inability to hear environmental sounds threatening to their safety and that of others. Mechanics, plumbers, and electricians who cannot hear the characteristic sounds of malfunctioning equipment are frustrated in their attempts to help customers who report mysterious problems with vehicles and appliances. These problems, often experienced secondary to mild hearing impairments, result in stress and fatigue from constant straining to hear and from worrying about the consequences of missing things. Efforts to compensate by keeping the volume on monitoring and signaling devices, radios, or telephones at a higher level can create problems with others who are in the vicinity or who use the same equipment. Hence, hearing impairment, viewed as a decrease in hearing acuity, also has auditory and nonauditory effects that, in a rehabilitative context, constitute potential disabilities and handicaps for individuals with hearing impairment. Counseling those with complaints related to an inability to hear or discriminate environmental and other nonspeech signals is equally responsive to problem-solving procedures and an empathic counseling relationship.

Conclusion

Despite evidence that hearing impairment is not a reliable predictor of hearing disability and handicap, the focus of intervention audiology has been slow to shift from documented hearing impairment to the disabling and handicapping problems that prompt patients to seek intervention. Ross (1987) admonishes fellow audiologists for not responding to clinical failures and for failing to implement service delivery models that ensure provision of appropriate rehabilitative intervention in the hearing aid dispensing process. Many of the perceived clinical constraints that preclude effective management of hearing disability and handicap can be blamed on the profession's failure to define its role as one that is truly rehabilitative in nature. Giolas (1990) also addresses the inadequacy of current service delivery in audiology relative to management of hearing handicap. He optimistically observes that the proliferation of self-report measurement tools in audiology is testimony to audiologists' awareness that assessment of hearing disability and handicap are prerequisites to appropriate intervention. Giolas (1990) and Jerger (1991) have reemphasized audiology's mission in management of hearing handicap, a mission all the more relevant among rehabilitative audiologists whose goal it is to facilitate adjustment to the auditory and nonauditory consequences of hearing impairment. Awareness of the inherent inadequacy in treating the audiogram has renewed emphasis on the role counseling necessarily plays in the management of hearing-impaired patients.

In summary, counseling, a facilitative problem-solving process, is the essence of successful rehabilitative intervention. Many aspects of affective, cognitive, and behavioral counseling methods have direct applications in management of patients with hearing impairment. An empathic counselor-client relationship and cognitive-behavioral problem-solving approaches are fundamental aspects of rehabilitation counseling that audiologists can adapt to address the auditory and nonauditory consequences of hearing impairment. The implications inherent in clinical management of hearing-impaired patients dictate a refocusing of service delivery models in audiology. Specifically, facilitating adjustment to hearing disability and handicap, that is, counseling, necessitates service delivery models that are rehabilitation oriented. Inasmuch as facilitating adjustment to hearing impairment is the goal of rehabilitative audiology, systematic incorporation of counseling into clinical practice is long overdue.

References

Adler, A., *The Practice and Theory of Individual Psychology.* Paterson, NJ: Littlefield, Adams (1963).

Alberti, P. W., Pichora-Fuller, M. K., Corbin, H., and Riko, K., Aural rehabilitation in a teaching hospital: evaluation and results. *Ann. Otol. Rhinol. Laryngol.,* 93(6), 589–594 (1984).

Alpiner, J. G., Evaluation of communication function. In J. G. Alpiner (Ed.), *Handbook of Adult Rehabilitative Audiology.* Baltimore: Williams & Wilkins (1982).

Alpiner, J. G., Chevrette, W., Glascoe, G., Metz, M., and Olsen, B., The Denver Scale of Communication Function. Unpublished manuscript, University of Denver (1974).

AMA/AAO, Guide for the evaluation of hearing handicap. *J. Am. Med. Assoc.,* 241, 2055–2059 (1979).

Americans with Disabilities Act of 1990 (Public Law 101-336), 42 USC Sec. 12101.

Anderson, T. P., An alternative frame of reference for rehabilitation: the helping process vs. the medical model. In R. P. Marinelli and A. E. Dell Orto (Eds.), *The Psychological and Social Impact of Physical Disability.* New York: Springer (1977).

Ansbacher, H. L., and Ansbacher, R., *The Individual Psychology of Alfred Adler.* New York: Harper Torchbooks (1964).

ASHA Committee on Rehabilitative Audiology, The audiologist: responsibilities in the rehabilitation of the auditorily handicapped. *Asha,* 16(2), 68–70 (1974).

ASHA Committee on Rehabilitative Audiology, Definition of and competencies for aural rehabilitation. *Asha,* 26(5), 37–41 (1984).

ASHA Task Force on the Definition of Hearing Handicap, On the definition of hearing handicap. *Asha,* 23(4), 293–297 (1981).

Bally, S. J., and Kaplan, H., The Gallaudet University aural rehabilitation elderhostels. *J. Acad. Rehab. Audiol.,* 21, 99–112 (1988).

Bandura, A., *Principles of Behavior Modification.* New York: Holt, Rinehart and Winston (1969).

Bandura, A., *Social Learning Theory.* Englewood Cliffs, NJ: Prentice-Hall (1977).

Bandura, A., *Social Foundations of Thought and Action: A Social Cognitive Theory.* Englewood Cliffs, NJ: Prentice-Hall (1986).

Barlow, D. H., Hayes, S. C., and Nelson, R. O., *The Scientist Practitioner: Research and Accountability in Clinical and Educational Settings.* New York: Pergamon Press (1984).

Barrett, C., and Wright, J., Therapist variables. In M. Hersen, L. Michelson, and A. Bellak (Eds.), *Issues in Psychotherapy Research.* New York: Plenum (1984).

Beck, A. T., *Cognitive Therapy and Emotional Disorders.* New York: International Universities Press (1976).

Beck, A. T., and Emery G., *Anxiety Disorders and Phobias.* New York: Basic Books (1985).

Beck, A. T., Rush, A. J., Shaw, B., and Emery, G., *Cognitive Therapy of Depression.* New York: Guilford Press (1979).

Belenchia, T. A., and Crowe, T. A., Prevalence of speech and hearing disorders in a state penitentiary population. *J. Commun. Dis.*, 16, 279–285 (1983).

Berne, E., *Transactional Analysis in Psychotherapy*. New York: Grove Press (1961).

Berne, E., *Games People Play: The Psychology of Human Relationships*. New York: Grove Press (1964).

Berne, E., *Principles of Group Treatment*. New York: Oxford University Press (1966).

Beaudry, J., and Hétu, R., Measurement of attitudes of those with unimpaired hearing towards the hearing impaired: a critical examination of the available scales. *J. Speech Lang. Path. Audiol.*, 14(2), 23–32 (1990).

Blechman, E. A., and Dannemiller, E. A., Effects on performance of perceived control over noxious noise. *J. Consult. Clin. Psychol.*, 44(4), 601–607 (1976).

Bohart, A. C., and Todd, J., *Foundations of Clinical and Counseling Psychology*, New York: Harper & Row (1988).

Brainerd, S. H., and Frankel, B. G., The relationship between audiometric and self-report measures of hearing handicap. *Ear Hear.*, 6, 89–92 (1985).

Brammer, L. M., *The Helping Relationship: Process and Skills*. Englewood Cliffs, NJ: Prentice-Hall (1985).

Brearley, G., and Birchley, P., *Introducing Counselling Skills and Technique: With Particular Application for the Paramedical Professions*. London: Faber and Faber (1986).

Brooks, D. N., Counselling and its effect on hearing aid use. *Scand. Audiol.*, 8, 101–107 (1979).

Brooks, D. N., Factors related to the under-use of post-aural hearing aids. *Br. J. Audiol.*, 19, 211–217 (1985).

Brooks, D. N., The effect of attitude on benefit derived for hearing aids. *Br. J. Audiol.* 23, 3–11 (1989).

Brooks, D. N., and Johnson, D. I., Pre-issue assessment and counselling as a component of hearing-aid provision. *Br. J. Audiol.*, 15, 13–19 (1981).

Caccavo, M. T., and Geist, P., Adjustment strategies for hearing-impaired people. *Hear. Instr.* 37(11), 46–52 (1986).

Cook, D., Psychosocial impact of disability. In R. M. Parker (Ed.), *Rehabilitation Counseling: Basics and Beyond*. Austin, TX: Pro-Ed (1987).

Corsini, R. J., Introduction. In R. J. Corsini and D. Wedding (Eds.), *Current Psychotherapies*. Itasca, IL: F. E. Peacock Publishers (1989).

Corsini, R. J., and Rosenberg, B., Mechanisms of group psychotherapy. *J. Abnorm. Soc. Psychol.*, 51 406–411 (1955).

Corsini, R. J., and Wedding, D., *Current Psychotherapies*, 4th ed. Itasca, IL: F. E. Peacock Publishers (1989).

Crowe, T. A., and Jackson, P. D., Hearing loss in a Mississippi penitentiary. *Hear. Instr.* 41(2), 7–10 (1990).

Davis, A. C., Hearing disorders in the population: first phase findings of the MRC National Study of Hearing. In M. E. Lutman and M. P. Haggard (Eds.), *Hearing Science and Hearing Disorders*. London: Academic Press (1983).

Demorest, M. E., and Erdman, S. A., A database management system for the Communication Profile for the Hearing Impaired. *J. Acad. Rehab. Audiol.*, 17, 87–96 (1984a).

Demorest, M. E., and Erdman, S. A., Clinical applications of self-assessment inventories. *Hear. Instr.*, 35(11), 32–38 (1984b).

Demorest, M. E., and Erdman, S. A., Scale composition and item analysis of the Communication Profile for the Hearing Impaired. *J. Speech Hear. Res.*, 29, 515–535 (1986).

Demorest, M. E., and Erdman, S. A., Development of the Communication Profile for the Hearing Impaired. *J. Speech Hear. Dis.*, 52, 129–143 (1987).

Demorest, M. E, and Erdman, S. A., Retest stability of the Communication Profile for the Hearing Impaired. *Ear Hear.*, 9, 237–242 (1988).

Demorest, M. E., and Erdman, S. A., Relationships among behavioral, environmental, and affective communication variables: a canonical analysis of the CPHI. *J. Speech Hear. Dis.*, 54, 180–188 (1989a).

Demorest, M. E., and Erdman, S. A., Factor structure of the Communication Profile for the Hearing Impaired. *J. Speech Hear. Dis.*, 54, 541–549 (1989b).

Demorest, M. E., Lansing C., Henoch, M. A., Jons, C. R., and Erdman, S. A., Research for the practicing clinician: exploiting clinical databases for research [Abstract]. *Asha*, 30(10), 159 (1988).

Demorest, M. E., and Walden, B. E., Psychometric principles in the selection, interpretation, and evaluation of communication self-assessment inventories. *J. Speech Hear. Dis.*, 49, 226–240 (1984).

DiMichael, S. G., *Assertiveness Training for Persons Who Are Hard of Hearing*. Rockville, MD: SHHH Publications (1985).

Dusay, J., *Egograms: How I See You and You See Me*. New York: Harper & Row (1977).

Dusay, J., *Egograms*. New York: Harper & Row (1978).

D'Zurilla, T. J., and Goldfried, M. R., Problem solving and behavior modification. *J. Abnorm. Psychol.*, 78, 107–126 (1971).

Egan, G., *The Skilled Helper: A Systematic Approach to Effective Helping*, 3rd ed. Pacific Grove, CA: Brooks/Cole (1986).

Ellis, A., *Reason and Emotion in Psychotherapy*. New York: Lyle Stuart (1962).

Ellis, A., and Grieger, R., *Handbook of Rational-Emotive Therapy*. New York: Springer (1977).

English, R. W., The application of personality theory to explain psychological reactions to physical disability. In R. P. Marinelli and A. E. Dell Orto (Eds.), *The Psychological and Social Impact of Physical Disability*. New York: Springer (1977).

Erdman, S. A., The use of assertiveness training in adult aural rehabilitation. *Audiol. (Audio J. Cont. Ed.)*, 5(12) (1980).

Erdman, S. A., History and current status of the Army's Aural Rehabilitation Program [Abstract]. *Asha*, 25(10), 128 (1983).

Erdman, S. A., Crowley, J. M., and Gillespie, G. G., Considerations in counseling the hearing impaired. *Hear. Instr.*, 35(11) (1984).

Erdman, S. A., and Demorest, M. E., Comparisons of husbands' and wives' perceptions of adjustment to hearing loss. Paper presented at the Academy of Rehabilitative Audiology Summer Institute, Lake Geneva, WI (1986a).

Erdman, S. A., and Demorest, M. E., Self-acceptance: correlates in the Communication Profile for the

Hearing Impaired [Abstract]. *Asha,* 28(10), 160 (1986b).

Erdman, S. A., and Demorest, M. E., *CPHI Manual: A Guide to Clinical Use.* Simpsonville, MD: CPHI Services (1990).

Erdman, S. A., Demorest, M. E., Wark, D. J., et al., Factors affecting adjustment to hearing loss [Abstract]. *Asha,* 32(10), 171 (1990).

Eriksson-Mangold, M., Ringdahl, A., Björklund, A.-K., and Wåhlin, B., The active fitting (AF) programme of hearing aids: a psychological perspective. *Br. J. Audiol.,* 24, 277–285 (1990).

Ewertsen, H. W., and Birk-Nielsen, H., Social Hearing Handicap Index: social handicap in relation to hearing impairment. *Audiology,* 12, 180–187 (1973).

Falvo, D. R., *Effective Patient Education: A Guide to Increased Compliance.* Rockville, MD: Aspen Systems (1985).

Gaeth, J. H., A history of aural rehabilitation. In M. A. Henoch (Ed.), *Aural Rehabilitation for the Elderly.* New York: Grune & Stratton (1979).

Gallagher, G., Returns for credit: fact of life or fuel for change. *Hear. J.,* 43(7), 13–18 (1990).

Garrity, T. F., Medical compliance and the clinician-patient relationship: a review. *Soc. Sci. Med.,* 15E, 215–222 (1981).

Geis, H. J., The problem of personal worth in the physically disabled patient. In R. P. Marinelli and A. E. Dell Orto (Eds.), *The Psychological and Social Impact of Physical Disability.* New York: Springer (1977).

Gellman, W., Projections in the field of physical disability. In R. P. Marinelli and A. E. Dell Orto (Eds.), *The Psychological and Social Impact of Physical Disability.* New York: Springer (1977).

Gerrard, B. A., Boniface, W. J., and Love, B. H., *Interpersonal Skills for Health Professionals.* Reston, VA: Reston Publishing (1980).

Giolas, T. G., "The measurement of hearing handicap" revisited: a 20-year perspective. *Ear Hear.,* 11(5), 2S–5S (1990).

Giolas, T. G., Owens, E., Lamb, S., and Schubert, E., Hearing Performance Inventory, *J. Speech Hear. Dis.,* 44, 169–195 (1979).

Glass, D. C., and Singer, J. E., Behavioral aftereffects of unpredictable and uncontrollable aversive events. *Am. Scient.,* 60, 457–465 (1972).

Golightly, C. K.,*Creative Problem Solving for Health Care Professionals.* Rockville, MD: Aspen Systems (1981).

Hall, J. A., and Dornan, M. C., Meta-analysis of satisfaction with medical care: description of research domain and analysis of overall satisfaction levels. *Soc. Sci. Med.,* 27, 637–644 (1988).

Hallberg, L. R.-M., and Carlsson, S. G., A qualitative study of strategies for managing a hearing impairment. *Br. J. Audiol.,* 25, 201–211 (1991a).

Hallberg, L. R.-M., and Carlsson, S. G., Hearing impairment, coping and perceived hearing handicap in middle-aged subjects with acquired hearing loss. *Br. J. Audiol.,* 25, 323–330 (1991b).

Hawes, N. A., and Niswander, P. S., Comparison of the Revised Hearing Performance Inventory with audiometric measures. *Ear Hear.,* 6(2), 93–97 (1985).

Heppner, P. P., A review of the problem-solving literature and its relationship to the counseling process. *J. Counsel. Psychol.,* 25(5), 366–375 (1978).

Heppner, P. P., and Petersen, C. H., The development and implications of a personal problem-solving inventory. *J. Counsel. Psychol.,* 29(1), 66–75 (1982).

Hétu, R., Lalonde, M., and Getty, L., Psychosocial disadvantages associated with occupational hearing loss as experienced in the family. *Audiology,* 26, 141–152 (1987).

Hétu, R., Riverin, L., Getty, L., Lalande, N. M., and St-Cyr, C., The reluctance to acknowledge hearing difficulties among hearing-impaired workers. *Br. J. Audiol.,* 24, 265–276 (1990).

Hétu, R., Riverin, L., Lalande, N., Getty, L., and St-Cyr, C., Qualitative analysis of the handicap associated with occupational hearing loss. *Br. J. Audiol.,* 22, 251–264 (1988).

High, W. S., Fairbanks, G., and Glorig, A., Scale for self-assessment of hearing handicap. *J. Speech Hear. Dis.,* 29, 215–230 (1964).

Hogan, R., Development of an empathy scale. *J. Consult. Clin. Pychol.,* 33, 307–316 (1969).

Illich, I., *Medical Nemesis.* New York: Pantheon (1977).

Jacobson, C. A., Jacobson, J. T., and Crowe, T. A., Hearing loss in prison inmates. *Ear Hear.,* 10(3), 178–183 (1989).

Jerger, J., Milestones and boundaries. *Am. J. Audiol.,* 1(1), 6 (1991).

Kaplan, H., Elderhostel for the hearing impaired. *Asha,* 25(7), 46–49 (1983).

Karasu, T., The specificity versus nonspecificity dilemma: toward identifying therapeutic change agents. *Am. J. Psychiatry,* 143, 695–698 (1986).

Kielinen, L. L., and Nerbonne, M. A., Further investigation of the relationship between hearing handicap and audiometric measures of hearing impairment. *J. Acad. Rehab. Audiol.,* 23, 89–94 (1990).

King, M., Novik, L., and Citrenbaum, C., *Irresistible Communication: Creative Skills for the Health Professional.* Philadelphia: W. B. Saunders (1983).

Knutson, J. F., and Lansing, C. R., The relationship between communication problems and psychological difficulties in persons with profound acquired hearing loss. *J. Speech Hear. Dis.,* 55, 656–664 (1990).

Kochkin, S., One more time . . . what did the 1984 HIA market survey say? *Hear. Instr.,* 41(11), 10–20 (1990).

Kyle, J. G., Jones, L. G., and Wood, P. L., Adjustment to acquired hearing loss: a working model. In H. Orlans (Ed.), *Adjustment to Adult Hearing Loss.* San Diego, CA: College-Hill Press (1985).

Lalande, N. M., Riverin, L., and Lambert, J., Occupational hearing loss: an aural rehabilitation program for workers and their spouses, characteristics of the program and target group (participants and nonparticipants). *Ear Hear.,* 9(5), 248–254 (1988).

Lamb, S. H., Owens, E., and Schubert, E. D., The revised form of the Hearing Performance Inventory. *Ear Hear.,* 4, 152–159 (1983).

Lazarus, A. A., *Multimodal Behavior Therapy.* New York: Springer-Verlag (1976).

Lazarus, A. A., *The Practice of Multimodal Therapy.* New York: McGraw-Hill (1981).

Lazarus, A. A., Multimodal therapy. In R. J. Corsini and D. Wedding (Eds.), *Current Psychotherapies.* Itasca, IL: F. E. Peacock Publishers (1989).

Lazarus, R. S., and Folkman, S., *Stress, Appraisal, and Coping.* New York: Springer (1984).

Libby, E. R., Asking the non-buyer "why?" *Hear. Instr.*, 41(11), 26 (1990).

Maguire, P., Communication skills and patient care. In A. Steptoe and A. Mathews (Eds.), *Health Care and Human Behaviour.* London: Academic Press (1984).

Markides, A., Brooks, D. N., Hart, F. G., and Stephens, S. D. G., Aural rehabilitation of hearing impaired adults: official policy of the British Society of Audiology. *Br. J. Audiol.*, 13, 7–14 (1979).

May, R., *Existential Psychology.* New York: Random House (1961).

May, R., *The Meaning of Anxiety* (rev. ed.). New York: Norton (1977).

May, R., and Yalom, I., Existential psychotherapy. In R. J. Corsini and D. Wedding (Eds.), *Current Psychotherapies.* Itasca, IL: F. E. Peacock Publishers (1989).

McCarthy, P. A., and Alpiner, J. G., An assessment scale of hearing handicap for use in family counseling. *J. Acad. Rehab. Audiol.*, 16, 256–270 (1983).

McCarthy, P. A., Culpepper, N. B., and Lucks, L., Variability in counseling experiences and training among ESB-accredited programs. *Asha*, 28(9), 49–52 (1986).

Meadow-Orlans, K. P., Social and psychological effects of hearing loss in adulthood: a literature review. In H. Orlans (Ed.), *Adjustment to Adult Hearing Loss.* San Diego, CA: College-Hill Press (1985).

Mehrabian, A., and Epstein, N., A measure of emotional empathy. *J. Personal.*, 40, 525–543 (1972).

Meichenbaum, D., *Cognitive Behavior Modification.* Morristown, NJ: General Learning Press (1974).

Meichenbaum, D., *Cognitive Behavior Modification: An Integrative Approach.* New York: Plenum (1977).

Meier, S. T., *The Elements of Counseling.* Pacific Grove, CA: Brooks/Cole (1989).

Menaghan, E. G., Individual coping efforts: moderators of the relationship between life stress and mental health outcomes. In H. B. Kaplan (Ed.), *Psychosocial Stress: Trends in Theory and Research.* New York: Academic Press (1983).

Mosak, H. H., Adlerian psychotherapy. In R. J. Corsini and D. Wedding (Eds.), *Current Psychotherapies.* Itasca, IL: F. E. Peacock Publishers (1989).

Newman, C. W., and Weinstein, B. E., Judgments of perceived hearing handicap by hearing impaired elderly men and their spouses. *J. Acad. Rehab. Audiol.*, 19, 109–115 (1986).

Newman, C. W., and Weinstein, B. E., Test-retest reliability of the Hearing Handicap Inventory for the Elderly using two administrative approaches. *Ear Hear.*, 10(3), 190–191 (1989).

Newman, C. W., Weinstein, B. E., Jacobson, G. P., and Hug, G. A., The Hearing Handicap Inventory for Adults: psychometric adequacy and audiometric correlates. *Ear Hear.*, 11(6), 430–433 (1990).

Noble, W., Correspondence, evaluation of hearing handicap: a critique of Ward's position. *Audiology*, 27, 53–61 (1988).

Noble, W. G., and Atherly, G. R. C., The Hearing Measure Scale: A questionnaire for the assessment of auditory disability. *J. Aud. Res.*, 10, 229–250 (1970).

Patterson, C. H., *Theories of Counseling and Psychotherapy.* New York: Harper & Row (1986).

Pavlov, I. P., *Conditional Reflexes.* London: Oxford University Press (1927).

Pavlov, I. P., *Lectures on Conditioned Reflexes.* New York: International Publishers (1928).

Perls, F. S., *Gestalt Therapy Verbatim.* Lafayette, CA: Real People Press (1969).

Perls, F. S., *The Gestalt Approach.* Palo Alto: Science and Behavior Books (1973).

Perls, F. S., Hefferline R., and Goodman, P., *Gestalt Therapy.* New York: Julian Press (1951).

Pettegrew, L. S., and Turkat, I. D., How patients communicate about their illness. *Human Communic. Res.*, 12(3), 376–394 (1986).

Pollack, M. C., The remediation process: psychological and counseling aspects. In J. G. Alpiner (Ed.), *Handbook of Adult Rehabilitative Audiology.* Baltimore: Williams & Wilkins (1978).

Purtilo, R., *Health Professional/Patient Interaction.* Philadelphia: W. B. Saunders (1978).

Raskin, N. J., and Rogers, C. R., Person-centered therapy. In R. J. Corsini and D. Wedding (Eds.), *Current Psychotherapies.* Itasca, IL: F. E. Peacock Publishers (1989).

Roberts, S. D., and Bouchard, K. R., Establishing rapport in rehabilitative audiology. *J. Acad. Rehabil. Audiol.* 22, 67–73 (1989).

Rogers, C. R., *Counseling and Psychotherapy.* Boston: Houghton Mifflin (1942).

Rogers, C. R., *Client-Centered Therapy.* Boston: Houghton Mifflin (1951).

Rogers, C. R., The necessary and sufficient conditions of therapeutic personality change. *J. Consult. Psychol.*, 21, 95–103 (1957).

Rogers, C. R., *On Becoming a Person.* Boston: Houghton Mifflin (1961).

Rogers, C. R., Empathic: an unappreciated way of being. *Counsel. Psychol.*, 5, 2–10 (1975).

Rogers, C. R., *A Way of Being.* Boston: Houghton Mifflin (1980).

Rogers, C. R., Client-centered therapy. In I. L. Kutash and A. Wolf (Eds.), *Psychotherapist's Handbook: Therapy and Technique in Practice.* San Francisco: Jossey-Bass (1986).

Ross, M., Aural rehabilitation revisited. *J. Acad. Rehab. Audiol.*, 20, 13–23 (1987).

Rowland, J. P., Dirks, D. D., Dubno, J. R., and Bell, T. S., Comparison of speech recognition-in-noise and subjective communication assessment. *Ear Hear.*, 6(6), 291–296 (1985).

Rupp, R. R., Higgins, J., and Mauer, J. F., A feasibility scale for predicting hearing aid use (FSPHAU). *J. Acad. Rehab. Audiol.*, 10, 81–104 (1977).

Sanders, D. A., Hearing aid orientation and counseling. In M. C. Pollack (Ed.), *Amplification for the Hearing Impaired.* New York: Grune & Stratton (1975).

Sanders, D. A., Hearing aid orientation and counseling. In M. C. Pollack (Ed.), *Amplification for the Hearing Impaired,* 2nd ed. New York: Grune & Stratton (1980).

Scadden, L. A., Psychosocial implications of technological advances for sensorially disabled persons. In B. W. Heller, L. M. Flohr, and L. S. Zegans (Eds.),

Psychosocial Interventions with Sensorially Disabled Persons. Orlando, FL: Grune & Stratton (1987).

Schow, R. L., and Gatehouse, S., Fundamental issues in self-assessment of hearing. *Ear Hear.,* 11(5), 6S–16S (1990).

Schow, R. L., and Nerbonne, M. A., Communication screening profile: use with elderly clients. *Ear Hear.,* 3(3), 135–147 (1982).

Sedge, R. K., Aural rehabilitation for individuals with high frequency hearing loss. *J. Acad. Rehab. Audiol.,* 12, 47–61 (1979).

Sedge, R. K., and Walden, B. E., An Army residential aural rehabilitation program for military personnel with high-frequency hearing losses. *Audiol. (Audio J. Cont. Ed.),* 4(9) (1979).

Shontz, F. C., Physical disability and personality: theory and recent research. In R. P. Marinelli and A. E. Dell Orto (Eds.), *The Psychological and Social Impact of Physical Disability.* New York: Springer (1977).

Skinner, B. F., *The Behavior of Organisms.* New York: Appleton-Century (1938).

Skinner, B. F., *Science and Human Behavior.* New York: Macmillan (1953).

Skinner, B. F., *Beyond Freedom and Dignity.* New York: Knopf (1971).

Skinner, M. W., *Hearing Aid Evaluation.* Englewood Cliffs, NJ: Prentice-Hall (1988).

Smedley, T. C., and Schow, R. L., Frustrations with hearing aid use: candid observations from the elderly. *Hear J.,* 43(6), 21–27 (1990).

Speaks, C. S., Jerger, J., and Trammell, J., Measurement of hearing handicap. *J. Speech Hear. Res.,* 13(4), 768–776 (1970).

Squier, R. W., A model of empathic understanding and adherence to treatment regimens in practitioner-patient relationships. *Soc. Sci. Med.,* 30(3), 325–339 (1990).

Stephens, D., and Hétu, R., Impairment, disability and handicap in audiology: towards a consensus. *Audiology,* 30(4), 185–200 (1991).

Surr, R. K., Schuchman, G. I., and Montgomery, A. A., Factors influencing use of hearing aids. *Arch. Otolaryngol.,* 104, 732–736 (1978).

Susser, M. W., and Watson, W., *Sociology in Medicine,* 2nd ed. London: Oxford University Press (1971).

Swan, I. R. C., and Gatehouse, S., Factors influencing consultation for management of hearing disability. *Br. J. Audiol.,* 24, 155–160 (1990).

Thomas, A. J., *Acquired Hearing Loss: Psychological and Psychosocial Implications.* London: Academic Press (1984).

Thomas, A. J., Rehabilitation of adults with acquired hearing loss: the psychological dimension. *Br. J. Audiol.,* 22, 81–83 (1988).

Thomas, A. J., and Gilhome Herbst, K. R., Social and psychological effects of acquired deafness for adults of employment age. *Br. J. Audiol.,* 14, 76–85 (1980).

Thomas, A., Lamont, M., and Harris, M., Problems encountered at work by people with severe acquired hearing loss. *Br. J. Audiol.,* 16, 39–43 (1982).

Thomas, K., Butler, A., and Parker, R., Psychosocial counseling. In R. M. Parker (Ed.), *Rehabilitation Counseling: Basics and Beyond.* Austin, TX: Pro-Ed (1987).

Thomas, K., and Parker, R., Counseling interventions. *J. Applied Rehab. Counsel.* 15, 15–19, 47 (1984).

Traynor, R. M., Adult aural rehabilitation in the 1980's. *Hearsay (J. Ohio Speech Hear. Assoc.),* 12–21 (Spring 1987).

Truax, C. B., A scale for the rating of accurate empathy. In C. R. Rogers, E. T. Gendlin, D. J. Kiesler, and C. B. Truax (Eds.), *The Therapeutic Relationship and Its Impact.* Madison: University of Wisconsin Press (1967).

Truax, C. B., and Carkhuff, R. R., *Toward Effective Counseling and Psychotherapy: Training and Practice.* Chicago: Aldine-Atherton (1967).

Truax, C. B., and Mitchell, K. M., Research on certain therapist skills in relation to process and outcome. In A. E. Bergin and S. L. Garfield (Eds.), *Handbook of Psychotherapy and Behavior Change: An Empirical Analysis.* New York: Wiley (1971).

Turk, D., Meichenbaum, D., and Genest, M., *Pain and Behavioral Medicine: A Cognitive-Behavioral Perspective.* New York: Guilford Press (1983).

Turner, R. J., Direct, indirect, and moderating effects of social support on psychological distress and associated conditions. In H. B. Kaplan (Ed.), *Psychosocial Stress: Trends in Theory and Research.* New York: Academic Press (1983).

Tye-Murray, N., Repair strategy usage by hearing-impaired adults and changes following communication therapy. *J. Speech Hear. Res.,* 34, 921–928 (1991).

Ventry, I. M., and Weinstein, B. E., The Hearing Handicap Inventory for the Elderly: a new tool. *Ear Hear.,* 3, 128–134 (1982).

Ward, W. D., The American Medical Association/American Academy of Otolaryngology formula for determination of hearing handicap. *Audiology* 22, 313–324 (1983).

Ward, W. D., Correspondence: answer to Noble. *Audiology,* 27, 61–64 (1988).

Weinstein, B. E., Spitzer, J. B., and Ventry, I. M., Test-retest reliability of the Hearing Handicap Inventory for the Elderly. *Ear Hear.,* 7, 295–299 (1986).

Weinstein, B. E., and Ventry, I. M., Audiologic correlates of hearing handicap in the elderly. *J. Speech Hear. Res.,* 26, 148–151 (1983a).

Weinstein, B. E., and Ventry, I. M., Audiometric correlates of the Hearing Handicap Inventory for the Elderly. *J. Speech Hear. Dis.,* 48, 379–384 (1983b).

WHO, *International Classification of Impairments, Disabilities and Handicaps: A Manual of Classification Relating to the Consequences of Disease.* Geneva: World Health Organization (1980).

Wolpe, J., *Psychotherapy for Reciprocal Inhibition.* Stanford, CA: Stanford University Press (1958).

Wolpe, J., *The Practice of Behavior Therapy,* 3rd ed. New York: Pergamon Press (1982).

Wright, B. E., *Physical Disability: A Psychosocial Approach.* New York: Harper & Row (1983).

Wylde, M. A., Psychological and counseling aspects of the adult remediation process. In J. G. Alpiner and P. A. McCarthy (Eds.), *Rehabilitative Audiology: Children and Adults.* Baltimore, MD: Williams & Wilkins (1987).

Yontef, G. M., and Simkin, J. S., Gestalt therapy. In R. J. Corsini and D. Wedding (Eds.), *Current Psychotherapies.* Itasca, IL: F. E. Peacock Publishers (1989).

4

TECHNOLOGY IN
REHABILITATIVE AUDIOLOGY

15

Cochlear Implants

ANNE L. BEITER, M.S., JUDITH A. BRIMACOMBE, M.A.

••

Cochlear implants are biomedical electronic devices that convert sound into electrical current for the purpose of directly stimulating remaining auditory nerve fibers to produce hearing sensations. Research in the area of electrical stimulation of the auditory system has an extensive history (see Simmons, 1966, for a review of early investigations); however, it has been only in the last 20 years that implantable devices have been developed for the purpose of long-term electrical stimulation in humans. During this relatively short period of time, cochlear implants have evolved from single-channel systems to more complex multichannel devices. A number of authors have summarized these developments (Luxford & Brackmann, 1985; House & Berliner, 1991; Mecklenburg & Lehnhardt, 1991; Mecklenburg & Shallop, 1988; Shallop & Mecklenburg, 1987; Staller, 1985; and Tyler & Tye-Murray, 1990).

Today, cochlear implantation is considered a safe and effective medical treatment for profound bilateral hearing loss in appropriately selected adults and children.* As such, cochlear implants are no longer viewed as strictly within the realm of clinical investigation; rather, their application is regarded as an important part of routine clinical practice in the management of pro-

found deafness. Otologists, audiologists, speech-language pathologists, educators of the hearing impaired, and other interested professionals are collaborating to provide the services that will enable cochlear implant recipients to maximize benefit from their devices.

Currently, there are a number of different cochlear implant systems under development and/or investigation; however, the two systems that have been used most extensively are the 3M/House single-channel and the Nucleus 22 channel cochlear implant systems.* Although the design features of specific devices may exhibit some very elemental differences (see Tyler & Tye-Murray, 1991), there are some general principles that characterize cochlear prostheses. All systems are composed of an implantable, internal component and an externally worn microphone and processor. Acoustic signals picked up by the microphone are electrically transduced and sent via cabling to the processor so that they may be filtered, analyzed, or processed in some manner. The electrical output from the processor is then delivered to the electrode(s) implanted within or in close proximity to the cochlea. The application of electrical current at the electrode site results in direct stimulation of remaining neural elements. The resultant electrical discharge of auditory neurons proceeds up through the central auditory

---

*In November 1984, the Food and Drug Administration (FDA) approved the 3M/House single-channel device for commercial use in adults. The FDA approved commercial distribution of the Nucleus multichannel cochlear implant in adults and children in October 1985 and June 1990, respectively. Other cochlear implants are classified as investigational in the United States.

---

*The 3M Company ceased manufacturing of their system in 1987, and this device has not been implanted in adults or children for the past several years.

system, reaches the brain, and is interpreted as sound.

Nucleus 22 Channel Cochlear Implant System

The Nucleus 22 channel cochlear implant system was developed with continued collaboration between the University of Melbourne, Melbourne, Australia, and Cochlear Proprietary Limited, Sydney, Australia. Historical reviews of this multichannel cochlear implant may be found in Clark et al. (1987a) and Patrick and Clark (1991). The cochlear implant consists of the implantable receiver/stimulator and a banded electrode array. The receiver/stimulator is an electronic device composed of a custom-designed integrated circuit and a small number of passive components. This circuitry is hermetically sealed within a titanium and ceramic capsule. A platinum receiving coil and a rare-earth magnet are external to the hermetically sealed capsule and are embedded in biocompatible, medical-grade silicone rubber that is used to encase the entire package. Connected to the receiver/stimulator by ceramic feedthroughs within the package is the smooth, flexible electrode array, which has 22 evenly spaced platinum electrode bands supported on a silicone rubber carrier. The electrodes vary in a smooth taper from 0.6 to 0.4 mm and are spaced equally along the distal 17 mm of the silicone carrier. A separate, insulated platinum-iridium wire is welded to each of the electrodes, and these wires run through the carrier, connecting each band separately to the receiver/stimulator. On the proximal 8 mm of the silicone carrier are 10 additional nonstimulating platinum bands that provide extra mechanical stiffness to the array to aid in its insertion into scala tympani.

The cochlear implant is seated under the skin in a surgically created depression in the mastoid bone, and the electrode array can be inserted up to 25 mm into the cochlea. Surgical considerations and technique are discussed by Clark et al. (1987b), Clark et al. (1991a), Clark et al. (1991b), and Webb et al. (1990).

An ear-level, directional, electret microphone, transmitting coil, cables, and a body-worn speech processor compose the external portion of the system. The system is powered by a single rechargeable AA battery. The transmitting coil is kept against the skin by a rare-earth magnet that attracts to the companion magnet in the implant. The speech processor receives the electrical signals sent from the microphone, performs an analogue-to-digital (A-D) conversion, then digitally extracts and encodes specific speech parameters. The resulting digital code is routed to the transmitting coil and then on to the implanted receiver/stimulator via radio frequency (RF) transmission.

The cochlear implant receives power and the digital code from the speech processor, decodes the digital pulses, and sends biphasic electrical current pulses to selected electrodes along the implanted array. For a more detailed description of the transmission of digital signals to the cochlear implant, see Brimacombe and Beiter (in press).

The speech processor is a miniature personal computer. It contains a random access memory (RAM), which stores a patient-specific program, or MAP. An IBM PC-compatible computer, two multibit interface computer cards, a specialized interface unit, and customized software make up the programming system that the clinician uses to obtain the necessary information to create each individualized MAP and program the speech processor for daily use. Specifically, measurements of the amount of current needed to obtain a threshold and a maximum comfortable loudness level for electrical hearing are made for each electrode pair. These values will vary within an individual across the electrode array, as well as from patient to patient. The psychophysical data are digitized and compiled as part of the MAP and transmitted across the skin as part of the digital instruction code to the cochlear implant. The programming system is very flexible, which allows the clinician to easily make adjustments to the program as the cochlear implant user becomes a more experienced listener. The RAM within the speech processor can be updated almost instantaneously with a new MAP.

Coding Strategies for the Nucleus Multichannel Cochlear Implant

In cochlear implant systems, the principal function of the processor is to prepare and code the incoming acoustic information for delivery to the implant. When the signal of interest is speech, the signal processing must ultimately deliver electrical stimulation to the auditory system that reproduces percepts that are speech-like for the cochlear implant recipient. For a review of speech perception relating to signal processing, see Millar et al. (1990).

The Nucleus system uses a digital speech feature extraction technique of signal processing. This approach assumes that there are known features in the speech signal that are more important than others for perception. The original speech feature coding strategy extracted and encoded three parameters that were known to be important for speech recognition. These are the amplitude of the ongoing speech envelope, the fundamental frequency (F0), and second formant frequency (F2) in the range of approximately 800 to 4000 Hz (Tong et al., 1979; Tong et al., 1980; Tong et al., 1982). Ongoing changes in the amplitude of the acoustic signal are coded as the amount of electrical current (between the measured threshold and maximum comfortable loudness level) delivered to the electrode pair. For a given input, the actual site of stimulation within the cochlea varies, depending on the measured spectral peak in the F2 frequency range. For a sound with a relatively high F2, a more basally placed electrode is stimulated, and conversely, an input with a low F2 results in electrical stimulation toward the apical end of the cochlea. Thus, the strategy is designed to take advantage of the tonotopic organization of the cochlea to elicit different pitch sensations for the listener. The rate of pulsatile stimulation to the selected electrode pair represents the fundamental or voice pitch. For sounds that are aperiodic, the rate is random around 100 Hz, producing a noise-like percept (Blamey et al., 1987a). This strategy, referred to as the F0/F2 speech coding scheme, was used in the first wearable speech processor.

Research aimed at developing other speech feature extraction strategies that could provide additional information continued at the University of Melbourne. One of the outcomes of this research was a coding scheme that included an estimate of the first-formant frequency (F1) and amplitude in the range of 280 to 1000 Hz (Blamey et al., 1987a; Blamey et al., 1987b; Blamey & Clark, 1990; Dowell et al., 1987). This strategy, referred to as the F0/F1/F2 speech coding scheme, presents two biphasic current pulses in rapid succession to two different electrode pairs for each glottal pulse. The more basally placed electrodes track F2 and are assigned frequency boundaries within the range of 800 to 4000 Hz. The more apically placed electrodes track F1 and are assigned frequency boundaries within the range of 280 to 1000 Hz. The rate of stimulation represents the F0 estimate, as in the F0/F2 strategy. For aperiodic sounds, the rate is random around 100 Hz.

Continued research into advanced coding strategies led to the development of a scheme that extracts additional high-frequency information from the acoustic signal. This strategy, referred to as Multipeak (MPEAK), extracts, codes, and delivers the F1 and F2 estimates in addition to the amplitudes in three high-frequency bands: 2000 to 2800 Hz (Band 3), 2800 to 4000 Hz (Band 4), and 4000 Hz and above (Band 5). Three fixed basal electrodes, one for each band, are stimulated according to the amount of energy in each of these bands.

The MPEAK scheme delivers four biphasic current pulses at the F0 rate. For aperiodic signals, the rate is random between 200 and 300 Hz. In the case of voiced phonemes and environmental sounds with a low-frequency periodic component, the electrodes representing F1 and F2, as well as the electrodes assigned to track Bands 3 and 4, are stimulated. The fixed electrode representing Band 5 is not stimulated, as there is little energy above 4000 Hz for such sounds. For voiceless phonemes and environmental sounds with little periodicity, the energy in the F1 range

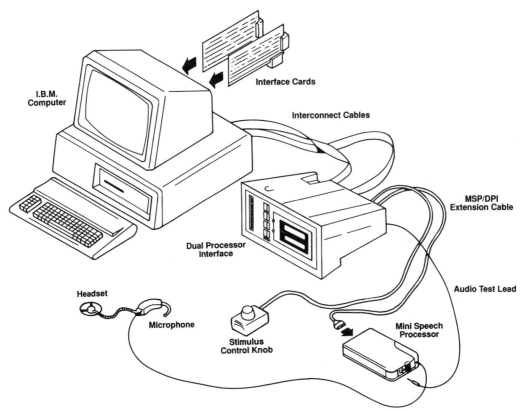

Figure 15.1. The programming system includes an IBM PC-compatible computer, two computer interface cards, an interface unit, the necessary cabling, and customized software.

is effectively zero. Consequently, the electrodes assigned to Bands 3, 4, and 5, as well as the electrode representing F2, are stimulated in rapid succession. Sequential stimulation of the electrode pairs occurs in a basal to apical direction. More information on the coding strategies used with the Nucleus system can be found in Blamey et al. (1987a, 1987b), Brimacombe and Beiter (in press), Dowell et al. (1987), Dowell et al. (1990), Koch et al. (1990), Patrick and Clark (1991), and Skinner et al. (1991).

Programming the Device

Following the surgical placement of the cochlear implant, there is typically a 4- to 6-week recuperative period prior to the programming of the speech processor. Once the surgical incision has healed and swelling over the area of the receiver/stimulator has reduced, the cochlear implant recipient returns to the clinic for the fitting of the external equipment. The first step in the fitting process is to program the speech processor. The programming system is illustrated in Figure 15.1.

Customized software is used to perform specific psychophysical tests, and an individualized MAP is configured that defines the parameters of electrical stimulation. The most important measurement is the determination of the electrical dynamic range of hearing for each electrode pair. This is accomplished by establishing the threshold and the maximum comfortable loudness level for electrical stimulation; these measures define the endpoints of the loudness growth function. This function defines how the ongoing loudness variations in speech and environmental sounds will be mapped onto the individual's electrical dynamic range and, therefore, how important loudness cues will be perceived. Electrical dynamic ranges are narrow, typically on the order of 6 to 25 dB (Shannon, 1983;

Simmons, 1966; White et al., 1984), while the amplitude variations in speech may be on the order of 30 dB.

After dynamic ranges for each stimulating electrode have been established, the software automatically assigns a frequency range to each electrode that will be used in the MAP. This assignment is made in an orderly fashion, with the high frequencies allocated to the more basally placed electrodes and the lower frequencies assigned to the more apically placed electrodes. Stimulation of the electrodes normally results in perceptions that follow the tonotopic organization of the cochlea, wherein the lowest place-pitch percept will be the most apical electrode, and the highest place-pitch percept will be the most basal electrode. Electrodes are differentially stimulated in rapid succession based on the speech processor's extraction of spectral information as described earlier in the section entitled "Coding Strategies for the Nucleus Multichannel Cochlear Implant." More information on programming the speech processor can be found in Beiter et al. (1991), Roberts (1991), and Staller et al. (1991a).

Candidate Selection

The National Center for Health Statistics has estimated that there are approximately 367,000 adults and children over the age of 3 years who are presumed to be profoundly deaf (Ries, 1982). Of those diagnosed with profound hearing loss, many will obtain varying degrees of benefit from traditional amplification (Fujikawa & Owens, 1978, 1979). While hearing aid benefit can be more difficult to objectively quantify in this population, simple audiological measures of pure-tone sensitivity are insufficient to predict those profoundly deaf individuals who may benefit from powerful, appropriately fit amplification (Boothroyd, 1989; Geers & Moog, 1989; Moeller, 1982; Owens & Raggio, 1988; Owens et al., 1985; Sims, 1982). Thus, the two general audiological criteria for selection of cochlear implant candidates—profound, bilateral sensorineural hearing loss and no significant benefit from well-fit amplification—are not always as straightforward as they might seem. An additional complicating factor is that

Table 15.1
Preoperative Patient Selection Criteria for Postlinguistically Deafened Adults

1. Profound sensorineural hearing loss, bilaterally
2. Postlinguistically deafened (as defined by acquired deafness after the age of 5 years)
3. Eighteen years of age or older
4. Little or no benefit from a hearing aid (as defined by no open-set speech discrimination when using standardized, recorded tests)
5. No radiological contraindications
6. Psychologically and motivationally suitable
7. Medical examination should show no contraindications for undergoing the operative or training procedure
   a. No deafness due to lesions of the acoustic nerve or central auditory pathway
   b. No active middle ear infection
   c. No absence of cochlear development

the degree of benefit an individual might expect to receive from a cochlear implant cannot be accurately predicted preoperatively (Fritze & Eisenwort, 1989; Gantz et al., 1988; National Institutes of Health, 1988). Having said this, one of the main objectives of the preoperative evaluation is to select those candidates who are most likely to benefit from receiving an implant. It is also important to note that the indications for prescribing a cochlear implant for both adults and children continue to evolve as devices improve and additional experience with implant recipients accumulates.

ADULT PREOPERATIVE SELECTION AND EVALUATION PROCESS

The recommended patient selection criteria, found in Table 15.1, are guidelines to the selection of those individuals who are most likely to benefit from cochlear implantation. Adults who are prelinguistically deafened do not fall under the indications for general use of a cochlear implant. The safety and efficacy of the Nucleus device in the prelinguistically deafened adult population is under clinical investigation with the FDA.

The preoperative evaluation consists of medical/surgical and audiological assessments as well as evaluations by other professionals, such as a speech-language pathologist, psychologist, or social-worker, as needed on a case-by-case basis. Several appointments will be required before a decision regarding candidacy can be made. Throughout the evaluation the prospective candidate and family receive educational counseling from the surgeon and audiologist regarding the risks and benefits of the procedure (Pope et al., 1986). It is important that the candidate be familiarized with the external hardware, counseled regarding the need for long-term repair maintenance, and told of the remote risk of internal device failure. For the Nucleus multichannel device, the internal device failure rate is less than 2%.

It is critical that adequate time be devoted to answering any questions the candidate or family has and to probing them regarding their expectations for use of the device. A series of Expectations Questionnaires have been developed for use with adults who are considering a cochlear implant (Cochlear Corporation, 1992). The intent of these questionnaires is to quantify both the prospective candidate's (Appendix 15.1) and the family member's (Appendix 15.2) expectations of device benefit. If expectations are unrealistically high, a decision regarding candidacy should be delayed until further counseling is completed to bring expectations into line. In this respect, it is extremely helpful if the prospective implant recipient and members of the family can meet and talk privately with a cochlear implant user and his or her family.

Medical/Surgical Evaluation

During the initial clinical visits a detailed medical history and thorough otologic examination are completed. One of the aims of the evaluation is to determine the etiology of the deafness and establish the age at onset and duration of profound hearing loss. Although individual patient variables in isolation have not been shown to be good predictors of postoperative performance, certain patient characteristics in combination (e.g., early onset and long duration of deafness) do affect the degree of postoperative benefit. In a recent update from the University of Iowa Cochlear Implant Project, Gantz (1992) found that 21% of the variance in postoperative open-set speech perception scores was accounted for by the variable of duration of deafness. Other variables accounted for considerably less variance; however, a number of factors were identified that, when taken in combination, may allow better prediction of postoperative performance.

During the physical examination, it is important to note any potential complicating factors, such as any previously created surgical defects, congenital anomalies, or other conditions that could require alterations to the surgical plan. In general, preexisting ear conditions should be treated prior to final determination of candidacy (Gray, 1991). In addition to profound deafness, some candidates may be blind (Martin et al., 1988), report vestibular problems, experience tinnitus, or have some other medical condition that needs to be taken into consideration during the evaluation. A general physical examination and necessary laboratory tests must be performed to establish that the patient is healthy enough to undergo surgery without undue risk.

Careful radiologic assessment of the cochleae is one of the most important components of the medical evaluation. High-resolution computerized tomography (CT) scans are essential for studying the structures of the inner ear, specifically the basal turn of the cochlea, and identifying any malformations or disease processes, such as cochlear otosclerosis. The results of imaging will be important from the standpoint of candidate exclusion, ear selection, presurgical counseling, and general surgical planning and management (Balkany & Dreisbach, 1987; Balkany et al., 1986; Pyman et al., 1990). Cochlear agenesis and absence of an auditory nerve are contraindications to cochlear implantation (Jackler et al., 1987). Other conditions such as cochlear dysplasia and partial or complete obliteration of the basal turn of the cochlea are considered relative contraindications. When osteoneogenesis is present, usually the surgeon can drill forward several millimeters in scala tympani through the new bone and achieve a partial insertion of the electrode array (Balkany & Dreisbach, 1987; Balkany et al., 1988). In some instances, surgeons have found an obliterated scala tympani but an open scala vestibuli and have placed the array into that scala (Steenerson et al., 1990).

When the physical or radiographic evaluations suggest the presence of a preexisting condition, the candidate must be fully informed and agree to proceed in light of the possibility of a less than complete insertion of a multichannel electrode array. Prior to surgery, the candidate should sign an informed consent document once the procedure, with its potential risks, has been thoroughly discussed with the surgeon.

The status of the auditory nerve can be evaluated preoperatively using electrical stimulation of the promontory or round window. This procedure involves the transtympanic placement of a needle electrode onto the area of the promontory or, alternatively, placement of a ball electrode into the round window niche. A small amount of electrical current is passed between the stimulating electrode and a surface electrode that is placed on the ipsilateral cheek or earlobe. The patient should report a consistent hearing sensation that is time-locked to the presentation of the stimulus and increases in intensity as current is increased. Individuals who do not exhibit responses to promontory or round window stimulation are generally not considered candidates for cochlear implantation, as a negative result suggests there are an insufficient number of remaining auditory nerve fibers to elicit a hearing percept (Cochlear Corporation, 1989; Lambert et al., 1987; Pyman et al., 1990). Promontory or round window stimulation may not be indicated in all cases. If a candidate demonstrates low-frequency auditory thresholds that are described as hearing rather than tactile, it may not be necessary to perform a promontory test. Whenever there is concern regarding the integrity of the auditory nerve when the patient exhibits a total hearing loss in the ear that is being considered for implantation, promontory stimulation should be performed. Promontory testing is essential when the deafness is due to head trauma, as it is possible that fracture of the temporal bone could be concomitant with severing of the acoustic nerve (Gray, 1991).

Audiological Evaluation
Level I: Air/Bone Conduction Audiometry and Immittance Testing.
The audiological assessment consists of measurements of residual hearing and middle ear function. Residual hearing is assessed using standard techniques for obtaining air- and bone-conducted pure-tone thresholds, bilaterally. Air-conduction thresholds should be determined for the frequencies ranging from 125 to 8000 Hz using a calibrated audiometer that has an output greater than 115 dB at 500 through 4000 Hz. Bone-conduction and immittance testing are performed to rule out a significant conductive component. Stapedial reflex test findings should be consistent with a profound sensorineural hearing loss. Most commonly, reflexes will be absent at frequencies above 250 Hz for those with profound sensorineural hearing loss, bilaterally. If reflexes are obtained at frequencies above 250 Hz, auditory brainstem response testing should be performed to rule out a nonorganic component to the hearing loss. Stimuli should consist of both unfiltered clicks and frequency-specific tone pips to ascertain the general configuration of the hearing loss.

Level II: Aided Audiometric and Speech Testing.
Once a profound bilateral sensorineural hearing loss has been determined, the degree of benefit obtained from amplification should be measured. First, a hearing aid evaluation should be conducted to establish whether the candidate's hearing aids are appropriate for the degree of hearing loss. If it is determined that alternative amplification would be more appropriate, a trial period is recommended. For postlinguistically deafened adults, a trial with a tactile device is not recommended because of the limited benefit derived by currently available technology (Skinner et al., 1988). The hearing aid evaluation should consist of standard electroacoustic measurements, soundfield warble-tone thresholds, and an assessment of speech discrimination ability. For a thorough discussion of hearing aid selection and evaluation, see Pollack, 1980, and Skinner, 1989.

Soundfield testing should be carried out in a monitored environment, using a measuring microphone attached to a sound-level meter. The candidate is seated facing a loudspeaker in a sound-treated room at a distance of 1 meter. The measuring probe microphone should be placed in close proximity to the hearing aid microphone. Warble-tone thresholds are assessed at frequencies ranging from 250 to 4000 Hz, and a speech detection threshold is obtained.

The speech discrimination test battery is administered in the best-aided condition, unless there is more residual hearing in one ear, warranting a monaural workup to assess the contribution of each ear to the binaural listening condition. In this case, a screening test that measures monaural and binaural open-set sentence recognition is recommended prior to the complete evaluation (Shallop, personal communication).

The speech perception battery typically includes closed- and open-set measures and an assessment of speech reading ability. Recorded materials are recommended over live-voice presentations so that results can be compared across cochlear implant centers and for a give patient over time. A thorough test battery, referred to as the Minimal Auditory Capabilities (MAC) battery, was designed by Owens and his colleagues (1985) for postlinguistically deafened adults with profound hearing loss. It includes 14 subtests that evaluate the perception of suprasegmental and segmental aspects of speech, environmental sounds recognition, and speechreading enhancement. The battery includes both easier closed-set and more difficult open-set measures. Another audiologic battery developed at the University of Iowa incorporates tests from the MAC battery and other measures devised by Tyler and his colleagues (1983). Some of the subtests in the Iowa test battery are available on video laserdisc (Tyler et al., 1986).

Although the above-mentioned batteries are excellent for research purposes, they may be impractical in a routine clinical setting. For this reason, a shorter test battery was devised that incorporates portions of the MAC and Iowa batteries. The tests included in this battery are listed in Table 15.2 (Cochlear Corporation, 1989). Mean preoperative scores on these measures for patients implanted with the Nucleus multichannel system are shown in Figures 15.2 to 15.4. The average candidate might score near chance on the closed-set Vowel and Medial Consonant tests and near or at zero on the more difficult open-set test measures. It is not uncommon for a profoundly deafened adult to score above chance on the easier closed-set Four-Choice Spondee test and show some enhancement in speechreading abilities.

Table 15.2
Recommended Audiologic Test Battery for Evaluation of Adult Candidates

Level I	Air/bone conduction audiometry and immittance testing
	Pure-tone thresholds under headphones
	Bone conduction thresholds
	Tympanomety
	Middle ear reflexes
	Auditory brainstem response testing (optional)
Level II	Aided audiometric and speech testing
	Initial hearing aid evaluation
	Trial with an appropriate hearing aid (when indicated)
Level III	Speech recognition testing
	Closed-Set
	Four-Choice Spondee
	Vowel
	Medial Consonant
	Open-Set
	Monosyllabic Words (NU #6)
	Word score
	Phoneme score
	CID Sentences
	Iowa Sentences Without Context
	Speechreading Enhancement
	CID Sentences
	Speech reading only
	Speech reading with sound

Once the medical and audiologic assessments have been completed, the cochlear implant team should discuss the candidate's preoperative profile. The medical findings are reviewed, paying close attention to the results of the high-resolution CT scans. The audiologic findings are discussed in relation to the potential for postoperative benefit based on findings from a large pool of implant recipients (Berliner, 1985).

PEDIATRIC PREOPERATIVE SELECTION AND EVALUATION PROCESS

The clinical evaluation of potential pediatric cochlear implant candidates involves professionals from otolaryngology, audiology, speech-language pathology, psychology, and education. Additionally, other disciplines may be added to the team as necessary on a case-by-case basis. The family also plays an integral role on the team.

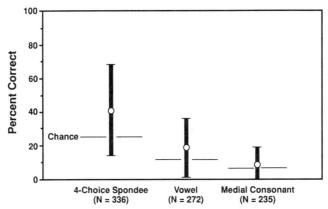

Figure 15.2. Preoperative means and standard deviations for selected closed-set speech identification tests. Chance performance also is indicated for each measure.

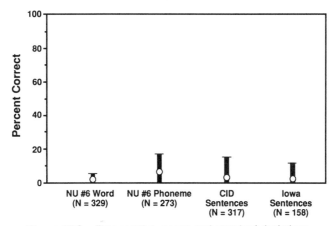

Figure 15.3. Preoperative means and standard deviations for selected open-set speech recognition tests.

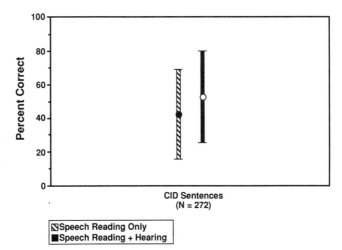

Figure 15.4. Preoperative means and standard deviations on the Visual Enhancement subtest of the MAC Battery for 272 postlinguistically deafened adults.

When the candidate is a young child, the parents assume the responsibility of deciding whether to pursue cochlear implantation as an option for their child. Ideally, the parents have accepted their child's deafness, have been informed regarding the various treatment options available, understand the long-term commitment to the child's habilitation, and support it fully. When the child is an adolescent or teenager, the team members must carefully examine the child's own feelings, expectations, and desires surrounding implantation. Older children who are going through the evaluation process solely because of parental wishes are not good cochlear implant candidates.

Sample questionnaires have been developed to assess the expectations of the pediatric candidate (Appendix 15.3) and the parents (Appendix 15.4). If expectations for device benefit are unrealistic, additional counseling is needed. One common unrealistic expectation is that the child will begin to speak intelligibly following implantation. Although this goal may be realized long term, it is important to counsel parents that this is a secondary benefit of implantation and that it may take many months or years of intervention before it is achieved. When counseling regarding the long-term commitment to habilitation, an effective strategy is to arrange for the family to meet with another family who has gone through the same decision-making process and who has an implanted child. Written material should be provided to the family. It should include information on the impact of deafness, how a cochlear implant functions, how children are evaluated prior to implantation, the surgery, the device fitting process, equipment troubleshooting suggestions, and the postimplantation habilitation (Cochlear Corporation, 1991).

The educator plays an important role on the team during the preoperative evaluation as well as during the postoperative habilitation and long-term management of the child. Early in the selection process, the school system and the child's teacher should be informed that the child is being considered for a cochlear implant and be invited to the team meetings. Specific information about the cochlear implant must be provided and any misconceptions the teachers have must be resolved. Preoperatively, the teacher provides information to the team regarding the child's functional use of amplification, his or her general learning style, the existence of any learning difficulties, and his or her overall communication abilities within the classroom. Prior to surgery, the child's teacher should introduce the entire class to the concept of what a cochlear implant is and how it works. Such materials are available for the classroom teacher (Cochlear Corporation, 1990). This will help the child successfully integrate into the class following the surgery and the initial fitting of the external equipment. Postoperatively, the classroom teacher will be responsible for verifying that the external equipment is functioning and for performing basic troubleshooting of the equipment.

The recommended selection criteria for children considered for cochlear implantation are found in Table 15.3. They are somewhat nonspecific, allowing the pediatric cochlear implant team to evaluate each child within a more individualized context. Currently, children under 2 years old are not considered candidates; however, both prelinguistically and postlinguistically deaf children are appropriate candidates for the procedure. Prior to age 2 years, it may be difficult to verify profound bilateral deafness or quantify the amount of benefit the child receives from amplification. From a surgical perspective, the implantation of children under 2 years may be technically feasible; however, it is considered a relative contraindication because of potential problems that may result from maturation of the skull (Mangham & Luxford, 1986).

The recommendation that the child be enrolled in an educational program that places strong emphasis on the development of auditory/oral communication underscores the fact that such abilities will not develop without the appropriate habilitation. This may suggest modifications to the individualized educational plan. In some cases it may be necessary to implement changes in the child's educational placement before proceeding with cochlear implantation (Beiter et al., 1991; Boothroyd et al., 1991).

Table 15.3
Recommended Audiologic Test Battery for Evaluation of Pediatric Candidates

Level I	Air/bone conduction audiometry and immittance testing
	Pure-tone thresholds under headphones
	Typanomety
	Middle ear reflexes
	Auditory brainstem response testing (optional)
	Hearing aid evaluation
	Hearing aid and/or vibrotactile aid trial (when indicated)[a]
	Pretraining (when indicated)[b]
Level II	Speech perception evaluation
	Closed-Set
	CID Early Speech Perception Battery
	Low Verbal Version (use only with those children who do not have enough language to take the standard version)
	Standard Version
	NU-CHIPS
	Open-Set
	GASP Words
	MAC Spondee Recognition
	CID Sentences
	PBK Words
	Measure of Speechreading (with and without sound)
	Craig Lipreading Inventory word subtest
	Visual Enhancement Subtest of the MAC Battery

[a] If the child has not been fitted with appropriate amplification, a minimum 6-month trial with hearing aids and/or a vibrotactile device is recommended under most conditions. An exception would be in the case of a postmeningitic child who is showing evidence on CT scans of ongoing ossification of the cochlea.
[b] Children who demonstrate minimal attending skills or who are not under stimulus/response control should be given pretraining to develop these skills prior to beginning the speech perception evaluation.

Medical/Surgical Evaluation

The preoperative medical evaluation consists of a comprehensive history, physical examination, all necessary laboratory tests, and high-resolution CT scans. The history should include information regarding the pregnancy, developmental milestones, any postnatal problems, additional handicaps, and a family history related to hearing loss. During the medical examination, any malformations of the ear should be noted. The incidence of otitis media should also be reviewed. High-resolution CT scans are essential for the evaluation of any inner ear malformations such as Mondini's dysplasia (Jackler et al., 1987a). the finding of a very narrow internal auditory canal may be a contraindication to cochlear implantation, as it may indicate that only the facial nerve is present (Jackler et al., 1987b). In older children, the viability of the auditory nerve can be assessed behaviorally using the promontory or round window stimulation procedure. Objective measures of eighth-nerve viability have been studied by Kileny and Kemink (1987) using electrophysiological techniques during preoperative promontory stimulation testing. As these procedures are refined, they may prove useful in the assessment of very young children when there is concern regarding the status of the auditory nerve.

Audiological Evaluation

The audiological evaluation of children for a cochlear implant follows many of the same steps described for adults, with the exception that the test materials for the assessment of benefit from amplification will be different and the evaluation process may take longer. In addition, if the child has never worn appropriate amplification, an extended trial (i.e., 6 months) is recommended. For very young children, pretraining may be an important component of the trial period (Beiter et al., 1991; Staller et al., 1991a). During the pretraining, basic auditory concepts are taught, leading to the development of conditioned responses to acoustic stimuli. In addition, the child should be enrolled in a program that stresses the meaningful use of audition. If progress with traditional amplification is noted, the decision regarding implant candidacy may be postponed until a more thorough evaluation of benefit from hearing aids can be completed (Northern, 1986).

Once a pediatric candidate has been determined to be profoundly deaf bilaterally using standard behavioral audiometry, immittance testing should be performed to identify any conductive component and to confirm the profound nature of the deafness through stapedial reflex testing. Electrophysiological measures may be used to substantiate the diagnosis but should not be used exclusively to determine candidacy. That is, some behavioral audiometric testing must be performed under headphones so that frequency-specific information can be obtained for each ear.

The speech perception tests used to evaluate the benefits obtained from traditional amplification will vary depending on the age and language abilities of the child. A hierarchy of tests is shown in Table 15.3. For the very young child with extremely limited receptive vocabulary, the low-verbal version of the CID Early Speech Perception (ESP) Battery (Moog & Geers, 1990) may be the most appropriate measure. For children with a richer receptive vocabulary, the standard version of the same test is used. The battery consists of three closed-set subtests that evaluate the child's ability to use suprasegmental and segmental information. The ESP Battery has several strengths: *(1)* It incorporates a hierarchy of skill levels; *(2)* the vocabulary is appropriate for young deaf children; *(3)* pictures or objects depict the auditory stimuli; and *(4)* stimuli are recorded but may be presented live voice if necessary (Staller et al., 1991a).

The Northwestern University Children's Perception of Speech (NU-CHIPS) test is a standardized, recorded, closed-set test (Elliott & Katz, 1980) consisting of monosyllabic words. It is appropriate only for children with more extensive vocabularies.

Tests of open-set word or sentence recognition range in difficulty and include the Glendonald Auditory Screening Procedure (GASP) (Erber, 19892), Spondee Recognition subtest from the MAC Battery, CID Sentences, and the phonetically balanced kindergarten list of monosyllabic words (PBKs) (Haskins, 1949). The GASP word and sentence subtests are the easiest of the open-set measures, primarily because of the use of simple vocabulary.

A measure of speechreading ability should be obtained also. This may prove difficult, especially with young children, given their short attention spans and the difficulty of the task. The Craig Lipreading Inventory (Jeffers & Barley, 1977) uses a picture-pointing task and relatively simple vocabulary. Older children with late-onset deafness may be tested using adult material such as the Visual Enhancement subtest of the MAC Battery.

Other test measures, devised by Osberger and colleagues (1991), include the Change/No Change test, the Screening Inventory of Perception Skills, the Minimal Pairs test, the Hoosier Auditory Visual Enhancement test, and the modified open-set Common Phrases test. In addition, the Monosyllable Trochee Spondee (MTS) test (Erber & Alencewicz, 1976), the Discrimination After Training task (Thielemeir, 1982), and the Word Intelligibility by Picture Identification (WIPI) (Lerman et al., 1965) have been used to assess suprasegmental and segmental discrimination abilities.

Children who demonstrate open-set auditory-only word or sentence recognition abilities are not considered to be candidates for a cochlear implant at this time. In addition, children who score significantly above chance on closed-set tasks that require the perception of spectral cues (e.g., NU-CHIPS test) also are not candidates. Poor performance on open-set speech recognition tasks may not reflect the child's ability to use spectral information. Rather, poor performance on these measures may be related to the limited receptive and expressive language skills demonstrated by many profoundly deaf children. For this reason, only children who perform at chance levels on closed-set word identification tests are considered for implantation (Beiter et al., 1991).

Auditory Training

Following the fitting of the external equipment, an individualized program of auditory training should be initiated. The length of this training will vary for each individual, extending from 4 to 10 weeks for a postlinguistically deafened adult, to long-term habilitation for a prelinguistically deafened child. It is important to begin auditory training at a level wherein the tasks are not too difficult for the individual.

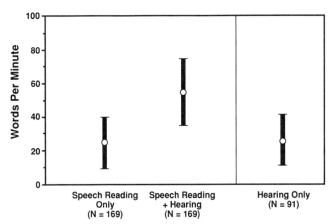

Figure 15.5. Means and standard deviations for speech tracking in three conditions postoperatively: speechreading only, speechreading plus hearing, hearing only.

In this way, progress can be based on achievements, and discouragement on the patient's part can be minimized. Screening tests can be used to determine the level where an individual should begin his or her training (Mecklenburg et al., 1987).

A multisensory approach to auditory training is recommended, as individuals will use all cues available to them in their everyday environment. For this reason training often begins with speech stimuli presented in an auditory-visual context. After success at this level, auditory-only speech material may be introduced. Initially, this material is presented in a closed-set format; later, contextually based open-set material can be used. Mecklenburg and colleagues (1987) provide an excellent hierarchy of materials.

Historically, both analytic and synthetic speech materials have been employed. The most common analytic materials have been vowels and consonants presented in a nonsense syllable paradigm in three conditions: speechreading only, speechreading plus hearing, and hearing only. The most commonly used synthetic task has been continuous discourse speech tracking (De Filippo & Scott, 1978). It is an interactive technique wherein the clinician verbally sends contextual material to the patient, who is required to repeat it back verbatim with 100% accuracy. A number of prompts and strategies are used to assure 100% reception of the information by the listener. Results are described as the number of words per minute correctly received by the listener. Ac-

cording to De Filippo and Scott, continuous discourse or speech tracking more closely mimics a true communication process, as compared to merely repeating unrelated sentences. Speech tracking provides a measure of communication efficiency. Several investigators have noted weaknesses with the tracking technique. The tracking rate can be influenced by the familiarity with and level of difficulty of the material, the speaking rate of the clinician and the patient, and the types of strategies and prompts used (Matthies & Carney, 1988; Tye-Murray & Tyler, 1988).

Figure 15.5 presents the mean speech tracking scores achieved by a group of postlinguistically deafened adult Nucleus multichannel cochlear implant recipients during their rehabilitation period (average number of sessions was five). For these individuals, scores in the speechreading plus hearing condition were significantly better ($p < 0.001$) than in the speechreading-only condition. Some patients could perform the speech tracking task in the hearing-only condition, achieving a mean score of 26 words per minute (wpm). It is interesting to note that for these subjects, scores in the hearing-only condition were very similar to those obtained in the speechreading-only condition.

For children, the type and frequency of auditory training must be based on the needs of the child. Factors such as age at onset of hearing loss, length of sensory deprivation, and dependence on spoken language affect the course of training and the

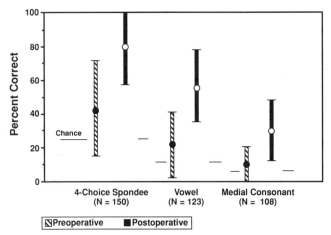

Figure 15.6. Preoperative and postoperative paired comparisons for selected closed-set speech identi-fication tests. Means and standard deviations are displayed.

rate of progress that can be expected for a given child. Brackett (1991) has divided children into four training categories based on these factors affecting progress. The categories are *(1)* postlinguistic, short-term deafness, age-appropriate language; *(2)* congenital or prelinguistic, short-term deafness (2 to 4 years old), limited-to-poor language; *(3)* postlinguistic, long-term deafness (greater than 4 years old), fair-to-good language; and *(4)* congenital or prelinguistic, long-term deafness (greater than 4 years old), limited-to-poor spoken language. Each of these groups will make progress over time, but the rates will vary. In general, Brackett recommends a synthetic, inte-grated approach that incorporates listening into all daily activities. Specific activities for auditory skill development in children have been developed by Erber (1982), Low-ell and Stoner (1960), Schuyler et al. (1985), and Stout and Windle (1986). A relatively complete listing of aural rehabilitation ma-terials for adults and children can be or-dered from the American Speech-Lan-guage-Hearing Association (1990).

Results

POSTLINGUISTICALLY DEAFENED ADULTS

Over 7000 adults and children have been implanted with various types of cochlear implants worldwide; 5000 have received the Nucleus multichannel system. The ben-efit obtained from cochlear implants has been found to vary depending on the type of device, for example, single-channel ver-sus multichannel systems (Brimacombe et al., 1989a; Gantz et al., 1988; Mangham & Kuprenas, 1989; Tyler et al., 1989). Benefit has also been variable across the population of patients implanted (Cohen et al., 1985; Dorman et al., 1989; Gantz, 1992, Gantz et al., 1988; Staller et al., 1991a, 1991b). Fac-tors affecting this interpatient variability may include the age at implantation, the age at onset of profound deafness, the years of sensory deprivation, the degree of auditory nerve survival, and the cognitive processing abilities of the individual.

Figures 15.6 and 15.7 present the pre- and postoperative scores obtained on sev-eral closed- and open-set tests of speech per-ception by postlinguistically deafened adults using the Nucleus multichannel cochlear implant system. Figure 15.8 pre-sents the means and standard deviations for the test of speechreading enhancement.

A number of researchers have reported similar findings for other postlinguistically deafened adult multichannel cochlear im-plant recipients. In general, these investi-gators have found that adults demonstrate a range of speech perception abilities. Typ-ically, an enhancement in speechreading ability is noted, and performance on closed- and open-set speech perception measures improves postoperatively, with a great deal of interpatient variability observed (Bri-macombe et al., 1989a; Cohen et al., 1985;

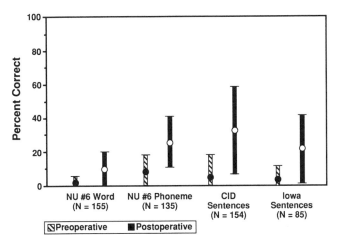

Figure 15.7. Preoperative and postoperative paired comparisons for selected open-set speech recogni- tion tests Means and standard deviations are dis- played.

Dorman et al., 1989; Dowell et al., 1987; Dowell et al., 1990; Gantz et al., 1988; Skinner et al., 1988; Skinner et al., 1991; Spivak & Waltzman, 1990; Tyler & Tye-Murray, 1991). Several investigators have also studied the range of abilities of adult Nucleus multichannel recipients when using the telephone (Brimacombe et al., 1989b; Brown et al., 1985; Cohen et al., 1989; Gissey, 1988). In one study of 102 adults (Brimacombe et al., 1989b), performance varied as a function of the difficulty of the test material administered over both long-distance and local telephone lines. Average scores were 84% for number identification, 53% for letter identification, 50% for overlearned speech, and 28% for the Psychoacoustic Laboratory (PAL) sentences (Hudgins et al., 1947).

CHILDREN

An FDA-approved, multisited clinical investigation to study the safety and effectiveness of the Nucleus multichannel cochlear implant in children commenced in 1986 and was completed in June 1990 (Staller, 1991c). As with adults, the demonstration of effectiveness of the prosthesis was related primarily to improvements in speech perception abilities in the listening-only condition and to speechreading enhancements. Preoperatively, each child was administered a set of speech discrimination measures that was appropriate for his or her age and linguistic level. Individual performance in the best aided condition was

compared to the child's postoperative performance with the cochlear implant on the same tests after 1 year of device use. The data from 80 children were analyzed and submitted to the FDA to establish the effectiveness of the implant in profoundly deaf children. However, as a part of the conditions of approval for use of the device, the postoperative performance of 178 children is monitored annually. Children must demonstrate a profound bilateral sensorineural hearing loss to qualify for cochlear implantation.

One of the simplest tests administered to children is the Discrimination after Training (DAT) test. This test has 12 levels that are ordered hierarchically from simple detection through the identification of one spondee word from four alternatives. Preoperatively, group mean performance with amplification reached level 5, indicating the perception of nonspectral, suprasegmental cues (e.g., duration, rhythm, syllable number). After 1 year of device use, the mean performance reached level 9, the discrimination of one spondee from two alternatives. Success at this level requires the perception of some spectral information. In addition, at the 1-year postoperative follow-up, 34% of the children tested passed level 12. By 2 years, 51% of the children passed the highest level, indicating that this test was now too easy for many of the children.

The Monosyllable Trochee Spondee (MTS) test consists of 12 pictured stimuli: four monosyllabic, four spondaic, and four

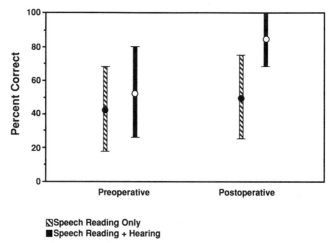

Speech Reading Only
Speech Reading + Hearing

Figure 15.8. Preoperative and postoperative paired comparisons on the Visual Enhancement subtest of the MAC Battery for 117 postlinguistically deafened adults.

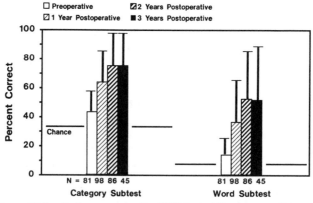

□ Preoperative   ⧄ 2 Years Postoperative
⧄ 1 Year Postoperative   ■ 3 Years Postoperative

Figure 15.9. Performance on the MTS test at the preoperative and three annual postoperative intervals. Means and standard deviations are displayed.

trochaic words. In the category subtest, a response is scored as correct if it falls within the correct syllabic category. For the more difficult word subtest, a response is correct only if the correct stimulus is chosen. Figure 15.9 presents preoperative, and 1-, 2-, and 3-year postoperative data for all children who have been administered this test. Preoperatively, as a group, the children did not score significantly above chance on either subtest. At the 1-year postoperative evaluation, mean performance increased to 63% on the category subtest and to almost 40% on the word subtest. On average, performance continued to improve with longer use of the device. Figure 15.10 presents paired comparisons for a group of 31 children who have been tested at the three annual postoperative evaluations. Significant

increases in performance were noted for both subtests over time.

The GASP administered as an open-set task has been used to record the beginnings of open-set word recognition in young children with cochlear implants, for whom more standardized tests are inappropriate because of their limited spoken language abilities. The word subtest of the GASP consists of 12 common words that typically would be within the vocabulary of most young children. Preoperatively, the children scored 0% on open-set word or recognition tests. Mean postoperative scores for all children administered the word subtest of the GASP at the 1-, 2-, and 3-year evaluations are displayed in Figure 15.11. Performance ranged from 24% after 1 year of experience to 41% at the 3-year evalua-

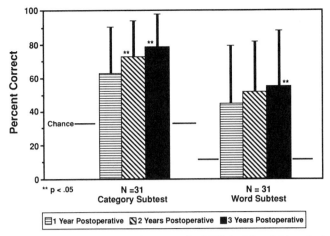

Figure 15.10. Paired comparisons on the MTS test for children tested at three postoperative intervals. Means and standard deviations are displayed.

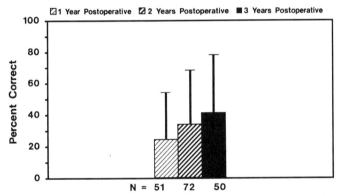

Figure 15.11. Performance on the GASP word subtest at three postoperative intervals. Means and standard deviations are displayed.

tion. Considerable variability in performance was noted across children, as indicated by the standard deviations. The GASP paired comparison data are found in Figure 15.12. Thirty-two children have been tested at both the first and second annual evaluations, and 11 children have been administered this test at all three postoperative intervals. Significant increases in performance were observed at each postoperative evaluation. Mean scores improved from 26% at 1 year to 56% after 3 years of device use.

To summarize, children using this cochlear implant have demonstrated significant improvements on both easy and more difficult closed-set speech perception measures. Many of the children, including some prelinguistically deafened children, have the ability to recognize simple words in an auditory-only, open-set format. Finally, continued monitoring of children's performance over time suggests that these children do improve as they gain more experience and training with the device.

Future Directions

Within the last decade a number of improvements in cochlear implant design have been introduced. The addition of more sophisticated speech coding strategies has led to improvements in performance for many cochlear implant recipients (Dowell et al., 1987; Dowell et al., 1990; Skinner et al., 1991; Tye-Murray et al., 1990). Research is currently underway to determine whether patient performance can be improved by using a greater number of chan-

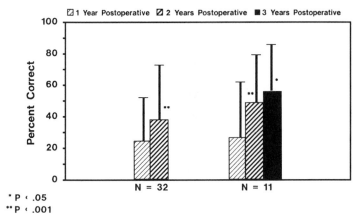

Figure 15.12. Paired comparisons on the GASP word subtest for two groups of subjects: those tested at the first and second annual postoperative intervals and those tested at all three annual postoperative intervals. Means and standard deviations are displayed.

nels of electrical stimulation and higher stimulation rates to preserve the temporal fine structure of speech and environmental sounds (McKay et al., 1991, 1992; Wilson et al., 1991). Preliminary results from these two groups of investigators are encouraging. In their studies, remarkably high scores were achieved by a small number of research subjects using experimental speech processors. The tests used were the most difficult in any battery, that is open-set monosyllabic words and sentences presented in noise.

In the future, improvements in digital signal processing may enable better preservation of important amplitude cues in speech and environment sounds, such as music. Improved noise reduction techniques may permit cochlear implant recipients to better understand in difficult listening environments. As microelectronic technology develops, devices will become smaller.

Further applications of cochlear implant technology to individuals who have small amounts of residual hearing are currently underway. Preliminary results of a clinical trial with postlinguistically hearing-impaired adults with a severe-to-profound loss have shown that these subjects' speech perception abilities can be significantly improved with the use of a multichannel cochlear implant (Arndt et al., 1991). It has also been suggested that some children who achieve marginal benefit from traditional amplification may benefit from current multichannel cochlear implant technology (Osberger et al., 1991). As cochlear implant technology improves, providing better levels of speech recognition, more patients with severe hearing losses and marginal benefit from amplification may be considered cochlear implant candidates.

References

American Speech-Language-Hearing Association, *Aural Rehabilitation: An Annotated Bibliography*, 32 (Suppl. 1) (1990).

Arndt, P.L., Brimacombe, J.A., Staller, S.J., and Beiter, A.L., Multichannel cochlear implantation in adults with residual hearing. Presented at American Academy of Otolaryngology Head and Neck Surgery, Kansas City, MO (September 24, 1991).

Balkany, T.J., Dreisbach, J.N., and Seibert, C.E., Radiographic imaging of the cochlear implant candidate: preliminary results. *Otolaryngol. Head Neck Surg.*, 95, 592–597 (1986).

Balkany, T.J., and Dreisbach, J.N., Surgical anatomy and radiographic imaging of cochlear implant surgery. *Am. J. Otol.*, 8, 195–200 (1987).

Balkany, T.J., Gantz, B.J., and Nadol, J.B., Multichannel cochlear implants in partially ossified cochleas. *Ann. Otol. Rhinol. Laryngol.*, 97 (Suppl. 135) 3–7 (1988).

Beiter, A.L., Staller, S.J., and Dowell, R.C., Evaluation and device programming in children. In S.J. Staller (Ed.), Multichannel Cochlear Implants in Children. *Ear Hear. Suppl.*, 12(4), 25S–33S (1991).

Berliner, K.I., Selection of cochlear implant patients. In R.A. Schindler and M.M. Merzenich (Eds.), *Cochlear Implants*. New York: Raven Press, pp. 395–402 (1985).

Blamey, P.J., and Clark, G.M., Place coding of vowel formants for cochlear implant patients. *J. Acoust. Soc. Am.*, 88, 667–673 (1990).

Blamey, P.J., Dowell, R.C., Brown, A.M., Clark, G.M., and Seligman, P.M., Vowel and consonant recognition of cochlear implant patients using formant-estimating speech processors. *J. Acoust. Soc. Am.*, 82, 48–57 (1987b).

Blamey, P.J., Dowell, R.C., Clark, G.M., and Seligman, P.M., Acoustic parameters measured by a formant-estimating speech processor for a multiple-channel cochlear implant. *J. Acoust. Soc. Am.*, 82, 38–47 (1987a).

Boothroyd, A., Hearing aids, cochlear implants, and profoundly deaf children. In E. Owens and D.K. Kessler (Eds.), *Cochlear Implants in Young Deaf Children*. Boston: College Hill Press, pp. 81–100 (1989).

Boothroyd, A., Geers, A.E., and Moog, J.S., Practical implications of cochlear implants in children. In S.J. Staller (Ed.), Multichannel Cochlear Implants in Children. *Ear Hear. Suppl* 12,(4),81S–89S (1991).

Brackett, D., Rehabilitation/education strategies for children with cochlear implants. *Cochlear Corp. Clin. Bull.*, 1–5 (November 1991).

Brimacombe, J.A., Beiter, A.L., Barker, M.J., Mikami, K.A, and Staller, S.J, Comparative results with speech recognition testing with subjects who have used both a single-channel and a multichannel cochlear implant system. In B. Fraysse and N. Cochard (Eds.), *Cochlear Implants: Acquisitions and Controversies*. Toulouse: Paragraphic, pp. 427–444 (1989a).

Brimacombe, J.A., Beiter, A.L., Barker, M.J., Mikami, K.A., O'Meilia, R.M., and Shallop, J.K., Speech recognition abilities over the telephone for Nucleus 22 channel cochlear implant recipients. In B. Fraysse and N. Cochard (Eds.), *Cochlear Implants; Acquisitions and Controversies*. Toulouse: Paragraphic, pp. 345–359 (1989b).

Brimacombe, J.A., and Beiter, A.L., The application of digital technology to cochlear implants. In R.E. Sandlin (Ed.), *Digital Hearing Aid Systems*. San Diego: Singular Press (in press).

Brown, A.M., Clark, G.M., Dowell, R.C., Martin, L.F.A., and Seligman, P.M., Telephone use by a multi-channel cochlear implant patient. *J. Laryngol. Otol.*, 99, 231–238 (1985).

Clark, G.M, Blamey, P.J., Brown, A.M., et al., The engineering of the receiver-stimulator and speech processor. In C.R. Pfaltz (Ed.), The University of Melbourne—Nucleus multi-electrode cochlear implant. *Advances in Oto-rhinolaryngology*, Vol. 38. Basel: Karger, pp. 63–84 (1987a).

Clark, G.M, Blamey, P.J., Brown, A.M., et al., The surgery. In C.R. Pfaltz (Ed.), The University of Melbourne—Nucleus multi-electrode cochlear implant. *Advances in Oto-rhinolaryngology*, Vol. 38. Basel: Karger, pp. 93–112 (1987b).

Clark, G.M., Cohen, N.L., and Shepherd, R.K., Surgical and safety considerations of multichannel cochlear implants in children. In S.J. Staller (Ed.), Multichannel Cochlear Implants in Children. *Ear Hear. Suppl.*, 12(4), 15S–24S (1991a).

Clark, G.M., Franz, B.K.-H., Pyman, B.C., and Webb, R.L., Surgery for multichannel cochlear implantation. In H. Cooper (Ed.), *Cochlear Implants: A Practical Guide*. London: Whurr Publishers Ltd., pp. 169–200 (1991b).

Cochlear Corporation, *Promontory Stimulation Manual*. Englewood, CO: Cochlear Corporation (1989).

Cochlear Corporation, *How You Hear with a Cochlear Implant*. Englewood, CO: Cochlear Corporation (1990).

Cochlear Corporation, *Parent Guide of the Mini System 22 Cochlear Implant*. Englewood, CO: Cochlear Corporation (1991).

Cochlear Corporation, *Mini System 22 Procedures Manual*. Englewood, CO: Cochlear Corporation (1992).

Cohen, N.L., Waltzman, S.B., and Shapiro, W.H., Clinical trials with a 22-channel cochlear prosthesis. *Laryngoscope*, 91, 1448–1454 (1985).

Cohen, N.L., Waltzman, S.B., and Shapiro, W.H., Telephone speech comprehension with use of the Nucleus cochlear implant. *Ann. Otol. Rhinol. Laryngol.*, 98(Suppl. 142), 8–11 (1989).

De Filippo, C.L., and Scott, B.L., A method for training and evaluating the reception of ongoing speech. *J. Acoust. Soc. Am.* 63, 1186–1192 (1978).

Dorman, M.F., Hannley, M.T., Dankowski, K., Smith, L., and McCandless, G., Word recognition by 50 patients fitted with the Symbion multichannel cochlear implant. *Ear Hear.*, 10, 44–49 (1989).

Dowell, R.C., Seligman, P.M., Blamey, P.J., and Clark, G.M., Speech perception using a two-formant 22-electrode cochlear prosthesis in quiet and in noise. *Acta Otolaryngol.*, 104, 439–446 (1987).

Dowell, R.C., Whitford, L.A,. Seligman, P.M., Franz, B.K.-H., and Clark, G.M., Preliminary results with a miniature speech processor for the 22-electrode Melbourne/Cochlear hearing prosthesis. *Otorhinolaryngol. Head Neck Surg.*, 1167–1173 (1990).

Elliott, L., and Katz, D., Northwestern University Children's Perception of Speech. St. Louis: Auditec (1980).

Erber, N., *Auditory Training*. Washington, DC: Alexander Graham Bell Association (1982).

Erber, N., and Alencewicz, C., Audiologic evaluation of deaf children. *J. Speech Hear. Disord.*, 41, 256–267 (1976).

Fritze, W., and Eisenwort, B., Statistical procedure for the preoperative prediction of the result of cochlear implantation. *Br. J. Audiol.*, 23, 293–297 (1989).

Fujikawa, S., and Osens, E., Hearing aid evaluation for persons with total postlingual hearing loss. *Arch. Otolaryngol.*, 104, 446–450 (1978).

Fujikawa, S., and Owens, E., Hearing aid evaluation for persons with postlingual hearing levels of 90 to 100 dB. *Arch. Otolaryngol.*, 105, 662–665 (1979).

Gantz, B.J., Iowa cochlear implant project. Presented at Colorado Otology Audiology Conference, Breckenridge, CO (March 4, 1992).

Gantz, B.J., Tyler, R.S., Knutson, J.F., et al., Evaluation of five different cochlear implant designs: audiological assessment and predictors of performance. *Laryngoscope*, 98, 1100–1106 (1988).

Geers, A.E., and Moog, J.S., Evaluating speech perception skills: tools for measuring benefits of cochlear implants, tactile aids, and hearing aids. In E. Owens and D.K. Kessler (Eds.), *Cochlear Implants in Young Deaf Children*. Boston: College Hill Press, pp. 227–256 (1989).

Gissey, D.M., Telephone listening abilities of cochlear implant recipients. Unpublished Master's thesis, The University of Florida, 1988.

Gray, R.F., Cochlear implants: the medical criteria for patient selection. In H. Cooper (Ed.), *Cochlear Im-*

plants: A Practical Guide. London: Whurr Publishers Ltd., pp. 146–154 (1991).

Haskins, J., Kindergarten phonetically balanced word lists (PBK). St. Louis: Auditec (1949).

House, W.F., and Berliner, K.K., Cochlear implants: from idea to clinical practice. In H. Cooper (Ed.), Cochlear Implants: A Practical Guide. London: Whurr Publishers Ltd., pp. 9–33 (1991).

Hudgins, C.V., Hawkins, J.E., Karlin, J.E., and Stevens, S.S., The development of recorded auditory tests for measuring hearing loss for speech. Laryngoscope, 47, 57–89 (1947).

Jackler, R.K., Luxford, W.M., and House, W.M., Congenital malformations of the inner ear: a classification based on embryogenesis. Laryngoscope, 90 (Suppl. 40), 2–14 (1987a).

Jackler, R.K., Luxford, W.M,. and House, W.M., Sound detection with the cochlear implant in five ears of four children with congenital malformations of the cochlea. Laryngoscope, 90 (Suppl. 40), 15–17 (1987b).

Jeffers, J., and Barley, M., Speech Reading "Lipreading." Springfield, IL: Charles C. Thomas (1977).

Kileny, P.R., and Kemink, J.L., Electrically evoked middle-latency auditory potentials in cochlear implant candidates. Arch. Otolaryngol. Head Neck Surg., 113, 1072–1077 (1987).

Koch, D.B., Seligman, P.M., Daly, C., and Whitford, L., A multipeak feature extraction coding strategy for a multichannel cochlear implant. Hear. Instru, 41, 28–32 (1990).

Lambert, P.R., Ruth, R.A., and Hodges, A.V., Meningitis and facial paresis. Arch. Otolaryngol. Head Neck Surg., 113, 1101–1103 (1987).

Lerman, J., Ross, M., and Mclauchin, R., A picture-identification test for hearing-impaired children. J. Aud. Res., 5, 273–278 (1965).

Lowell, E., and Stoner, M., Play it by ear. Los Angeles: John Tracy Clinic (1960).

Luxford, W.M., and Brackmann, D.E., The history of cochlear implants. In R.F. Gray (Ed.), Cochlear Implants. San Diego: College Hill Press, pp. 1–26 (1985).

Mangham, C.A., and Luxford, W.M., Cochlear prosthesis surgery in children. In D.J. Mecklenburg (Ed.), Cochlear Implants in Children. Sem. Hear., 7(4). New York: Thieme Medical Publishers, pp. 361–369 (1986).

Mangham, C.A., and Kuprenas, S.V., Open-set minimum auditory capability scores for House and Nucleus cochlear prostheses. Am. J. Otol., 10, 263–266 (1989).

Martin, E.L., Burnett, P.A., Himelick, T.E., Phillips, M.A., and Over, S.K., Speech recognition by a deaf-blind multichannel cochlear patient. Ear Hear., 9, 70–74 (1988).

Matthies, M.L., and Carney, A.E., A modified speech tracking procedure as a communicative performance measure. J. Speech Hear. Res., 31, 394–404 (1988).

McKay, C.M., McDermott, H.J., Vandali, A.E., and Clark, G.M., Preliminary results with a six spectral maxima sound processor for the University of Melbourne/Nucleus multiple-electrode cochlear implant. J. Otolaryngol. Soc. Australia, 6, 354–359 (1991).

McKay, C.M., McDermott, H.J., Vandali, A.E., and Clark, G.M., A comparison of speech perception of cochlear implantees using the spectral maxima sound processor (SMSP) and the MSP (MULTI-PEAK) processor. Acta Otolaryngol., 112, 752–761 (1992).

Mecklenburg, D.J., Dowell, R.C., and Jenison, V.W., Nucleus 22 Channel Cochlear Implant System Rehabilitation Manual. Englewood, CO: Cochlear Corporation (1987).

Mecklenburg, D.J, and Shallop, J.K., Cochlear implants. In N.J. Lass, L.V. McReynolds, J.L. Northern, and D.E. Yoder (Eds.), Handbook of Speech-Language Pathology and Audiology. Toronto: B.C. Decker, pp. 1355–1368 (1988).

Mecklenburg, D.J, and Lehnhardt, E., The development of cochlear implants in Europe, Asia, and Australia. In H. Cooper (Ed.), Cochlear Implants: A Practical Guide. London: Whurr Publishers Ltd., pp. 34–57 (1991).

Millar, J.B., Blamey, P.J., Tong, Y.C., Patrick, J.F., and Clark, G.M., Speech perception. In G.M. Clark, Y.C. Tong, and J.F. Patrick (Eds.), Cochlear Prostheses. Edinburgh: Churchill Livingstone, pp. 41–68 (1990).

Moeller, M.P., Hearing and speechreading assessment with the severely hearing-impaired child. In D.G. Sims, G.G. Walter, and R.L. Whitehead (Eds.), Deafness and Communication Assessment and Training. Baltimore: Williams & Wilkins, pp. 127–140 (1982).

Moog, J.S., and Geers, A.E., Early Speech Perception Battery. St. Louis: Central Institute for the Deaf (1990).

National Institutes of Health Consensus Development Conference Statement on Cochlear Implants, 7(2) (1988).

Northern, J.L., Selection of children for cochlear implantation. In D.J. Mecklenburg (Ed.), Cochlear Implants in Children. Sem. Hear., 7(4). New York: Thieme Medical Publishers, pp. 341–347 (1986).

Osberger, M.J., Miyamoto, R.T., Zimmerman-Phillips, S., et al., Independent evaluation of the speech perception abilities of children with the Nucleus 22-channel cochlear implant system. In S.J. Staller (Ed.), Multichannel Cochlear Implants in Children. Ear Hear. Suppl., 12(4), 66S–80S (1991).

Owens, E., Kessler, D.K., Raggio, M.W., and Schubert, E.D., Analysis and revision of the minimal auditory capabilities (MAC) battery. Ear Hear., 6, 280–290 (1985).

Owens, E., Kessler, D.K., Telleen, C.C., et al., The Minimal Auditory Capabilities Battery. St. Louis: Auditec (1985).

Owens, E., and Raggio, M.W., Performance inventory for profound and severe loss (PIPSL). J. Speech Hear. Disord., 53, 42–56 (1988).

Patrick, J.F., and Clark, G.M., The Nucleus 22-channel cochlear implant system. In S.J. Staller (Ed.), Multichannel Cochlear Implants in Children. Ear Hear. Suppl., 12(4), 3S–9S (1991).

Pollack, M.C. (Ed.), Amplification for the Hearing Impaired. New York: Grune & Stratton (1980).

Pope, M.L., Miyamoto, R.T., Myres, W.A., et al., Cochlear implant candidate selection. Ear Hear., 7, 71–73 (1986).

Pyman, B.C., Brown, A.M., Dowell, R.C., and Clark, G.M., Preoperative evaluation and selection of adults. In G.M. Clark, Y.C. Tong, and J.F. Patrick (Eds.), *Cochlear Prostheses*. Edinburgh: Churchill Livingstone, pp. 125–134 (1990).

Ries, P.W., Hearing ability of persons by socio-demographic and health characteristics. *U.S. Vital and Health Statistics*, Series 10, #140, Hyattsville, MD: U.S. Department of Health and Human Services (1982).

Roberts, S., Speech-processor fitting for cochlear implants. In H. Cooper (Ed.), *Cochlear Implants: A Practical Guide*. London: Whurr Publishers Ltd., pp. 201–218 (1991).

Schuyler, V.S., Rushmer, N., Arpan, R., et al., Parent-Infant Communication. Portland, OR: Infant Hearing Resource (1985).

Shallop, J.K., and Mecklenburg, D.J., Technical aspects of cochlear implants. In R.E. Sandlin (Ed.), *Handbook of Hearing Aid Amplification*. San Diego: College Hill Press, pp. 265–280 (1987).

Shannon, R.V., Multichannel electrical stimulation of the auditory nerve in man. I. Basic psychophysics. *Hear. Res..*, 11, 157–189 (1983).

Sims, D.G., Hearing and speechreading evaluation for the deaf adult. In D.G. Sims, G.G. Walter, and R.L. Whitehead (Eds.), *Deafness and Communication Assessment and Training*. Baltimore: Williams & Wilkins, pp. 141–154 (1982).

Simmons, F.B., Electrical stimulation of the auditory nerve in man. *Arch. Otolaryngol.*, 84, 2–54 (1966).

Skinner, M.W., *Hearing Aid Evaluation*. Englewood Cliffs, NJ: Prentice-Hall (1988).

Skinner, M.W., Binzer, S.M., Fredrickson, J.M., et al., Comparison of benefit from vibrotactile aid and cochlear implant for postlinguistically deaf adults. *Laryngoscope*, 98, 1092–1099 (1988).

Skinner, M.W., Holden, L.K., Holden, T.A., et al., Performance of postlinguistically deaf adults with the wearable speech processor (WSPIII) and mini speech processor (MSP) of the Nucleus multi-electrode cochlear implant. *Ear Hear.*, 12, 3–22 (1991).

Spivak, L.G., and Waltzman, S.B., Performance of cochlear implant patients as a function of time. *J. Speech Hear. Res.*, 33, 511–519 (1990).

Staller, S.J., Cochlear implant characteristics: a review of current technology. In G.A. McCandless (Ed.), Cochlear Implants, *Sem. Hear.*, New York: Thieme-Stratton, pp. 23–32 (1985).

Staller, S.J., Beiter, A.L., Brimacombe, J.A., Children and multichannel cochlear implants. In H. Cooper (Ed.), *Cochlear Implants: A Practical Guide*. London: Whurr Publishers Ltd., 283–321 (1991a).

Staller, S.J., Dowell, R.C., Beiter, A.L,. and Brimacombe, J.A., Perceptual abilities of children with the Nucleus 22-channel cochlear implant. In S.J. Staller (Ed.), Multichannel Cochlear Implants in Children. *Ear Hear. Suppl.*, 12(4), 34S–47S (1991b).

Staller, S.J. (Ed.), Multichannel Cochlear Implants in Children. *Ear Hear. Suppl.*, 12(4) (1991c).

Steenerson, R.L., Gary, L.B., and Wynens, M.S., Scala vestibuli cochlear implantation for labyrinthine ossification. *Am. J. Otol.*, 11, 360–363 (1990).

Stout, G., and Windle, J., Developmental approach to successful listening. Houston: DASL, Ltd. (1986).

Thielemeir, M., *The Discrimination after Training Test*. Los Angeles: House Ear Institute (1982).

Tong, Y.C., Black, R.C., Clark, G.M., et al., A preliminary report on a multiple-channel cochlear implant operation. *J. Laryngol. Otol.*, 93, 679–695 (1979).

Tong, Y.C., Clark, G.M., Seligman, P.M., and Patrick, J.F., Speech processing for a multiple-electrode cochlear implant prosthesis. *J. Acoust. Soc. Am..*, 1897–1899 (1980).

Tong, Y.C., Clark, G.M., Blamey, P.J., Busby, P.A., and Dowell, R.C., Psychophysical studies for two multiple-channel cochlear implant patients. *J. Acoust. Soc. Am.*, 71, 153–160 (1982).

Tye-Murray, N., and Tyler, R.S., A critique of continuous discourse tracking as a test procedure. *J. Speech Hear. Disord*, 53, 226–231 (1988).

Tye-Murray, N., Lowder, M., and Tyler, R.S., Comparison of the F0F2 and F0F1F2 processing strategies for the Cochlear Corporation cochlear implant. *Ear Hear.*, 11, 195–200 (1990).

Tyler, R., Preece, J., and Lowder, M., The Iowa cochlear implant tests. Iowa City: University of Iowa, Department of Otolaryngology–Head and Neck Surgery (1983).

Tyler, R., Preece, J., and Tye-Murray, N., The laser videodisc sentence test. Iowa City: University of Iowa, Department of Otolaryngology–Head and Neck Surgery (1986).

Tyler, R.S., Moore, B.C., and Kuk, F.K., Performance of some of the better cochlear implant patients. *J. Speech Hear. Res.*, 32, 887–911 (1989).

Tyler, R.S., and Tye-Murray, N., Cochlear implant signal-processing strategies and patient perception of speech and environmental sounds. In H. Cooper (Ed.), *Cochlear Implants: A Practical Guide*. London: Whurr Publishers Ltd., pp. 58–83 (1991).

Waltzman, S.B., Cohen, N.L., Shapiro, W.H., and Hoffman, R.A., The prognostic value of round window electrical stimulation in cochlear implant patients. *Otolaryngol. Head Neck Surg.*, 103, 102–106 (1990).

Webb, R.L., Pyman, B.C., Franz, B.K.-H., and Clark, G.M., The surgery of cochlear implantation. In G.M. Clark, Y.C. Tong, and J.F. Patrick (Eds.), *Cochlear Prostheses*. Edinburgh: Churchill Livingstone, pp. 158–180 (1990).

White, M.W., Merzenich, M.M., and Gardi, J.N., Multichannel cochlear implants. *Arch. Otolaryngol.*, 110, 493–501 (1984).

Wilson, B.S., Finley, C.C., Lawson, D.T., Wolford, R.D., Eddington, D.K., and Rabinowitz, W.M., Better speech recognition with cochlear implants. *Nature*, 352, 236–238 (1991).

APPENDIX 15.1 *Sample Expectations Questionnaire for an Adult Candidate*

NAME: _____

DATE: _____

NO. 1

CANDIDATE

ADULT EXPECTATIONS QUESTIONNAIRE

(Answer TRUE or FALSE)

When I am using the Nucleus Cochlear Implant . . .

_____ 1. Conversation over the telephone will be easy to understand.

_____ 2. Lipreading will always be a major part of my communication.

_____ 3. If there is background noise, it may always be a problem.

_____ 4. Most television programs will be easy to understand with hearing alone.

_____ 5. Sounds around me will be different from how I remember them.

_____ 6. It will be impossible for me to separate one word from another when listening to normal conversation.

_____ 7. I will be able to understand all speech without lipreading, once I have received training.

_____ 8. In an auditorium, it will usually be very difficult to understand the speaker.

_____ 9. It will be possible to hear my own voice.

_____ 10. I can be assured of better job opportunities because of better hearing.

_____ 11. Music will sound as I remember.

_____ 12. Others will not know that I have a hearing disability.

_____ 13. Speech will sound natural to me.

_____ 14. It will be necessary to undergo some training time in order to make use of the new sound sensation.

_____ 15. I will be able to tell the difference between some, but not all, voices.

APPENDIX 15.2 *Sample Expectations Questionnaire for the Family Member of an Adult Candidate*

NAME: _____

RELATION: _____

DATE: _____

NO. 1

FAMILY/FRIEND

ADULT EXPECTATIONS QUESTIONNAIRE

(Answer TRUE or FALSE)

Once my family member/friend receives the Nucleus Cochlear Implant . . .

_____ 1. It will be possible to carry on normal conversations when there is average noise at the dinner table.

_____ 2. Music will sound normal to him/her.

_____ 3. (S)he will need further training to make the best use of the new sounds.

_____ 4. (S)he will be able to understand all speech without lipreading.

_____ 5. We will be able to have a normal conversation over the telephone.

_____ 6. (S)he should be able to better control the loudness of his/her voice.

_____ 7. Background noise may still make communications more difficult.

_____ 8. (S)he should be able to recognize a number of environmental sounds after some use and training.

_____ 9. Lipreading will no longer be a major part of his/her communications.

_____ 10. Sounds will be different than what (s)he remembers.

_____ 11. It will be difficult for him/her to follow a conversation when several people are talking at once.

_____ 12. His/her deafness will no longer be a disability.

_____ 13. (S)he will be assured of better job opportunities because of improved hearing.

APPENDIX 15.3 Sample Expectations Questionnaire for a Pediatric Candidate

NAME: _____   NO. 1

AGE: _____   CANDIDATE

DATE: _____

CHILDREN'S EXPECTATIONS QUESTIONNAIRE

(Answer TRUE or FALSE)

When I am using the Nucleus Cochlear Implant . . .

_____ 1. I will be able to talk on the phone right away.

_____ 2. I will usually have to see someone's face to understand words.

_____ 3. Noise will always make hearing and understanding harder.

_____ 4. I will understand people talking on TV.

_____ 5. I will be able to notice many everyday sounds.

_____ 6. All words will sound clear to me.

_____ 7. I will be able to understand all speech without lipreading, once I have received training.

_____ 8. At school, it will usually be very difficult to understand the teacher if I can see her face.

_____ 9. I will be able to hear my own voice.

_____ 10. I won't be able to hear better in school.

_____ 11. Music will sound good to me.

_____ 12. Others will not know that I have a hearing problem.

_____ 13. Speech will sound natural to me.

_____ 14. I will have to have some training so that I can learn new sounds.

_____ 15. I will be able to tell the difference between some, but not all, voices.

APPENDIX 15.4 *Sample Expectations Questionnaire for the Family Member of a Pediatric Candidate*

NAME: _____   NO. 1
DATE: _____   PARENTS

CHILDREN'S EXPECTATIONS QUESTIONNAIRE

(Answer TRUE or FALSE)

Once my child receives the Nucleus Cochlear Implant . . .

_____ 1. It may be possible to have a normal conversation with our child when there is average noise at the dinner table—only if (s)he is looking at me.

_____ 2. Music will sound normal to him/her.

_____ 3. (S)he will need further training to make the best use of the new sounds.

_____ 4. (S)he will be able to understand speech without lipreading.

_____ 5. We will be able to have a normal conversation over the telephone.

_____ 6. (S)he should be able to better control the loudness of his/her voice.

_____ 7. Background noise may still make communication more difficult.

_____ 8. (S)he should be able to recognize a number of environmental sounds after some use and training.

_____ 9. Lipreading will no longer be a major part of his/her communications.

_____ 10. Learning to identify all sounds may be difficult.

_____ 11. It will be difficult for him/her to follow a conversation when several people are talking at once.

_____ 12. His/her deafness will no longer be a problem.

_____ 13. (S)he will be assured of better school performance because of improved hearing.

16

Assistive Technology for Deaf and Hard-of-Hearing People

CYNTHIA L. COMPTON, M.S.

All people, including those who are hearing impaired, have communication needs in three basic areas: *(1)* face-to-face communication and the enjoyment of broadcast media, *(2)* telephone communication, and *(3)* communication of the occurrence of alerting signals and situations. Historically, the profession of audiology has depended on the personal hearing aid to meet these needs—and not always with success. In the last decade, however, technological advances in the personal hearing aid, coupled with improved fitting and rehabilitative techniques, have provided us with solutions to communication problems that, in the past, could not have been resolved. Hearing aid selection considerations now include a variety of electroacoustic parameters, such as frequency response, gain, and saturation sound pressure level (SSPL), and a myriad of special features such as type of microphone (directional or omnidirectional), type of compression circuit, noise suppression circuits, type of earmold plumbing, and programmability. Still, even today, this arsenal of hearing aid technology cannot always be counted on to solve every client's receptive communication difficulties (Beck & Nance, 1989).

For example it is common for a hearing aid user to experience difficulty understanding speech in noise, from a distance, and on the telephone. A person with even a mild to moderate hearing impairment might be functionally deaf to a smoke alarm located down the hall and behind a closed door if she is in a deep sleep and has removed her hearing aids. The same person might miss the doorbell if she is listening to the television in a room located away from the doorbell chime—regardless of the fact that she is wearing her hearing aids. Finally, a child with normal hearing, but with recurrent middle ear infections or a central auditory processing disorder, is at a definite educational disadvantage when seated in a typical classroom characterized by poor room acoustics and excessive ambient noise.

Numerous auditory and nonauditory technologies—assistive devices—are available to meet these communication needs. As important as the personal hearing aid, these devices may be used in addition to or in place of the personal hearing aid, cochlear implant, or tactile device. As a profession, we must be prepared not only to fit and recommend personal amplification systems and assistive devices appropriately but also to be able to evaluate their place within the larger framework of maximizing the communication skills of the hearing-impaired person in *all* aspects of his or her daily life. Accordingly, we must also be prepared to provide the ongoing training and counseling necessary to assure successful use of the technology.

The purpose of this chapter is threefold: *(1)* to review the various types of assistive technologies, *(2)* to provide the reader with a framework for identifying the potential assistive device user and his or her specific equipment needs, and *(3)* to discuss the role of the professional in the procurement of assistive technology.

Assistive Devices: An Overview

Historically, both auditory and nonauditory devices have been grouped under the label "assistive *listening* devices"; however, it is important to recognize that not all communication involves listening, nor can all hearing-impaired people benefit from auditory technologies. Many people benefit from devices that convey information using visual and/or tactile stimuli. Thus, it is recommended that, as a group, these technologies be referred to as "assistive devices" or even "communication devices for deaf and hard-of-hearing people." These labels not only are more precise but also are more acceptable by culturally deaf individuals who may find the term "listening" offensive.

Assistive devices can be classified into three categories:

Systems to assist in face-to-face communication and in the enjoyment of broadcast media (radio, television, etc.)
Systems to assist in telephone communication
Systems to assist in the awareness and identification of environmental sounds and situations

Within each of these categories there exist auditory and nonauditory systems to accomplish these tasks.

SYSTEMS TO ASSIST IN FACE-TO-FACE COMMUNICATION AND THE RECEPTION OF BROADCAST MEDIA

Auditory Devices (Assistive Listening Devices)

Three environmental factors affect a listener's access to auditory communication—distance, background noise, and room acoustics.

Distance. Sound fades rapidly as distance increases. Even nominal distances can cause speech to become unintelligible for people with mild hearing loss.

Background noise. Classrooms and meeting areas tend to be noisy. This background noise can be generated from within the room (heating and cooling systems or movement of the occupants) or can originate from outside the room (hallway noise or traffic). For speech understanding ability to be maintained, hearing-impaired listeners need reduced background noise levels.

Room acoustics. When sound waves strike the wall of a room, they reflect off, repeatedly hitting other walls of the room. This multiple reflection or reverberation of sound disrupts speech understanding by causing multiple sound images or echoes to arrive at the listener's ears at slightly different times.

Poor listening environments are annoying to most of us, but the effect they have on hearing-impaired listeners is much more severe. Hearing aids amplify not only desired sounds but also noise. Because the hearing aid's microphone is located at the ear, and not at the sound source, it is more likely to pick up background noise as well as, or even better than, the desired sound. Assistive listening devices (ALDs) are designed to reduce the effects of distance, background noise, and reverberation. Microphones on ALDs are positioned a few inches from the speaker rather than several feet away. Like "binoculars for the ears" ALDs reach out and grab the desired sound and send it directly to the listener's ear minus the deleterious effects of distance, background noise, or poor room acoustics.

Speech loses energy as it travels from the speaker's mouth to the listener's hearing aid, and there is confusion with the background noise (Fig. 16.1A). A hardwired remote microphone system attached to a hearing aid can preserve the loudness and the integrity of the speech signal (Fig. 16.1B). As speech leaves the speaker's lips, some of it travels through the air to the hearing aid, losing energy as in Figure 16.1A. However, with a remote microphone, most of the speech enters the microphone, travels through the cord as an electrical signal, and enters the hearing aid (or earphone) of the listener, where it is changed back to sound and sent to the ear

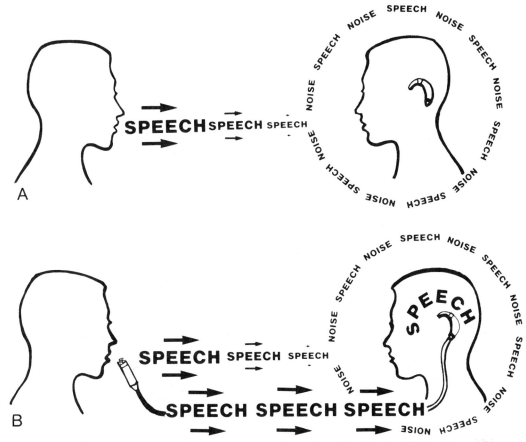

Figure 16.1. How assistive listening devices improve speech understanding. (With permission from Compton, C.L., *Assistive Devices: Doorways to In-dependence*. Washington, DC: Academy of Dispensing Audiologists [1991].)

without a loss of energy. Speech is therefore much louder than the surrounding noise, and understanding ability is improved.

Hardwired Systems. Hardwired systems physically tether the listener to the sound source (Figs. 16.2 and 16.3). The sound source—a person talking, the television, a radio—may be picked up via a remote handheld, lapel, or velcro-attached microphone. For electronic sound sources, an electrical plug-jack connection can also be used. The signal is then delivered to the listener's ears via a headset or earbuds or to a personal hearing aid via direct audio input (DAI) or inductive coupling (neckloop or silhouette inductor). Separation from the sound source is limited by the length of the cord.

Hardwired systems are of two types: hearing aid dependent systems and hearing aid independent systems.

Hearing aid dependent systems. Hearing aid dependent systems simply mean that the listening system can only be used in connection with a hearing aid. This might occur in one of two ways: using direct audio input (DAI) (Fig. 16.2A and **B**) or using inductive coupling (Fig. 16.2C). *DAI systems*, available from most behind-the-ear (BTE) hearing aid companies and some custom in-the-ear (ITE) companies, plug directly into hearing aids via an audio shoe or a plug/jack interface. The technology is also available for cochlear implants, tactile aids, and some body-type hearing aids. Lightweight and inexpensive, these systems can be used to access broadcast media via a direct plug-in connection or remote microphone.

At this time, because of impedance variations, it cannot always be assumed that any DAI system can be used with any brand

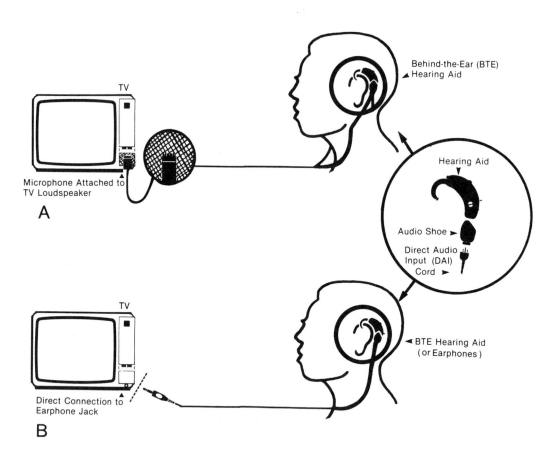

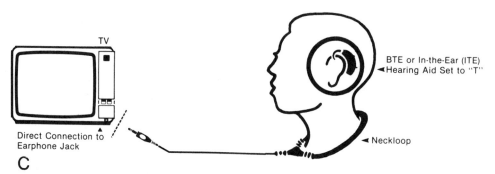

Figure 16.2. Use of hearing aid dependent hardwired systems with television. (With permission from Compton, C.L., *Assistive Devices: Doorways to In-* *dependence.* Washington, DC: Academy of Dispensing Audiologists [1991].)

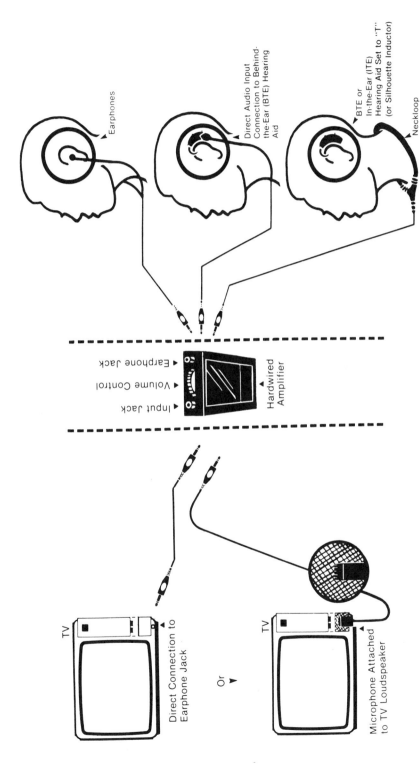

Figure 16.3. Use of hardwired personal amplification system (PAS) with television. (With permission from Compton, C.L., *Assistive Devices: Doorways to Independence.* Washington, DC: Academy of Dispensing Audiologists [1991].)

of hearing aid. Although there are exceptions and custom modifications are possible, in general, Brand "A" hearing aid must be used with its own audio shoe, cord, and microphone. Hearing aid dependent *inductive systems* include plug-in neckloops and silhouette inductors that connect directly into the earphone jack of televisions, radios, dictaphones, and other electronic devices and are powered by the voltage from the device (Fig. 16.2C).

Hearing aid independent systems. Also called personal amplification systems (PAS) or stand-alone systems, these battery-powered hardwired systems have their own microphone, amplifier, and earphone headset. However, if necessary, the system can also be used with a hearing aid, through the use of a DAI cord, neckloop, or silhouette inductor (Fig. 16.3).

PAS can serve as part-time or full-time amplification systems for those people who for one reason or another do not use a hearing aid. For those who do, PAS offers the only way a hearing aid equipped with a telecoil, but without a DAI connection, can be coupled to a remote microphone system. Several brands of PAS are available, some with built-in telecoils that allow them to also be used as induction loop receivers (discussed later). PAS can be ordered with corded microphones and extension cords for use with neckloops or headphones to allow for remote microphone placement. Some brands on the market do not have separate microphones that can be placed remotely at the sound source. Instead, the microphone and volume control are built into the amplifier. However, if an extension cord is added between the headset and the amplifier and the amplifier is placed close to the desired sound source, then an enhanced signal-to-noise ratio can be provided—the purpose of an ALD. The problem with this arrangement is that the volume control is then at the sound source (e.g., at the TV) instead of in the listener's lap where it would be more convenient.

Wireless Systems. Wireless systems consist of a battery- or AC-powered transmitter that sends some type of radio signal to a battery-powered receiver, avoiding the need for a cord between the sound source and the listener. Although more expensive than hardwired systems, wireless systems are superior when mobility and versatility are concerns. Applications include large areas such as concert and lecture halls, classrooms, courtrooms, churches and temples, theaters, museums, theme parks, arenas, sports stadiums, ports of transportation, and retirement and nursing homes. They also work well in public transportation vehicles and tour buses. Wireless systems can also be used successfully at home, in the car, in the office, at service counters, and in other situations involving small-group, one-to-one, or listenening-alone situations (e.g., TV, radio, and stereo) where a hardwired system could be used but the user prefers not to be tethered to the sound source. Each type of wireless system has its pros and cons. No one system is superior to the others. Which system is best depends on the situation in which it is to be used as well as many other factors such as personal preference, available funding, maintenance and security requirements, interference, and available technical expertise and service.

Induction loop. Induction loop technology has been used in hearing assistance applications for more than four decades. Having its roots in Europe, it is now enjoying increased popularity in the United States. The basic component of an induction loop system is a loop of wire encircling a room and connected to the output of an audio power amplifier (Fig. 16.4).

The signal fed into the amplifier can originate from a microphone, a tape recorder, a television, or a similar source. Once sound enters the system, it is converted into electrical signals. The signals are then amplified and sent through the loop, which broadcasts them to the entire room in the form of electromagnetic energy. This magnetic field varies in direct proportion to the strength and frequency of the signal being passed through the loop. The receiver for this system is the telecoil circuit in an individual's hearing aid (Fig. 165.5A and B). If a listener does not have a hearing aid, or has a hearing aid not equipped with a telecoil, reception from a loop system is impossible unless the listener uses a special telecoil receiver (Fig. 16.5C).

There are three types of telecoil receivers. One is pocket-sized and equipped with earphones, another is encased in a hand-

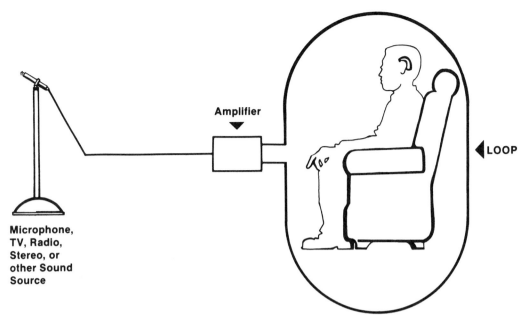

Figure 16.4. Use of an induction loop system with a behind-the-ear (BTE) hearing aid set to "T" (telecoil) position. (With permission from Compton, C.L., *Assistive Devices: Doorways to Independence*. Washington, DC: Academy of Dispensing Audiologists [1991].)

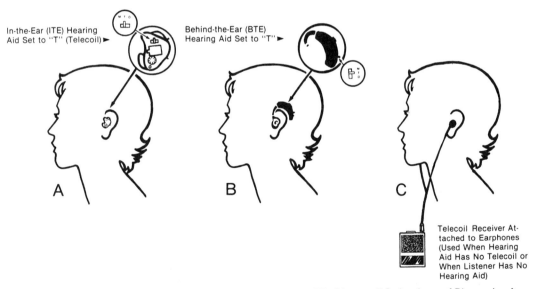

Figure 16.5. Methods of sound pickup from an induction loop system. (With permission from Compton, C.L., *Assistive Devices: Doorways to Independence*. Washington, DC: Academy of Dispensing Audiologists [1991].)

held wand (this type is often used at service counters and in museums and other public areas), and the third type is encased inside a plastic chassis that looks like either a behind-the-ear, in-the-ear, or in-the-canal type hearing aid.

Induction (or audio) loop systems are relatively inexpensive and work well when properly installed. A big advantage of loop systems is that they do not require maintenance of separate receivers, provided the listeners have telecoil-equipped hearing

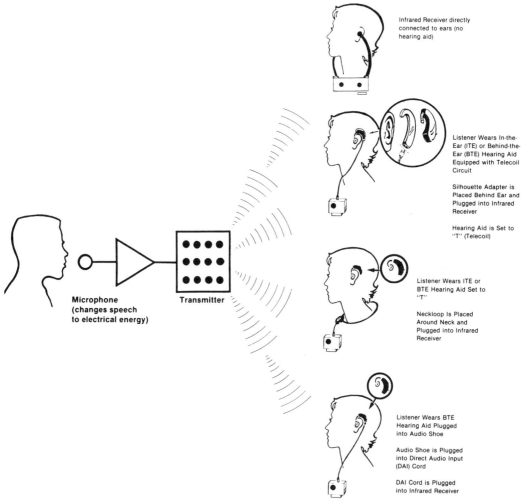

Figure 16.6. Use of an infrared transmission system. (With permission from Compton, C.L., *Assistive Devices: Doorways to Independence*. Washington, DC: Academy of Dispensing Audiologists [1991].)

aids. With the other wireless systems, a separate receiver and maintenance program are required—even if the listener uses a hearing aid, it must be connected to an infrared or FM receiver. Use of the hearing aid telecoil as a wireless receiver is also cosmetically appealing to many people. Again, if a listener does not have a hearing aid or has a hearing aid without a telecoil, then a separate receiver can be used but must be maintained.

Induction loop systems are vulnerable to electromagnetic interference (60-cycle hum) from various sources such as fluorescent light, transformers, and electrical power wiring within a building. In addition, electromagnetic energy from a loop system

can travel through solid surfaces, causing spillover of the signal into adjacent rooms. Another problem is that the strength of the magnetic signal decreases sharply with distance. Finally, sensitivity of hearing aid telecoil reception is often dependent on the spatial positioning of the coil within the hearing aid chassis. Reduction in output can occur simply by changing the plane of the telecoil in relation to the induction source. In 1988 (Gilmore & Lederman), Oval Window Audio developed a three-dimensional induction system that consists of a prefabricated configuration of three audio loops, varying in amplitude and phase, embedded in a flexible foam mat that is placed under a carpet. This design has reportedly resulted in excellent signal uniformity throughout the room in which it is placed, irrespective of hearing aid telecoil positioning. In addition, spillover of the signal between rooms has been decreased to the point that, in many cases, unlike with traditional loop systems, adjacent rooms can be looped.

When using a loop system, hearing-impaired listeners must sit within or next to the loop. Many times it is not practical or even possible to loop an entire room. Thus, hearing-impaired listeners may be required to sit within a designated looped area. If a portion of a room is looped, it usually will be toward the front of the room so that the listeners can take advantage of visual cues (e.g., speechreading) from the speaker. However, some people might not appreciate being required to sit in an assigned area. This issue should be addressed when deciding among wireless listening systems. Finally, it has often been said that the installation of a loop system can be difficult or impossible in some buildings because of the architectural characteristics and/or historic value of the buildings. It should be pointed out that, although there are exceptions, it is possible to install a loop system in most buildings, regardless of their structure or historic value, without adversely affecting structural or aesthetic integrity. For example, in Europe, where loop technology has existed for many years, it is not uncommon for ancient churches and other structures to contain induction systems.

Infrared. Infrared systems transmit sound in the form of harmless light waves that are invisible to the human eye. After the desired sound is picked up, a special transmitter/emitter sends the signal on invisible light waves to individual wireless receivers that must be worn by each listener. These receivers contain a photo detector diode or "eye" that picks up the infrared light and changes it into sound. The receiver can be worn connected to earphones or earbuds or can be used with a hearing aid via inductive pickup (neckloop or silhouette inductor) or direct audio input (Fig. 16.6).

There are no seating restrictions with infrared transmission, provided the room has a sufficient number of properly positioned infrared transmitters. In addition, because infrared light will not penetrate solid barriers, it can be used simultaneously in adjacent rooms without interference and is ideal for use in the legitimate theater, courtrooms, larger conference rooms, cinema houses, and other areas where security of the signal is a concern. Currently, most (but not all) large-area infrared systems designed for use by the hearing impaired are mono and transmit on a carrier frequency of 95 kHZ. Small transmitters are available in monaural and stereo configurations for television listening at home as well as at business meetings and other group or one-to-one situations. Because most systems used with hearing-impaired people use a 95-kHz carrier frequency,* an infrared user can usually (but not always) take his or her receiver from home and use it at the theater in order to avoid waiting in line for the theater's receivers. The limitations of infrared technology are as follows: Infrared systems cannot be used outside because they are subject to interference from sunlight. Infrared light also travels in a straight line, meaning that the strongest and clearest signal is obtained when received from direct line of transmission. In most applications, the infrared signal is also reflected by walls, ceilings, furnishings, clothing, and so on, and the reception of the signal is not completely direction. However, in large-area applications where the coverage area of the emitters may be pushed to its maximum, the infrared signal may prove to be more directional, requiring the user to face in the direction of the emitters in order to receive a clear signal.

Infrared transmitters cannot be efficiently operated by battery power because of their comparatively high power needs. Even personal transmitters must be powered by a wall outlet, limiting their use as a portable ALD. Finally, the performance of an infrared transmitter in larger rooms without the addition of remote emitters may provide a limited signal and a potentially inferior performance.

---

*Infrared systems used in locations for language translation (e.g., United Nations) or in studio recording may employ up to 12 different frequencies, or channels, of transmission. Stereo infrared systems are also available for home use by people who want to listen to music or stereo television with wireless headphones. These broadcast on two frequencies: 95 Hz and 250 kHz (Beaulac, 1991).

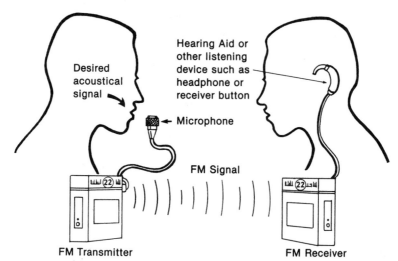

Figure 16.7. Use of an FM transmission system. (With permission from Compton, C.L., *Assistive De-* *vices: Doorways to Independence.* Washington, DC: Academy of Dispensing Audiologists [1991].)

Frequency modulation (FM). FM systems transmit the desired signal using a frequency modulated (FM) radio wave. FM systems are authorized by the Federal Communications Commission (FCC) to broadcast on a special hearing assistance band of 72.025 MHz to 75.975 MHz on either 40 narrowband (NB) or 10 wideband (WB) channels.

As with the other two wireless systems, the FM transmitter can be coupled directly to a sound source via a plug/jack connection or can pick up sound by means of a microphone. The signal is changed into an electrical signal and then into an FM radio wave that is broadcast through the air. As with infrared, each listener must wear a receiver that picks up the radio transmission and sends it to earphones or a hearing aid (via induction or DAI (Fig. 16.7).

FM systems are perhaps the most versatile of all listening systems. Easy to install, they can be used indoors or outdoors, in large areas or in small groups, in one-to-one listening situations, or while listening to media. Through the use of separate frequencies, several groups of FM users can function in the same room without interfering with each other's transmission. The transmission range of personal FM systems is approximately 150 to 200 feet, but more powerful systems are available for large areas such as auditoriums and outdoor stadiums. As with loop and infrared sys-

tems, FM systems can be connected to existing public address systems to provide communication access to both normal-hearing and hearing-impaired listeners.

Some FM systems contain hearing aids (auditory trainers), and some do not (personal FM). FM technology is being employed in the education of hearing-impaired children as well as children with central auditory processing disorders. It, like all ALDs, is also becoming popular with adults to assist in communication at home, in the workplace, and while recreating.

Limitations of FM systems include the fact that they are expensive to maintain and are subject to sporadic interference from other radio transmissions that are allowed to use the same broadcast bands (pagers, etc.). In some cases, interference is so pronounced that it limits the number of usable frequencies available. As a result, some large educational institutions cannot operate a sufficient number of FM systems to cover all of their classrooms. In an attempt to alleviate this situation, in 1992, the Federal Communications Commission (FCC) increased the total number of channels available for FM transmission from 32 to 40 (narrowband) and from 8 to 10 (wideband).

Another problem involves the fact that so many different frequencies can be used to transmit the signal. NB and WB systems operate on different channels from each other, use different frequency spacing, and possess different transmission characteristics. Because of these differences, they are essentially incompatible with each other. For example, the signal produced by an NB transmitter may not be detected by a WB receiver or may not produce the same output signal as when used with the complementary NB receiver. Conversely, depending on the channel used, a small portion of the signal produced by a WB transmitter might happen to align with an NB receiver. However, depending on the selectivity of the NB receiver, reception could be distorted. Because of this, it is not necessarily true that a user of FM transmission at home can necessarily use his or her personal FM receiver in an FM-equipped theater.

Microphone Placement and the Use of Environmental Microphones. At the beginning of this section on assistive listening devices, the importance of placing the remote microphone at the desired sound source was stressed. This is crucial for the successful use of all ALDs, hardwired or wireless. But, it is not always possible, or desirable, to clip a microphone to just one speaker. While this may be possible, and appropriate, for a lecture situation, various types of communication situations lend themselves to a variety of microphone applications.

Microphones of various types (omnidirectional, directional, directional boom, pressure zone [PZM]) may be used when listening in one-to-one or group conversations. For example, in a business meeting where everyone is seated around a table, a PZM can be conveniently placed in the center of the table and used with any of the assistive listening systems. As long as people take turns talking and the conversation occurs in a quiet room, there is usually no need to pass a microphone around. This not only speeds up conversation but may be less intrusive than asking each person to take turns using and passing a microphone. Multiple microphones can also be placed around the table for people to share.

A good quality directional boom microphone is designed to reach out and grab the desired sound in front of it in a relatively narrow range and can be a good choice for meetings or parties. But, its use requires that the listener maintain control of the microphone, pointing it directly at the person he or she desires to hear. Even in noisy rooms, this type of microphone does a very good job of picking up the speech rather than the background noise.

When used with hearing aids, ALDs can be used with the hearing aid's environmental microphone (EM) activated or deactivated. Depending on the manufacturer's philosophy, control of the EM is accomplished via the hearing aid's switch, audio shoe, or DAI cords. Sometimes it is desirable to keep the hearing aid's environmental microphone on, and sometimes it is not. For example, when a hearing-impaired person is listening to TV using an infrared system, she might also want to be able to hear her spouse's comments. However, at a noisy party, the user of a directional boom microphone might want to deactivate his hearing aid's microphone and rely on the boom mike only to pick up the desired sound.

Visual Devices

Visual devices for face-to-face communication and for television reception are used by both deaf and hard-of-hearing people and may or may not be used in conjunction with auditory technology, speechreading, or sign, oral, or cued speech interpreters.

Real-Time Captioning. Captioning of live lectures has grown in popularity in recent years and will continue to do so. Like live captioning of television, real-time captioning of lectures can be done in two ways. In the first, a transcript of the person's speech is fed into a computer system and then displayed on a projection screen (in sub- or surtitles), either alone or along with a live picture of the lecturer. In the second method, verbatim captioning of unscripted material is done by a trained court reporter, using a special computerized system that can generate the full text of the proceedings with only slight time delays.

Real-time captioning service can be purchased from a captioning vendor or provided by organizations that have purchased the necessary captioning systems. Costs of real-time captioning include the cost of the equipment plus the hourly fee of a captioner (Compton, 1992; Harkins, 1991).

Projection Techniques for Notetaking. Whereas real-time captioning provides a full, verbatim text of the proceedings of meetings, less expensive technologies can provide a lower level of output that may suffice in certain situations.

Notetaking. For example, a copy of a person's speech might be obtained ahead of time, transferred onto a transparency, and then projected on a screen during the actual lecture. An assistant can indicate with a pointer the speaker's place in the text. This technique is very inexpensive and can be helpful, particularly to hard-of-hearing people and late-deafened adults who are using auditory technologies and speechreading but who may still have difficulty understanding what is being said. If a script is not available, a competent notetaker can sit at an overhead projector and write notes as the speech is spoken. This helps people keep track of the topic at hand.

Computer-assisted notetaking. Using computer technology and a skilled typist, the same process can be carried out with even more satisfactory results. When displaying notes for a large group, the necessary equipment includes a laptop or personal computer, a projection pad, a transmissive overhead projector, and a projection screen or wall. The projection pad is connected to the computer so that what is being typed appears on the projector pad window in a liquid crystal display. The projection pad is placed on top of the platen of the overhead projector. A typist takes notes during the lecture, which then appear on the screen for the audience to read. As with real-time captioning, high-resolution projection systems are available, as is software that allows for various sizes of text. For smaller groups, the notes can be displayed on a computer monitor. This technique is quickly gaining in popularity for meetings involving deaf and hard-of-hearing people.

An important side benefit of both real-time and computer-assisted notetaking is that a hard copy of the lecture can be saved on a disk for editing and subsequent dissemination.

Notewriting. Many times situations occur where a person desires to communicate with a deaf or hard-of-hearing person who cannot understand spoken language. If, for whatever reason, an interpreter is not used, some low-tech, commonsense methods can be used to facilitate communication.

One option is for both people to simply write notes back and forth to each other. Or, a TDD or nearby computer keyboard can be used to speed up the process of writing notes back and forth.

Closed Captioning. Closed-captioned decoders provide television access to deaf as well as hard-of-hearing individuals. For many hard-of-hearing individuals, closed captioning can fill in the gaps of comprehension that amplification and speechreading cannot.* And, even people who use amplification for awareness only can often enjoy the music tracks of movies, music videos, and other shows by using an ALD along with the decoder. The Television Decoder Circuitry Act of 1990 (PL 101–431) requires that all new televisions with screens 13 inches and larger contain decoder circuitry. This eliminates the need for a separate decoder box and will make captioning accessible to millions of Americans.

Telephone Devices and Systems

Auditory Telephone Devices. ALDs for the voice telephone can be used with or without a hearing aid. When used with a hearing aid, they can be used in conjunction with the hearing aid's microphone circuit (acoustic coupling) or with the hearing aid's telecoil circuit (inductive coupling). The appropriateness of each coupling method is largely dependent on the individual's hearing impairment.

Replacement handsets. Available with round (G-style or 500-type) or square (K-style) ear and mouth pieces, these devices can be used with modular handset telephones only and must be electronically matched to the telephone to avoid distortion and to provide adequate gain. Replacement handset amplifiers can be used with or without a hearing aid, depending on the user's preference and particular hearing impairment. When used with a hearing aid telecoil, the handset must, of course, be hearing aid compatible. A person with even profound hearing impairment can often use

---

*Clients who plan to use captioning as well as speechreading and audition to receive television programming should be warned that captioned and spoken words do not occur simultaneously. Initially, this may create confusion and frustration for the television viewer.

a voice telephone successfully if fitted with a hearing aid with an adequate telecoil and a hearing aid compatible amplified replacement handset. Handsets are available with rotary volume controls as well as volume controls that turn themselves down on hang-up. Noise-canceling microphones or mute switches are also available on some handsets. These devices make telephone listening amid background noise easier.

In-line amplifiers. As with replacement handsets, in-line amplifiers must be used with modular phones. These devices attach between the body of the phone and the curly cord of the handset. On some electronic (as opposed to carbon bell ringers) phone systems, line-powered, in-line amplifiers will reduce the loudness of the user's voice to the person on the other end of the line because of power drain. In this case, a transformer- or battery-powered in-line amplifier can be employed to alleviate the problem.

Portable amplifiers. There are two types of battery-powered portable amplifiers—those that couple magnetically to the telephone and those that couple acoustically. Magnetically coupled amplifiers can be used only on hearing aid compatible phones. The Hearing Aid Compatibility Act of 1988 (PL 394) decrees that all telephones manufactured or imported for use in the United States after August 16, 1991 be hearing aid compatible. However, this legislation exempts phones used with public mobile services, private radio services, and secure telephones—telephones used for the transmission of classified or sensitive information. In addition, this legislation does not require homeowners to replace their nonhearing aid compatible telephones with compatible models. Consequently, to ensure a consumer telephone access, it is prudent to recommend a portable amplifier that couples acoustically. As of this writing, there is only one device on the market, the AT&T Portable Amplifier, which couples to the phone acoustically and can be used without a hearing aid (up to a moderate loss) or with a hearing aid's microphone or telecoil.

Portable induction systems. As of this writing, two battery-powered, acoustic-to-magnetic adapters are available that couple acoustically to any phone. The Rastronics TA-80 is an acoustic-to-magnetic (A/M)

adapter that attaches to the telephone handset's earpiece, picks up an acoustic telephone signal, and changes it to electromagnetic energy for pickup by a hearing aid's telecoil. It also can be ordered with a monaural cord terminating in a silhouette inductor. By putting both hearing aids to "T" and by holding the handset and adapter to one hearing aid and placing the silhouette over the ear next to the other hearing aid, the listener can use both hearing aids for diotic telephone reception. This device can also be used as a remote microphone system by wearing the silhouette on one ear and holding out the microphone or attaching it to a television or other sound source using an extension cord. Having no loudspeaker, this device can only be used with a hearing aid's telecoil. The second device, the AT&T Portable Amplifier, can be used with the unaided ear or coupled acoustically or inductively to a hearing aid.

Interpersonal ALDs with telephone interface. One device on the market, the Phonak TC-100 consists of a disk-shaped microphone that is attached to the earpiece of a telephone handset. A listener picks up the sound from the telephone by using a direct audio input connection from his or her hearing aid to the device. This device can also be used as a remote microphone. Although it looks similar to the Rastronics TA-80, this device does not create an electromagnetic field.

Several other hardwired and wireless interpersonal ALDs contain modular telephone interfaces, enabling the user to listen to the telephone monotically or diotically, and can be used with earphones or hearing aids (DAI or inductively). All of the devices mentioned in this section can be particularly useful for hearing-impaired people who rely on heavy telephone usage for occupational reasons; these devices can make the difference between retaining or losing such employment. The direct audio input devices are particularly helpful in situations where, because of electromagnetic interference from computers, fluorescent lighting, and so on, use of the hearing aid's telecoil for telephone listening is rendered useless.

Acoustic telepads/couplers. The feedback that occurs when coupling a hearing aid acoustically to the telephone can often be eliminated through the use of an inexpensive foam telepad or plastic coupler that slips over the telephone receiver speaker. A shortened styrofoam cup minus its bottom can also be used for this same purpose.

Telephones designed for the hearing impaired. As of this writing, two companies, Walker Sound and Williams Sound, market hearing aid compatible telephones that provide significantly increased amplification over that of traditional telephone amplifiers via an adjustable gain control built into the body of the telephone. These specialty phones also provide enhanced high-frequency responses, much like a hearing aid. Williams Sound markets two models with *adjustable* frequency responses and signal processing circuitry. Because of the power requirements of their amplifiers, the Williams Sound telephones operate in half-duplex, causing the user's voice to fade slightly if interrupted by the person on the other end of the line. Thus, communication strategies must be used to avoid this situation. The more powerful model also allows the connection of a hearing aid via DAI or induction. Both brands of telephones also contain built-in low-frequency ringers.

Nonauditory Telephone Devices. The primary means of telephone communication by people who cannot understand even amplified speech on the telephone is the Telecommunication Device for the Deaf (TDD).* The term TDD, although ostensibly a generic term for any device used by deaf, hard-of-hearing, or speech-impaired people for telephone communication, actually applies only to a narrow category of devices. Descendants of teletypewriters, today's TDDs are small terminals approximately 9″ by 12″ in size and weighing between 2 and 5 pounds. Standard TDDs transmit letters and numbers in Baudot code, which uses a five-bit character and transmits at 45.45 baud. There is normally no difficulty in communication between standard TDDs. The maximum rate of transmission is about 60 words per minute, which is consistent with a reasonable typing speed.

Many people now use personal computers (PCs) at home and in the workplace. PCs can communicate with each other over telephone lines, which make them useful as visual telephone devices. However, PCs use the American Standard Code for Information Interchange (ASCII), which is not compatible with the Baudot code used by traditional TDDs. That is, the TDD and the PC "speak" different languages and at different speeds.

TDDs are available with both Baudot and ASCII capability. ASCII TDDs can communicate at a faster rate (300 baud) with another similarly equipped TDD. However, the real advantage of an ASCII TDD is that it will allow the TDD user to communicate directly with any PC that is equipped with a modem and appropriate telecommunications software. Some PCs are equipped with "smart" modems and software that allow them to communicate with both Baudot and ASCII TDDs.

Dual-party relay systems are also available that allow the user of a voice telephone to communicate with a person using a TDD or computer via a TDD/computer-using operator. The Americans with Disabilities Act (PL 101–336) mandates that all telephone companies provide intra- and interstate relay services by July 26, 1993.

Other visually based telephone technologies include touch-tone technology, message relay systems, and facsimile (FAX) transmission. Research is also being done toward the eventual introduction of video telephones that would permit the use of sign language and speechreading over phone lines (Harkins, 1991).

Alerting Devices
Electronic. Alerting devices are often thought of as being used by only severely to profoundly hearing-impaired people. However, this technology is gaining in popularity with hard-of-hearing people who want to function independently as well as with normal-hearing individuals who need help in detecting warning sounds because of ambient noise and architectural barriers.

The first alerting devices developed focused on common signals to be monitored, such as the telephone ring, the doorbell ring, the fire alarm, the wake-up alarm, and the baby's cry. While these are still the most common requests, normal-hearing or mildly hearing-impaired people may need assistance in monitoring the increasing number of soft auditory signals used today.

---

*In 1992, the Federal Communications Commission (FCC) adopted the term "Text Telephone" (TT). Both terms, as well as the term "TTY" (teletypewriter), will probably continue to be used for some time.

These include microwave timers, telephone ring "chirps," computer prompts, intercom prompts, and apartment intercom buzzers.

Because of the great variety of sounds used in our environment, the audiologist is often involved in the recommendation of an appropriate signaling system. In many instances, a hearing aid enables a person to hear most sounds. But, if a person is not wearing his or her hearing aid (e.g., while sleeping), is in another room, is amid background noise, or is hooked up to the television with ALD, then, at these times, visual or vibrotactile alerting systems may serve as a backup system to the hearing aid.

Alerting devices monitor sounds using a microphone, a direct electrical connection, or inductive pickup. Signal transmission occurs using hardwired or wireless technology. Types of alerting stimuli include visual (bright incandescent light, strobe light), auditory (signal that is louder and/or lower in pitch), or kinesthetic (vibration [e.g., bed shakers, pocket pagers] or air stream [e.g., fan]).

Wireless systems are available that can monitor various signals in an entire home or office from within any room of the building.

Portable vibratory pagers are also available. Some of these pagers transmit over short distances (100 feet), whereas others can reach out thousands of miles, using sophisticated telecommunications systems composed of telephone lines, satellite downlinks, and local power antennas. Some paging systems are also available that alert the wearer via sound or vibration and display an alphanumeric message.

Wake-up systems include small, portable, battery-powered clocks that shake a person awake as well as AC-powered clocks that can be connected to a lamp, a strobe, a bed shaker, or a fan. A very inexpensive system consisting of a lamp, a lamp timer, and a flasher button placed in the lamp socket also can be recommended.

The monitoring of computer prompts can be accomplished through the use of a hearing aid or special visual display that can be programmed to appear on the computer monitor.

Research at the Graduate Center of the City University of New York (CUNY) and Gallaudet University is being done toward the eventual development of a visual alerting system that, using a signal processor, warns hearing-impaired drivers of important sounds such as sirens from emergency vehicles and closeby car horns but ignores all other normal traffic noise. This type of technology may eventually be used in all microphone pickup alerting systems, virtually eliminating the occurrence of false-positive warning signals (Singer, 1992; Weiss, 1991).

Visual alerting technology that meets National Fire Protection (NFPA) criteria is available to warn hearing-impaired people in the event of a fire or other emergency. This life-saving protection is accomplished using signaling devices such as strobe lights or vibration units with various intensities, often combined with compatible smoke detectors. The required signal intensity of these devices is determined by local fire protection authorities having jurisdiction. NFPA provides installation standards that are used by the local authorities and provides information as to the proper use and installation of these products. Underwriters Laboratories (UL) evaluates the product for its applicable safety requirements and signal intensity rating only (DeVoss, 1992).

If a product is found to comply with the applicable safety requirements, the company name and product identification are shown in one of UL's product directories. In the case of fire alarm signaling equipment, UL has a Fire Protection Equipment Directory (the "Brown Book") that lists the different product categories and the products listed within them. The directory is used by inspection authorities to confirm that the product has been evaluated in the category that addresses its intended use (DeVoss, 1992).

By reviewing the installation standard (NFPA) and the listing information provided in the UL product directories, an inspection authority can determine the acceptability of the final field installation. The NFPA committee responsible for the installation requirements for visual and audible signal appliances is referred to as the "Committee on Notification Appliances for Signaling Systems." Work is now underway by both UL and NFPA to improve and clarify requirements for signaling devices used by people with hearing impairment. This is extremely important, since many fire warning systems currently being marketed do not meet NFPA and UL standards yet are being purchased and are giving a false sense of security to consumers. Clearly written standards will enable us, as well as others, to recommend products that are safe as well as effective.

Mammalian. The hearing ear dog is a viable alternative to electronic alerting technology. Warm and fuzzy, a hearing ear dog is powered by food, water, and love and can provide important companionship as well as communication access and safety to its owner. Hearing ear dogs are trained professionally to alert their owners to various pertinent sounds. Almost all states have hearing dog legislation. Although the vast majority of states may give legal status equivalent to seeing eye dogs, many require some form of certification and have some limitations. For more information, contact the National Information Center on Deafness (NICD) at Gallaudet University, 800 Florida Avenue, Washington, DC 20002–3695 (202–651–5051).

SUMMARY OF OVERVIEW

As discussed, a person's communication needs may not necessarily be met through a hearing aid. In addition to the personal hearing aid, there are numerous auditory and nonauditory technologies available to help deaf and hard-of-hearing people communicate. For a more detailed, generously illustrated review of these technologies, a monograph (Harkins, 1991), and videotape and companion book (Compton, 1991) are recommended. For ordering information, see Appendix 16.1.

The Needs Assessment/ Selection Process

Audiologic assessment and the selection of appropriate technology must occur within the context of a comprehensive, individualized, reality-based communication needs assessment that looks at life-style, hearing level, speech recognition, and numerous other factors before determining which type or types of technologies are best for a client. Knowledge of the technology, coupled with a thorough case history focusing on these factors, will determine not

only whether a hearing aid or assistive devices are necessary but *what specific type of technology* should be recommended.

LIFE-STYLE

A patient's life-style plays a crucial role in deciding which type of technology is best or whether technology is needed at all. Analysis of interpersonal, telephone, and alerting communication needs should be carried out in every situation the person may encounter. These situations commonly include communication at home (private or group [e.g., retirement home]), at work, while traveling, while recreating, and at school. Let's look at these situations individually, as technology requirements often vary with each situation.

Communication Needs at Home

Communication needs at home include:

Telephone communication
TV reception
Radio, stereo reception
One-to-one conversation
Group conversation (family, relatives, friends, associates)
Reception of warning signals (e.g., telephone ring, doorbell/door knock, fire alarm, wake-up alarm, appliance signals, monitoring of children's or mate's activities from another room, and security signals)

Communication at home will necessitate technologies that are compatible with the client's, as well as his or her family's, habits. For example, an amplified handset that turns itself down on hang-up might prove to be a prudent recommendation, especially when normal-hearing family members might also use the amplifier-equipped telephone. Television listening devices equipped with remote microphones might also be desired over plug-in models where family members want to enjoy TV programming as well. Wireless alerting devices for various sounds around the home can be monitored from any room in the house having a receiver. Introducing hearing-impaired children to the use of alerting devices at an early age helps them learn cause and effect (e.g., light flashing five times means someone is at the door) as well as independence (e.g., young children can learn to wake up by themselves using visual or vibrotactile wake-up systems).

Communication Needs in a Group Home

Communication needs in a group home situation (retirement home, nursing home, half-way house, etc.) may be similar to those in the home with the addition of the following:

Communication may involve receptive conversation in common dining areas, game rooms, media rooms, and the chapel and may include conversation with medical personnel and other caregivers.

Reception of warning signals also apply unless the individual is under 24-hour supervision (wherein group home personnel would be responsible for the client's safety and security and for admission of visitors to the client's room or apartment).

In addition to hearing aids and ALDs, acoustical treatment of common areas, especially dining rooms, can do much to reduce the negative effects of noise and reverberation on communication.

Communication Needs at Work

When querying a client about communication on his or her job, one must examine the following areas:

Telephone communication (in office, while traveling)
Office conversation (one to one, meetings within office)
Lectures/seminars within or outside of office
Casual conversation with colleagues, clients (office, car, restaurants, etc.)
Speech recognition from a dictaphone or telephone answering machine
Reception of important warning signals in the office and while traveling (e.g., fire alarm, telephone ring, pager, doorbell/door knock, computer prompts)

Selecting an amplifier for an office telephone is usually more difficult than selecting one for a home phone. Numerous types of office telephones are available. Most of these phones are electronic and cannot be used with just any amplified handset. One must be aware of which handsets will work with which phones as well as of the availability of externally powered in-line amplifiers that do work with most office phones. Further, the use of a hearing aid's telecoil with the telephone might prove to be impossible in an office beset with electromagnetic interference from computers and fluorescent lighting. In this case, it might be more appropriate to couple the hearing aid to the phone by using its microphone (if loss is mild enough) and a noise-canceling handset or by using direct audio input.

The need to hear on a dictaphone may point out the need for a hearing aid equipped with a DAI connection or telecoil to allow the hearing aid to be used with a DAI or neckloop interface to the dictaphone. Difficulty hearing incoming messages on an answering machine (even with a hearing aid) may point out the need for an answering machine retrofitted with a hearing aid compatible telephone receiver (and telecoil-equipped hearing aid). Wireless listening devices such as FM, infrared, and induction loop systems are more appropriate for long-distance listening (e.g., seminars and group meetings) than would be hardwired systems that limit movement and distance from the sound source.

Communication Needs at School/College

Communication needs here may include:

Speech recognition in classrooms, lecture halls
Speech-language therapy
Auditory training
Meetings with teachers and other personnel
One-to-one or group conversation in dormitory, apartment, etc.
Telecommunications in dormitory, apartment, on and off campus
Reception of warning signals as mentioned previously, including local (client's room, apartment) and general (hallway, common areas) fire alarm systems in dormitory and/or apartment

Reception of speech and music can be improved through the use of ALDs. Traditionally, FM systems have been used in grades K through 12 in the United States for the education of hearing-impaired children. However, this technology is also finding popularity in higher education as well as in the education of children with central auditory processing problems. FM systems lend themselves nicely to classroom usage in a college setting, allowing the listener complete freedom of movement and the added advantage of being able to tape record the lecture as it is being listened to. The tape recording can then be reviewed and compared to notes at a later date. Induction loop systems are also becoming more popular in education because of their low maintenance, low cost, and cosmetic acceptability. Finally, amplified classrooms are also gaining favor with educators.*

All schools and colleges should be equipped with hearing aid compatible, amplified telephones as well as TDDs so that students have access to each other, to their parents, and to others. It is also important that parents and others be able to contact the students. The use of telephone relay systems should also be taken advantage of when needed.

Recreation and Travel

Recreational and travel activities include:

Telephone conversation (pay phone, hotel, car)

One-to-one, small- or large-group conversations in hotels, lecture halls, restaurants

Speech recognition while on indoor and outdoor tours (bus, train, plane, boat, on foot, bicycles, horses, skis, etc.)

Instruction (any type of hobby or activity where the hearing-impaired person must be able to hear instructor/guide)

Access to the telephone while traveling can be provided through the use of portable

amplifiers and small, portable TDDs. More and more airports are equipped with pay phone TDDs and FAXes. As more and more theaters, movie houses, houses of worship, and other large areas install wireless listening systems, accessibility to these locations becomes increased. However, it becomes even more important that hearing aid users be fitted with hearing aids that can be used in conjunction with these large-area systems. Regardless of how well a hearing aid is fitted, if it does not contain a telecoil, it cannot be used with a large-area listening system. This is not to say that all clients will need telecoils in their hearing aids. Nevertheless, when fitting personal amplification, one must ensure that the client can benefit from large-area listening systems in his or her community—either via a telecoil circuitry or by removing the hearing aid and using a headset. Many hearing-impaired people can benefit from ALDs when engaging in recreational activities. The listening device of choice can simply be determined by the type of activity. For example, skiing, horseback riding, hiking, and golfing occur outdoors and are mobile activities. Therefore, a personal FM system would be a convenient and effective choice for the transmission of an instructor's voice to the hearing-impaired student (or vice versa). On the other hand, quilting, usually an indoor and stationary activity, could be handled with an infrared or induction loop system. One-to-one instruction in a foreign language might be handled with a less expensive hardwired system, since the activity could occur across a table and the student's hands would not be in danger of becoming tangled in the cord connecting the teacher's microphone to the student's personal amplifier (as might occur with quilting).

Alerting devices may also be needed in all of the communication situations mentioned. Paging systems can be beneficial at home and especially on the job. Systems that alert one to the doorbell or door knock are important in all situations. Wake-up devices are important for home use as well as for business and pleasure travel. Visual, vibrotactile, or enhanced audio time reminders can be used for cooking, chemical experiments, test taking, or sports competition. Emergency alerting devices, such as

---

*An amplified classroom is simply a portable public address (PA) system. The teacher uses a wireless microphone (FM) that transmits his or her voice to an amplifier that powers several speakers placed around the room. At this writing, classroom amplification systems are available from three companies (Comtek, Telex, Phonic Ear). Classroom amplification systems can be used with normal-hearing children who must learn in classrooms characterized by poor room acoustics. In addition, children with central auditory processing difficulties or unilateral hearing loss with recurrent otitis media can benefit from the enhanced signal-to-noise ratio provided by these systems. Finally, because the transmitter broadcasts on an FM frequency, individual FM receivers also can be used to pick up the teacher's voice directly by those students who have more severe hearing difficulties and are using FM receivers with earphones or hearing aids.

smoke detectors, are a must in all situations. Proper installations of UL-approved alerting systems must be carried out in private homes, retirement homes, office buildings, schools, hotels, or other accommodations. Alerting stimuli (enhanced auditory, visual, or vibrotactile stimuli or a combination thereof) that meet the needs of occupants must be chosen. These stimuli must be effective whether the person is sleeping or awake and must be detected regardless of where the person is located. For example, a flashing strobe light, no matter how bright, will not alert a deaf-blind person to danger. Accordingly, a sighted deaf person would not be able to detect a bright strobe light if he or she is in a restroom of an office building, but the flashing signal is located in his or her office. Appropriately placed remote signalers must be installed in all locations that building occupants could possibly be—or occupants must be provided with effective body-worn emergency pagers.

COUNSELING

Following a thorough communication and audiologic assessment, the clinician should have a good foundation on which to base specific decisions concerning the need for personal amplification, assistive devices, and aural rehabilitation. Unfortunately, there are currently no empirical data (related to degree of hearing loss, speech-recognition scores, etc.) on which to base decisions concerning personal hearing aids and assistive technology. However, based on our experience at the Gallaudet Audiology Clinic, some clinical observations are offered that might be helpful in the decision-making process:

Often, clients with pure-tone averages of 40 dB HL may require telecoil circuitry. Telephone listening is probably the biggest concern of clients, next to one-to-one and TV listening. To decide on whether to install a telecoil, observe how well the client performs on the telephone, both without and with an amplifier. If the client experiences difficulty without one, install a telecoil.
There is not always a positive correlation between degree of hearing impairment and the need for assistive listening devices. While this is generally true, life-style often determines the need for an ALD. For example, clients with very mild hearing impairment who work may need the assistance of a remote microphone in staff meetings or in other difficult listening situations. On the other hand, a retired person with a very mild hearing impairment and a quiet life-style may not even require a hearing aid.
In general, there is a negative correlation between the need for ALDs and speech recognition ability. But life-style plays an important role here too. An active life-style seems to call for ALDs more often, even for people with better speech-recognition scores. Clients with mild high-frequency hearing impairment with good aided speech recognition scores can sometimes benefit from the use of a hearing aid coupled to a remote microphone system in staff meetings. Furthermore, clients who use hearing aids for speech awareness only can sometimes find ALDs beneficial, as in the case of deaf clients who use DAI and neckloop interfaces with portable tape players to enjoy music.
In general, there is a positive correlation between degree of hearing impairment and the need for alerting devices. However, even people with mild hearing impairment may need enhanced auditory or visual signaling systems when their hearing aids are not being worn or when they are using an ALD to listen to media (TV, stereo, etc.).

HEARING AID/ASSISTIVE DEVICE EVALUATION

If a hearing aid is to be recommended, the clinician must determine whether it will need to be used with an assistive device. This decision will be based on the communication needs assessment as well as the performance of the hearing aid. Although final decisions do not necessarily need to be made during the hearing aid evaluation, it is a good place to decide on what type of hearing aid to fit. The client should be shown models of BTE, ITE, and ITC hearing aids, and the pros and cons of each type should be explained. If assistive listening devices appear to be needed, then this should be discussed at this time. It is also important to address the fact that telecoil circuitry and DAI can be readily incorporated into some types of hearing aids but not others. We have found that clients are often willing to sacrifice cosmetics for better hearing, once they understand the advantages and disadvantages of the various hearing aid technologies.

Selection of Appropriate Hearing Aid(s)

Although it is not always possible to achieve, hearing aids should be selected with the goal of solving as many of the client's communication difficulties as possible. One of the most common difficulties experienced by hearing aid users is listening amid background noise. This problem may be solved using special circuitry. If the problem is not solved through special circuitry, then the hearing aid should be equipped with features to allow it to be coupled to ALDs. Telecoil circuitry may also be needed specifically for telephone communication.

Use of Hearing Aid(s) with the Telephone. A client's ability to recognize speech through a telephone should be a major concern of the clinician during the hearing aid selection process. For many people, the telecoil is the single most important hearing aid option, allowing access not only to the telephone but also to interpersonal and large-area ALDs. Some considerations for each type of hearing aid include the following:

1. BTE hearing aids offer stronger telecoil circuits and more sophisticated switching systems than do other hearing aids. They are therefore easier to use with ALDs and the telephone and provide many more listening options than do ITE hearing aids.
2. ITE hearing aids may be more cosmetically acceptable and may be the only hearing aid of choice in certain cases because of pinna malformation, activity level (e.g., sports), and so on. If an ITE hearing aid is chosen, the clinician must decide whether to install a telecoil circuit. Depending on the degree of the hearing impairment, the ITE may be coupled to the telephone in one of two ways, inductively or acoustically.
   A. Inductive Coupling
      Because of the occurrence of feedback with acoustic coupling and because

the installation of a telecoil circuit will allow for ALD interface in large areas such as theaters, inductive coupling is recommended for clients with moderate to severe hearing impairment. When installing a telecoil, one must consider proper strength and orientation.

Telecoil performance in ITE hearing aids can be improved by several methods: by adding a preamplifier circuit, by adding additional coils of wire to the telecoil, by wiring two telecoils together, by increasing the size of the telecoil's ferriferous core, and by orienting the telecoil perpendicular to the magnetic field it is trying to receive. If the hearing aid is to be used with an ALD, the telecoil should be mounted vertically to allow for the best reception from a room loop, neckloop, or silhouette inductor. If the hearing aid's telecoil is to be used to pick up electromagnetic leakage from the telephone *directly*, then the telecoil should be mounted horizontally, although this is not as crucial, since the hearing aid is held so close to the telephone. If the client desires to use the telecoil next to the telephone receiver, but will also be using ALDs in interpersonal communication situations, then the telecoil can be mounted vertically and the client can be taught to compensate on the telephone by angling the telephone receiver for the best reception. One must also consider whether switch modifications are necessary (e.g., does the client need a combination microphone/telecoil [M/T] switch?). The client must also be instructed on proper use of the telecoil.

   B. Acoustic Coupling
      Acoustic coupling may be necessary because of ear size or client preference for an ITC hearing aid. To eliminate feedback when the hearing aid microphone is held next to the telephone handset, a foam telepad, plastic acoustic coupler, or handset amplifier (amplifier turned up, hearing aid microphone turned down) can be tried. It also may be possible for the client to simply remove the hearing

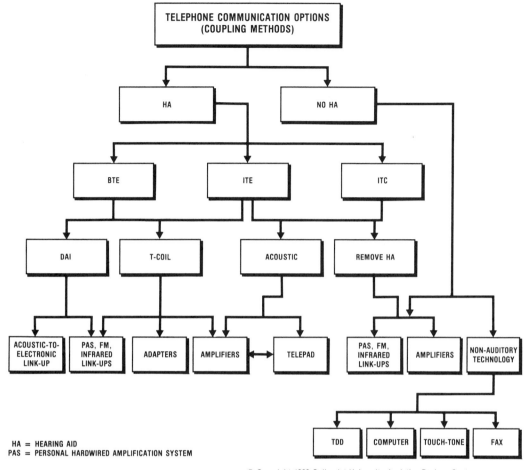

TELEPHONE COMMUNICATION OPTIONS
(COUPLING METHODS)

HA

NO HA

BTE

ITE

ITC

DAI

T-COIL

ACOUSTIC

REMOVE HA

ACOUSTIC-TO-ELECTRONIC LINK-UP

PAS, FM, INFRARED LINK-UPS

ADAPTERS

AMPLIFIERS

TELEPAD

PAS, FM, INFRARED LINK-UPS

AMPLIFIERS

NON-AUDITORY TECHNOLOGY

TDD

COMPUTER

TOUCH-TONE

FAX

HA = HEARING AID
PAS = PERSONAL HARDWIRED AMPLIFICATION SYSTEM

© Copyright 1989 Gallaudet University Assistive Devices Center

Figure 16.8. Telephone communication options (coupling methods). (With permission from Compton, C.L., Assistive Devices Center, Department of Audiology and Speech-Language Pathology, School of Communication, Gallaudet University, Washington, DC. Copyright, 1989.)

aid and use a telephone amplifier. If acoustic coupling (with or without a hearing aid) does not result in satisfactory telephone performance, then a hearing aid with an appropriate telecoil must be considered.

C. Direct Audio Input

It is also possible to install a DAI circuit on some brands of ITE hearing aids, allowing them to be coupled to ALDs, which can then be interfaced to the telephone. This might be warranted in the rare case of a cosmetics-conscious ITE user who cannot couple his or her hearing aid to the telephone—either inductively (due to magnetic interference) or acoustically

(due to feedback, etc.)—and who cannot use the naked ear with the telephone.

Various ways the ear can be coupled to the telephone are shown in Figure 16.8. Note that the use of a hearing aid telecoil increases one's telephone listening options.

Use of Hearing Aids with ALDs. If it appears that a client's interpersonal communication difficulties are not being solved through the use of a personal hearing aid only, then one must consider interfacing the hearing aid with an ALD. In fact, some clients' needs may be best met through the use of an ALD only, as in the case of an elderly, hospital-bound person. Communication options provided by using an ALD

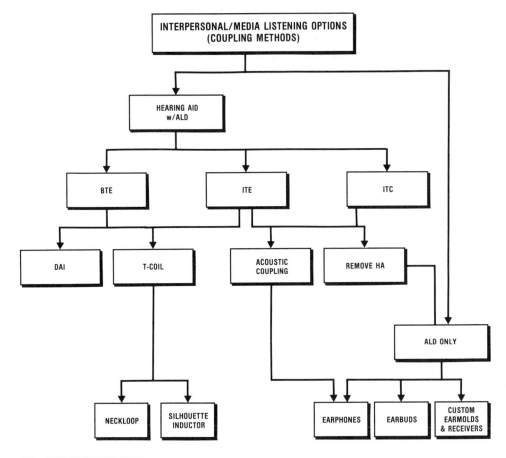

ALD = ASSISTIVE LISTENING DEVICE

© Copyright 1989 Gallaudet University Assistive Devices Center

Figure 16.9. Interpersonal/media listening options (coupling methods). (With permission from Compton, C.L., Assistive Devices Center, Department of Audiology and Speech-Language Pathology, School of Communication, Gallaudet University, Washington, DC. Copyright, 1989.)

with and without a hearing aid as well as with the various types of hearing aids are presented in Figure 16.9.

Some issues to consider are as follows:

1. BTE hearing aids provide the most flexibility with ALDs. Switching systems offer various modes for control of the hearing aid environmental microphone. Because of the larger hearing aid chassis, stronger telecoils are available for use with large-area induction loops, neckloops, and silhouette inductors.

2. If an ITE hearing aid is chosen, it should be equipped with a proper telecoil. If not, the client should also be counseled concerning his or her future ability to hear and understand speech in face-to-face and broadcast media listening situations. The following questions must be considered:

If the client continues to have difficulty listening in noise and from a distance, how will he or she use the hearing aid with an ALD?

Will it be possible for the person to *remove* the hearing aid and use a hard-wired ALD or wireless ALD receiver with earphones, earbuds, or custom earmold receivers?

3. Does the client need a way of controlling the hearing aid's external microphone? BTE hearing aids allow for more flexible manipulation of the hearing aid's external microphone. A combination M/T or

M/DAI mode might be desired for people who want to maintain contact with the outside world while using ALDs. T- and DAI-only modes are desired for especially noisy situations or for people whose speech recognition ability deteriorates significantly in the presence of any background competition.

ITE hearing aids can be ordered with M/T toggle switches or combination M/T switches. As mentioned previously, telecoil performance in ITE hearing aids can be improved. Adjustments must be done on a case-by-case basis by consulting with each manufacturer's engineering department.

Finally, as mentioned in the section on using hearing aids with the telephone, DAI is also available from some manufacturers.

Selection of Appropriate Assistive Devices

Often, the hearing aid is fitted and the client is given an opportunity to use it in the real world prior to a final decision being made concerning the need for assistive devices. During the hearing aid trial, the needs assessment process can be repeated. If the client continues to have difficulty in certain listening situations, then assistive devices may be indicated. In addition to the lifestyle considerations already discussed, several other issues need to be weighed when selecting appropriate assistive technology. Each issue is listed below and is accompanied by several examples:

Effectiveness. Clients should be fitted with technology that is effective. Although this may seem obvious, all too often technology is recommended that is too complicated for the client to use. Or, the client has not received sufficient instruction in use of the technology to make it effective.

Affordability. Affordability of technology will always be an issue, especially if the client has been instructed to purchase hearing aids in addition to assistive devices. However, it is important to present the assistive device(s) and the hearing aid(s) as a "total communication system." If the client understands that, for example, the hearing aid by itself cannot be expected to solve the three basic communication needs, then he or she will be more accepting of the need to purchase additional technology.

Is the system too complicated for the client to manage? Will additional training/counseling be needed? If so, this service and the time it commands must be built into the audiologist's or speech-language pathologist's fee structure. Physical design of the device is also important. Are the batteries easy to remove/replace? Is a raised volume control wheel needed? Can the device be recharged without removing the batteries?

Quality/Dependability. Clients demand technology that will perform for them when needed and will last. Prices for technology vary, and each client should be counseled regarding which is the best technology for the money. In this day and age of slick advertising, clients should be made aware that, in most cases, dependable technology will cost more. Dependability becomes an even more important issue in the area of emergency alerting systems such as smoke detectors.

Some systems are easier to carry around than others. For example, a DAI remote microphone system is lighter in weight and easier to set up than is an FM system (although an FM system is more versatile). A battery-powered portable telephone amplifier is easier to put in one's pocket or purse than is a replacement handset amplifier (which can be used only with a modular telephone).

Versatility. Some systems are more versatile than others. Although they may cost more, they avoid the need for a different system for each application—and the training that goes with it. For example, FM is more versatile than other interpersonal listening systems. It works well indoors or outdoors and can be used for TV or telephone listening or for listening to a lecture or meeting. If, however, a client has only TV listening needs, then an inexpensive hardwired system might be the system of choice. All interpersonal listening systems can be equipped with various types of microphones, making them applicable to a variety of listening situations. Similarly, some alerting systems allow the user to select the most effective way of alerting him or her to the sound.

Mobility. Distance and mobility needs will often determine the choice between hardwired and wireless systems. For example, short-distance and immobile activities (e.g., TV listening, one-to-one conversation, or small-group conversation) can be met with both hardwired or wireless systems. Short-distance, mobile, and indoor and outdoor activities (e.g., sports, hobbies) can best be met with FM technology, although some short-distance, mobile activities, such as "working a room" at a party can be met via a hardwired remote microphone system (e.g., a DAI directional boom microphone).

Long-distance, immobile, and indoor or outdoor (e.g., lectures) needs can best be met with FM or loop technology (although infrared and loop technology would be appropriate for indoor activities). A wireless system such as FM would be most appropriate for a person with both mobile and immobile receptive communication needs. A person with a limited budget and mostly indoor, immobile needs might be best served with hardwired technology, provided that his or her large-area listening needs can be met with wireless systems available in the community.

Durability. Clients want technology that will last, especially because they have paid a significant amount of money for it.

Compatibility. If a person must wear a hearing aid all the time, care should be taken to assure its compatibility with telephones as well as with personal ALD receivers in the home and community. This is most easily accomplished by including a telecoil circuit, although DAI circuitry can be added if necessary. In some cases, acoustic coupling of the hearing aid to the telephone can be successfully carried out, and use of ALDs can be accomplished by removing the hearing aid and using earphones or earbuds.

Compatibility of TDDs with each other and with computers is also an issue that must be addressed.

Cosmetics. Clients may require reassurance and possibly assertiveness training to use certain ALDs. In general, it is best to first demonstrate the equipment before discussing cosmetics. Often the client is so impressed with the assistance provided by the technology that the issue of cosmetics becomes less important. Sometimes "more is less"—that is, equipment such as an FM

system can be less obvious than a small, hardwired DAI remote microphone because of the ability to hide the FM receiver and the neckloop under clothing. Audio loop systems are particularly cosmetically acceptable, since they allow the listener to use his or her hearing aid telecoil as the ALD receiver. Some people may associate hardwired amplifiers and wireless receivers with portable radios or tape players and may therefore not be adverse to using assistive listening technology.

Previous Experience. Previous experience with technology and/or hearing health care professionals can have a positive, negative, or neutral effect. It is important to find out where the patient is "coming from" so that his or her preconceptions can be understood and handled in a positive way.

Need for Nonauditory Telecommunications Systems. TDDs, computers, FAX machines, and decoders may be needed to augment or even replace auditory devices. One must consider standard and optional features in terms of the client's communication needs in the various situations.

Need for Alerting Devices. Alerting devices can augment or replace hearing aids. Alerting devices might be needed in the home or office while the client is using an ALD to couple to a desired sound source (e.g., dictation machine or TV). Alerting devices can also be indicated when a hearing aid is used in noise or reverberation, is used from a distance or in another room, or is not being used at all (e.g., while sleeping). While vibrotactile devices can maintain privacy, some people may, at first, consider them an intrusion into their physical space.

Alerting devices should not be recommended unless they have appropriate UL listing and meet safety and housing codes. When selecting a device for a client's home, office, or other setting in which the device(s) will be used, a floor plan is helpful. Coverage and mobility needs must be addressed: For example, if the sender and the receiver must be mobile, then a phone-activated alphanumeric pager might be best. If both the sender and the receiver are confined to a particular building, then an AC- or battery-powered interoffice paging system might work, depending on the transmission range required and the amount of metal support beams in the building. Alerting devices offer various options in terms of the way they monitor, transmit, and signal. The advantages and disadvantages of hardwired and wireless systems should be considered and explained.

Cultural Issues. Although hearing impairment is often treated from a medical model point of view, many hearing-impaired people also view it from a cultural perspective. Cultural orientation can have an important impact on a person's acceptance or rejection of technology. Clients who have lost their hearing gradually usually consider themselves "hard of hearing" and from an auditory world. Consequently, they may be reticent, and even fearful, to use nonauditory technologies representative of deaf culture (TDDs, decoders, and visual and vibrotactile alerting devices). Similarly, clients who, despite their significant auditory skills, identify themselves with the deaf culture are often fearful of using auditory technologies. This may be due to negative past experiences as well as current conceptions that the use of auditory technology will cause them to be labeled by their peers as "hearing minded."

It is critical to provide a comfortable, supportive, and nonjudgmental atmosphere in which a client can examine his or her technology options. It is important to communicate to the client that assistive devices are simply tools for communication access and that the use of these tools does not suggest that one must abandon his or her cultural identity.

The support of the client's family, friends, and colleagues is often instrumental in the successful use of assistive devices. As such, it is important to involve them in counseling sessions. Introduction to clients to support groups such as Self-Help for Hard of Hearing People (SHHH) is also helpful.

Demonstration/Evaluation of Equipment

Behavioral Evaluation. When demonstrating assistive technology, it is important to provide the client with "ears-on" and "hands-on" experience so that he or she can gain an appreciation and a comfort level for it. The demonstration should be made as relevant as possible to the client's real-life communication needs. Some examples follow:

If a client is experiencing difficulty on the telephone, then the hearing aid telecoil, telephone amplifier, or other device should be demonstrated using telephone recordings or actual telephone conversations.

A client desiring to once again enjoy music can be shown how to connect his or her hearing aid to a portable stereo tape player via a binaural, stereo DAI cord or a neckloop connected to a stereo-to-mono adapter.

Demonstration of television as played through an ALD or closed-captioned decoder can be made using recordings of interesting programs. A library of relevant audio- and videotapes can be developed. For example, music may include classical to jazz, and television may include "Sesame Street" for kids, music videos for teens, and "Wall Street Week" for bankers.

If desired, a hardwired or wireless remote microphone system can be demonstrated in a test booth in background noise or in a room set aside for assistive device demonstrations. This room might be equipped with a loudspeaker system through which various types of background noise could be played.

A small display of selected alerting devices is helpful in explaining their setup and usage.

Objective Measurement. Choosing an assistive listening device for a client involves an analysis of that client's hearing impairment and listening needs in a variety of relevant everyday situations. Once the type of device is determined, then a brand must be selected. A serious impediment to the objective selection of assistive listening devices is the lack of standardized protocols for electroacoustic and probe tube measurement.

Although *electroacoustic measurement* procedure have been suggested (Gravel & Konkle, 1982; Hawkins & Van Tasell, 1982; Lewis et al., 1989; Lewis et al., in press; Sinclair, Freeman, & Riggs, 1981; Thibodeau, 1990a), until there is a national standard,* we will not see unity of measurement across the various brands of products, making it difficult to judge the quality of the various types of systems. Clinical test equipment and protocols are also needed for electroacoustic evaluation of telephone amplifiers, adapters, and specialty telephones. Finally, although there is a standard for the electroacoustic measurement of telecoils (ANSI 53.22, 1987), it uses only one frequency (1000 Hz) for measurement, which may misrepresent the overall telecoil gain across frequencies of the hearing aid. Additionally, the standard uses an input field strength of 10 ma/m, which is significantly weaker than that provided by many telephones and ALDs (Gilmore & Lederman, 1989). Finally, 2-cm³ measures often do not accurately reflect the telecoil response that is present in the real ear when the hearing is being worn.

If *probe tube measurement* is considered important in the hearing aid fitting process, then a comparable protocol must be developed for the evaluation of assistive listening devices. ALDs can be used alone or in conjunction with a personal hearing aid. Either way, objective measurement of the system (ALD and/or hearing aid telecoil) must be made if one is to ascertain that an appropriate frequency response, without the risk of excessive harmonic distortion, uncomfortable and/or overamplification, or underamplification is being provided.

Research has shown that when hearing aids are coupled to FM systems, the hearing aid characteristics are not necessarily maintained (Hawkins & Schum, 1985; Thibodeau, 1990b; Thibodeau, McCaffrey, & Abrahamson, 1988). Currently, there are very limited assessment techniques being developed to look at the real-ear performance of ALDs (Grimes & Mueller, 1991; Hawkins, 1987; Lewis, et al., 1989; Thibodeau, 1990a). The establishment of a national measurement protocol is essential for clients to be fitted in a scientific and safe manner. This is particularly important for young children or others who cannot provide subjective feedback regarding potentially inappropriate fittings.

Speech Perception Testing. Once appropriate coupling method and settings have been chosen, speech recognition or discrimination testing may be carried out to determine the performance of the ALD or to compare performance between the personal hearing aid and the ALD. Lewis et al. (1989) provide a step-by-step method for documenting the advantage of an FM system. This protocol could also be adapted for other assistive listening devices as well. Holmes and Frank (1984) and Wallber, MacKenzie, and Clyme (1987) have developed formalized behavioral assessment procedures for documenting telecoil performance with the telephone.

Documentation of the ALD performance may be needed for educational purposes, for third-party and/or employer financial support for ALDs, or to simply prove to a client that he or she can be assisted by the technology.

Follow-Up/Aural Rehabilitation

Just as with personal hearing aid fittings, follow-up counseling and evaluation are essential following the recommendation of assistive technology. Additional orientation and training may also be necessary. For example, some clients may require repeated instruction on how to use their hearing aid telecoil circuit with the telephone and ALDs. Others may need intensive practice in setting up, using, troubleshooting, and maintaining auditory and nonauditory assistive devices. Speechreading, auditory training (face to face and telephone), training in the use of communication/environmental strategies, and counseling may also be needed. Furthermore, assertiveness training may be required, as the use of assistive technology often requires the cooperation of others. For example, it can be especially anxiety producing to have to ask a lecturer to wear an FM transmitter, to request that colleagues at a staff meeting take turns talking into a microphone, or to ask a speaker to slow down for the real-time captioner. For these reasons, it is important to assist the client, via instruction and role playing, in developing the skills and psy-

---

*In May 1991, the American National Standards Institute (ANSI) S3 Committee on Acoustics authorized the establishment of a new writing group on assistive listening devices. One of the tasks of this group is to develop a national measurement standard for assistive listening devices.

chological strength necessary to assure successful, long-term assistive device usage.

The Role of the Professional

In the last decade, the area of assistive technology has matured from an academic curiosity to a legitimate clinical specialty. Several forces have contributed to this transformation, with two being the most influential—consumer activism and legislative mandates. Consumers who are hearing impaired are becoming increasingly aware of their right to communication access. Third-party providers are beginning to recognize and pay for this technology. What does all this mean to the audiologist or speech-language pathologist in training?

Although each professional's role will differ slightly, it is critical that future audiologists and speech-language pathologists be able to recognize when assistive technology is needed, to evaluate it, to recommend it, to advocate for it, to secure funding for it, and to train clients to use it. This training will extend to school officials, employers, and others who affect the lives of people with reception communication problems. Work in the area of assistive technology will also demand excellent networking skills. Audiologists and speech-language pathologists need to be prepared to work effectively with consumers, acoustical engineers, attorneys, employers, teachers, state and local government officials, and managers of public accommodations.

Both audiologists and speech-language pathologists should have a good working knowledge of the various types of auditory and nonauditory assistive technologies and when they are appropriate. With proper training, it may be appropriate for both professionals to recommend nonauditory technology (alerting and visual telephone and television systems). However, the fitting and recommendation of assistive *listening* devices (as with hearing aids and cochlear implants) fall within the scope of practice of an audiologist. In many cases, an audiologist should be consulted before nonauditory technology is recommended so that it can be determined whether auditory technology might be more appropriate in some instances. For example, a patient fitted with an inappropriately adjusted hearing aid might assume he needs a television decoder when, in fact, he may only need an adjustment of his hearing aid.

Because both audiologists and speech-language pathologists engage in aural rehabilitation training, both should be familiar with the use of telecoils, remote microphones, amplified handsets, and auditory as well as nonauditory technology in this process. Furthermore, practitioners in both professions should be comfortable with including assistive technology in individual educational plans (IEPs) for children.

Summary

A broad assortment of auditory and nonauditory technology is available to assist in removing the communication barriers that can prevent deaf and hard-of-hearing people of all ages from leading independent and productive life-styles.

By carefully evaluating our clients' communication needs and by having a good working knowledge of today's hearing aids and other equally important assistive technologies, we can select systems to effectively meet these needs and can incorporate them into appropriate and comprehensive rehabilitative programs that will improve our clients' communication skills and empower them to function in today's society with independence and dignity. To do less would be a disservice to our patients as well as to our professions.

References

Beaulac, D., Siemens Hearing Instruments, Inc., personal communication (1991).

Beck, L.B., and Nance, G.C., Hearing aids, assistive listening devices, and telephones: issues to consider. In C.L. Compton (Guest Ed.) and J.L. Northern and W.H. Perkins (Eds.-in-Chief), *Sem. Hear.*, 10(1), 78–89 (1989).

Compton, C.L., Assistive Devices: Doorways to Independence (videotape and companion book). Washington, DC: Gallaudet University. Available from Academy of Dispensing Audiologists, Columbia, SC, 1–800–445–8629 (1991).

Compton, C.L., Assistive listening devices: videotext displays. *Am. J. Audiol.*, 1(2), 19–20 (1992).

DeVoss, Ferdinand, Underwriters Laboratories, personal communication (1992).

Gilmore, R., and Lederman, N., Induction loop assistive listening systems: new designs and techniques. Paper presented at the annual meeting of the American Speech-Language-Hearing Association, Boston, MA (November 1988).

Gilmore, R., and Lederman, N., Induction loop assistive listening systems: back to the future? *Hear. Instru.*, 40:3 (1989).

Gravel, J., and Konkle, D., Electroacoustic hearing aid performance with neckloop inductive coupling. Presented at the American Speech-Language-Hearing Association Convention, Toronto, Canada (1982).

Grimes, A.M, and Mueller, H.G., Using probe-microphone measures to assess telecoils and ALDs. *Hear. J.*, 44(6),. 16–21.

Harkins, J.E., Visual devices for deaf and hard of hearing people: state-of-the-art. *GRI Monograph Series*, Washington, DC: Gallaudet Research Institute, Series A, No 2 (1991).

Hawkins, D.B., Assessment of FM systems with an ear canal probe tube microphone system. *Ear Hear.*, 8:301–303 (1987).

Hawkins, D.B., Methods of improving speech recognition in the presence of noise and reverberation. *Audiolog. Acoust.*, 9(10) (1985).

Hawkins, D.B., and Schum, D.J., Some effects of FM coupling on hearing aid characteristics. *J. Speech Hear. Disord.*, 50:132–141 (1985).

Hawkins, D., and Van Tasell, D., Some effects of FM-system coupling on hearing aid characteristics, *J. Speech Hear. Disord.*, 47:355–362 (1982).

Holmes, A., and Frank, T., Telephone listening ability for hearing impaired individuals. *Ear Hear.*, 5:96–100 (1984).

Lewis, D., Feigin, J., Karasek, A., and Stelmachowicz, P., Evaluation and assessment of FM systems. Presented at the American Speech-Language-Hearing Association Convention in St. Louis, MO (1989).

Lewis, D., Feigin, J., Karasek, A., and Stelmachowicz, P., 1989. Evaluation and assessment of FM systems. *Ear Hear.* (in press).

Sinclair, J.S., Freeman, B.A., and Riggs, D.E., Appendix: the use of the hearing aid test box to assess the performance of FM auditory training units. In Bess, F.H., Freeman, B.A., and Sinclair, J.S. (Eds.), *Amplification in Education*, Washington, DC: A.G. Bell Association, pp.. 381–383 (1981).

Singer, B., Gallaudet University, personal communication (1992).

Thibodeau, L., Clinical considerations in using classroom amplification systems. Paper read at the Second Annual Meeting of the American Academy of Audiology, New Orleans, LA (April 1990a).

Thibodeau, L., Electroacoustic performance of direct-input hearing aids with FM amplification systems. *Lang. Speech Hear. Serv. Schools*, 21:49–56 (1990b).

Thibodeau, L., McCaffrey, H., and Abrahamson, J., Effects of coupling hearing aids to FM systems via neckloops. *J. Acad. Rehabil. Audiol.*, 21:49–56 (1988).

Wallber, M., MacKenzie, D., and Clyme, E., Telecoil Evaluation Procedure. *National Technical Institute for the Deaf, RIT*, Rochester, New York, by agreement with the U.S. Department of Education. Auditec of St Louis (1987).

Van Tasell, D., and Landin, D., Frequency response characteristics of FM mini-loop auditory trainers. *J. Speech Hear. Disord.*, 45:247–258 (1980).

Weiss, M., Graduate Center of the City University of New York, personal communication (1991).

APPENDIX

16.1 *Resources*

American Speech-Language-Hearing Association
10801 Rockville Pike
Rockville, MD 20852
(301) 897–5700
(*For literature and assistance with ADA legislation*)

National Center for Law and Deafness
Gallaudet University
800 Florida Avenue NE
Washington, DC 20002–3695
(202) 651–5373 (Voice/TDD)
(*For advocacy issues related to hearing impairment*)

Underwriters Laboratories, Inc.
Publications Stock
333 Pfingsten Road
Northbrook, IL 60062
(708) 272–8800
(*For information on UL listing for alerting devices and for research results related to visual and vibrotactile fire alerting devices*)

SUGGESTED PROFESSIONAL LIBRARY

Assistive Devices: Doorways to Independence

Compton, C.L., Assistive Devices: Doorways to Independence (videotape and companion book). Washington, DC: Gallaudet University. Available from Academy of Dispensing Audiologists, Columbia, SC, 1–800–445–8629 (1991).

This 65-minute, open-captioned videotape and booklet discusses assistive devices in depth at the consumer level and is also appropriate for professionals interested in learning about the various technologies for receptive communication. Designed to be used in waiting rooms, professional libraries, graduate training programs, senior centers, nursing homes, and so on, the extensively illustrated booklet serves as a detailed reference for topics discussed in the video and contains a comprehensive section on large-area ALD applications and nonauditory technologies—topics often overlooked. To order, call the Academy of Dispensing Audiologists, Columbia, SC, at 1–800–445–8629.

Legal Rights: The Guide for Deaf and Hard-of-Hearing People

DuBow, S., Geer, S., Peltz Strauss, K., *Legal Rights: The Guide for Deaf and Hard of Hearing People*. Washington, DC: Gallaudet Press (1992).

Authored by Gallaudet's National Center for Law Deafness, this excellent book features complete information on the ADA, the Television Decoder Circuitry Act, and full updates on all other laws that affect deaf and hard-of-hearing people. Written for the layperson, it is an excellent guide for compliance with federal legislation requiring removal of communication barriers in all aspects of our society.

17

Computers in Hearing Rehabilitation

JOSEPH SMALDINO, Ph.D., SHARON SMALDINO, Ph.D.

Most audiologists intuitively agree with the proposition that hearing-impaired individuals can significantly benefit from habilitative and rehabilitative services. It is frequently the case, however, that these services are not offered to the individuals most likely to benefit from them. Many reasons can be suggested for this service gap, including questionable effectiveness of the services provided and a limited number of adequately trained service providers (Lieberth & Martin, 1991).

Closing the Service Gap

Audiologists have struggled with methods to increase the effectiveness of the rehabilitative process. One approach has been to develop procedural models that promise to focus the audiologist on the components of the entire process and to force consideration of sequences and interactions of the components. The underlying assumption of these models is that individual audiologists often do not practice the entire process, overlook important interactions, and so are less effective than they could be. Another approach has been to develop computer programs that in some way augment the role of the professional. Programs have been developed that enhance the quality of information about a hearing-impaired patient, help organize the information about a patient, automate treatment schemes, or analyze results and effectiveness of treatment.

Procedural Models

Procedural models are a means of organizing thoughts about a process. In this sense, models describe a professional's philosophy and shape the evaluation and treatment schemes used in the rehabilitative process (Goldstein & Stephens, 1981). Computers can be used as tools to implement a rehabilitative philosophy, and this has happened in recent years. In this way, computer applications really reflect procedural philosophies and ways of thinking about the rehabilitative process. Procedural models can be classified on a continuum from unidimensional to multidimensional.

The Procedural Continuum

Unidimensional models focus primarily on one or two components of the rehabilitative process. While components other than the focus are considered, they are not tightly integrated together. A common unidimensional model is shown in Figure 17.1. This rehabilitative model focuses on the hearing aid as the primary component for successful rehabilitation. While there is implied consideration of counseling and validation, these additional aspects are not central to the procedural intervention. We are not suggesting that successfully fitting a hearing aid is a simple endeavor; in fact, the complexities of doing it in a valid fash-

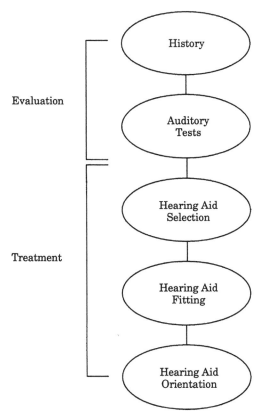

Evaluation

Treatment

Figure 17.1. Example of a unidimensional procedural model.

gest that clarification of these aspects for the professional is one reason for multidimensional models. They serve to help establish a philosophy of intervention and therefore can be used to educate others in effective rehabilitation procedures. There are advantages and disadvantages to multidimensional models. The most obvious advantage over unidimensional models is that more than one aspect of the rehabilitative process is evaluated and treated. The most significant disadvantage of current multidimensional models is that, although salient components are identified, the linkages and interactions between components are not clearly outlined. Because of this, multidimensional models are frequently used in a linear fashion. This mode of use is shown in Figure 17.2. When considered this way, a linearly applied multidimensional model is equivalent to a series of unidimensional models applied in sequence and so inherits the same disadvantages of the unidimensional models.

A third type of model is both nonlinear and multidimensional and is shown in Figure 17.3 The meaning of "multidimensional" has already been considered, but "nonlinear" requires further explanation. A nonlinear application assumes that all components have equal relevance and that consideration of one component does not necessarily lead to another known component; in fact it may lead to the creation of an entirely new component. The most significant disadvantage is the complexity. The most important advantage is that it provides a vehicle for evaluating the effectiveness of rehabilitative intervention and promotes learning about the rehabilitative process by the user.

ion are probably why it is often a central component in rehabilitative models. There are advantages and disadvantages to unidimensional models. In our view, the main disadvantages are that these models discourage a global view of the rehabilitative process, do not consider effectiveness outside the focus of the intervention, cannot use other significant facts to shape the rehabilitative process, and limit the professional learning that can occur from clinical intervention. On the advantage side, unidimensional models are easy to conceive and can be most readily adapted for use in a computer program.

The proponents of multidimensional models argue that for the process to be effective, all the salient aspects need to be considered. An example of a multidimensional model is shown in Figure 17.2.

To establish a multidimensional model, one must be aware of the aspects that significantly affect the rehabilitative process. Builders of multidimensional models sug-

Some Current Computer Applications in the Rehabilitative Process

Regardless of the model used, the rehabilitative process can be most simply described as a process of evaluation and treatment. In this next section we will try to identify the major areas in which computers and/or computer programs have

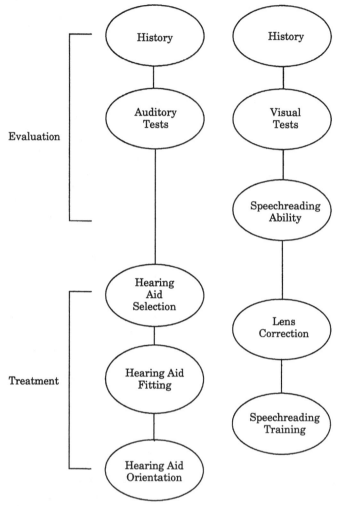

Figure 17.2.   Example of a linear multidimensional procedural model.

been used to enhance the effectiveness and/ or productivity of professionals engaged in the process.

EVALUATION

Digital or computer-based audiological equipment is commonplace in the modern diagnostic audiology clinic. The advantages of computers in the clinic include the following: A larger number of test parameters can be evaluated; the parameters that are assessed can be evaluated with greater precision and refinement; test results can be efficiently organized and stored; and test results can be clerically managed and reports produced (Ball, Anderson, & Schweitzer, 1986; Stach & Jerger, 1986). In terms of the rehabilitative process, digital audiometric equipment offers the promise of a more detailed description of how the auditory system breaks down, resulting in hearing loss. It is hoped that the increased detail can be used to understand more fully the breakdown and point the way to more effective rehabilitation.

The development of computer-based applications in audiology is an ongoing process. Certain applications that are under development or that do not yet have widespread use may especially affect the rehabilitative process. One of these areas is the use of sophisticated psychometric procedures in the gathering and evaluation of subjective responses. Many of these procedures handle issues relating to the reliability and validity of subject responses bet-

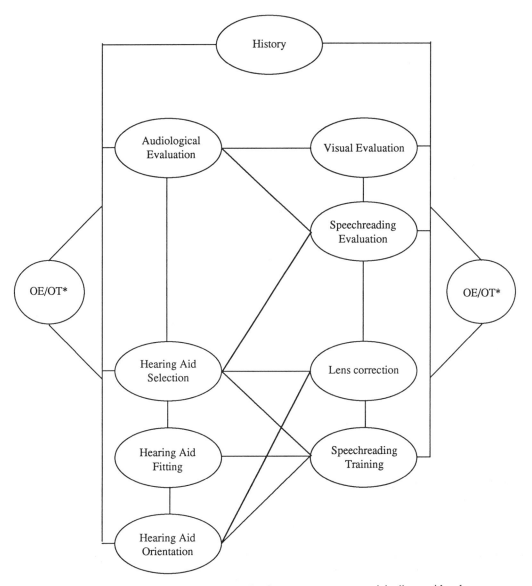

*OE/OT – Leads to another evaluation or treatment not originally considered

Figure 17.3. Example of a nonlinear multidimensional procedural model.

ter than more commonly used procedures and may provide less bias and thus a more accurate picture of important independent variables in the rehabilitative process. Another area is linkage of computers to optical discs to allow innovative materials and presentation formats for speech tests, as well as scoring programs that permit detailed analysis of patient responses (Cox & McDaniel, 1984, 1989). A third area includes computer-digitized/synthesized speech. Several audiometers already pro-

vide the option to present standard speech materials from digital storage. Not only does this improve the standardization of delivery of the speech tests, but it allows the user greater variety in test selection and flexibility in presentation format. Although computer-synthesized speech is not commonly available in current audiometers, computer programs exist to generate speech in this way (LaRiviere & Sherblom, 1986). Speech synthesis programs will permit the audiologist to generate speech stimuli at the very boundaries of our knowledge of speech perception.

The subjective hearing handicap scale has become an important evaluative tool in the rehabilitative process. A psychometrically constructed handicap scale can be used to identify patient strengths and weaknesses and can also be used as a gauge of treatment effectiveness (Demorest & Walden, 1984). Some of the scales are simple and do not benefit greatly from computer programming, but other comprehensive scales benefit from the computer's ability to sort and categorize with great efficiency (Demorest, 1987; Demorest & Erdman, 1984). In these cases, the professional is saved a great deal of time, which can then be applied to the interpretation of the results and use of the results in constructing a treatment plan.

TREATMENT

One of the first applications of computer programs in audiology was in the area of helping the audiologist to select hearing aids with electroacoustic characteristics that would benefit the hearing-impaired individual (Curran & Preves, 1986; DeJonge, 1991).

Given adequate information about a hearing-impaired individual and rules for making decisions about how to rehabilitate an individual with certain characteristics, it would be possible for a computer program to advise the audiologist as to treatment approaches that may be most effective for rehabilitation. One such program, described by Traynor and Smaldino (1988), produced treatment plan outlines from patient history, audiometric data, and results from a hearing handicap scale. While no other programs are known to accomplish this task at this time, planning programs of this type could dramatically enhance the effective treatment options available to professionals with limited rehabilitative training.

Tye-Murray and Tyler (1991) have described a computer-based interactive videodisc arrangement for use in hearing rehabilitation. Although the equipment costs are currently high, the technology suggests that in the future, some aspects of hearing rehabilitative treatment can be automated. One advantage to the professional of automation of this type includes very efficient analysis of effectiveness of treatment that triggers changes in treatment to improve effectiveness. Also, because direct professional time is reduced, there is the real potential for improving the cost/benefit ratio for hearing rehabilitative services. Since cost of rehabilitative services hinders widespread delivery of these services, automation reduces or eliminates the hindrance.

One other area where computers have affected the rehabilitative process is computer-aided instruction. Sims and Clymer (1986) have described a computer-based interactive video system that has been used to teach hearing-impaired individuals.

Problems with the Procedural Model

More and more audiologists are discovering the professional enhancements provided by computer programs and are beginning to use them in everyday practice. However, if the computer applications just described were lumped into a procedural model for the rehabilitative process, the model would have several serious flaws:

1. The model would not be very multidimensional. Many important aspects of the evaluation and remediation of the hearing-impaired individual would be omitted, simply because there is no software available for a component.
2. The model would not be well integrated because the information from one program is frequently not available for input into another program. The professional is left with detailed information about a particular component but little opportunity to allow that information to influence decisions about other components.
3. The model would not encourage evaluation of the efficacy of the entire process, since many components would be missing.
4. The model would not provide a learning opportunity for the professional because details of success or failure would not be easily available.

Table 17.1
Expert System Example

Problem: What is the best hearing handicap scale to use with patient A?

Facts/Rules	User Input	Input from Other Rules
IF school age THEN use handicap scale 1.	Is patient school age?	IF age >5 but $<$ or $=18$ THEN patient is school age.
IF work age THEN use handicap scale 2.	Is patient work age?	If age >18 but $<$ or, $=65$ THEN patient is work age.
IF retired THEN use handicap scale 3.	Is patient retired?	If age >65 THEN patient is retired.

5. Most of the programs are based on a single point of view, which cannot be easily adapted to individual professionals or patients.

Toward a Solution to the Dilemma

EXPERT SYSTEMS

When faced with a complex problem, professionals naturally seek out an expert for possible solutions and advice. Computer scientists have attempted to develop computer programs that can encapsulate knowledge of an expert and make the knowledge available to a nonexpert. These programs, called expert system shells, have not been generally applied to the rehabilitative process but can be useful in helping an individual professional think about constructing a process. An expert system shell permits a professional with some expertise in the rehabilitative process to outline the steps needed to solve a rehabilitative problem. The outline used to solve the problems is represented as facts in the form of "if . . . then" rules. *If* a set of statements is true, *then* the final statements are also true. The expert system uses what is called an "inference engine" to select the rules that need to be proved. Each fact in a rule can be shown to be true by inferring correctness based on other rules or by asking the program used to provide information. The program is interactive in that the rules chosen will depend on the information provided by the program user. The sum of the facts in the expert system program is referred to as the "knowledge base" (Duda & Gashing,

1981; Thompson & Thompson, 1985). A simple example of these principles is shown in Table 17.1. In this simple example the expert system program is designed to help the user decide which hearing handicap scale is most suited for a particular patient. The recommended hearing handicap scale is based on rules constructed by an expert in choosing appropriate scales. The inference engine part of the expert system either asks the user for needed information to use the appropriate rules or gleans the information needed from facts established by other rules.

We stated earlier that expert systems are not readily available in the rehabilitative audiology. This fact stems from the major developmental disadvantages of expert systems. The multidimensional set of problems that compose the rehabilitative process require development of a massive interconnected knowledge base. Development of such a knowledge base would require a major time commitment and the developer to possess advanced programming skills. Massive amounts of time and advanced programming skills are not common among clinicians. An expert system also requires a set of unambiguous rules. Because there is a good deal of variation among professionals, unambiguous universally accepted rule development would be difficult.

There are major disadvantages to the user of an expert system as well. Figure 17.4 diagrams the relationship between an expert system stored knowledge base and the user knowledge base. The program knowledge base is only as comprehensive as the expert who developed it. A unidimensional linear mode of thinking can be pro-

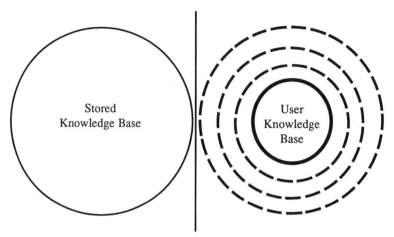

Figure 17.4. Example of a multidimensional expert system.

grammed into an expert system and not reflect the nonlinear multidimensional aspects of most rehabilitative problems. The user in the worst case would be limited to the advice of a single, not very thoughtful, expert. Probably the biggest disadvantage is that there is an interface boundary between the expert system knowledge base and the user knowledge base. The user cannot influence the expert system knowledge base, and so the program cannot be changed because of the experiences of the user. The information flow is entirely from the program to the user. This dependency on an external knowledge base does not promote creativity or development of a personal philosophy. These, of course, are the very elements necessary for the creation of a rehabilitative strategy.

HYPERMEDIA

One traditional complaint of the technology gurus has been that most of the applications did not truly use the capacity of the computer. Criticisms of software are that it does not provide the user with enough control and that the design of the software is little better than being an electronic page turner. For years, most software publishers have created drill and practice and tutorial types of software, often trying to incorporate a game-like approach to encourage the learner. These approaches, however, have fallen short. That the user is not able to manipulate the software to reflect his or her particular way of thinking or reacting has been a concern of those in-

volved in use of the technology in instructional situations.

In addition, application software—for example, word processing, database, or spreadsheets—is often created to be as generic as possible. The time invested in developing this type of software necessitates that it be as commercially viable as possible. Thus, software that is of interest to a small number of professionals is less likely to be developed. Often there is an effort to use the generic software to create specialized templates. Again, this may fall short of the professional's specific needs. For these reasons, hypermedia holds a potential for the professional.

In his landmark book entitled *Mindstorms: Children, Computers and Powerful Ideas*, Seymour Papert (1980) described computer programs that allowed the user to learn from the program by teaching the program to accomplish specific tasks. This is a different concept from computer-aided instruction, because computer-aided instruction is based on the premise that the user will learn from the computer program, not the other way around. Papert believed that if a learner is given a rich enough environment of choices, the learner will develop problem-solving and decision-making skills, as well as a pragmatic understanding of the knowledge necessary to solve problems. In this way, programs can be used to develop and nurture a learner's ability to construct strategies for solving problems. If programs like Papert described existed for use in learning about the hearing rehabilitative process, several distinct advantages might be noticed. First it would encourage creative thinking about how to solve problems in the rehabilitative process. Perhaps starting with unidimensional considerations, the user would soon move to multidimensionality as the number of problems that were considered and solved increased. The de facto result of this exercise would be a process model developed by the user, which addressed problems encountered in that learner's professional environment. Second, a rich environment of alternatives would encourage the user to experiment or test different sequences and interactions. Testing in this way, the user would tend to discard ineffective ways of thinking about interactions and accept those interactions that enhanced solution of the problem at hand. Third, the user would teach himself or herself about the rehabilitative process and understand how the learning occurred so that revision or addition of knowledge would be very easy.

Recently, there has been a trend in the literature which speaks to making software "hyper." The software is designed to provide the user with an array of possibilities to move about within a particular application, avoiding a predetermined organizational scheme. Each user chooses the pathway that is unique to his or her style of thinking and processing information. This new approach to designing computer-based software has created a whole new type of software termed "hypermedia."

Moving into Hypermedia

Hypermedia can be accomplished on the MS-DOS (using LinkWay or ToolBook), Macintosh DOS (using HyperCard), or Apple PRODOS (using HyperStudio) computer platforms that are readily available to the practicing hearing clinician. It is possible for the professional to develop materials that are unique to a particular need, creating them to be highly flexible and very usable and without having to be a computer "expert" to do it. A professional can become a software developer, thus assuring that the materials to be used will best reflect the type of learning desired, without relying on a software developer to create something

so generic that its application is limited as has been the case thus far.

Although it is far beyond the scope of this chapter to describe hypermedia in detail, our objectives are to introduce the principles underlying hypermedia, to describe the main elements of hypermedia, to provide examples of hypermedia applications that may encourage each professional to experiment with hypermedia, and to suggest an approach to hypermedia development. But first a conceptual basis for hypermedia must be established.

CONCEPTUAL BASIS OF HYPERMEDIA

Information management provided in hypermedia is based on cognitive psychological theories of how people structure knowledge and how they learn (Nelson, 1974, 1981). Hypermedia is designed to resemble models of memory and learning called active structural networks that are composed of a set of nodes (concepts) interconnected by relations (links). The entire set is known as a person's knowledge structure that is uniquely based on the individual's experiences and capacities (Jonassen, 1989). Each node is defined by the network of relations attached to it. Learning occurs when the knowledge structures are reorganized by constructing new nodes and interconnecting them with each other and with existing nodes. The more interconnections that are made, the better comprehended information will be and the easier it will be to learn or acquire new knowledge (Howard, 1983; Jonassen, 1989; Lachman, Lachman, & Butterfield, 1979). It follows that since the knowledge structures are individualistic, the manner in which an individual accesses, interacts with, and interrelates knowledge is also individualistic. In a hypermedia environment, information is made available to the learner by providing a malleable structure and sequence. How hypermedia accomplishes this is the subject of the next section.

HYPERMEDIA ORGANIZATION PRINCIPLES

Hypermedia can best be described as chunks or pieces of information that have some elements of association. These pieces of information can be in the form of text,

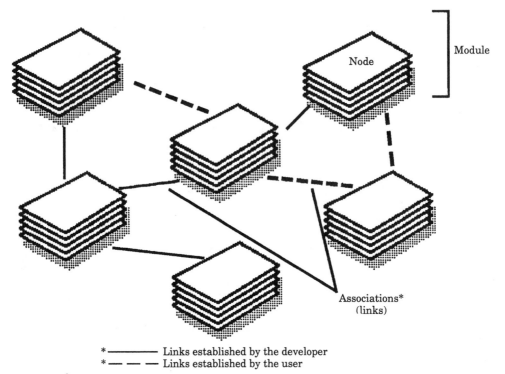

* ——————— Links established by the developer
* — — — — Links established by the user

Figure 17.5. Model of a hypermedia environment with random associations.

graphics, audio, or video. There is no continuous flow of text, like in a textbook or resource book. Rather the information is broken into small units or chunks. Each chunk, or basic unit of information, is termed a node. Each node is a module of information that can be accessed in any one of a variety of different ways by the user (Fig. 17.5).

The intent of the software, or hypermediaware, is to provide the user with possibilities to move about within a particular set of nodes without necessarily using a predetermined structure or sequence. The nodes themselves can be amended or added to, making the information in them more meaningful or complete (Jonassen, 1989). In this manner, hypermedia permits the user to use individualistic patterns of thinking and learning.

Modules of information in hypermedia are analogous to notecards in a collection of cards (Myers & Lamb, 1990). Each notecard contains a node of information. Subsequent cards or sets of cards may contain extensions of the information on the initial card or may contain other relevant or re-

lated information (Fig. 17.5). Hypermedia is usually set up so that each computer screen display is equivalent to one of the notecards with graphics and/or text.

Nodes of information are connected through the use of associations or links to other nodes of information (Fig. 17.5). The user may select from a directory of links or create new links to connect nodes. The selection or creation of a link allows the user to browse or examine the information in the set of nodes in many different ways and from many different perspectives. As the user browses, the choices made are reflective of the manner in which that user organizes information. Thus the program allows the user dynamic control of the information in the node set. Nelson (1974) argued that dynamic control is what differentiates the hypermedia learning environment from other instructional environments.

There are generally two type of association links available to the user in a hypermedia program (Jonassen, 1989). Structured links associate information nodes using an explicit organizational structure.

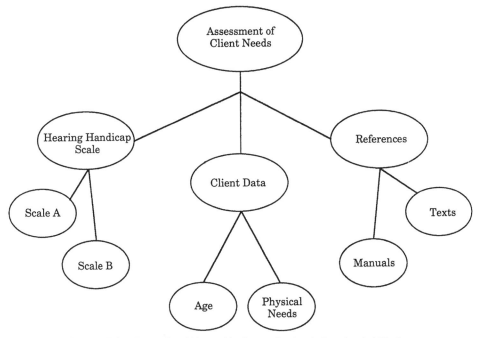

Figure 17.6. Example of hierarchical organization in hearing habilitation.

In this type of arrangement, the organization of the linkages implies a known or preferred manner in which to associate the informational nodes. Nonstructured links make no assumption about the underlying organization of the informational nodes. Because there is no preferred sequence or order in which to associate the informational nodes, the user browses freely through the node set.

A structured link allows the user to choose an option from a list that provides only a limited number of choices to the user. The user can move about within the material with the possibility of not returning to the other alternatives offered. Because the choices are limited and because a user can be caught in considerations of a single topic without returning to the alternatives, this type of hypermedia structure encourages unidimensional thinking or, at best, limited multidimensional thinking. An example of a structured link might be a menu of choices that refer to specific tests or assessment tools the clinician might use when trying to determine the extent of the hearing handicap. Such links are shown in Figure 17.6. The choices available direct the user to subsets of modules that are related.

The user is free to select the particular subsets in a nonsequential manner and is also free to not select some of the choices.

An unstructured link provides the user the opportunity to more freely within the hypermediaware to any location. The user can obtain the specific information needed, then return to the original place in the material (Fig. 17.7). Thus the user can decide within the context of the situation with a particular client which of the potential approaches might be the most appropriate. The unstructured link provides the professional the opportunity to move about in the hypermediaware in a manner most like the way knowledge is structured for him or her.

The unstructured link demonstrates the potential of hypermedia in providing the user with links that are unique to the user. Not every user will make use of these potential links. Each time a user interfaces with the material may mean the use of different unstructured links, the earlier choices not seeming to be necessary during the subsequent use. The unstructured link then can move the user beyond the developer's pattern of thinking and into the realm of considering alternative ways of researching a solution to a problem. An unstructured link

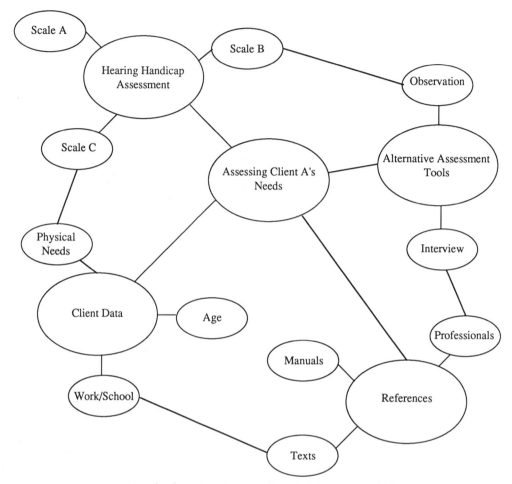

Figure 17.7. Example of hypermedia web in hearing habilitation.

can open up the opportunity for the user to interface with the original knowledge base in an expanded manner (Fig. 17.8). The user can begin to interact with the stored knowledge base in a unique manner. To the clinician this means that there is an opportunity to learn from the stored knowledge base and also to add to that same knowledge base. In a truly multidimensional scheme, both knowledge bases are expanded through use.

MOVING ABOUT IN HYPERMEDIA

Hypermedia requires that the user must make decisions about where to go next within the material (Myers & Lamb, 1990). The user navigates through the information using linking devices termed "buttons." Buttons promote a quick and easy way for the user to access information, hence the

interactive nature of hypermedia. A button can be a graphic or a textual object that suggests pathways for the user to select. The user, with the aid of a mouse device, points to the button and clicks on the mouse. The hypermedia button then activates the link between the cards, moving the user from the current node to the selected new node (Fig. 17.9). The use of the button interface or link between cards speeds up the process of moving about within the hypermedia environment.

HYPERMEDIA IN REHABILITATION

A hypermedia model takes on the appearance of a web of ideas or alternatives rather than a listing of choices or rules. Starting with the problem of assessing hearing handicap as the central focus, or center of the web, it is possible then not only to

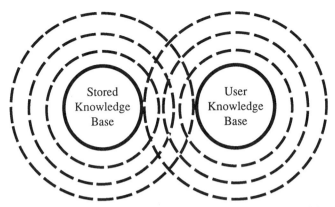

Figure 17.8. Example of a multidimensional hypermedia model.

examine the traditional alternatives but to recognize there might be additional choices or nodes to address in solving the problem. Choices might include specific hearing handicap scales, alternative approaches to assessing hearing handicap scales, alternative approaches to assessing hearing handicap, data about the client, and referential materials of importance to the rehabilitation professional. Being able to select a single alternative or many of the different choices helps the professional in making the decision about how to best assess the client's hearing handicap.

HYPERMEDIA ELEMENTS

The foundation of all hypermedia programs is found in several consistent elements (Myers & Lamb, 1990). The first element is the screen unit. In HyperCard and HyperStudio this is termed the "card." In LinkWay and ToolBook the term is "page." Each screen on the computer is analogous to a 3×5 card with graphics, text, and visual and auditory effects. A collection of cards or pages constitutes a "stack" or "folder."

The second element is the stack or folder. Most users are familiar with the term "file" when referring to word-processed documents as files. The collection of cards or pages constitutes a hypermedia document, which is termed a stack or folder. One of the unique features of hypermedia is the ability to connect the cards or pages within the stack or folder. The developer can even create subsections of instructional material into units that can be connected, thus connecting several stacks or folders together.

A third element of hypermedia is the button. To get the user to move about within the hypermedia, there needs to be a way for the user to indicate a selection. By providing an object that the user can point to with a mouse and click on with the mouse button, the user can select the pathway in which to continue interacting. Buttons are the easiest way for the user to move quickly about in a hypermedia environment. Buttons can use graphics (icons), words, or special symbols to guide the user in locating the specific area to touch.

The final element of hypermedia is the field. Fields are areas for entering, storing, and displaying text. A variety of fonts, styles, and sizes can be used to enhance the text. Fields can vary in size and style. Fields are a way of inputting information by both the developer and the user.

HYPERMEDIA DEVELOPMENT

Use of hypermediaware for development of computer-based materials is an emerging area within nearly all of the professions that have used microcomputer-based training heretofore. The challenge for the professional is to create materials that are innovative and unique while maintaining some consistency. It is essential that certain considerations be brought into play when developing hypermedia applications. One thrust of this chapter is to provide guidelines for hypermediaware development that can be easily incorporated into the development of HyperCard, HyperStudio, and LinkWay stacks and folders. By incorporating these guidelines it is possible to create "hyper" drill and practice, tutorials,

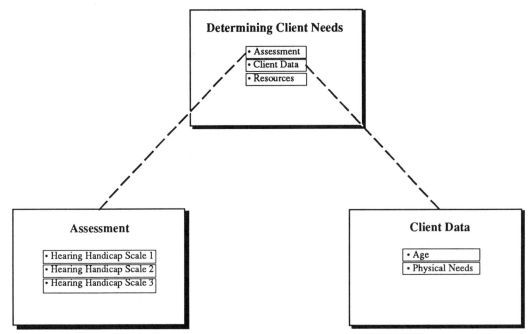

Figure 17.9. Linking via buttons within hypermedia.

simulations, and other types of instructional materials quickly and easily. It is also possible to create specific application utility materials for the professional.

DEVELOPMENT GUIDELINES

There are some general guidelines for developing software that follow a standardized procedure. When creating software, it is essential to plan carefully. The process that is suggested here is termed the Instructional Development Process. It is not limited to the development of instructional materials and can be applied to computer-based material development (Criswell, 1989; Dick & Carey, 1990).

The first phase of the process is analysis. The first step in analysis is to assess the need for the software. Looking at existing software can often be very helpful in preventing a reinvention of the wheel. It is also very helpful to examine the strengths and limitations of existing software to be certain that the software that is to be developed will be optimally designed.

Another aspect of the assessment of the need is to consult with potential users of the planned software. These professionals can provide insight into elements that need to be included in the software. They also can provide some suggestions as to the or-

ganization and supplementary materials that might be needed.

The second step of the analysis phase is the analysis of the content. The person who is developing the software needs to have a clear understanding of the material to be included in the software. Whether the software is to be of an instructional or a utility type, the content of the material needs to be accurate and up to date.

The third step of the analysis phase is consideration of the probable user. The software developer needs to consider the potential user when designing the product. If the user is kept in mind during the development of the software, then the product will more likely be readily used.

The final step of the analysis phase of the process is to establish goals and objectives. The software developer needs to have a clear idea of the direction that the software is to go. If the materials being developed are instructional in nature, then the goals and objectives are directed at the learner outcomes. If the software is to be used as a utility package, then the outcomes need to be directed toward the achievement of the end product for the user.

The second major phase of the development process is the design phase. The developer uses the information gathered in the needs assessment, the content analysis, and the learner analysis to prepare usable software. There are certain considerations that need to be recognized in the development of computer-based software. First is that the materials are designed in such a way as to make the computer and the software appear "transparent" to the user. The user is not impeded by the need to use the computer, nor is the user limited in accomplishing the task because of complexity in the software manipulations.

It is also very important that the software be as flexible as possible for the user. To gain the greatest market for software, the more versatile it is the better. However, it is important not to make the software so generic as to become incomplete in the eyes of the user.

The final phase in the development process is evaluation. Before a developer of software begins to market a product, field testing is essential. Asking a few professionals to look over the software can make the difference in the success or failure of a product. Having colleagues examine the software, or "beta" test it, can provide the developer with insight as to strengths and possible improvements that might be made. Having gathered this information, the developer can then make any improvements in the materials, thus producing a software package that is impressive and of which the developer can be proud.

These guidelines are essential for the development of quality software. However, there are some special considerations when developing hypermedia.

HYPERMEDIA GUIDELINES

There are certain considerations that a hypermediaware developer must keep in mind when developing stacks or files (Cook, 1991). The considerations mentioned in the development process are important to the development of quality software. With the arrival of hypermedia, certain special considerations must be included.

Important to the user is an ability to anticipate that certain responses or actions will lead to expected or predictable responses. The user needs to be assured that when a certain key stroke is made, the software will respond accordingly. For exam-

ple, if the user wishes to discontinue using the software, an initial response would be to press the ESC key. The anticipated response is that the user will be able to get out of the software easily. If pressing the ESC key does not lead the user out of the software but to another location within the software that is nowhere near the end, then the user may be at a loss as to how to leave. The same can be said for pressing certain iconic buttons and expecting to go to specific places within the hypermedia. An example would be to press the "home" icon button and expect to go to the home card in HyperCard. If by pressing the "home" button, the user moves onto the next screen in the series of screens, then it is possible that the user will become confused and unable to maneuver successfully through the hypermediaware.

Within this same framework is the idea of consistency. Certain types of key strokes or buttons will be the same no matter what stack or folder is being used. It can be expected that the arrow in the lower right-hand corner of the screen that points to the right might move the user onto the next card or screen. It this is the symbol used throughout the hypermedia world, then the user does not need an explanation of the right arrow; it is understood that an icon indicates the choice of the next screen. There is a need to make certain that the icons used are apparent to the user.

Cook (1991) entitled his article "Lost (and Found) in Hyperspace." His choice of title is clear to anyone who has tried to use hypermedia without a clear understanding of the expected outcomes or the type of links that have been extablished within the stack or file. It is easy for a user, especially a novice, to become hopelessly lost within the hypermedia. To provide a cue for the user is relatively easy and keeps the user from becoming totally confused and distracted from the task. For example, if the developer has created several subskill areas within the hypermediaware, it would be relatively easy to indicate on the card or screen that the user is on a particular number of a total, for example, screen 5 of 20. Then the user has assurance that he or she is still within the unit of instruction and is not lost or confused.

We have one final suggestion for the development of hypermediaware. In the past,

Table 17.2
Characteristics of Computer Approaches in Hearing Rehabilitation

	Traditional Computer Programs	Expert Systems	Hypermedia
Multidimensional	− (+)	− (+)	+
Informational feedback to user	− (+)	− (+)	+
Enables user evaluation	+	+	+
Integration of databases possible	−	−	+
Ease of use	+	+ (−)	+ (−)
Ease of development	+	− (+)	+ (−)
Functions as learning tool	−	− (+)	+

− = limitation, + = strength, ( ) = potential.

software developers were encouraged to draw flowcharts or flow diagrams of how the software will operate, creating a type of blueprint. These were not complex to do, just time consuming. Often with very linear software, it seemed unnecessary for the developer to take the time to draw these charts or diagrams. When working in a hypermedia environment, it is essential for the software developer to complete a blueprint.

One very effective way of creating the hypermedia blueprint to guide the developer is to use 3×5 or 5×7 index cards. Each screen in the program is represented by one card. All of the elements on the screen are sketched out, including the buttons, graphics, and text fields. Whenever a button is created, it is easy to color code it to the card or stack to which it is connected. Scripts, the directions to the computer, can be written in advance to ensure consistency and accuracy. By having these cards available, the developer can lay out on a tabletop, or the floor, all of the cards, to be certain the cards or pages are connected in a logical pattern. In addition, considerable time is saved by working all of the "bugs" out first on the cards. When the developer sits down to the computer to begin the actual development of the computer-based hypermediaware, many of the potential problems have been identified. Thus, the developer can more efficiently use the time for writing the software.

BEYOND THIS CHAPTER

Current computers and computer program designs have already influenced the effectiveness and productivity of the hearing clinician. Computers and programs under development will surely continue the trend in the future as more and more professionals use these products. Some of the "hyper" programs engage the user into a sort of informational dialogue or odyssey that encourages the professional to produce changes in or new knowledge about the rehabilitative process. By using these tools, each professional can become less of a consumer of information and more of a producer of knowledge. In the end, the impact of computer technology will depend on the number of individuals in the profession who use the technology on a regular basis.

Table 17.2 summarizes some of the characteristics of computer approaches described in the chapter. The seven topics covered in the table emphasize those areas that are characteristic of programs that accommodate the complexity of the rehabilitative process yet provide flexibility for the user to learn from established knowledge and create knowledge that is yet unknown. Program approaches have different strengths and weaknesses. These are indicated in the table. If used as a guide, the hearing health care professional can use the table to help choose an approach that best meets his or her needs. Some of the newer computers and program designs are very "user friendly" and encourage the neophyte to become involved. We have included a small resource guide (see Appendix 17.1) at the end of the chapter to aid you in your initial quest for computer usage in the hearing rehabilitative process.

We started this chapter indicating that hearing rehabilitation services were not widely available because of unproven effectiveness and because there were a limited number of adequately prepared professionals. We believe computers and judiciously chosen programs can change the situation, but professionals need to engage themselves in the computer age. Sometimes people view learning to use a computer in professional practice as an elephant-sized task. As someone once said "The best way to eat an elephant is one byte at a time." Bon appetit!

References

Ball, L., Anderson, L. and Schweitzer, C., Microcomputers in office management of speech and hearing facilities. In J. Northern (Ed.), *The Personal Computer for Speech, Language, and Hearing Professionals.* Boston: Little, Brown (1986).

Cook, D.A., Lost (and found) in hyperspace. *CBT Directions*, 10–17 (July, 1991).

Cox, R., and McDaniel, D., Intelligibility ratings of continuous discourse: application to hearing aid fitting. *J. Acoust. Soc. Am.*, 76, 758–766 (1984).

Cox, R., and McDaniel, D., Development of Speech Intelligibility Rating (SIR) Test for hearing aid comparisons. *J. Speech Hear. Res.*, **32,** 347–352 (1989).

Criswell, E.L., *The Design of Computer-Based Instruction.* New York: Macmillan Publishing (1989).

Curran, J., and Preves, D., Microcomputers and hearing aids. In J. Northern (Ed.), *The Personal Computer for Speech, Language, and Hearing Professionals.* Boston: Little, Brown (1986).

DeJonge, B., *Hearing Aid Selection Program.* Pittsburgh, PA: Support Syndicate for Audiology (1991).

Demorest, M., *User's Guide to the CPHI Database System.* Washington, DC: CPHI Services (1987).

Demorest, M., and Erdman, S., A database management system for the Communication Profile for the Hearing Impaired. *J. Acad. Rehabil. Audiol.*, 17, 87–96 (1984).

Demorest, M., and Walden, B., Psycholmetric principles in the selection, interpretation, and evaluation of communication self-assessment inventories. *J. Speech Hear. Disord.*, 49, 226–240 (1984).

Dick, W., and Carey, L., *The Systematic Design of Instruction* (3rd ed.). Glenview, IL: Scott, Foresman/Little, Brown Higher Education (1990).

Duda, R., and Gaschnig, J., Knowledge-based expert systems come of age. *Byte.*, 6, 9 (1981).

Goldstein, D., and Stephens, S., Audiological rehabilitation: management model I. *Audiology,* 20, 432–452 (1981).

Howard, D., *Cognitive Psychology.* New York: Macmillan (1983).

Jonassen, D., *Hypertext/Hypermedia.* Englewood Cliffs, NJ: Educational Technology Publications (1989).

Lachman, R., Lachman, J., Butterfield, E., *Cognitive Psychology and Information Processing.* Hillsdale, NJ: Lawrence Erlbaum Associates (1979).

LaRiviere, C., and Sherblom, J., Speech synthesis and speech recognition by microcomputer. In J. Northern (Ed.), *The Personal Computer for Speech, Language, and Hearing Professionals.* Boston: Little, Brown (1986).

Lieberth, A., and Martin, D., Hyperehab. Paper presented to the Summer Insititute of the Academy of Rehabilitative Audiology, Breckenridge, CO (1991).

Myers, D., and Lamb, A., *HyperCard Authoring Tool for Presentations, Tutorials and Information Exploration.* Orange, CA: Career Publishing (1990).

Nelson, T., *Dream Machines.* South Bend, IN: The Distributors (1974).

Nelson, T., *Literary Machines.* Swarthmore, PA: The Author (1981).

Papert, S., *Mindstorms: Children, Computers, and Powerful Ideas.* New York: Basic Books (1980).

Sims, D., and Clymer, E.W., Computer-assisted instruction for the hearing impaired. In J. Northern (Ed.), *The Personal Computer for Speech, Language, and Hearing Professionals.* Boston: Little, Brown (1986).

Stach, B., and Jerger, J., Microcomputer applications in audiology. In J. Northern (Ed.), *The Personal Computer for Speech, Language, and Hearing Professionals.* Boston: Little, Brown (1986).

Thompson, B., and Thompson, W., *MicroExpert.* New York: McGraw-Hill (1985).

Traynor, R., and Smaldino, J., *Computerized Adult Aural Rehabilitation.* State College, PA: Parrot Software (1988).

Tye-Murray, N., and Tyler, R., Home-based aural rehabilitation therapy for cochlear implant patients. Paper presented to the Summer Institute of the Academy of Rehabilitative Audiology, Breckenridge, CO (1991).

APPENDIX
17.1 *Suggested Readings*

Curtis, J., *An Introduction to Microcomputers in Speech, Language and Hearing.* Boston: Little, Brown (1987).

Northern, J., *The Personal Computer for Speech, Language and Hearing Professionals.* Boston: Little, Brown (1986).

Silverman, F., *Microcomputers in Speech-Language Pathology and Audiology.* Englewood Cliffs, NJ: Prentice-Hall (1987).

Hypermedia Programs and Suggested Readings

HyperCard	HyperCard Developers Kit
Claris Corp.	Claris Corp.
5201 Patrick Henry Drive	5201 Patrick Henry Drive
Box 58168	Box 58168
Santa Clara, CA 95052-8168	Santa Clara, CA 95052-8168

Beekman, G., *Hypercard in a Hurry.* Belmont, CA: Wadsworth (1990).

Beekman, G., *Hypercard 2 in a Hurry.* Belmont, CA: Wadsworth (1992).

Maran, R., *HyperCard Quickstart: A Graphics Approach.* Carmel, IN: Que Corporation (1988).

Myers, D., and Lamb, A., *HyperCard Authoring Tool.* Orange, CA: Career Publishing (1990).

> Linkway
> IBM Corp.
> Box 1328-W
> Boca Raton, FL 33429-1328

Kheriaty, L., *Getting a Quick Start with IBM LinkWay.* Boca Raton, FL: IBM Corporation (1991).

> ToolBook
> Asymetrix Corp.
> 110–110th Ave. N.E.
> Suite 717
> Bellevue, WA 98004

Catalogs of Computer Programs and Shareware

Educorp Computer Services [Shareware]. Educorp, 531 Stevens Ave., Suite B, Solana Beach, CA 92075.

HyperCard ToolBox [Shareware]. User Magazine, P.O. Box 56986, Boulder, CO 80321.

Journal for Computer Users in Speech and Hearing. CUSH Business Office, P.O. Box 2160, Hudson, OH 44236.

MPG [Shell Shareware]. Modern Learning Aids, New York, NY.

Parrot Software. P.O. Box 1139, State College, PA 16804.

Support Syndicate for Audiology. 1739 E. Carson Street, Pittsburgh, PA 15203.

5

FUTURE DIRECTIONS

18

Needs of the Geriatric Population

BARBARA E. WEINSTEIN, Ph.D.

Currently, approximately 25 million persons over 65 years of age reside in the United States, and the number is expected to rise to 55 million by the year 2020. One in every five individuals, or 20% of the total U.S. population, will be over the age of 65 by the year 2050 (Gambert, 1987). As we move into the 21st century, the population likely to experience the greatest growth will be persons 55 years of age and older (Hartke, 1991). Individuals age in two ways: chronologically or physiologically (Gambert, 1987). The term "chronological age" refers to one's age on the birth certificate, whereas physiological age connotes the way in which our bodies are functioning (Gambert, 1987). These two types of aging are often at odds with one another, and the relationship is further complicated by psychological and socioeconomic factors that influence the aging process in complex ways. As aging is a dynamic, individualized aspect of human development, the term "older" rather than "old" will be used in this chapter when describing later life (Hartke, 1991).

The evaluation and rehabilitation of older adults require a perspective different from that adopted for younger individuals, on both a conceptual and a practical level (Hartke, 1991; Kane, Ouslander, & Abrass, 1989). Rehabilitation of the older adult requires a "biopsychosocial approach" with an emphasis on restoring "functional ability" (Brummel-Smith, 1990; Kane et al., 1989). The clinician must consider the im-

plications of diagnostic and laboratory findings for overall health and well-being, with the goal being assisted independence and maintenance of a satisfying quality of life (Brummel-Smith, 1990; Hartke, 1991; Weinstein, 1991). The goals of geriatric rehabilitation are best achieved via an interdisciplinary team approach accomplished by administering comprehensive functional assessment and treatment services to the older adult and his or her support system (Hartke, 1991). In light of this philosophy of rehabilitation with older adults, this chapter attempts to provide a perspective that differs from the traditional. The goal will be to provide the reader with an understanding of the contribution audiologic intervention (e.g., hearing aids) can make to the functional well-being of older adults and how we can focus our rehabilitation efforts at obtaining such outcomes.

Psychological Considerations

A number of psychosocial variables should be considered when designing and implementing a rehabilitation program for the older hearing-impaired adult. These include emotional status in general, the psychosocial impact of acquired hearing loss in particular, and the motivational level of the individual. Emotional status such as affective state (e.g., anger, sadness) or mood (e.g., anxiety, depression) can influence the client's ability to learn new skills and to form therapeutic relationships and can have an impact on rehabilitation potential and rehabilitation outcomes (Trezona, 1991). In addition, functionally significant changes in cognitive status may interfere with sustained and selective attention and may compromise procedural learning memory, and the ability to imitate the behavior of the clinician or other hearing-impaired age cohorts (Rentz, 1991). Chronic conditions such as hearing loss often trigger or exacerbate some of the aforementioned emotional reactions or conditions such as senile dementia. Accordingly, when designing a client-centered rehabilitation program, clinicians should have an understanding of the contribution of unremediated hearing loss to psychosocial status.

PSYCHOSOCIAL CONSEQUENCES OF HEARING LOSS

A number of recent studies have demonstrated that hearing loss has an adverse effect on functional status, on quality of life, on cognitive function, and on emotional, behavioral, and social well-being (Bess et al., 1989; Mulrow et al., 1990a; Uhlmann et al., 1989). Mulrow et al. (1990a) conducted a cross-sectional study of 204 elderly male veterans selected for a primary care clinic designed to assess the association between hearing impairment and quality of life. Quality of life was defined according to two disease-specific and three generic measures that have been standardized on older adults (Mulrow et al., 1990a). The disease-specific measures were the Hearing Handicap Inventory for the Elderly (HHIE), which assesses the self-perceived emotional and social effects of hearing loss, and the Quantified Denver Scale of Communication Function (QDS). The QDS quantifies the perceived communication difficulties secondary to hearing impairment (Mulrow et al., 1990a). The generic measures included the Short Portable Mental Status Questionnaire (SPMSQ), which yields information about cognitive function; The Geriatric Depression Scale (GDS), which assesses affect; and the Self-Evaluation of Life Function (SELF), which assesses function in several domains including physical disability, social satisfac-

tion, aging, depression, self-esteem, and personal control.

Hearing loss in the sample of older hearing-impaired adults was associated with significant social, emotional, and communication handicaps, as mean scores on the HHIE and QDS were significantly higher for the hearing-impaired group than for the unimpaired group. In contrast, mean scores on the GDS and the SELF did not differ for the groups with and without a hearing impairment. Similarly, mental status was intact for both groups of subjects. As the extent of the perceived social and emotional dysfunction was considerable for their sample (i.e., 66% had HHIE scores >42, indicative of severe handicap, and 16% had mild to moderate handicaps or HHIE scores between 18 and 40), the authors concluded that hearing loss has an adverse effect on quality of life. A follow-up randomized trial of hearing aid rehabilitation indicated that hearing aid intervention was effective at reducing the communication and psychosocial handicaps, as well as depressive and cognitive symptoms experienced by the majority of hearing-impaired older males in their sample (Mulrow et al., 1990b). Their findings underscore the importance of quantifying the specific emotional and social consequences of hearing loss to ensure that intervention is successful at remediating the behaviors that were most probably instrumental in the decision to seek rehabilitative assistance.

Data are beginning to accumulate documenting a link between hearing loss and cognitive status in persons diagnosed with senile dementia. The major findings of studies of hearing loss in persons with dementia include the following:

1. Hearing loss is more prevalent in older adults with dementia (Weinstein & Amsel, 1986).
2. Older adults with dementia are likely to have more severe hearing loss than those without dementia (Uhlmann et al., 1989; Weinstein & Amsel, 1986).
3. The risk of dementia increases as a function of increasing hearing loss, after adjusting for potentially confounding variables such as depression, number of primary prescriptions, and age (Uhlmann et al., 1989).

4. Unremediated hearing loss lowers performance on aurally administered diagnostic tests used to quantify the severity of senile dementia (Weinstein & Amsel, 1986).
5. Hearing aids lower scores on tests of cognitive function, suggesting improved mental status with hearing aid use (Mulrow et al., 1990b).

Given the high prevalence of senile dementia among older adults, especially those residing in institutions, and the high prevalence of hearing loss, it is likely that the two disorders will co-occur in a large portion of older adults. Further unremediated hearing loss can confound the diagnosis of dementia and often exacerbates the behavioral manifestations of senile dementia. Similarly, the lack of familiarity with the behavioral characteristics of persons with dementia can jeopardize the validity of the audiologic assessment and interfere with the benefits to be derived from audiologic interventions, such as hearing aids and assistive listening devices. Accordingly, audiologists should informally assess mental status in persons being considered for intervention by asking simple questions that yield information regarding memory and orientation or by administering a validated instrument such as the Short Portable Mental Status Questionnaire (SPMSQ) (Pfeiffer, 1975). Evidence of impaired cognition will influence the type, nature, and outcome of the intervention (e.g., a hearing aid versus an assistive device).

In sum, in light of the link between hearing loss, social, emotional, and communication function, affect, and cognition and the positive quality of life changes and functional status benefits of hearing aids, it behooves audiologists to incorporate selected measures of function into the decision-making process regarding the need for hearing aids and the outcomes obtained with hearing aids. Further, information about the effects of hearing loss on quality of life, and the potential improvements in quality of life associated with hearing aid use, can be incorporated into the counseling process to motivate resistant older adults to consider a trial period with hearing aids (Kricos, Lesner, & Sandridge, 1991; Weinstein, 1991).

AGING AND MOTIVATION

The aging process influences one's motivational level, especially in regard to the purchase of rehabilitation services. In short, motivation is "one of the most important factors that affects rehabilitation and adaptation to disability" (Kemp, 1990, p. 295). Motivation influences one's capacity to overcome adversity and one's desire to participate in social activities and to improve function (Kemp, 1990). The clinician must have a complete understanding of motivational dynamics so that it does not interfere with the audiological rehabilitation program. The four variables that interact to determine one's level of motivation include (Kemp, 1990):

1. Wants, including goals, desires, or needs as they relate to audiologic rehabilitation
2. Beliefs, including expectations, assumptions, or perceptions regarding the virtues of the audiologic rehabilitation process
3. Rewards, including the benefit, outcome, or payoff for participating in rehabilitation
4. Costs including the physical, psychologic, and social costs of participating in an audiologic rehabilitation program

The audiologist who takes the time to understand the client's emotional status and motive system will be in a better position to proceed and succeed at audiologic rehabilitation. Kemp (1990) recommended that the rehabilitation worker examine and analyze each of the components of motivation in the context of aging, of the disability (i.e., hearing loss), and of the rehabilitative intervention (i.e., hearing aid). When assessing and attempting to manipulate one's motivation for using a hearing aid, the audiologist should consider the following points (Kemp, 1990; Weinstein, 1991):

1. One's subjective viewpoint about each of the components of motivation will influence both the decision to purchase rehabilitation services and the outcome of rehabilitation. Table 18.1 lists examples of what hearing-impaired individuals may want from hearing aids and lists possible expectations and beliefs older

---

Table 18.1
Motivating Factors Behind Hearing Aid Use in Older Adults

Potential Wants, Needs, and Goals Relative to Hearing Aids

1. Improved television/radio hearing and understanding
2. Improved speech understanding in quiet and noise
3. Maintenance of independence
4. Reduction of emotional and social consequences of hearing loss
5. Restoration of quality of life, self-esteem, and life satisfaction

Beliefs, Expectations, and Perceptions Regarding Hearing Aids

1. Easier to hear and understand speech[a]
2. Comfortable and easy to use, insert, and remove[a]
3. More comfortable in a greater number of situations than without a hearing aid.[a]
4. Improved ability to hear environmental noises (e.g., telephone ringing, doorbell, car horn).
5. Improved hearing and understanding in group situations and at a distance.

---

[a] *Source:* Kricos, P., Lesner, S., and Sandridge, S., Expectations of older adults regarding the use of hearing aids. *J. Am. Acad. Audiol.,* 2, 129–133 (1991).

Table 18.2
Rewards Associated with Hearing Aid Use

---

1. Excellent aided word recognition ability in quiet and noise
2. Frequency-gain functions that meet prescribed targets
3. Reduction in the perceived emotional and social handicap associated with hearing impairment
4. Improved communication with family
5. Improved affect

---

hearing-impaired adults may have regarding hearing aids.
2. It is crucial to uncover the rewards necessary to encourage and sustain hearing aid use. Table 18.2 lists potential rewards the hearing impaired may seek from hearing aid use.
3. There are unique physical, social, psychological costs associated with hearing loss. The cost-related variables in Table 18.3 can be used to motivate individuals to pursue audiologic rehabilitation. According to Kemp (1990), motivated dy-

namics are especially applicable to older adults, where health problems and social losses often pose obstacles to compliance with health/rehabilitative procedures. Kemp (1990) postulated that proper understanding of motivation can help the clinician in his or her attempt at promoting the well-being of disabled individuals and, in the case of the hearing impaired, in increasing the pool of successful older hearing aid users.

In sum, a host of biologic, environmental, and psychosocial variables interact to influence candidacy for and outcomes with audiologic rehabilitation. Table 18.4 provides a summary of the biopsychosocial variables to be considered when deciding on the rehabilitation potential (i.e., candidacy) of an older hearing-impaired adult. Understanding each has practical implications for treatment of the hearing-impaired older adult.

Outcome Indicators in Audiologic Rehabilitation

Clinicians and researchers have long been collaborating on definitive criteria against which to judge outcomes (e.g., benefit/success) from hearing aid rehabilitation. The desired outcomes for hearing-impaired individuals should be closely linked to the consequences of unremediated hearing loss. Unfortunately, no consensus exists regarding definitive criteria for measuring or predicting outcomes. The choice of an appropriate outcome indicator should depend on a number of variables. First, the goal of audiological rehabilitation influences, to a large extent, the outcomes the clinician wishes to measure. The goals should be based on the hearing-impaired consumer's buying behavior (Kotler & Clarke, 1987). That is, what needs are the consumers hoping to satisfy by purchasing audiologic rehabilitation services?

Maslow's hierarchy of needs typology can be very helpful in pinpointing consumer needs. Maslow theorized that people tend to satisfy their more basic needs first and then seek to realize higher level needs. Therefore, in audiologic terms, one might speculate that individuals would attempt to

Table 18.3
Potential Psychologic and Social Costs
Associated with Unremediated Handicapping

Hearing Loss

Psychologic Costs

1. Decreased self-esteem
2. Loss of independence
3. Depressed affect
4. Reduced enjoyment of leisure activities

Social Costs

1. Avoidance of previously enjoyed activities
2. Inappropriate responses during conversations
3. Difficulty communicating over the telephone
4. Personal safety jeopardized by inability to hear warning signals
5. Inability to function with maximal efficiency at work

satisfy their basic level of hearing first and gradually progress to the higher levels of hearing. According to Ramsdell (1960), the most fundamental level of hearing is the primitive level, which constitutes an unconscious link between the individual and a constantly changing environment. The ability to hear background sounds contributes to our sense of being part of an alive world (Ramsdell, 1960). Using Maslow's typology, satisfying the primitive level might be conceived of as satisfying one's basic physiologic needs. For persons with severe to profound hearing loss, the ability to hear background noise is often a priority because of the psychosocial consequences of deprivation at this level.

According to Maslow (1954), the next need people will attempt to satisfy is that of safety. This need dovetails with the second level of hearing, namely the signal/warning level. Ramsdell (1960) postulated that at this level, sound serves as an indicator of an outside stimulus or event and assists us in locating the source of sound. In a sense, at this level, hearing serves to inform persons of dangers in the environment, including the presence of smoke in the home, an oncoming vehicle, or a knock at the door. Having realized the basic needs necessary for survival, people will seek to satisfy higher social, self-esteem, and self-

actualization needs (Kotler & Clarke, 1987). The ability to hear signals in the environment is an especially important goal for most hearing-impaired older adults, especially for those who live alone. The availability of assistive listening devices is an important step toward ensuring that older adults continue to live in a safe environment.

The function subserved by the third level of hearing, namely the symbolic level, is the ability to communicate. For the most part, hearing-impaired individuals deprived of hearing at the third level may suffer from a loss of social independence. Further, inability to communicate may interfere with life satisfaction and may have an impact on one's self-esteem (Kemp, 1990). According to Kemp (1990), the latter issues are of greatest concern to persons with disability, and thus rehabilitation efforts must target these as outcomes of rehabilitation. Therefore, a primary goal of audiologic rehabilitation should be to restore each of these levels of hearing so that our efforts can improve daily function and preserve and promote self-esteem. A series of studies have recently been reported in the literature that demonstrate how hearing aids fulfill each of these needs, providing significant benefit to older adults soon after they obtain a hearing aid.

Hearing Aid Benefit in the Elderly

Henoch (1991) recently reported that in addition to the traditional goals of the hearing aid fitting, namely to improve the audibility and intelligibility of speech and nonspeech stimuli without degrading speech perception, a primary goal should be to decrease the self-perceived handicap of the hearing-impaired individual. McCarthy (1991) also acknowledged that self-report measures of hearing aid benefit are proving to be valid criterion measures. She speculated that their increasing acceptance may grow out of two factors: (*1*) traditional psychophysical and electracoustic measures used to quantify hearing aid benefit are limited in terms of their predictive validity. In short, results obtained using traditional

Table 18.4
Variables Affecting Hearing Aid Candidacy/Rehabilitation Potential in Older Adults

Sociological	Psychological	Cognitive	Physiological
Economics	Motivation	Cognitive reserve	Age
Life-style	Self-reported handicap	Memory	Hearing status
Level of independence/ dependence	Emotional status		Manual dexterity
			Visual status
Availability of a motivated caregiver interested in implementing treatment regimens			

Table 18.5
Perceived Benefits from Hearing Aids as Reported by Older Hearing-Impaired Adults

Improvements in Communication[a]

1. Improved communication in easy listening conditions
2. Ease of communication enhanced with a hearing aid
3. Improved speech understanding in reverberant conditions, with background noise, and with reduced visual cues

Improvements in Psychosocial Function

1. Improved emotional function[b]
2. Improved social function[b]
3. Improved psychosocial function as perceived by the spouse of the hearing impaired[b]
4. Improved cognition[c]
5. Improved affect[d]

[a] Assessed the Profile of Hearing Aid Benefit (PHAB) and the Intelligibility Rating Scale (IRIS) post hearing aid fitting (Cox, Gilmore, & Alexander, 1991).
[b] Assessed using the Hearing Handicap Inventory for the Elderly (pre and post hearing aid fitting).
[c] Assessed using the Short Portable Mental Status Questionnaire (pre and post hearing aid fitting).
[d] Assessed using the Geriatric Depression Scale (pre and post hearing aid fitting).

evaluation techniques in the clinic cannot be generalized to everyday communication. (*2*) Information gleaned from self-report measures have proved to be valid indicators of success and can be used to modify the response of hearing aids, thereby enhancing overall benefit.

The works of Newman and Weinstein (1988), Newman et al. (1991), Mulrow et al. (1990b) and Cox, Gilmore, and Alexander (1991) have set the stage for the use of self-assessment tools as indices of hearing aid benefit in older hearing-impaired adults. Their data have demonstrated how

quality of life can be improved with rehabilitation and also show that older hearing-impaired adults have the capability of making functional gains with rehabilitation soon after (i.e., 3 weeks) purchasing a hearing aid (Rentz, 1991). The beneficial treatment effects include: reduction in the psychosocial handicaps associated with hearing loss, significant improvement in cognitive function and depression, and improved familial relations as documented indirectly by spousal assessments of hearing aid benefit experienced by the hearing impaired. Mulrow et al. (1990b) were able to demonstrate the cost benefit of audiologic rehabilitation with the elderly, as well.

Table 18.5 summarizes the benefits of hearing aid use achieved by older hearing aid users. It is clear from the table that hearing aids satisfy the needs expressed by Maslow (1954) and restore the levels of hearing described by Ramsdell (1960).

Cox, Gilmore, and Alexander (1991) described the sensitivity of two analytic inventories for assessing daily life experiences with hearing aids, namely the PHAB and the IRIS. The PHAB is a 66-item inventory, consisting of seven subscales that profile performance in several listening conditions—in reverberant rooms, with reduced visual cues, and in the presence of background noise (Cox et al., 1991). Further, the PHAB provides an estimate of the perceived effort involved in communication, of reactions to environmental sounds, and of the perceived quality of voices and other sounds (Cox et al., 1991). The IRIS is composed of 47 items and yields an estimate of the proportion of speech the hearing-impaired individual understands with and without the hearing aid. The two questionnaires were sent to a group of hearing aid users, with 42 individuals completing both. The mean age of their subjects was 69 years, and the majority presented with mild hearing loss (Cox et al., 1991). Both questionnaires yielded substantial benefit on the subscales assessing perceived communication benefit from hearing aids in a variety of disparate listening conditions, and the PHAB also demonstrated improved ability on the part of the respondents to perceive environmental sounds with a hearing aid. Based on a variety of analyses, the authors concluded that the PHAB questionnaire holds considerable promise as an outcome measure of the relative efficacy of hearing aid treatments and as a tool for determining the best frequency response for a given hearing aid (Cox et al., 1991). Responses to the PHAB may also be helpful during counseling sessions to offer strategies for improved communication in the situations that are the most difficult for the hearing-impaired individual. The data of Cox et al. (1991) provide evidence that older adults derive significant benefit from hearing aids, especially in the domain of communication function. The relation between improved communication function assessed using the PHAB and self-assessed handicap is an area worthy of investigation.

Data on the impact of hearing aid use on perceived handicap also demonstrate that older adults do in fact derive substantial benefit from hearing aids. Newman and Weinstein (1988) were among the first investigators to adapt the HHIE as a baseline against which to judge success or failure of rehabilitative intervention with hearing aids in older adults. A sample of 18 new hearing aid users completed the HHIE prior to and after 1 year of hearing aid use. The spouses of the new hearing aid users also judged their handicap prior to and 1 year after hearing aid use. Statistically significant differences between scores on the HHIE before and after the hearing aid fitting emerged in both samples, suggesting that after 1 year, hearing aids continue to reduce the perceived emotional and social consequences of hearing loss.

Because a 1-year time interval is often too long for clinical purposes, and because the HHIE may be considered too time consuming an instrument to complete in a busy clinical practice, Newman et al. (1991) ad-

ministered the HHIE-S to a sample of 91 new hearing aid users prior to and 3 weeks after the hearing aid fitting. Once again, a statistically significant reduction in the perceived emotional and social consequences of hearing loss emerged. The reduction in handicap was quite dramatic, such that 78% of the subjects demonstrated a true change in perceived handicap based on a 95% confidence interval (CI) of 10 points. Another interesting outcome of their study was that across all hearing level categories (mild to severe), the majority of subjects had an HHIE-S score of 16 to 18 prior to obtaining a hearing aid, which improved to an HHIE-S score of 3 to 4 after hearing aid use. Similarly, when subjects were divided according to word recognition ability, a score of 16 to 18 emerged as the typical HHIE-S score prior to hearing aid use. A major implication of the aforementioned findings is that a handicap score of 16 to 18 may be predictive of hearing aid candidacy and success in older adults.

Mulrow et al. (1990b) recently completed a randomized trial of hearing aid rehabilitation in older males with mild to moderate levels of impairment. One-half of the subjects in their sample obtained hearing aids, and the remaining subjects (matched for hearing loss, age, medication status, etc.) were placed on the waiting list for hearing aids. All subjects completed five scales designed to assess quality of life, defined as a multidimensional concept encompassing social, affective, cognitive, and physical domains (Mulrow et al., 1990b). Quality of life was assessed at baseline and at follow-up at 6 weeks and 4 months. Two disease-specific measures, namely the HHIE and the Quantified Denver Scale of Communication Function, were completed by all subjects. Three generic instruments including the Short Portable Mental Status Questionnaire (SPMSQ), the Geriatric Depression Scale (GDS), and the Self-Evaluation of Life Function (SELF) were also completed at three separate intervals by all subjects. The majority of subjects (98%) in the experimental group were fit with in-the-ear hearing aids monaurally, and 70% of all subjects had mild levels of hearing loss. Subjects in both groups obtained comparable scores at baseline on all quality of life measures; however, only the hearing aid users obtained improved scores on the baseline measures after 6 weeks of hearing aid use. The authors therefore concluded that hearing aids are successful treatments for reversing the social, emotional, and communicative dysfunction caused by hearing impairment. In addition, in light of improvements in cognitive function and depression, they reasoned that hearing aids lead to improvements in cognition and lessening of depression. It was notable that the improvements in quality of life demonstrated after 6 weeks of hearing aid use, were sustained at 4 months. These data suggest that hearing aids are beneficial and effective treatments and that the functional status benefits are evident in older adults with mild to moderate levels of hearing loss soon after they begin to use a hearing aid.

In sum, despite anecdotal reports that older adults are not good hearing aid candidates and that they derive limited benefit from hearing aids, a number of investigators have documented the ability of hearing aids to reverse communication dysfunction, social/emotional handicaps, depression, and impaired cognition. Audiologists are encouraged to experiment with some of the tools that have been described, as the data that emerge from administration of many of the measures can be used in rehabilitation planning, counseling, and in-service training. The measures can also be used during the hearing aid orientation to modify the response of hearing aids that do not appear beneficial in selected listening conditions. Further, the ability to objectively quantify functional improvements from hearing aid intervention can be especially useful for quality assurance studies to actually document rehabilitative outcomes. Finally, it is especially important to provide frequent feedback to older adults regarding the benefits they perceive from hearing aids, as this will encourage the hearing-impaired individual to continue to use the hearing aid. Perceived self-efficacy or achievement of a certain level of performance is an especially important principle in geriatric rehabilitation (Trezona, 1991). High perceived self-efficacy leads to greater persistence even in the face of tasks that seem difficult.

The data emanating from the aforementioned outcome studies suggest that there is considerable variability in the response of older adults to a given hearing impairment and that handicap data, rather than impairment data, may assist in the selection of candidates for successful hearing aid fittings. That is, rather than relying on the audiogram, audiologists must factor the client's subjective appraisal of the consequences of the hearing loss into the equation when deciding on whether to recommend a hearing aid to an older hearing-impaired individual and when deciding on the most appropriate device.

Counseling Implications of Data on Hearing Aid Use and Benefit

Kricos, Lesner, and Sandridge (1991, p. 129) contend that "the older adult's satisfaction with, use of, and perceived benefits from amplification may be greatly influenced by the original attitudes and expectations of the older adult toward hearing aids prior to the actual hearing aid fitting." Similarly, Madell et al. (1991) reported that the major reason for rejection of hearing aids was that the consumer's performance with the hearing aid did not meet his or her expectations. Brooks (1989) concurred that a negative attitude toward hearing aids is a significant factor in hearing aid use yet can be modified with counseling. In fact, expectations-performance theory holds that consumer satisfaction is a function of the consumer's product expectations and the product's perceived performance (Kotler & Clarke, 1987). Specifically, if performance with the hearing aid matches expectations, the hearing-impaired consumer will be satisfied, whereas if it falls short he or she will be dissatisfied. The latter appears to be the case with large numbers of older hearing-impaired adults.

To ensure that hearing-impaired consumers are satisfied with their purchase of audiologic rehabilitation services (e.g., a hearing aid)—that is, that their performance with the hearing aid meets with their expectations—we must first be clear on what their expectations are. The counseling process should be aimed at understanding what motivated the hearing-impaired individual to seek audiologic services; that is, what were the triggering factors prompting the interest that gave rise to the purchase of a hearing aid (Kotler & Clarke, 1987)? The internal cues or triggering factor is often a physiologic stimulus, such as the inability to hear or understand in noisy situations. The stimulus may be psychological, such as feelings of anxiety or frustration because of an inability to function in the manner previously enjoyed (Kotler & Clarke, 1990). An external cue may have been a stimulus such as a commercial for a particular style or size of hearing aid, such as a "miracle ear" hearing aid. In the latter case, the product must have the attributes promised in the commercial if the consumer is to be satisfied.

The challenge faced by the audiologist is making sure that he or she thoroughly explores the factors triggering the hearing-impaired consumer to act. To identify the specific situations in which the client experiences speech understanding difficulties, a self-assessment scale such as PHAB or the Denver Scale of Communication Function may be appropriate. To uncover the emotional and social consequences possibly triggering the decision to purchase a hearing aid, one might administer the HH[T]E or the HHIE-S. The goal of the hearing aid selection should then be to ensure that the hearing aid is effective in minimizing the listening situations in which the individual is experiencing difficulty and to reduce the emotional/social consequences associated with difficulty understanding, which were revealed through the self-assessment. When the client returns for the hearing aid check, the scales administered at baseline should be readministered, and responses elicited should be based on experience with the hearing aid. If the fitting is successful, the data reported in earlier sections suggest that benefit can be apparent merely 3 weeks after initiating hearing aid use. The audiologist should review responses to the questionnaires with the new hearing aid user and demonstrate how the hearing aid seems to have reversed the handicaps or communication difficulties that prompted the person to purchase a hearing aid. If "unaided" expectations do not match with "aided" performance, modifications can be made in the frequency response of the hearing aid, a trial period with a different hearing aid may be recommended, or additional rehabilitation (e.g.,

environmental manipulation training, speechreading) may be advocated. Additional counseling to establish more realistic expectations is important as well. At all times, the emphasis of the counseling sessions should be to satisfy the hearing-impaired individual's hierarchy of wants as revealed in the initial and follow-up assessments (Kotler & Clarke, 1987).

During the counseling sessions, the audiologist must strive to establish the traits conducive to positive outcomes. These include assertiveness, wherein the hearing-impaired consumer is encouraged to manipulate the environment and persons in the environment so that communication function is maximized. Further, the audiologist must ensure that a family member or caregiver is closely involved in the rehabilitation process to ensure carryover of new information and to facilitate use of the hearing aid. The audiologist must understand that in geriatric rehabilitation, even small gains are important and should be communicated to the hearing-impaired consumer. The audiologist must ensure that successes are rewarded and that reinforcement is closely linked to the desired behavior (Kemp, 1990). Finally, the clinician must continually assess the motivational level of the older adult and at times work to improve the level of motivation by using the motivation model presented in an earlier section of this chapter. Throughout the counseling process, it is critical that the audiologist remember that improvement in rehabilitation tasks correlates with the patient's own appraisal of his or her potential for recovery. This consideration points out the importance of always uncovering the subjective viewpoint rather than only relying on your own appraisal of the situation (Kemp, 1990). In fact, a number of specialists in geriatric rehabilitation have demonstrated that "what a person wants and how specific and realistic their goals are help to determine overall performance" (Kemp, 1990, p. 301).

Summary

In summary, many older adults suffer from a multiplicity of age-related changes and prejudices. Socially, they often experience a loss of family, loss of income, and loss of work role. They are also the target of societal prejudice, such that chronological age in and of itself can be a factor preventing them from meeting criteria of eligibility for rehabilitation services (Brummel-Smith, 1990). In the biologic or physiologic sphere, nearly 80% suffer from at least one chronic condition/disability, and a large proportion experience multiple chronic conditions. Many disabled older adults consider the major impact of acquired disability to be adjusting to the social and psychologic consequences (Brummel-Smith, 1990). That is, disabilities such as hearing loss are often associated with cognitive deficits, affective disorders, and emotional, communicative, and social handicaps. Overcoming the consequences of disability is often difficult because they have doubts about their ability to recover from a disabling condition, and society and health care professionals also question the value of interventions with older adults. The major psychologic obstacle to use of rehabilitation services is, however, low motivation. Older persons suffer from low motivation because they are unclear as to the benefits of specific interventions and because they tend toward the status quo, are not risk takers, and try to avoid the cost of failure (Brummel-Smith, 1990).

We must understand and use some of the rehabilitation principles unique to geriatrics. These include the fact that a functional orientation, that is preservation of function, should be the ultimate goal. Clinicians must work with the older adult to develop goals that are functional and that will promote independence, as defined by the disabled individual (Brummel-Smith, 1990). For example, if an older adult merely wants a device to improve understanding of the television, he or she should be made aware of the options and should be encouraged to make the selection in line with his other specific goals. If the older adult must be convinced that the hearing aid promotes understanding in selected situations, we must demonstrate this, often prior to the decision to purchase a device. Similarly, older adults are more likely to purchase rehabilitation services, including an amplification device, if they are convinced that it will reverse the changes they encounter as a result of the disability (Kemp, 1990). Dis-abilities tend to decrease social independence, reduce life satisfaction, and compromise self-esteem because the disability may affect how the person is viewed and affects what the person can do (Kemp, 1990). To the extent that rehabilitation promotes independence, restores self-esteem, and contributes to enhanced life satisfaction, it will be considered worth the physical and financial commitment (Kemp, 1990). We, therefore, must link hearing aid use to these rehabilitative outcomes, which are key to older adults and fundamental to geriatrics.

The needs of the geriatric population, as they relate to audiology, are simple. Older adults need to be able to communicate effectively so that they can function independently and live satisfying lives. As audiologists we can help them realize these goals if we emphasize and demonstrate that our interventions are designed to achieve these ends.

References

Bess, F., Lichtenstein, M., and Logan, S. Making hearing impairment functionally relevant: linkages with hearing disability and handicap. *Acta Otolaryngol. (Stockh)*, Suppl., 476, 226–231 (1991).

Brooks, D., The effects of attitude on benefit obtained from hearing aids. *Br. J. Audiol.*, 23, 3–11 (1989).

Brummel-Smith, K., Introduction. In B. Kemp, K. Smith, and J. Ramsdell (Eds.), *Geriatric Rehabilitation*. Boston: College Hill Publication (1990).

Cooper, J., and Gates, G., Hearing in the elderly—The Framingham cohort, 1983–1985. Part II. Prevalence of central auditory processing disorders. *Ear Hear.*, 12, 304–312 (1991).

Cox, R., Gilmore, C., and Alexander, G., Comparison of two questionnaires for patient assessed hearing aid benefit. *J. Am. Acad. Audiol.*, 2, 134–144 (1991).

Gambert, S., Aging—The medical perspective. In *State of the Art Perspectives in Geriatrics*. New York: Hunter-Mt. Sinai Geriatric Education Center (1987).

Hartke, R., Introduction. In R. Hartke (Ed.), *Psychological Aspects of Geriatric Rehabilitation*. Maryland: Aspen Publication (1991).

Henoch, M., Speech perception, hearing aid technology and aural rehabilitation: future perspective. *Ear Hear.*, Suppl. 12, 187S–191A (1991).

Jerger, J., Oliver, T., and Pirozzolo, F., Impact of central auditory processing disorder and cognitive deficit in the self-assessment of hearing handicap in the elderly. *J. Am. Acad. Audiol.* 1, 75–80 (1990).

Kane, R., Ouslander, J., and Abross, I., *Essentials of Clinical Geriatrics,* 2nd edition. New York: McGraw Hill Information Services Co. (1989).

Kapetyn, T., Satisfaction with fitted hearing aids. II. An investigation in the influence of psycho-social factors. *Scand. Audiol.*, 6, 171–177 (1977).

Kemp, B., Motivational dynamics in geriatric rehabilitation toward a therapeutic model. In B. Kemp, K. Smith, and J. Ramsdell (Eds.), *Geriatric Rehabilitation*. Boston: College Hill Publication (1990).

Kohler, P., and Clark, R. *Marketing for Health Care Organizations*. New Jersey: Prentice-Hall (1987).

Kricos, P., Lesner, S., and Sandridge, S., Expectations of older adults regarding the use of hearing aids. *J. Am. Acad. Audiol.*, 2, 129–133 (1991).

Loebel, J., and Eisdorfer, C., Psychological and psychiatric factors in the rehabilitation of the elderly. In T. F. Williams (Ed.), *Rehabilitation in the Aging*. New York: Raven Press (1984).

Madell, J., Pfeiffer, E., Ross, M., and Chellappa, M., Hearing aid returns at a community hearing and speech agency. *Hear. J.*, 44, 18–23 (1991).

Maslow, A., *Motivation and Personality*. New York: Harper & Row (1954).

McCarthy, P., Clinical observations of self-report and global measures of hearing aid benefit. In G. Studebaker, F. Bess, and L. Beck (Eds.), *The Vanderbilt Hearing Aid Report II*. Maryland: York Press (1991).

Mulrow, C., Aguilar, C., Endicott, J., et al., Association between hearing impairment and the quality of the life of elderly individuals. *J. Am. Geriatr. Soc.*, 38, 45–50 (1990a).

Mulrow, C., Aguilar, C., Endicott, J., et al., Quality of life changes and hearing impairment: results of randomized trial. *Ann. Intern. Med.*, 113, 188–194 (1990b).

Newman, C., and Weinstein, B., The hearing handicap inventory for the elderly as a measure of hearing aid benefit. *Ear Hear.*, 9, 81–85 (1988).

Newman, C., Jacobson, G., Hug, G., Weinstein, B., and Malinoff, R., A practical method for quantifying hearing aid benefit in older adults. *J. Am. Acad. Audiol.*, 2, 70–75 (1991).

Pfeiffer, E., A short portable mental status questionnaire for the assessment of organic brain deficit in elderly patients. *J. Am. Geriatr. Soc.*, 23, 433–441 (1976).

Ramsdell, D., The psychology of the hard of hearing and deafened adult. H. Davis and S. Silverman (Eds.), *Hearing and Deafness*. New York: Holt, Rinehart & Silverman (1960).

Rentz, D., The assessment of rehabilitation potential: cognitive factors. In R. Hartke (Ed.), *Psychological Aspects of Geriatric Rehabilitation*. Maryland: Aspen Publication (1991).

Roth, E., The aging process: physiological changes. In R. Hartke (Ed.), *Psychological Aspects of Geriatric Rehabilitation*. Maryland: Aspen Publication (1991).

Trezona, R., The assessment of rehabilitation potential: emotional factors. In R. Hartke (Ed.), *Psychological Aspects of Geriatric Rehabilitation*. Maryland: Aspen Publication (1991).

Uhlmann, R., Larson, E., Rees, T., Koepsell, T., and Dukert, L., Relationship of hearing impairment to dementia and cognitive dysfunction in older adults. *JAMA* 261, 1916–1919 (1989).

Weinstein, B., Hearing aids at my age: Why bother? *Am. Speech Hear. Assoc.*, 33, 38–40 (1991).

Weinstein, B., Hearing aids and the elderly: audiologic and psychologic considerations. In G. Studebaker, F. Bess, and L. Beck (Eds.), *The Vanderbilt Hearing Aid Report II*. Maryland: York Press (1991).

Weinstein, B., and Amsel, L., Hearing loss and senile dementia in the institutionalized elderly. *Clin. Gerontol.*, 4, 3–15 (1986).

Weinstein, B., and Ventry, I., Audiometric correlates of the hearing handicap inventory for the elderly. *J. Speech Hear. Discord.*, 48, 379–384 (1983).

19

Research Needs in Rehabilitative Audiology

BRIAN E. WALDEN, Ph.D., KEN W. GRANT, Ph.D.*

It is clear from the preceding chapters that rehabilitative audiology is a diverse field involving various sensory aids, clinical methodologies, and client populations. Rehabilitative audiologists are responsible for providing such varied services as fitting digitally programmable hearing aids, assessing performance and providing training with cochlear implant patients, advising clients regarding assistive listening devices, assessing the disruption to communication performance that accompanies hearing impairment, and counseling. Their clients range from infants to the elderly. Nowhere is the diverse nature of rehabilitative audiology more apparent, however, than when one considers the state of research in the field.

Whereas some aspects of the field are receiving considerable research attention, others are almost totally neglected. Currently, there are active research programs around the world studying signal processing methods for improving speech understanding by persons with impaired hearing. Hearing aid technology is changing at a rapid rate. As of this writing, the first large-scale attempt to market a fully digital hearing aid has failed; noise-suppression hearing aids based on adaptive filtering seem not to have withstood the test of clinical research and

evaluation; digitally programmable analogue circuitry is growing rapidly in popularity; and present-day multichannel methods of output limiting seem to be demonstrating benefit after several earlier attempts largely failed (Braida et al., 1982). The "state of the art" in hearing aid technology, however, may be quite different in the very near future. Similarly, research efforts to improve cochlear implant technology are advancing at a rapid rate. New methods of coding speech information are under investigation, as are improvements in electrode design to provide greater specificity in place-frequency mapping.

In contrast to current research efforts in the area of sensory aids, few systematic attempts are being made to improve traditional aural rehabilitation methodologies such as speechreading training, auditory training, and auditory-visual integration training. It is noteworthy that this text does not include any chapters specifically devoted to these traditional methodologies, which defined the field for all but its most recent history. This lack of research into traditional aural rehabilitative techniques reflects the current clinical practice of the profession. With the exception of those rehabilitative audiologists involved in training programs using cochlear implants or tactile devices, relatively few clinicians appear to be providing traditional speechreading training, auditory training, or auditory-visual integration training to their adult clients.

---

*The opinions and assertions contained herein are the private views of the authors and are not to be construed as official or as reflecting the views of the Department of the Army or the Department of Defense.

One could argue that the lack of clinical research into traditional methodologies simply reflects the current relative unpopularity of those techniques among rehabilitative audiologists. The same argument cannot be made for the general lack of systematic research regarding counseling-oriented approaches. During much of the past 15 to 20 years, there was a steady movement away from traditional clinical procedures toward counseling-oriented methods such as information counseling, environmental control training, assertiveness training, and adjustment counseling. These methods are intended to help the client adjust to hearing loss and minimize the impact of impaired communication rather than to deal directly with the impaired sensory input. Despite the widespread use of such techniques, there exists an almost total lack of systematic clinical research to determine the efficacy of these methods. Given the amount of time devoted to these techniques by rehabilitative audiologists, one could easily argue that the lack of such research represents the single greatest research need in rehabilitative audiology.

Even in the area of communication self-assessment, where a number of inventories have been introduced for clinical use in recent years, relatively little research has been conducted to demonstrate the actual utility of these measures in ongoing clinical programs. It is not clear whether this reflects a general lack of use of these inventories by rehabilitative audiologists or some other factor. In any case, it is unlikely that clinicians will be persuaded of the value of such inventories until their clinical utility has been clearly demonstrated through systematic clinical observation and research.

One consequence of the present state of research activities in the field of rehabilitative audiology is that some unresolved questions have a much higher probability of being answered in the next few years than others. For example, it is inevitable that in the very near future rehabilitative audiologists will be able to match almost any target gain derived from prescriptive formulas in hearing aid fitting, given digitally programmable circuitry. Similarly, interactive methods of prescriptive fitting of modern hearing aids involving many variables are almost sure to be refined within the next few years (Newman et al., 1987). It is much less likely, however, that we will know with any degree of certainty if or when traditional speechreading training can result in a real improvement in the daily communication ability of an adult with an acquired, high-frequency hearing impairment. Yet, the latter issue is just as important to resolve as the former issues regarding hearing aid fitting.

Given current research efforts in the field, it would serve little purpose to review research needs that are highly likely to be filled in the foreseeable future. Consequently, this chapter focuses on selected research needs that have proved to be particularly resistant to experimentation and/or that have been largely ignored by researchers in the past. Although the chapter is divided into two major sections (sensory aids and traditional aural rehabilitation techniques), there is a common thread running throughout the various issues discussed—that is, validation and clinical efficacy. Clearly, the related problems of validating clinical methodologies and demonstrating their clinical utility are at the core of the most critical research needs in the field of rehabilitative audiology.

Given that this text is intended primarily for practitioners, this chapter is written from that perspective. Although some of the issues to be discussed may appear to be basic research needs and somewhat theoretical, all are highly relevant to the clinical practice of rehabilitative audiology. To make the connection between these research needs and clinical practice more apparent, the focus of this chapter will be on *fundamental assumptions underlying clinical practice.* These clinical assumptions will be highlighted throughout the chapter by bold italics. By clearly delineating such fundamental assumptions, it is hoped that practitioners will be stimulated to look carefully at the rationale for their current clinical practices. Researchers may find such a discussion useful in further defining essential research needs that must be addressed in order for the clinical practice of the profession to advance. Finally, the authors acknowledge that the issues to be dis-

Table 19.1.
Categories of Sensory Aids

Type Processing	Auditory	Visual	Tactile	Direct Electrical
Nonspeech-specific	Early hearing aids	Oscilloscope, envelope displays	Single-channel vibrator	Single-channel stimulator
Spectrum analysis	Modern hearing aids	Spectrographic displays	Tactile vocoder	Multichannel stimulation
Feature extraction	Speech-feature translation	Feature displays	Feature displays	Feature extraction prior to stimulation
Speech recognition	Speech recoding	Captioning, TDD	Speech to braille	

Reprinted with permission from Levitt, H., Signal processing for sensory aids: a unified view. *Am. J. Otol.*, 12 (suppl.), 52–55 (1991).

cussed reflect, in large measure, their particular research interests. Inevitably, some important issues and research needs in the field of rehabilitative audiology are not addressed.

Sensory Aids

The majority of ongoing research in the field of rehabilitative audiology deals with sensory aids for persons with impaired hearing. Although sensory aids are usually categorized according to the modality of stimulation (i.e., auditory, visual, tactile, auditory-neural), Levitt (1991) has recently suggested an alternative method of categorizing sensory aids that focuses on the nature of the signal processing that is accomplished by the device. Table 19.1 summarizes this categorization of sensory aids.

The simplest view of sensory aids is that we need to provide some transformation of the speech signal that is clearly perceptible to the client (nonspeech-specific processing). Early hearing aids and some single-channel cochlear implants are examples. Such sensory aids make little effort to process the speech signal beyond making it easily detectable. Implicit in this approach are the assumptions that *all aspects of the signal are equally useful to the client* and that *no parts of the signal will have a harmful effect on speech perception.* There is overwhelming experimental and clinical evidence that the first of these two assumptions is not true (see below). Similarly, there is considerable experimental evidence to suggest that the second assumption is also unfounded. Mar-

tin and Pickett (1970) and many subsequent investigators have demonstrated that persons with impaired hearing experience more upward spread of masking than do normal-hearing listeners, suggesting that low-frequency parts of the signal may actually interfere with processing the higher frequency portions. Further, nonspeech-specific signal processing largely ignores the reduced channel capacity (i.e., ability to process information) that results from hearing impairment. Even so, the benefit provided to clients with such rudimentary processing often has been remarkable.

The next level of complexity in signal processing is represented by sensory aids that assume that *parts of the speech signal are more critical for accurate speech perception than others* (spectrum analysis). The validity of this assumption is both highly intuitive and well established in the literature (Levitt, 1982). The majority of contemporary sensory aids, including most modern hearing aids, tactile vocoders, and multichannel cochlear implants, incorporate this type of signal processing. Most of the focus of these sensory aids has been on spectral considerations. For example, modern hearing aids and spectrum-based cochlear implants use spectrum shaping and amplitude control to place as much of the critical parts of the speech spectrum as possible into the client's residual hearing area or range of neural stimulation. Additional examples of more experimental approaches of this type of processing include attempts to alter the consonant-vowel ratio and/or segmental durations (Freyman & Nerbonne, 1989; Freyman, Nerbonne, & Cote,

1991; Montgomery & Edge, 1988; Montgomery et al., 1987).

Another kind of processing that has been incorporated into some experimental sensory aids are algorithms that extract certain phonetic characteristics of the speech signal (feature extraction). Most of the focus of these efforts has been on coding articulatory/phonetic features (e.g., frication, nasalization) and are based on the assumption that *feature recognition is fundamental to the speech perception process.* Early theories that speech perception involved a series of sequential binary decisions with regard to feature attributes (Jakobson, Fant, & Halle, 1952) have not been entirely abandoned (Stevens, 1986). However, a number of issues concerning the transformation from acoustic properties to phonetic features have never been addressed adequately by such theories (Klatt, 1989). Still, there have been some successful experimental applications of this type of speech processing (see Levitt, 1991, for a review). Most notable are multichannel cochlear implant processors that detect and code speech features.

The most complex level of signal processing would be sensory aids that actually recognized speech. Such processors would recognize the speech message and either present it to an unimpaired modality (e.g., acoustic recognition to printed text) or recode it to better suit the residual capacity of the impaired auditory system. To date, no signal processing algorithm is available that can automatically recognize an unrestricted speech message with a high degree of accuracy. Only a cursory consideration of automatic speech recognition is required to appreciate the problems involved. Two issues are particularly problematic. First, the acoustic representation of the various sounds of speech can differ considerably depending on the phonetic context and talker. Second, recognition of the speech message requires knowledge of the language. Although there is still not a unified theory of speech perception that is universally accepted (Klatt, 1989), recent advances in artificial intelligence encourage the belief that the problem of automatic speech recognition can be solved.

The system of categorizing sensory aids described by Levitt (1991) and reproduced in Table 19.1 focuses attention on the most fundamental research issues that must be addressed in the design of signal processing aids to improve speech understanding in persons with impaired hearing. With this as a framework, we will proceed with a discussion of selected issues regarding sensory aids currently in use with this population.

HEARING AIDS

Although comparative methods of hearing aid evaluation using monosyllabic word recognition (Carhart, 1946) were used by rehabilitative audiologists for nearly 40 years, few audiologists today use speech materials as the basis for hearing aid selection. Rather, as was suggested earlier, the primary intent of contemporary hearing aid selection and fitting procedures is to place as much of the amplified speech spectrum as possible into the client's residual hearing area. The 1990 Vanderbilt/VA Hearing Aid Conference consensus statement (Hawkins et al., 1991) stipulates that hearing aid selection procedures for adults should include the following seven essential components:

1. Determine hearing aid candidacy.
2. Determine initial electroacoustic characteristics (i.e., SSPL90, gain/frequency response).
3. Determine important hearing aid features (e.g., style, telecoil, directional microphone).
4. Select hearing aid that meets desired electroacoustic characteristics.
5. Verify electroacoustic characteristics.
6. Assess performance of hearing aid characteristics on the client.
7. Perform counseling and follow-up procedures.

It is noteworthy that relatively little consideration is given to direct tests of speech recognition according to these recommended procedures. Yet, unquestionably, the primary purpose for fitting a hearing aid to the vast majority of clients is to improve speech understanding! It is clear, therefore, that contemporary methods of hearing aid selection are based on the assumption that *the primary effect of hearing impairment on speech recognition is reduced audibility.* A corollary of this assumption is that *hearing impairment can be accurately modeled by spectrum shaping.* Given that the primary focus of contemporary hearing aid selection procedures is to shape and amplify the speech spectrum into the client's residual hearing area, the reduced speech recognition ability that typically accompanies hearing impairment must be attributable to reduced audibility for this approach to make sense.

Audibility is, of course, critical to speech recognition and hearing aid fitting. Obviously, the distinctive cues of speech cannot be recognized if they are not audible. The issue, however, is whether making the distinctive cues of speech audible is sufficient for speech recognition. In a study of stop consonant recognition, Turner and Robb (1987) examined the effect of spectral-cue audibility with hearing-impaired subjects. Although the results suggested that audibility was essential for correct recognition as expected, complete audibility of the spectral cues did not guarantee correct consonant recognition. More recently, Zeng and Turner (1990) attempted to distinguish between the role of audibility and that of suprathreshold discriminability in voiceless fricative recognition. They observed that the reduced recognition observed for subjects with impaired hearing was due both to reduced audibility of the frication burst cue and to reduced discriminability of the consonant-vowel transition cue. Hearing-impaired subjects could not make optimal use of the formant transition cues even though these cues were audible.

Some investigators have attempted to test directly the extent to which hearing impairment can be modeled as spectrum shaping. Walden et al. (1981), for example, compared speech recognition under conditions of hearing impairment and acoustic filtering using persons with unilateral hearing impairments as subjects. A suprathreshold loudness balance procedure between the normal and impaired ears was used to adjust a multifilter to match the spectrum shaping imposed by the hearing loss. Consonant recognition was then measured in the impaired ear and in the normal ear listening through the multifilter. Mean consonant recognition was generally poorer in the impaired ear, although the patterns of feature recognition were quite similar between ears. More recently, Humes et al. (1987) compared nonsense syllable recog-

nition in persons with impaired hearing and in persons with normal hearing whose thresholds were masked with broad-band noise shaped to match the thresholds of the impaired listeners. For half of the subjects with hearing impairment, syllable recognition scores were comparable to that of the noise-masked normals. The remaining subjects with impaired hearing showed poorer performance than the noise-masked normals.

These and other investigations have yielded conflicting results regarding the extent to which impaired hearing can be modeled accurately by spectrum shaping alone. Characteristic of all of these studies has been substantial intersubject variability. In addition to the obvious filtering effects of sensorineural hearing impairment, it is clear that frequency and temporal resolution can be reduced in some persons with impaired hearing (Schorn & Swicker, 1990; Tyler, 1986; Tyler et al., 1982). It is not so clear, however, what effect the impaired frequency and temporal resolution may have on speech recognition ability (Dubno & Dirks, 1990; Festen & Plomp, 1983; Luttman & Clark, 1986; Moore & Glasberg, 1987).

Although the research literature may be equivocal regarding the extent to which impaired hearing can be modeled by spectrum shaping alone, clinical experience and intuition appear less uncertain on this matter. Despite the nearly universal adoption of hearing aid selection methods that assume that hearing impairment is fundamentally spectrum shaping, most rehabilitative audiologists probably do not question that phonemic regression may accompany presbycusis (Alpiner & McCarthy, 1987, p. 372). In any case, it is clear that research that further clarifies the effects of sensorineural hearing impairment on the auditory processing of speech and other complex acoustic stimuli is critical to validating current methods of hearing aid selection, as well as to designing future sensory aids. It will be especially important in future research to delineate the relative contribution of factors unrelated to audibility that may contribute to the effects of hearing impairment on speech recognition. If such factors play only a minor role, the amount of signal processing that may be required to alter the frequency and/or temporal cues of speech may not be warranted.

Perhaps the most fundamental assumption underlying all hearing aid selection methodologies to date is that *there is a "best" hearing aid fitting for each client.* The Carhart (1946) comparative hearing aid evaluation method, for example, involved selecting the aid that performed best among a set of preselected instruments, based on measures of speech recognition. Likewise, contemporary functional gain/probe-tube microphone methods select the instrument whose gain/frequency response characteristics come closest to that specified by a particular prescriptive formula.

The assumption that there is a single optimal hearing aid fitting for each client necessarily leads to a number of related assumptions, each of which will be discussed briefly.

The first assumption is that there is little or no interaction among electroacoustic characteristics, hearing impairment, and the listening environment. If one seeks to select a single "best" instrument for a client, it must be assumed that whatever frequency response, gain, and output limiting characteristics are selected will be the best possible for that client across varying listening environments. This is not to say that the instrument selected would provide equal or even significant benefit in every listening situation. It is clear that a hearing aid is not equally beneficial to the client in different listening environments (Cox & Alexander, 1991a; Walden, Demorest, & Hepler, 1984). The issue, rather, is whether the instrument that provides the best possible performance in one listening environment will also provide the best possible performance in a different listening environment. Is the performance hierarchy of a set of hearing aids constant across listening environments?

Given the fundamental nature of this assumption, remarkably little research has been published that is directly relevant to this issue. Two investigations have compared the performance hierarchy of a set of hearing aids in a sound-treated test suite with that in a normally reverberant room. Harris and Goldstein (1985) measured quality judgments of continuous discourse obtained from experienced hearing aid users for four hearing aids. Although the performance hierarchy of the aids differed considerably across listeners, the majority of subjects provided generally similar performance hierarchies for the two listening environments. In a second study comparing a sound-treated environment with a normally reverberant environment, Logan et al. (1984) obtained both quality judgments and relative intelligibility preference judgments from experienced hearing aid users listening to continuous discourse recorded through five hearing aids. For both the quality judgments and the subjective judgments of intelligibility, substantial interactions were observed between the performance hierarchy of the hearing aids and the listening environment. The instrument that was preferred in one environment was not the preferred instrument in the other environment.

More recently, Cox and Alexander (1991a) measured the improvement in sentence intelligibility provided by three hearing aids differing in frequency response slope, in three everyday listening environments representing quiet, reverberant, and noisy situations. Although the mean benefit provided by amplification differed significantly across the three listening environments, benefit did not interact significantly with the frequency response slope. Inspection of the individual data revealed that none of the three frequency response slope conditions consistently provided the most improvement in speech intelligibility for any of the three listening environments. In a companion paper, Cox and Alexander (1991b) measured preferred gain for the same three frequency response slopes and three everyday listening environments. The subjects were experienced hearing aid users. Significant differences in mean preferred gain were observed across listening environments and frequency response slopes. However, the interaction of these two variables again was not significant.

One of the deterrents to conducting research that explores possible interactions of electroacoustic characteristics with the listening environment is the difficulty in switching rapidly among different hearing aids. Although this problem has been at least partially surmounted in the past using certain laboratory recording methods, such techniques have limited flexibility and face validity. These difficulties have been largely overcome with the introduction of digitally programmable multiple memory hearing aids. With these instruments, the subject can switch quickly between electroacoustic settings within a given listening environment and/or as the listening environment changes. Recently, Ringdahl et al. (1990) used a clinical-trials paradigm to compare hearing aid preferences between a programmable hearing aid that provided seven different gain/frequency response settings and the subject's own hearing aid, in six specified listening environments (e.g., listening to television news, listening to music). They observed that most subjects chose to use different gain/frequency response settings in different listening environments.

It is clear that additional research is required to determine definitively the extent to which electroacoustic characteristics and listening environments may interact. Assuming that such interactions exist, considerable research will be required to define the essential acoustic characteristics of various listening environments and the specific set of electroacoustic characteristics that will optimize performance in a given listening environment. The implications of this research for the design of future sensory aids, however, are obvious.

The second assumption is that the hearing aid that performs best under auditory-only conditions will also perform best under auditory-visual conditions. It is likely that at least some visual speech cues are available to hearing aid wearers in most communication situations. However, in contrast to other sensory aids (i.e., cochlear implants and tactile devices), auditory-visual speech perception is rarely considered systematically in clinical evaluations of hearing aids. Clearly, aided speech recognition ability should improve with the addition of visual clues. The question is whether this improvement will be the same across a set of hearing aids that might be fit to a given client. If the improvement from visual cues is quite variable for different instruments, the hearing aid that provides the best performance under auditory-only conditions may not be the best instrument when visual cues are available.

Fundamental to the issue of whether there is an interaction between hearing aid electroacoustic characterics and the benefit of visual cues is the nature of auditory-visual speech perception. If the combination of auditory and visual information in bisensory perception were basically additive (i.e., Auditory-Visual Performance = Auditory Performance + Visual Performance), then the performance hierarchy of a set of hearing aids should be the same for both auditory and auditory-visual conditions. However, the relationship between the two modalities is not additive. Rather, there is an integration of auditory and visual information in bisensory speech perception (Massaro, 1987, Chap. 7). Generally, the extent to which visual cues will benefit auditory speech perception depends on the degree of redundancy between the information that is provided in each of the sensory modalities. To a first approximation, the more similar the information available in the two modalities, the more limited will be the improvement in speech recognition resulting from visual cues (Blamey et al., 1989; Braida, 1991; Walden, Prosek, & Worthington, 1974).

Earlier it was noted that not all parts of the spectrum are of equal importance in conveying speech cues. Miller and Nicely (1955), for example, demonstrated that cues for place of articulation are in the mid-to-high frequencies predominantly. Given that speechreading provides information primarily with regard to place of articulation, this would suggest that low-frequency cues should be more complementary to speechreading than high-frequency information. Although such a complementary relationship is widely assumed to exist, the only published report to date is not consistent with this view. Grant and Braida (1991) combined visual cues with six filtered speech bands that differed in center frequency but that were of the same approximate auditory intelligibility. Despite the widely varying spectral composition of the bands, auditory-visual speech recognition was approximately the same across the six conditions of bandpass filtering. This would suggest that the relatively more subtle differences in frequency response/gain characteristics that are likely to exist among a set of hearing aids preselected for a client will not result in large interactions between electroacoustic characteristics and benefit from visual cues.

Considerably more research is required to delineate the manner in which amplified speech and speechreading may combine in bisensory speech perception. Grant and Braida (1991) suggest that their failure to demonstrate that different spectral regions provide varying complementary and redundant cues to speechreading may relate to their use of sentences as the test materials. It is possible that such relationships would be more apparent if their experiment were repeated using syllable-length materials. Moreover, Summerfield (1987) has suggested that models of auditory-visual speech perception that attempt to predict bisensory performance on the basis of the complementary relationship between the features transmitted via audition and vision are overly simplistic. Additionally, numerous investigators have demonstrated that, when different speech sounds are presented simultaneously via audition and vision, some phoneme combinations will result in a single speech sound being perceived that is different from either of those being presented to the two modalities (see, for example, McGurk & MacDonald, 1976, and Walden et al., 1990). Finally, in a study intended to examine the possible complementary relationships between amplification and speech reading, Walden et al. (1987) observed that even high-frequency emphasis hearing aids seemed to provide primarily manner of articulation and voicing cues! Clearly, much more research is required.

The third assumption is that the hearing aid that performs best in the clinic evaluation will be the instrument that will perform best in daily communication. After the clinical hearing aid evaluation is completed and the patient has been fitted with "the best" instrument available (regardless of the selection criterion), the rehabilitative audiologist must assume that the client will obtain optimal benefit from that hearing aid in daily communication as well. That is, it must be assumed that the performance hierarchy of a set of hearing aids in a clinical evaluation will be the same as the perform-

ance hierarchy for those instruments in more realistic communication situations. Fundamentally, this is an assumption about the predictive validity of our clinical assessment techniques. It also is relevant to a related assumption that *the relative performance of a set of hearing aids does not change as the client adjusts to amplification.*

Walden et al. (1983) compared the performance hierarchy for a set of hearing aids obtained with NU-6 word lists in clinic to preference rankings for the same instruments in daily communication. When statistically significant differences in word-recognition scores (according to the binomial model; Thornton & Raffin, 1978) were observed in clinic, these differences were generally reflected in similar preference rankings in daily communication. The differences in electroacoustic characteristics among the test instruments that were required to obtain significant performance differences in clinic, however, were much greater than would typically be observed among a set of hearing aids preselected for a given client. In the same study, the retest stability of the performance hierarchy for a set of hearing aids obtained in clinic was measured after a week of trial use. Frequent changes were observed in the performance hierarchy based on NU-6 word-recognition scores. The tendency was for significant performance differences during the initial evaluation to disappear after a week of adjustment to amplification.

The results of Walden et al. (1983) are consistent with more recent investigations of contemporary prescriptive fitting methods that explore the predictive validity of these techniques (Cox & Alexander, 1991a; Sammeth et al., 1989; Stroud & Hammill, 1989). Generally, these studies have revealed that, when different prescriptive fittings are compared in daily communication, significant differences in benefit are not observed.

At the first Vanderbilt Conference on Amplification, validation of hearing aid selection procedures was identified as the most urgent research priority (Bess, 1982). It is likely that this is still the case today. Experiments designed to determine the predictive validity of clinical hearing aid selection and fitting procedures are difficult to conduct because of problems in defining, quantifying, and measuring the validation criterion, that is, success with amplification outside of the clinic environment. There is no single direct measure of hearing aid success because this criterion variable is multidimensional and dynamic. It is not immediately apparent, therefore, how best to represent everyday communication performance with a hearing aid. Walden (1982) suggested five possible validation measures:

1. *Frequency of Use.* This criterion measure assumes that the more benefit and success a client experiences from amplification, the more he or she will use the hearing aid (see Surr, Schuchman, & Montgomery, 1978, for example). In recent years, rehabilitative audiologists have begun to fit increasingly milder hearing losses with amplification. Many of these clients require amplification only in selected difficult listening situations. It is likely, therefore, that frequency of use is not a highly valid measure of everyday success with a hearing aid for these individuals.

2. *Frequency of Changes in Fitting.* This validation criterion assumes that, if the clinical hearing aid selection and fitting procedures are valid, they will result in an optimal fit for the client. Consequently, major modifications in the hearing aid fitting should rarely be required. Although this may be theoretically true, most rehabilitative audiologists regard the selection and fitting of amplification as a dynamic, interactive process, based on clinical test results and feedback from the client. Hence, such a validation criterion is not useful in practice.

3. *Specific Benefit Provided.* This criterion measure assumes that significant improvement on some aspect of the clinical evaluation should predict significant improvement in that aspect of daily use. Such a measure was relevant for speech-based comparative hearing aid evaluation procedures that had some degree of content validity and face validity. Using this criterion, significant improvement in the aided speech reception threshold or in word recognition in noise should predict a similar improvement in sensitivity to speech and in speech understanding in noisy listening environments. Such a criterion measure has little relevance, however, for contemporary prescriptive clinical methodologies.

4. *Observations of the Client.* In this approach, the success of a hearing aid fitting is determined by having the clinician observe the client in daily communication situations. Although the use of such an observation approach has been reported (Colton & Reeder, 1980), it would seem to have very limited usefulness because of the obvious difficulties in observing clients outside the clinic.

5. *Client Acceptability Ratings.* Valid clinical selection and fitting procedures should result in amplification that the client judges to provide optimal benefit in everyday communication. When the rehabilitative audiologist questions the client regarding success with the hearing aid following an initial trial period, this is an effort to validate the hearing aid fitting. More structured approaches to obtain client judgments of performance with a hearing aid have been introduced in recent years, including written questionnaires designed to assess hearing aid benefit. Walden et al. (1984), for example, developed a 64-item questionnaire, the Hearing Aid Performance Inventory (HAPI). The items of the HAPI were constructed to reflect 12 signal and situational features (e.g., familiarity of setting, level of environmental noise) that were assumed to be relevant to success with amplification. Based on the responses of 128 experienced users, the internal consistency reliability of the HAPI was found to be quite high (coefficient alpha = 0.96). Factor analysis revealed four types of listening situations that might be assessed separately: (*1*) noisy situations, (*2*) quiet situations with the talker in proximity, (*3*) situations with reduced signal information (e.g., no visual cues available), and (*4*) situations with nonspeech stimuli.

More recently, Cox and Gilmore (1990) introduced the Profile of Hearing Aid Performance (PHAP), a 66-item self-administered inventory of hearing aid performance in everyday life. Based on the responses of 225 experienced hearing aid users, the 66 items were organized into four scales and seven subscales representing different environmental sounds and listening conditions. In a separate group of 76 experienced hearing aid users, the internal consistency reliability of the scales and subscales was found to be generally high. In addition, 30 of these 76 subjects completed the PHAP a second time 10 to 20 days following the first administration to assess retest reliability. Moderate-to-high retest correlation coefficients were observed for each of the subscales. Statistically significant differences at the 0.90 and 0.95 confidence levels were provided for each scale and subscale.

The results of both Walden et al. (1984) and Cox and Gilmore (1990) suggest that a self-report methodology for measuring successful use of amplification in daily life is a useful criterion measure in predictive validation studies of hearing aid selection procedures. Although the statistical properties of these inventories have been well defined, considerable additional research is required to determine their clinical utility. These efforts should be directed at determining a clinically significant difference (in contrast to a purely statistically significant difference), both for clinical hearing aid evaluation measures and for self-report measures of hearing aid success in daily life. For example, how large a difference in the gain/frequency response of a hearing aid is required to produce a significant performance change on a self-assessment inventory? Similarly, how much of a score change on a self-assessment inventory is required to create a noticeable change in success with amplification in daily life?

COCHLEAR IMPLANTS

Given the relatively small population of hearing-impaired persons who are candidates for a cochlear implant, the interest among hearing health care professionals in these sensory aids has been phenomenal. Boothroyd, Geers, and Moog (1991) estimated that, of the approximately 4000 babies born in the United States each year with hearing loss so severe as to prevent the spontaneous development of spoken language, only about 200 are candidates for a cochlear implant. The pool of postlingually deafened children and adults is similarly limited. (Cochlear implants have been fit to prelingually deafened adults on a very limited basis, and the general candidacy of these individuals is quite controversial, both among health care practitioners and within the adult deaf community.)

In view of the limited population of implant candidates, the allocation of medical resources to implant programs is remarkably large, and the amount of basic and clinical research that has been published is truly amazing. There are several reasons for this high level of interest and research activity, including the following:

1. Cochlear implants represent new technology. They are not simply a different kind of hearing aid. Rather, they represent a new approach (i.e., electrical stimulation of auditory nerve fibers) to aural rehabilitation.
2. Cochlear implants provide auditory researchers with a unique opportunity to explore the processing mechanisms of the central auditory pathways in response to electrical stimulation of the auditory nerve and, potentially, to investigate coding of sensory information in the brain.
3. Cochlear implants restore "hearing." Unlike tactile devices, cochlear implants produce a sensation of sound in most cases of postlingual deafness. For this reason, they have appeal to these clients who are accustomed to hearing, as well as to rehabilitative audiologists who are accustomed to dealing with audition.
4. Cochlear implants require surgical intervention. Much of the early research and development, as well as the clinical expansion of cochlear implant programs, is attributable to physicians. Cochlear implants represent a new arena in the medical management of hearing-impaired persons who, heretofore, could not be helped by medical treatment.
5. To date, cochlear implant research has been well supported by funding agencies.
6. Cochlear implants are generally successful (in a few cases, amazingly so) in pro-

viding usable speech information to clients who otherwise have little or no residual acoustic sensitivity. This is especially so when the implant is used in conjunction with speechreading. Further, the potential exists for clients with more residual hearing to be candidates for cochlear implants as this technology is refined.

Because of the high level of clinical and research activity in cochlear implants, this area of aural rehabilitation is changing quite rapidly. A discussion of research needs in this area is further complicated by the diversity of the population of hearing-impaired persons who are potential candidates. Four different groups of hearing-impaired clients have been fit with cochlear implants: (1) postlingually deafened adults, (2) prelingually deafened adults, (3) postlingually deafened children, and (4) prelingually deafened children. Each group represents a somewhat unique set of rehabilitative problems, with different sets of linguistic, social, and other resources available to them in using the electrical stimulation provided by the implant.

Despite the relative newness of this technology and the diversity of the population of hearing-impaired persons who are potential candidates for cochlear implants, some tentative assumptions have emerged that appear to form the basis for current clinical practice with these clients. One such fundamental assumption is that *the electrical transformation of the acoustic speech signal should be readily interpreted as speech.* Perceptual models of acoustic speech decoding have generally guided processor designs. Consequently, signal processing to code electrically important acoustic/articulatory parameters of speech (e.g., formant frequencies, voicing) has been incorporated into some designs (Patrick & Clark, 1991). The implication of this assumption is that clients will receive benefit from the cochlear implant to the extent that it restores a sensation of hearing. If the electrical stimulation can be interpreted as speech, it will allow the implant user to draw on highly learned perceptual and cognitive speech and language skills acquired prior to the onset of deafness. This naturally suggests a second assumption that *training in the use of implants need not be extensive for postlingually deafened clients* because they are not required to learn a completely novel perceptual code. The prevalence of this assumption is reflected by the fact that few implant centers employ a long-term structured training program that has been evaluated for its effectiveness.

The implications of these assumptions for adult clients who are prelingually deaf are quite different. It is assumed that these individuals have learned language through nonauditory pathways (e.g., sign language) and that the presentation of speech cues through an implant represents a completely new speech code for the client. To date, this group has received the least amount of benefit from implants, and most centers do not consider prelingually deafened adults suitable candidates for implantation. Whether the relatively limited success of these clients reflects the general lack of long-term structure training with the implant or other factors requires additional research.

A third fundamental assumption that seems to have emerged in implant technology and clinical practice is that, because the channel capacity of the implant user's auditory system is drastically reduced, *some preprocessing of the speech waveform is necessary in order to simplify the task of extracting relevant speech information.* Two basic strategies have been used to address the processing limitations imposed by the implanted ear. The first is to decompose the speech spectrum into different frequency bands and to present the outputs of these bands (or their amplitude envelopes) to different electrodes distributed along the cochlea (Gantz et al., 1988; Wilson et al., 1991). The goal is to encode the distribution of speech energy in the frequency dimension as variations along a spatial dimension, thus creating a place-frequency map in the implanted cochlea. The second basic processing strategy is to extract selected speech features in an attempt to reduce the amount of information transmitted to the client (Patrick & Clark, 1991). This is accomplished by converting some attributes of the original speech signal into binary cues (e.g., voicing) or by transforming continuous variables in the speech signal (e.g., formant frequencies, fundamental frequency) into a small number of discrete values.

The degree of preprocessing required from the implant depends on the processing capabilities of the implanted ear and on whether the device is to be used as a substitute for normal cochlear processing or simply as an aid to speechreading. For a device to function as a substitute for normal cochlear processing, substantial amounts of information about the segmental and suprasegmental aspects of speech must be conveyed. This requirement appears to be rarely met by current implant designs, with the exception of a few "star" implant patients. Considerably more research will be required to improve the performance of cochlear implants as substitutes for normal cochlear processing.

If the more modest goal of functioning as an aid to speechreading is selected for the device, relatively small amounts of supplementary information are required from the implant. Previous results on auditory supplements to speechreading have shown that simple acoustic signals derived from speech (e.g., presence or absence of voicing, variations in the fundamental or formant frequencies, variations in the speech envelope extracted from selected frequency regions), when combined with speechreading, yield remarkably good speech reception performance (Grant et al., 1985; Rosen & Fourcin, 1983). Thus, by using the implant as an aid to speechreading, the electrocochlear channel capacity of the client need not be very great.

Psychophysical data obtained from implant users reveal that frequency and intensity resolution are substantially poorer, and the dynamic range of the electrical stimulation is much smaller, than normal hearing (Pfingst, 1984; Pfingst, Burnett, & Sutton, 1983; Shannon, 1983; Simmons, 1966). These basic psychophysical limitations have led researchers and clinicians alike to expect limited levels of speech recognition performance from the implant alone. According to a recent review (CHABA, 1991), only 5 to 10% of implant users may be expected to use the implant effectively without the benefit of speechreading. For example, the recognition of open-set single words typically is near chance performance with the implant alone. When combined with visual cues, however, the typical implant user shows an improvement in word recognition of up to 30% over speechreading alone (CHABA, 1991).

Based on these performance expectations, an emerging view of cochlear implants is that, in all but a very few cases, *cochlear implants function primarily as an aid to speechreading rather than as a substitute for hearing.* Obviously, this assumption implies a related assumption that *persons with profound hearing impairments can effectively integrate the electrical stimulation provided by the implant with speech cues available through vision.* Braida (1991) developed and evaluated models for multimodal integration that can provide quantitative criteria for assessing the ability of cochlear implant clients to use the cues provided through their implant and through speechreading optimally. These models make predictions both for overall accuracy and for the pattern of residual confusions in the bimodal condition, based on the confusion matrices obtained separately in the unimodal conditions (i.e., implant only and speechreading only). Preliminary applications of these models to implant users suggest that many, but not all, clients can optimally integrate the cues derived from the implant with those obtained from speechreading (Braida, 1991).

A final fundamental assumption underlying cochlear implant technology is that *multiple channels of stimulation are capable of transmitting more useful information than a single channel of stimulation.* By definition, single-channel devices provide relatively undifferentiated or unidimensional information about the acoustic signal. Consequently, these devices should not be well suited to tasks such as phoneme identification that require more detailed information. Many of the limitations imposed by single-channel stimulation can be at least partially obviated through the use of multichannel electrode arrays. Most often, the array is organized with frequency encoded as the place of stimulation and intensity encoded as current amplitude. Most studies comparing the performance of single-channel and multichannel implants have reported that the multichannel devices provided generally superior performance (Gantz et al., 1988; Gantz et al., 1989; Tye-Murry & Tyler, 1989). However, some implant subjects have obtained excellent results with a single implanted electrode (e.g., Hochmair-Desoyer, Hochmair, & Stiglbrunner, 1985). Likewise, clients fitted with multichannel devices have not always performed better than single-channel users (e.g., Tyler, Moore, & Kuk, 1989). Notwithstanding such exceptions, future implant designs are almost certain to involve multichannel processing and electrodes. Identification of the number and nature of channels necessary to obtain optimal performance will require considerable additional research.

TACTILE DEVICES

Unlike cochlear implant technology, which is relatively new, attempts to code and transmit speech through tactile displays on the skin began more than 60 years ago (Gault, 1924). Interest in tactile devices seemed to increase in the 1970s, when a number of basic research studies were conducted to determine the discriminative capacities of the skin (see Sherrick, 1984, for a review). Relatively few concerted attempts, however, were made during this time to produce wearable tactile aids or to train hearing-impaired persons for extended periods in the use of tactile cues. In recent years, there has been renewed interest in tactile devices among sensory aids researchers, perhaps stimulated by the extensive attention given to cochlear implants. Given that (1) tactile devices are capable of providing roughly similar cues of speech as cochlear implants, and (2) cochlear implants involve surgery and are quite costly, tactile aids would seem to be a logical alternative. As a result, some wearable tactile aids have become commercially available.

Despite cochlear implants and tactile devices having the same purpose (i.e., to provide cues for speech and other sounds to profoundly hearing-impaired persons), there are several very important differences:

1. Whereas cochlear implants stimulate the neural pathways of the auditory system (after "bypassing" the damaged end organ), tactile devices rely on complete sensory substitution.

2. Although cochlear implants have achieved relatively widespread acceptance among health care professionals as an effective rehabilitative measure for certain clients, tactile devices generally are not regarded as such.
3. There has been a high level of commercial interest and involvement in cochlear implants as compared to a modest commercial interest in tactile devices.
4. On average, hearing-impaired persons have achieved less success in recognizing speech via tactile displays as compared to cochlear implants.*
5. The level of user satisfaction, on average, is higher for cochlear implants than for tactile devices, especially for postlingually deafened adults.

There are at least three possible explanations for the greater acceptance and success of cochlear implants as compared to tactile devices. First, it is clear that cochlear implants have enjoyed widespread backing by commercial interests and the medical community. Both groups have been persistent in refining this technology and its clinical implementation. As a result, the design of cochlear implants has improved significantly during the past decade, and there has been ample opportunity to demonstrate the efficacy of these devices in clinical trials. In contrast, interest in the development of tactile devices has been largely limited to the scientific/academic community. Although technological improvements have been made in these devices, the absence of commercially available, wearable, multichannel tactile aids until recent years, coupled with the relative lack of long-term clinical trials, has limited the expanded use and acceptance of tactile devices.

A second explanation for the greater success of cochlear implants versus tactile devices is that generally different populations of profoundly hearing-impaired persons have received each type of device. Although approximately equal numbers of patients have been fit with cochlear implants and tactile devices as of this writing, the ma-

---

*Although the most successful users of tactile devices have obtained superior performance to that achieved by the average cochlear implant user, no person fitted with a tactile device has achieved the same level of success in recognizing speech via their sensory aid as have the most successful implant users.

jority of implant patients are postlingually deafened adults who are implanted with multichannel systems. In contrast, the majority of tactile aid patients are prelingually deaf children, and the devices typically employ only one or two channels of stimulation (CHABA, 1991). Although the postlingually deafened adult represents a considerable rehabilitative challenge, the challenges are even more complex with the prelingually deaf child because there is no preexisting language base on which to build in therapy. The differences both in the degree of speech processing provided by the device and in the patient populations make direct comparisons between implant and tactile aid performance difficult, if not impossible. One might wish to argue, for example, that the difference in success between cochlear implants and tactile devices is a demonstration that auditory speech perception is inherently preferable to speech perception via another modality. However, the lack of long-term clinical trials with multichannel tactile devices fitted to postlingually deafened persons makes such a comparison nearly meaningless and represents a significant challenge to future research efforts comparing these two classes of sensory aids.

A third possible explanation for why cochlear implants have achieved a higher level of acceptance and use is simply that they may be inherently more effective than tactile displays as a substitute for normal auditory processing. A definitive explanation will require additional research and clinical experience. However, resolution of this issue will undoubtedly relate to the validity of certain basic assumptions that form the rationale for tactile sensory aids.

Perhaps most basic of these assumptions is that *speech perception is possible with complete sensory substitution.* That is, it must be assumed that *audition is not necessary for speech decoding.* Early theories of speech perception posited that humans are predisposed neurologically to decode speech via audition. Liberman et al. (1968), for example, stated that "the speech decoder is, we suspect, biologically linked to an auditory input and cannot be transferred or redeveloped for any other modality." Although this issue could be argued on a theoretical basis, as a practical matter, a va-

riety of nonauditory speech recognition methods have been demonstrated, including tactile speechreading (i.e., Tadoma), visual and tactile finger spelling, and visual and tactile signing. Each of these so-called "natural" nonauditory communication strategies is capable of transmitting information about speech and language with a high degree of accuracy and at near-normal rates of commuication (Reed et al., 1989).

Given the success of Tadoma and other nonauditory communication strategies, it would appear that hearing is not essential for speech perception. However, as speech codes, each of these methods of communication has serious limitations. Tactile signing and finger spelling, for example, require that the "talker" (sender) possess communication skills in producing manual signs. In the case of Tadoma, the "listener" (receiver) must touch the talker's face to monitor the speech movements associated with the jaw, lips, oral airflow, and laryngeal vibration, making speech perception at a distance impossible. These limitations have the obvious effect of severely restricting the number of people with whom a deaf signer or tactile speechreader can converse.

The limitations of natural tactile communication methods potentially are circumvented by electronic tactile devices that transform acoustic speech into patterns of cutaneous stimulation. Such tactile aids extract a variety of speech attributes from the acoustic signal and display them via one or more mechanical or electrocutaneous transducers placed on the surface of the skin.

The primary advantages of electronic tactile aids over the natural methods are that they do not require the talker and receiver to be in direct physical or (potentially) visual contact with one another, and they do not require special knowledge on the part of the talker. However, there are significant differences between the information provided by natural methods and the information provided by electronic tactile methods of representing speech. These differences may limit the potential of tactile aids, at least as they are currently designed. Unlike the natural tactile methods, which encode information along a variety of dimensions (e.g., hand shape, movement, hand orientation) and which actively engage proprioceptive as well as cutaneous receptors in the skin, muscles, and joints, current tactile aid designs passively stimulate only cutaneous receptors along the skin surface. Further, the natural tactile methods tend to operate as a unique language with morphology, syntax, and semantics appropriate to the receiving sense. In the case of Tadoma, information directly related to the articulatory gestures of speech is conveyed. In contrast, tactile aids operate on the acoustic waveform and do not provide direct information about articulatory gestures. Further research is required to determine whether the success of Tadoma is due primarily to the richness of its multidimensional display or to its articulatory nature.

The use of Tadoma by deaf-blind persons frequently has been cited as proof that tactile speech perception is possible (CHABA, 1991; Reed et al., 1985). Although this may be proof in principle, the success of natural tactile methods of communication does not provide a persuasive argument that passive mechanical or electrocutaneous tactile stimulation may serve as an adequate substitute for hearing, given the fundamental differences between the information provided by natural tactile speech communication methods and available electronic tactile aids. Rather, the efficacy of electronic tactile aids is based on the assumption that *the essential cues for speech recognition contained in the acoustic waveform can be encoded as passive cutaneous stimulation that, in turn, can be decoded as speech.* This assumption is reflected by the assertions of Reed et al. (1989, pp. 65–66) that:

1. The tactual sense is capable of receiving continuous speech at normal speaking rates with nearly zero error rates.
2. Subjects are capable of integrating a relatively impoverished tactual signal with visual speechreading to achieve essentially normal speech reception performance.
3. Limitations on the speech reception performance obtained with current tactual aids are due primarily to inadequacies in the design of the aids and/or in the training received with the aids.
4. There are no fundamental scientific obstacles to eliminating these inadequacies and achieving much improved speech

reception for individuals with profound hearing impairment.

Such an optimistic view of tactile aids has considerable intuitive appeal. When a person acquires a hearing impairment that is so severe that conventional amplification is not feasible, each of the two most popular alternatives (i.e., speechreading and cochlear implants) are far less than ideal. Speechreading alone does not provide sufficient cues to permit accurate speech recognition, except in rare cases. Likewise, cochlear implants are a poor substitute for the auditory processing performed by a normal cochlea. Further, the ability of available cochlear implants to stimulate different neural fibers in the cochlear nerve selectively is gross at best compared to a normal cochlea. In the case of tactile devices, however, it is theoretically possible to represent any aspect of the acoustic signal via a tactile display. Further, this stimulation is provided to an intact sensory system that is easily and broadly accessible. But, is the sense of touch adequate for the recognition of speech?

Although this question may seem straightforward at first glance, the answer depends on a number of complex variables, including the amount of signal processing performed by the aid and the characteristics of speech that are actually encoded as tactile stimulation, the nature of the transducer(s) used to present the tactile signal to the skin, the sensory capabilities of the skin, and whether visual speech cues are available. A complete discussion of each of these variables is beyond the scope of this chapter. Only a brief description of each, therefore, will be provided.

The first variable *is the nature and complexity of the signal processing performed by the aid.* If a sufficient amount of signal processing can be performed by the aid, there is little question that speech can be successfully conveyed via the tactile sense. For example, if the tactile aid were capable of actually recognizing the string of phonemes that makes up a speech message, this information could be presented in a number of ways to the receiver including, for example, as braille characters. Unfortunately, such automatic speech recognition is not possible at present. The amount and complexity of the signal processing actually accomplished by currently available tactile aids range from simple single-channel devices that convert the frequency intensity pattern of sound over time via linear amplification, to multichannel systems that extract various parameters of speech (e.g., voicing, fundamental frequency, spectral shape) and present them via arrays of mechanical or electrocutaneous stimulators. Obviously, the more simple and the less relevant to speech perception the signal processing provided by the sensory aid, the more "signal processing" must be assumed by the receiver. Whatever the processing involved, it must result in a perceptual code that the receiver can learn to recognize as speech. Until the problem of reliable automatic speech recognition for unrestricted messages and talkers is solved, considerably more research is required to determine the optimal set of acoustic parameters to be extracted from the acoustic waveform and the optimal encoding of those parameters as tactile stimulation.

The second variable is *the transducer(s) used to present the tactile stimulation.* Ultimately, the nature of the tactile stimulation that may be provided to the receiver is limited by the characteristics of the transducer. Currently available tactile transducers are passive in nature; that is, they present vibratory or electrocutaneous stimulation to the surface of the skin. Such stimulation does not take advantage of the full capabilities of the tactile sense, which involve proprioceptive feedback as well as active exploration. If, for example, a transducer were constructed that moved the fingers and hand of the receiver in the manner that the speech articulators do in Tadoma, the potential of touch to recognize speech might be more fully exploited. (This, of course, ignores the considerable problem of constructing the signal processor that would be capable of deducing the movement of the articulators from the acoustic waveform!) Even in terms of passive tactile stimulation, a number of transducer-related issues must be resolved, including mechanical characteristics, the number of stimulators and how to array them, and the optimal location on the body to place the transducer(s).

The third variable is *the sensory capabilities of the skin.* It seems evident that

speech evolved to fit the sensory capabilities of the human ear. The ear, for example, is most sensitive in the spectral region, which carries the most salient cues for speech recognition. Likewise, the ear is capable of following rapidly changing frequencies and intensities such as are encountered in speech. It is equally evident that the sense of touch is not nearly as well suited for sensing the frequencies, relative amplitudes, and rapid transitions involved in speech. Tactile sensitivity to changes in vibration frequency and amplitude are rather limited (Rothenberg et al., 1977; Sachs, Miller, & Grant, 1980). In contrast, the skin is quite sensitive to location of stimulation; that is, closely adjacent sites on the skin can be accurately discriminated (Weinstein, 1980). As a result, a common strategy in tactile aids is to code frequency and/or amplitude information as different points along the skin via an array of tactile stimulators. However, this transformation of the acoustic signal adds another layer of complex encoding that must be decoded by the receiver. Whether such complex transformations of the acoustic speech signal can be decoded with a high degree of accuracy must be the subject of considerably more clinical research.

The fourth variable is *the availability of visual cues.* The potential of tactile aids, particularly of passive cutaneous tactile devices, probably depends in large measure on whether they are considered as a complete substitute for hearing or as a supplement to speechreading. Obviously, the task of coding all of the essential cues for speech recognition is considerably more complex than disambiguating the visual speech signal. Because of the complex transformations that are required to code speech, the goal of complete sensory substitution of touch for hearing may simply be unrealistic until the fundamental problems of automatic speech recognition are solved. However, there are clear indications in the literature that tactile stimulation may serve as an effective supplement to speechreading (Boothroyd, 1989; Hanin, Boothroyd, & Hnath-Chisolm, 1988; Weisenberger, Craig, & Abbott, 1991). Constructing a tactile aid that is intended as a complete substitute for hearing versus one that is intended simply to supplement speechreading may require fundamentally different signal processing by the device. Considerable research is required to identify the speech cues that, when coded as tactile stimulation, are optimally complementary with speechreading. Investigations of auditory supplements to speechreading are likely to be relevant to this issue (Breeuwer & Plomp, 1984, 1985, 1986; Grant et al., 1985; Grant & Braida, 1991; Grant, Braida, & Renn, 1991).

Even if it is assumed that speech perception is possible with complete sensory substitution and that the essential cues for speech recognition can be encoded as passive cutaneous tactile stimulation, it probably must also be assumed that *a relatively long period of training is required for the client to interpret the vibratory patterns on the skin as speech.* As previously noted, for postlingually deafened cochlear implant clients, the perceived sensations may tap into a rich store of knowledge of previously heard sounds. Further, the client has a long history of simultaneously hearing and viewing speech cues. Because of this, the benefit obtained with implant stimulation may be immediate and dramatic, especially in combination with speechreading.* For clients receiving a tactile aid, the perceived sensations are quite novel. Not only must the client learn to distinguish one sensation from another, but he or she must also develop associations between these sensations coded in memory and the external acoustic environment. That is, the client must learn a completely new perceptual code. This process may take years to complete (Watson, 1980). The challenge that this presents to sensory aids researchers is obvious.

Few studies exist that permit meaningful assessment of the effects of long-term training and clinical experience with tactile sensory aids. One of the primary deterrents to meaningful long-term clinical trials to determine the full potential of tactile stimulation has been the unavailability of wearable multichannel aids. There have been some clinical reports of long-term use with single- and two-channel wearable tactile de-

vices (Geers, 1986; Goldstein & Proctor, 1985; Proctor & Goldstein, 1983). However, tactile aids showing the greatest potential benefits in research studies tend to employ several channels (10 or more) and are large and bulky. It is rare for a client to acquire much more than 60 hours of experience with such prototype laboratory devices. Most studies report results after only a few hours of training. Further advancements in transducer technology are necessary to produce a lightweight, powerful, and power-efficient wearable multichannel tactile aid. Notable progress in this area, however, has been reported by Blamey and Clark (1985) and, more recently, by the Audiological Engineering Corporation (1991).

In addition to the practical problems associated with transducer technology, future research efforts must investigate more thoroughly whether there is a critical leaning period early in life during which humans are neurologically "primed" to learn speech and language. It is standard clinical practice with conventional hearing aids to fit prelingually hearing-impaired children as early in life as possible. Because of the complex recording of the speech signal that is required, it may be even more critical in the case of sensory substitution aids that the child be provided with these novel sensory experiences during an early period of learning and neurological development. Even if a deaf child's experience with tactile speech begins as early as possible, substantial learning periods will be required before significant progress is obtained. Studies concerned with the acquisition of a tactile vocabulary in deaf children 2 years of age and older, as well as in adults, indicate very shallow learning curves of roughly 1 to 4 words per hour of training (Brooks et al., 1985; Engelmann & Rosov, 1975). Whether these rates would improve if the tactile stimulation were provided earlier in life is not known.

Despite the potential of tactile sensory aids as a substitute for hearing in deaf persons, one must still question whether the auditory system might not be inherently preferable as the primary input channel for speech and language. Additional research is required to resolve this issue definitively. Preliminary evidence suggests that this may be the case, at least for persons who had a

*A history of hearing and viewing speech, however, does not obviate the need for structured speech recognition training with newly implanted clients. A trial period of at least 3 to 6 months, which includes training and testing by an experienced therapist, has been recommended for these clients (CHABA, 1991).

previous sense of hearing, who learned language before the onset of deafness, and who, therefore, are able to draw on prior auditory experience in speech perception. Whether the relatively limited success in recognizing speech that has been obtained with tactile aids to date is due to inadequacies in the design of currently available devices and/ or in the training that has been provided to recipients of tactile aids (Reed et al., 1989), rather than to inherent limitations imposed by sensory substitution, awaits further research.

Traditional Aural Rehabilitation Techniques

The field of rehabilitative audiology traces its roots back to the first half of this century when a number of methodologies were introduced for teaching speechreading to deaf children and adults. Both analytic and synthetic approaches were advocated. In either case, these traditional methodologies involved presenting speech samples to the deaf client and eliciting recognition responses of some kind. These techniques were feedback oriented; that is, a speech stimulus was presented to the client for recognition, after which the clinician provided feedback regarding the correctness of the client's response. Gradually, these traditional feedback-oriented methods were adapted for use with clients having less severe adventitious hearing impairments, for auditory training and auditory-visual integration training, and for speechreading training.

Traditional feedback-oriented training methods dominated the field of rehabilitative audiology for more than half a century. During the mid-1970s, however, the popularity of these techniques diminished considerably, and counseling-oriented techniques replaced traditional training methods as the predominant aural rehabilitative approach. Although it is still the case today that traditional feedback-oriented training methods are used infrequently by rehabilitative audiologists with adult clients having mild or moderate acquired hearing impairments, the increasing popularity of cochlear implants and the renewed interest in tactile devices have resulted in a resurgence of interest in feedback-oriented training techniques. Unfortunately, in most cases, these techniques have been adapted and implemented for use with cochlear implant clients without consideration of the theoretical issues (with very practical clinical implications) that probably resulted in the original demise of these techniques in the 1970s. These issues, therefore, remain highly relevant today and are briefly addressed in the form of assumptions underlying clinical practice in the following sections on auditory training and speechreading/auditory-visual integration training.

AUDITORY TRAINING

The purpose of auditory training is to maximize the client's use of residual hearing. Obviously, then, this training is directed at a sense that is impaired. Further, in the case of adult clients with acquired hearing impairments, training is directed at the sensory modality through which the client originally learned to recognize speech and through which he or she has a lifetime of experience recognizing speech. These basic observations suggest several assumptions that underlie traditional feedback-oriented auditory training methods.

The most fundamental of these assumptions is that *it is possible to teach a client with impaired hearing to make better use of distorted auditory speech signals.* Although this assumption rarely has been questioned, at least in published reports of auditory training, the fundamental idea that we should be able to improve the client's use of the distorted auditory input might be questioned. This is most obvious when the hearing impairment has rendered the acoustic cues for the recognition of a particular speech sound inaudible to the client. If the audibility of those cues cannot be restored through amplification, there is little basis for attempting auditory training of that speech sound. The efficacy of feedback-oriented auditory training is less clear, however, when the speech cues are audible but distorted. To conceptualize this situation more clearly, it is necessary to consider the general process of speech perception.

It is clear that normal-hearing persons acquire the ability to understand speech primarily through audition during the first few years of life. Although many complex theories of speech perception exist, most models posit that a part of this process is the acquisition of internal representations of speech sounds (or some other short segment of speech) that are stored in long-term auditory memory. The process of decoding (i.e., perceiving) speech must involve segmentation and, at some level, a comparison of the incoming auditory speech segments with these templates. When the incoming sensory event provides a reasonable match with the internal representation, correct identification occurs.* On the other hand, when the essential characteristics of the incoming sensory event are not sufficiently similar to the target internal representation (because of some distortion that may be introduced by hearing impairment or the environment), the wrong internal representation will be selected as the best match. When this happens, correct identification is interrupted and a phonemic confusion takes place.

From this perspective, the rationale for feedback-oriented auditory training for the prelingually severely impaired child is clear: Because internal representations of the various speech sounds do not exist, the goal is to create associations between the distorted acoustic input, an internal representation of that input in long-term memory, and linguistic meaning. (Speech perception is impaired even after extensive auditory training because, presumably, the distortion introduced by the hearing impairment does not allow every speech sound to be unambiguously distinguished.) However, the rationale for auditory training is not as clear in the case of a person who acquires a sensorineural hearing impairment after the internal representations of speech sounds have been established normally in long-term auditory memory.

Clearly, the effect of an acquired sensorineural hearing loss is to distort the incoming auditory signal. Phonemic confu-

sions occur because of "mismatches" between the distorted auditory input and the internal representations of the speech sounds. Presumably, the goal of auditory training in such cases is to make new associations between the distorted auditory input and the existing internal representations of the speech sounds. Given that the original associations were formed naturally in the course of normal exposure to speech communication, why should structured training be required later in life when the original associations have been disrupted because of acquired hearing impairment? Might not new associations be formed without therapeutic intervention in the same way in which the original associations were formed?

Relatively few published reports exist to document the efficacy of traditional auditory training methodologies, especially for adults with acquired hearing impairments and substantial residual hearing. Walden et al. (1981), for example, investigated the effects of a concentrated program of feedback-oriented auditory consonant recognition training on speech recognition. They observed a significant improvement both in the auditory recognition of consonants and in the auditory-visual recognition of sentences. Further, improvement in the recognition of consonants was moderately correlated with improvement in the recognition of sentences, suggesting that the effects of auditory consonant recognition training generalized to more realistic speech stimuli. The possible long-term effects of this training were not explored.

Another potential effect of hearing impairment that has considerable implications for auditory training methodologies is the possibility that the internal representations of speech sounds themselves might be altered as a result of long-term hearing impairment to reflect the distorted auditory input. If the internal representations eventually are altered, the speech recognition difficulties encountered by a person with hearing impairment may be more than simply distortion of the auditory input. Rather, the phoneme boundaries of the internal representations of the speech sounds might be ambiguous as a result of long-term hearing impairment. If such is the case, the hearing-impaired listener may encounter problems

---

*A range of incoming sensory events all can be "matched" to a given template because of variations in phonetic context, talker differences, the acoustic background, and so on. Even though these variations in the input usually are discriminable by the listener under the right experimental circumstances, they typically are ignored in the perceptual process; that is, listeners typically *respond* "categorically" even though the perception may not be strictly categorical.

such as those faced when a normal-hearing person attempts to learn a foreign language for which the phoneme boundaries are different from his or her native language. The problem is not distortion of the auditory input but relative perceptual insensitivity to speech sound discriminations that are essential to the new language.

Walden et al. (1980) conducted a study that was intended to explore the possibility that acquired long-term hearing impairment might alter the internal representations of speech sounds. They obtained similarity judgments among pairs of consonants presented sequentially. The consonant pairs were presented under two test conditions: auditorily and orthographically (i.e., printed consonants presented visually). In the latter test condition, the subject was instructed to rate the similarity of the two consonants "as you think about them," rather than on the basis of the shapes of the letters (Walden et al., 1980, p. 167). The stimuli were presented to subjects with normal hearing, subjects with long-term acquired sensorineural hearing impairments, and subjects with severe congenital hearing impairments.

Because the orthographic condition bypassed the auditory system, it was assumed that responses to the visually presented stimuli would reflect the internal representations of the consonants in long-term memory, independent of any distortion that might be introduced by hearing impairment. The similarity judgments of the subjects with normal hearing under the orthographic condition were expected to be comparable to their responses under the auditory condition, given that the internal representations of the speech sounds are assumed to be based on auditory input. Likewise, the similarity judgments of the congenitally impaired subjects under the orthographic condition were expected to be like their responses under the auditory condition for the same reason, but different from normal because of their hearing impairments. The critical aspect of the experiment was the relationship between the auditory and the orthographic similarity judgments in the subjects with long-term acquired hearing impairments. If the orthographic data of these subjects were like those of the normal-hearing subjects, this

would suggest that long-term hearing impairment does not alter the internal representations of the speech sounds as they are established during the period of normal hearing. On the other hand, if the orthographic responses of the subjects with acquired hearing impairments were like their auditory judgments (which should reflect their hearing impairments), this would suggest that the internal representations of speech sounds can change due to long-term hearing impairment.

Although the design of this experiment seemed appropriate to exploring this question, the data provided unexpected results. The responses of all three subject groups under the orthographic test condition were remarkably similar to one another and to the auditory condition for the normal-hearing subjects. Consequently, there was little evidence of the effects of the hearing impairments on the internal representations of the speech sounds for *either* of the hearing loss groups. Although such a result could be explained for the subjects with acquired hearing impairments (i.e., acquired hearing impairment does not affect the normal internal representations of the speech sounds established prior to the hearing impairment), such an explanation was not possible for the data from the subjects with congenital hearing impairments who had never heard the speech sounds undistorted.

Because the auditory test condition required that subjects be able to respond to consonant-vowel syllables, it was necessary to select congenitally impaired subjects with a substantial amount of residual hearing. Further, each of the congenitally impaired subjects had received years of auditory training prior to participation in this experiment. If the experiment were repeated with congenitally impaired subjects with more severe impairments and/or a history of minimal auditory training, more definitive results might be obtained. In any case, research that explores the issue of how hearing impairment may affect the way in which speech sounds are conceptualized in auditory memory, as well as other possible changes in "top-down" auditory speech processing resulting from acquired hearing impairment, is highly relevant to designing auditory training methodologies for these clients.

A second basic assumption underlying traditional auditory training that is highly related to the preceding assumption is that *speech perception can be adapted or modified, even in adulthood.* Speech perception is regarded as a strategy of dealing with a particular class of acoustic signals that is learned and, therefore, flexible. An opposing view is that humans are "prewired" to decode speech in ways that reflect the nature of the speech signal. According to this view, linguistic experience during an early sensitive or "critical" period (Lenneberg, 1967) tunes the speech decoding mechanism to the distinctive contrasts of a given language, and later attempts to modify the decoding process will be unsuccessful once the critical period has passed (see Strange & Jenkins, 1978, for discussion). Although models of speech perception that assumed a prewired speech mode were prominent in early theories, they have become less popular in light of more recent research. Reports by Werker and Tees (1984) and Logan, Lively, and Pisoni (1991), for example, reveal that sensitivity to nonnative linguistic contrasts can be demonstrated in adult listeners if proper training and testing methods are employed. This suggests that speech decoding strategies may also be modifiable in hearing-impaired adults, given appropriate auditory training. Little research, however, has been conducted to explore the specific speech decoding strategies employed by hearing-impaired listeners and, particularly, how these strategies may be affected by training.

Fundamental to the notion of training the client's residual hearing is the acoustic and phonological redundancy of the speech signal. If the primary cue for distinguishing a particular speech sound has been made inaudible or otherwise distorted beyond recognition by hearing impairment, it must be assumed that *the listener can learn to make greater use of secondary cues to recognize speech.* Given the fundamental nature of this assumption, there is surprisingly little published research that documents its validity. In one of the few direct investigations of this issue, Summers and Leek (1991) recently examined the use of second-formant frequency and vowel duration information in vowel identification by hearing-impaired listeners. Using subjects with poorer-than-normal frequency resolution

in the F2 region (as measured by a notched-noise masking paradigm), these investigators observed a decreased reliance on formant frequency information in making vowel identification decisions. However, this decrease was not accompanied by an increased reliance on vowel duration. The authors suggested that these listeners may make more use of cues in the F1 frequency region as an adjustment to their impairments in processing at higher frequencies. F1 frequency cues, however, were neutralized so that this possibility could not be verified. These findings suggest that hearing-impaired listeners may make adjustments in the perceptual weighting assigned to various acoustic cues based on the salience of these cues after processing through the impaired ear. This research, however, did not address the extent to which such adjustments in weightings might be facilitated by training.

Although additional clinical research that directly investigates the possible effects of feedback-oriented auditory training on speech recognition is necessary, the relevance and efficacy of such training cannot be clearly established until additional research further delineates the specific effects of hearing impairment on speech perception. In other words, the rehabilitative audiologist must know what it is that is to be trained. If the effect of the hearing impairment is to reduce the audibility of the primary cues of speech, one might conceptualize the process of auditory training as getting the client to attend to more subtle differences in these cues than is ordinarily required of persons with normal hearing. If the effect of the hearing impairment is to make the primary cues inaudible, the goal of auditory training might be thought of as teaching the client to attend to secondary cues that may yet be available through audition. If the effect of the hearing impairment is to distort the cues for speech, but that distorted input is clearly audible, the goal may be to facilitate the formation of new associations between the distorted input and the internal representations of the speech sounds.

Feedback-oriented auditory training may provide minimal benefit to many hearing-impaired clients because the fundamental assumptions underlying these traditional methodologies may not be valid. It is also possible, however, that these techniques may not be highly successful because we have not developed optimal clinical strategies that are responsive to the specific and individual effects of hearing impairment on speech perception. Research that better defines these effects must remain a high priority for hearing scientists in the foreseeable future.

SPEECHREADING TRAINING AND AUDITORY-VISUAL INTEGRATION TRAINING

During the early part of this century and before, speechreading training was associated with deaf education, particularly in oral communication programs for the prelingually deaf. Although the focus of much of the early training efforts was to teach these persons to recognize speech from only visual cues, gradually rehabilitative audiologists became less involved with attempts to teach visual-only recognition of speech and more focused on training auditory-visual speech recognition. This reflects the fact that aural rehabilitative services were increasingly directed at adults with adventitious hearing impairments and substantial residual hearing. In addition, except for the exceedingly rare "superstar" lipreader, accurate visual-only recognition of speech produced at normal speaking rates generally was not achieved, even with extensive training.

Because the potential for accurate speech recognition from only visual cues is so limited, when contemporary rehabilitative audiologists provide speechreading (i.e., visual-only) training, it is almost always with the assumption that it will improve the contribution of visual cues in combination with some other sensory input (e.g., amplified auditory, electrocochlear, tactile). That is, visual-only speechreading training and auditory-visual speech recognition training typically have the same goal of improving speech recognition ability with sensory input for multiple sources. However, the more common rehabilitative strategy today is speech recognition training with multiple sources of input, rather than unimodal speechreading training.

Whether visual speech recognition training is provided only with visual cues or with visual cues in combination with some other sensory input, several basic assumptions

can be identified that form the rationale for such rehabilitative methodologies. Among the most fundamental of these assumptions is that *speech, as encoded in the movement of the articulators, is readily decoded as speech by the visual system and the brain.* Obviously, the ability to decode speech normally is significantly better via audition than via vision. This is usually attributed to the fact that substantially fewer speech cues are available from the visual signal as compared to the auditory signal. That is, visual speech recognition is generally thought to be more difficult than auditory speech recognition because of stimulus considerations such as increased phonemic ambiguity and segmentation problems. Clearly, such factors play a significant role in limiting visual-only speech recognition ability. However, it is also possible that visual-only speech recognition is inferior to auditory speech recognition because fundamentally different perceptual processes are involved. Specifically, the decoding of speech via hearing may be a "natural" process in which the sensory system is specialized to the signal (or, more likely, where the signal is specialized to the sensory system). In contrast, visual speech recognition may be quite unnatural and only "along for the ride" with auditory speech perception. If visual-only speech recognition is a fundamentally different process from auditory speech perception, the potential of speechreading as a substitute for impaired auditory speech recognition is quite limited, independent of any stimulus considerations that may limit visual speech recognition performance. An experiment addressing the issue of whether auditory and visual speech perception are fundamentally different processes was reported by Walden, Montgomery, and Prosek (1987). The purpose of that experiment was to determine if observers respond categorically to visually presented speech stimuli. It is well known that listeners tend to respond categorically to segment-length speech stimuli presented auditorily (see Repp, 1984, for a review).* In contrast, responses to nonspeech auditory stimuli tend to be continuous.

---

*Although it was originally assumed that the categorical responses of listeners to speech stimuli reflected categorical perception, more recent research suggests that the extent to which a stimulus continuum is perceived categorically is dependent on stimulus variables, tasks variables, and subject variables rather than on some basic sensory limitation.

The most frequently employed experimental paradigm for demonstrating categorical responding to auditory speech stimuli involves presenting a continuum of synthetic consonant-vowel stimuli individually to listeners for labeling as the exemplar consonants, and in triads for ABX discrimination. The results of such experiments are summarized as labeling functions that show the percentage of responses to each stimulus that was labeled as each of the possible exemplar consonants, and as discrimination functions that show the percentage of correct discriminations for stimulus pairs. The classic finding in such experiments is labeling functions with steep slopes at the points along the stimulus continuum corresponding to category boundaries, and discrimination functions with peaks for stimulus pairs that span a category boundary. Both of these results are consistent with categorical responding.

The experiment of Walden, Montgomery, and Prosek (1987) paralleled the traditional categorical perception experimental paradigm but used synthetic visual speech articulations rather than auditory stimuli. Specifically, animations of the syllables /ba/, /va/, and /wa/, as well as six linearly interpolated intermediate stimuli between each of the possible exemplar pairs, were generated on a computer-based graphics system. Three experimental tasks were performed for each of the three eight-item continua. The first two tasks were the traditional labeling and ABX discrimination tasks. The final task required subjects to assign a numerical rating to each animation, indicating the extent to which it was like one or the other exemplar syllable in each continuum. The results revealed labeling functions with abrupt transitions at the category boundaries. These results were quite consistent with labeling functions typically observed for auditory speech stimuli. However, the peaks in the ABX discrimination functions generally did not coincide with the category boundaries. Further, the mean rating functions were relatively linear. The results for the ABX discrimination task and the rating task, therefore, were more consistent with continuous rather than categorical responding.

Although the results of Walden, Montgomery, and Prosek (1987) are not completely consistent with the view that the same perceptual processes underlie both auditory and visual speech recognition, rather persuasive evidence that auditory and visual speech perception are not fundamentally different at higher levels in the decoding processes is provided by a number of recent experiments using the intersensory discrepancy paradigm to explore visual biasing of auditory speech perception. A substantial literature exists within perceptual psychology using the intersensory discrepancy paradigm to study bisensory perception (see Welch & Warren, 1980, for a review). Much of this literature has involved visual and proprioceptive specification of spatial localization. The general outcome of this research is that discrepant sensory information tends to bias the observer toward one of the two input stimuli.

The first investigation using the intersensory discrepancy paradigm with speech stimuli was reported by McGurk and MacDonald (1976). They presented discrepant auditory and visual stop consonants to normal-hearing observers. For certain combinations of consonants, a third consonant was heard that was different from the two stimuli! For example, when an audio /ba/ was combined with a video /ga/, subjects typically perceived /da/. This phenomenon has come to be known as the McGurk effect and has been replicated by numerous investigators for a variety of consonant combinations (Green & Kuhl, 1986; MacDonald & McGurk, 1978; Manuel et al. 1983; Massaro & Cohen, 1983; Roberts & Summerfield, 1981; Walden et al., 1990).

That a third consonant may be perceived that is different from either of the stimulus consonants is inconsistent with a view that speech perception is fundamentally auditory and that visual information is a serendipitous concomitant of the auditory signal. Rather, the McGurk effect reflects sensory integration, suggesting that at some point in the decoding process, auditory and visual speech perception share processes in common. Clearly, additional research is required to define more precisely the perceptual processes underlying speechreading. As in the case for auditory training, however, the design of optimal speechreading training methodologies is dependent on a considerably greater understanding of these processes than currently exists.

A second fundamental assumption underlying speechreading training is that, *until hearing impairment is incurred, visual speech recognition represents an unpracticed skill that is, for the most part, largely irrelevant to normal speech perception.* Whereas hearing impairment directly affects auditory speech recognition, it leaves visual speech recognition unimpaired. From this simple perspective, therefore, it may be clear why impaired auditory speech recognition should be trained, but it is not so apparent why unimpaired visual speech recognition should require "rehabilitation." However, if it is assumed that normal-hearing persons do not rely on visual cues for speech perception, then the need for speechreading training after hearing impairment is incurred becomes apparent.

There is a variety of indirect and direct evidence that visual cues play an important role in speech recognition by persons with normal hearing. Anecdotally, normal-hearing persons and hearing-impaired persons alike tend to look at a talker. Similarly, it is generally disconcerting to watch a movie where the sound track is not synchronized with the video frames. More directly, normal-hearing and hearing-impaired persons tend to perform approximately the same on speechreading tests even though normal-hearing persons, ostensibly, have little experience lipreading (e.g., Owens & Blazek, 1985). Further, normal-hearing persons, like persons with impaired hearing, tend to recognize speech much better in noisy environments when visual cues are available.

Perhaps the most persuasive (certainly the most elegant!) evidence that speech perception by persons with normal hearing is high influenced by visual cues comes from experiments referred to earlier that explore the biasing effect of discrepant visual cues on auditory speech recognition. The susceptibility of normal-hearing observers to the McGurk effect demonstrates quite clearly that visual speech cues play a highly significant role in their speech perception.

A third fundamental assumption underlying speechreading training is that *a person may learn to rely more on visual cues after incurring hearing impairment.* From the preceding discussion, it would appear unlikely that speechreading training with persons who have incurred a hearing impairment in adulthood would serve to introduce visual cues in speech perception. Rather such cues have always played a significant role in their speech perception ability. However, if visual cues acquire increased significance after hearing becomes impaired, then speechreading training may facilitate a greater reliance on these cues.

Rehabilitative audiologists have long observed clinically that hearing-impaired persons may become "visually oriented" (Alpiner & McCarthy, 1987, p. 333). Chermak, for example, states that "one of the diagnostic symptoms of impaired hearing is an individual's noticeable awareness and attentiveness to . . . visual stimuli" (Chermak, 1981, p. 40). Although the idea that a person may become more visually oriented as a result of hearing impairment seems to be generally accepted clinically, there is little empirical evidence to support this notion. Recently, however, Walden et al. (1990) provided experimental support for such a view. Using the intersensory discrepancy paradigm, they compared the susceptibility of normal-hearing and hearing-impaired observers to visual biasing of their auditory speech perception. Synthetic auditory stimuli that varied along a /ba-da-ga/ continuum were presented simultaneously with natural visual articulations of /ba/ and of /ga/. The subjects were instructed to both watch and listen to the stimulus items but to indicate if each sounded most like /ba/, /da/, or /ga/. Hence, the tasks measured the visual biasing effect of discrepant natural articulations on the auditory perception of the synthetic syllables. In contrast to the hearing-impaired subjects who listened to the auditory stimuli in quiet, the synthetic consonant-vowel stimuli were presented to the normal-hearing subjects in a low-level background noise. The level of the noise was adjusted such that it affected the auditory recognition of the normal-hearing subjects to the same extent as the hearing impairments affected the auditory recognition of the subjects with hearing loss. In essence, the two subject groups had comparable reductions in hearing ability. However, the hearing-impaired group had a number of years of experience adjusting to their hearing impairments, whereas the normal-hearing subjects had no prior experience with impaired hearing.

The results revealed that the hearing-impaired subjects showed substantially greater susceptibility to visual biasing of their auditory speech perception than did the normal-hearing persons listening in the background noise. Given the comparable reductions in auditory recognition imposed by the hearing impairments and the noise, these results suggest that hearing-impaired persons may develop a propensity to rely on visual cues as a result of long-term hearing impairment that is independent of any need for visual information that may exist in a specific communication situation. It appears, therefore, that the relative importance of auditory and visual cues in bisensory speech perception is dynamic and may be influenced by the occurrence of hearing impairment. Whether this increased reliance on visual information may be facilitated by training was not addressed by Walden et al. and requires additional research.

A final assumption to be considered that underlies speechreading training is that *it is possible to improve a hearing-impaired person's ability to use visual uses through feedback-oriented training beyond that which would occur naturally in the course of adjusting to the hearing impairment.* Even if one assumes that the use of visual cues in speech recognition is not optimized until a hearing impairment is incurred, it is still reasonable to question whether formal training should be required to maximize the contribution of visual information. It may be reasonable to assume that, because of their desire to communicate, persons with impaired hearing would learn to make optimal use of visual cues naturally in the course of adjusting to their hearing impairments. By analogy, hearing-impaired persons do not have to be taught to cup their hand behind their ears to get the few decibels of amplification provided!

Perhaps the most direct way in which to address the question of whether formal speechreading training is beneficial is to consider some of the published research studies that sought to determine the efficacy of such training. Given the clinical relevance of this question, relatively little research has been conducted to determine whether formal speechreading and auditory-visual integration training actually results in improved speech recognition ability. Early attempts to determine the effects of speechreading training generally suggested that it does improve overall speechreading ability (Black, O'Reilly, & Peck, 1963; Heider & Heider, 1940; Hutton, 1960; Lowell, Taaffe, & Rushford, 1959). Subsequent investigations also suggested the benefit of training. Specifically, feedback-oriented speechreading and auditory-visual integration training with consonants improved not only the recognition of consonants/visemes (Walden et al., 1977) but also auditory-visual sentence recognition ability (Montgomery et al., 1984; Walden et al., 1981). In a more recent investigation, Lesner, Sandridge, and Kricos (1987) examined the effects of analytic visual consonant recognition training on visual consonant and sentence recognition. They observed that visual consonant recognition improved significantly as a result of the training. However, the ability to speechread sentences did not change. Finally, Danz and Binnie (1983) examined the effect of auditory-visual training with continuous discourse, using the tracking method of De Filippo and Scott (1978). The results revealed a significant improvement in visual-only consonant recognition and in intelligibility estimates of visual-only and auditory-visual recognition of continuous discourse following the training.

Although the preponderance of available research suggests that speechreading training can improve visual and auditory-visual speech recognition ability, the results of this research cannot be considered definitive. Training studies are exceedingly difficult and time consuming to conduct and generally include a number of potentially confounding variables. Among the several limitations typical of the published research are the following:

1. A small number of subjects are included in the study, thereby limiting the extent to which the findings can be generalized.
2. The amount of training provided to each subject is quite limited (e.g., a few hours). Hence, asymptotic performance may not be achieved.
3. Similar or even identical speech materials are used for training and for the pre- and posttraining testing, thus raising the

possibility that any improvement in performance may be a result of increased familiarity with the test situation rather than an actual improvement in the ability to extract cues from the visual speech signal.

4. Posttraining testing is administered very shortly after the conclusion of the training, so the long-term effects of training cannot be assessed.

5. Little or no control is exerted over subject variables such as motivation and test-taking strategies. As a result, the experimental and control groups in training studies often are not comparable.

It should be apparent that considerably more research is required before the effect of speechreading and auditory-visual integration training on the speech recognition ability of hearing-impaired persons will be determined. There are many theoretical arguments for and against such training, some of which have been discussed in this section. Most of these arguments are far from being resolved. Further, the available empirical clinical research, as we have seen, is far from definitive in resolving this issue. Perhaps our best guide in judging the efficacy of speechreading and auditory-visual integration training is clinical experience. The general decline during the 1960s and 1970s in the use of traditional training methodologies by rehabilitative audiologists with adults having mild-to-moderate acquired hearing impairments may well reflect the general ineffectiveness of such techniques to make lasting changes in speech recognition ability of these clients. It remains to be seen whether the current interest in feedback-oriented training with patients receiving cochlear implants and tactile sensory aids will withstand the test of clinical practice. Nevertheless, as was observed for traditional auditory training methodologies, speechreading training may fail because the basic assumptions underlying these clinical techniques are not valid. It is also possible, however, that current methods are not optimal for the training requirements of the client.

Certainly, our clinical successes provide a useful guide for developing effective rehabilitative strategies. However, in the absence of integrated models of the effects of hearing impairment on speech recognition ability, our clinical failures probably do not constitute a reasonable basis for determining the validity of the most basic assumptions underlying traditional aural rehabilitation techniques. Progress in the clinical management of persons with impaired hearing awaits additional research.

References

Alpiner, J. G., and McCarthy, P. A., *Rehabilitative Audiology: Children and Adults.* Baltimore: Williams & Wilkins (1987).

Audiological Engineering Corporation, Tactaid 7 from Audiological Engineering. *Hear. J.,* 44(4), 53 (1991).

Bess, F. H., Amplification for the hearing impaired: research priorities. In G. A. Studebaker and F. H. Bess (Eds), *The Vanderbilt Hearing-Aid Report: State of the Art—Research Needs* (Monographs in Contemporary Audiology). Upper Darby, PA: E. R. Libby, pp. 217–218 (1982).

Black, J. W., O'Reilly, P. P., and Peck, L., Self-administered training in lipreading. *J. Speech Hear. Disord.,* 28, 183–186 (1963).

Blamey, P. J., and Clark, G. M., A wearable multi-electrode electrotactile speech processor for the profoundly deaf. *J. Acoust. Soc. Am.,* 77, 1619–1620 (1985).

Blamey, P. J., Cowan, R. S. C., Alcantara, J. I., Whitford, L. A., and Clark, G. M., Speech perception using combinations of auditory, visual, and tactile information. *J. Rehabil. Res. Develop.,* 26, 15–24 (1989).

Boothroyd, A., Developing and evaluating a tactile speechreading aid. In N. S. McGarr (Ed.), *Research on the Use of Sensory Aids for Hearing-Impaired People* (*Volta Rev.,* Vol. 91). Washington, DC: A. G. Bell Association (1989).

Boothroyd, A., Geers, A. E., Moog, J. S., Practical implications of cochlear implants in children. *Ear Hear.,* 12 (Suppl.), 81S–89S (1991).

Braida, L. D., Crossmodal integration in the identification of consonant segments. *Quart. J. Experiment. Psychol.,* 43, 647–677 (1991).

Braida, L. D., Durlach, N. I., De Gennaro, S. V., Peterson, P. M., and Bustamante, D. K., Review of recent research on multiband amplitude compression for the hearing impaired. In G. Studebaker and F. Bess (Eds.), *The Vanderbilt Hearing-Aid Report: State of the Art—Research Needs* (Monographs in Contemporary Audiology). Upper Darby, PA: E. R. Libby, pp. 133–140 (1982).

Breeuwer, M., and Plomp, R., Speechreading supplemented with frequency-selective sound-pressure information. *J. Acoust. Soc. Am.,* 76, 686–691 (1984).

Breeuwer, M., and Plomp, R., Speechreading supplemented with formant-frequency information from voiced speech. *J. Acoust. Soc. Am.,* 77, 314–317 (1985).

Breeuwer, M., and Plomp, R., Speechreading supplemented with auditorily presented speech parameters. *J. Acoust. Soc. Am.,* 79, 481–499 (1986).

Brooks, P. L., Frost, B. J., Mason, J. L., and Chung, K., Acquisition of a 250-word vocabulary through a tactile vocoder. *J. Acoust. Soc. Am.,* 77, 1576–1579 (1985).

Carhart, R., Tests for selection of hearing aids. *Laryngoscope,* 56, 780–794 (1946).

CHABA (Working Group on Communication Aids for the Hearing-Impaired, Committee on Hearing, Bioacoustics, and Biomechanics), Speech-perception aids for hearing-impaired people: current status and needed research. *J. Acoust. Soc. Am.,* 90, 637–685 (1991).

Chermak, G. D., *Handbook of Audiological Rehabilitation.* Springfield: Charles C. Thomas (1981).

Clark, G. M., Black, R., Forster, I. C., Patrick, J. F., and Tong, Y. C., Design criteria of a multiple-electrode cochlear implant hearing prosthesis. *J. Acoust. Soc. Am.,* 63, 631–633 (1978).

Colton, J. C., and Reeder, R. M., An observational approach to evaluating hearing aid performance. Paper presented to the Annual Convention of the American Speech-Language-Hearing Association, Detroit, MI (November 1980).

Cox, R. M., and Alexander, G. C., Hearing aid benefit in everyday environments. *Ear Hear.,* 12, 127–139 (1991a).

Cox, R. M., and Alexander, G. C., Preferred hearing aid gain in everyday environments. *Ear Hear.,* 12, 123–126 (1991b).

Cox, R. M., and Gilmore, C., Development of the Profile of Hearing Aid Performance (PHAP). *J. Speech Hear. Res.,* 33, 343–357 (1990).

Danz, A. D., and Binnie, C. A., Quantification of the effects of training the auditory-visual reception of connected speech. *Ear Hear.,* 4, 146–151 (1983).

De Filippo, C. L., and Scott, B. L., A method for training and evaluating the reception of ongoing speech. *J Acoust. Soc. Am.,* 63, 1186–1192 (1978).

Dubno, J. R., and Dirks, D. D., Associations among frequency and temporal resolution and consonant recognition for hearing-impaired listeners. *Acta Otolaryngol.,* 469 (Suppl.), 23–29 (1990).

Engelmann, S., and Rosov, R. J., Tactual hearing experiment with deaf and hearing subjects. *J. Exceptional Child.,* 41, 245–253 (1975).

Festen, J. M., and Plomp, R., Relations between auditory functions in impaired hearing. *J. Acoust. Soc. Am.,* 73, 652–662 (1983).

Freyman, R. L., and Nerbonne, G. P., The importance of consonant-vowel intensity ratio in the intelligibility of voiceless consonants. *J. Speech Hear. Res.,* 32, 524–535 (1989).

Freyman, R. L., Nerbonne, G. P., and Cote, H. A., Effect of consonant-vowel ratio modification on amplitude envelope cues for consonant recognition. *J. Speech Hear. Res.,* 34, 415–426 (1991).

Gantz, B. J., Tye-Murray, N., and Tyler, R. S., Word recognition performance with single-channel and multichannel cochlear implants. *Am. J. Otol.,* 10, 91–94 (1989).

Gantz, B. J., Tyler, R. S., Knutson, J. F., Woodworth, G., Abbas, P., McCabe, B. F., Hinrichs, J., Tye-Murray, N., Lansing, C., Kuk, R., and Brown, C., Evaluation of five different cochlear implant designs: audiologic assessment and predictors of performance. *Laryngoscope,* 98, 1100–1106 (1988).

Gault, R. H., Progress in experiments on tactual or oral speech. *J. Abnorm. Soc. Psychol.,* 14, 155–159 (1924).

Geers, A. E., Vibrotactile stimulation: a case study with a profoundly deaf child. *J. Rehabil. Res. Develop.,* 23, 111–118 (1986).

Goldstein, M. H., Jr., and Proctor, A., Tactile aids for profoundly deaf children. *J. Acoust. Soc. Am.,* 77, 258–265 (1985).

Grant, K. W., Ardell, L. H., Kuhl, P. K., and Sparks, D. W., The contribution of fundamental frequency, amplitude envelope, and voicing duration cues to speechreading in normal-hearing subjects. *J. Acoust. Soc. Am.,* 77, 671–677 (1985).

Grant, K. W., and Braida, L. D., Evaluating the articulation index for auditory-visual input. *J. Acoust. Soc. Am.,* 89, 2952–2960 (1991).

Grant, K. W., Braida, L. D., and Renn, R. J., Single band amplitude envelope cues as an aid to speechreading. *Quart. J. Experiment. Psychol.,* 43, 621–645 (1991).

Green, K. P., and Kuhl, P. K., The role of visual information from a talker's face in the processing of place and manner features in speech. Paper presented at the meeting of the Acoustical Society of America, Anaheim, CA (December 1986).

Hanin, L., Boothroyd, A., and Hnath-Chisolm, T., Tactile perception of voice fundamental frequency as an aid to the speechreading of sentences. *Ear Hear.,* 9, 335–341 (1988).

Harris, R. W., and Goldstein, D. P., Hearing aid quality judgments in reverberant and nonreverberant environments using a magnitude estimation procedure. *Audiology,* 24, 32–43 (1985).

Hawkins, D. B., Beck, L. B., Bratt, G. W., Fabry, D. A., Mueller, H. G., and Stelmachowicz, P. G., Vanderbilt/VA hearing aid conference 1990 consensus statement: recommended components of a hearing aid selection procedure for adults. *Asha,* 33, 37–38 (1991).

Heider, F. K., and Heider, G. M., An experimental investigation of lipreading. *Psychologic. Monographs,* 52, 124–153 (1940).

Hochmair-Desoyer, I. J., Hochmair, E. S., and Stiglbrunner, H. K., Psychoacoustic temporal processing and speech understanding in cochlear implant patients. In R. A. Schindler and M. M. Merzenich (Eds.), *Cochlear Implants.* New York: Raven, 291–304 (1985).

Humes, L. E., Dirks, D. D., Bell, T. S., and Kincaid, G. E., Recognition of nonsense syllables by hearing-impaired listeners and by noise-masked normal hearers. *J. Acoust. Soc. Am.,* 81, 765–773 (1987).

Hutton, C., A diagnostic approach to combined techniques in aural rehabilitation. *J. Speech Hear. Disord.,* 25, 267–272 (1960).

Jakobson, R., Fant, C. G. M., and Halle, M., *Preliminaries to Speech Analysis.* Cambridge, MA: MIT Press (1952).

Klatt, D. H., Review of selected models of speech perception. In W. Marslen-Wilson (Ed.), *Lexical Representation and Process.* Cambridge, MA: MIT Press, pp. 169–226 (1989).

Lenneberg, E., *Biological Foundations of Language.* New York: Wiley (1967).

Lesner, S. A., Sandridge, S. A., and Kricos, P. B., Training influences on visual consonant and sentence recognition. *Ear Hear.,* 8, 283–287 (1987).

Levitt, H., Signal processing for sensory aids: a unified view. *Am. J. Otol.,* 12 (Suppl.), 52–55 (1991).

Levitt, H., Speech discrimination ability in the hearing impaired: spectrum considerations. In G. Studebaker and F. Bess (Eds.), *The Vanderbilt Hearing-Aid Report: State of the Art—Research Needs* (Monographs in Contemporary Audiology). Upper Darby, PA: E. R. Libby, pp. 32–43 (1982).

Liberman, A. M., Cooper, F. S., Shankweiler, D. P., and Studdert-Kennedy, M., "Why are speech spectrograms hard to read?" *Am. Ann. Deaf,* 113, 127–132 (1968).

Logan, J. S., Lively, S. E., and Pisoni, D. B., Training Japanese listeners to identify /r/ and /l/: a first report. *J. Acoust. Soc. Am.,* 89, 874–886 (1991).

Logan, S. A., Schwartz, D. M., Ahlstrom, J. B., and Ahlstrom, C., Effects of the acoustic environment on hearing aid quality/intelligibility judgments. Presented at the Annual Convention of the American Speech-Language-Hearing Association, San Francisco, CA (1984).

Lowell, E. L., Taaffe, G., and Rushford, G., The effectiveness of instructional films on lipreading. *West. Speech,* 23, 158–161 (1959).

Luttman, M. E., and Clark, J., Speech identification under simulated hearing-aid frequency response characteristics in relation to sensitivity, frequency resolution, and temporal resolution. *J. Acoust. Soc. Am.,* 80, 1030–1040 (1986).

MacDonald, J., and McGurk, H., Visual influences on speech perception processes. *Perception Psychophys.,* 24, 253–257 (1978).

Manuel, S. Y., Repp, B. H., Studdert-Kennedy, M., and Liberman, A. M., Exploring the "McGurk effect." Paper presented at the meeting of the Acoustical Society of America, San Diego, CA (November 1983).

Martin, E. S., and Pickett, J. M., Sensorineural hearing loss and upward spread of masking. *J. Speech Hear. Res.,* 13, 426–437 (1970).

Massaro, D. W., *Speech Perception by Ear and Eye: A Paradigm for Psychological Inquiry* (Chap. 7). Hillsdale, NJ: Lawrence Erlbaum Associates (1987).

Massaro, D. W., and Cohen, M. M., Evaluation and integration of visual and auditory information in speech perception. *J. Experiment. Psychol.: Human Perception Perform.,* 9, 753–771 (1983).

McGurk, H, and MacDonald, J., Hearing lips and seeing voices. *Nature,* 264, 746–748 (1976).

Miller, G. A., and Nicely, P. E., An analysis of perceptual confusions among some English consonants. *J. Acoust. Soc. Am.,* 27, 338–352 (1955).

Montgomery, A. A., and Edge, R. A., Evaluation of two speech enhancement techniques to improve intelligibility for hearing-impaired adults. *J. Speech Hear. Res.,* 31, 386–393 (1988).

Montgomery, A. A., Prosek, R. A., Walden, B. E., and Cord, M. T., The effect of increasing consonant/vowel intensity ratio on speech loudness. *J. Rehabil. Res. Develop.,* 24, 221–228 (1987).

Montgomery, A. A., Walden, B. E., Schwartz, D. M., and Prosek, R. A., Training auditory-visual speech

reception in adults with moderate sensorineural hearing loss. *Ear Hear.,* 5, 30–36 (1984).

Moore, B. C. J., and Glasberg, B. R., Relationship between psychophysical abilities and speech perception for subjects with unilateral and bilateral cochlear hearing impairments. In M. E. H. Schouten (Ed.), *The Psychophysics of Speech.* Dordrecht: Martinus Nijhoff Publishers (1987).

Neuman, A. C., Levitt, H., Mills, R., and Schwander, T., An evaluation of three adaptive hearing aid selection strategies. *J. Acoust. Soc. Am.,* 82, 1967–1976 (1987).

Owens, E., and Blazek, B., Visemes observed by hearing-impaired and normal-hearing adult viewers. *J. Speech Hear. Res.,* 28, 381–393 (1985).

Patrick, J. F., and Clark, G. M., The Nucleus 22-channel cochlear implant system. *Ear Hear.,* 12 (4 Suppl.), 35–95, (1991).

Pfingst, B. E., Operating ranges and intensity psychophysics for cochlear implants: implications for speech processing strategies. *Arch. Otolaryngol.,* 110, 140–144 (1984).

Pfingst, B. E., Burnett, P. A., and Sutton, D., Intensity discrimination with cochlear implants. *J. Acoust. Soc. Am.,* 73, 1283–1292 (1983).

Proctor, A., and Goldstein, M. H., Development of lexical comprehension in a profoundly deaf child using a wearable, vibrotactile communication aid. *Lang. Speech, Hear. Serv. Schools,* 14, 138–149 (1983).

Reed, C. M., Durlach, N. I., Delhorne, L. A., Rabinowitz, W. M., and Grant, K. W., Research on tactual communications of speech: ideas, issues, and findings. *Volta Rev.,* 91, 65–78 (1989).

Reed, C. M., Rabinowitz, W. M., Durlach, N. I., Braida, L. D., Conway-Fithian, S., and Schultz, M. C., Research on the Tadoma method of speech communication. *J. Acoust. Soc. Am.,* 77, 247–257 (1985).

Repp, B. H., Categorical perception: issues, methods, findings. In N. J. Lass (Ed.), *Speech and Language: Advances in Basic Research and Practice,* Vol. 10. New York: Academic Press, pp. 243–335 (1984).

Ringdahl, A., Eriksson-Mangold, M., Isrealsson, B., Lindkvist, A., and Mangold, S., Clinical trials with a programmable hearing aid set for various listening environments. *Br. J. Audiol.,* 24, 235–242 (1990).

Roberts, M., and Summerfield, Q., Audiovisual presentation demonstrates that selective adaption in speech perception is purely auditory. *Perception Psychophys.,* 30, 309–314 (1981).

Rosen, S. M., and Fourcin, A. J., When less is more—Further work. *Speech, Hearing, Language,* 1, University College London, Department of Phonetics and Linguistics, pp. 3–27 (1983).

Rothenberg, M., Verrillo, R. T., Zahorian, S. A., Brachman, M. L., and Bolanowski, S. J., Jr., Vibrotactile frequency for encoding a speech parameter. *J. Acoust. Soc. Am.,* 62, 1003–1012 (1977).

Sachs, R. M., Miller, J. D., and Grant, K. W., Perceived magnitude of multiple electrocutaneous pulses. *Perception Psychophys.,* 28, 255–262 (1980).

Sammeth, C. A., Bess, F. H., Bratt, G. W., Peek, B. F., Logan, S. A., and Amberg, S. M., The Vanderbilt/Veterans Administration hearing aid selection study: interim report. Presented at the Annual Convention of the American Speech-Language-Hearing Association, St. Louis (November 1989).

Schorn, K., and Zwicker, E., Frequency selectivity and temporal resolution in patients with various inner ear disorders. *Audiology, 29*, 8–20 (1990).

Shannon, R. V., Multichannel electrical stimulation of the auditory nerve in man. I. Basic psychophysics. *Hear. Res., 11*, 157–189 (1983).

Sherrick, C. E., Basic and applied research in tactile aids for deaf people: progress and prospects. *J. Acoust. Soc. Am., 75*, 1325–1342 (1984).

Simmons, F. B., Electrical stimulation of the auditory nerve in man. *Arch. Otolaryngol., 84*, 2–54 (1966).

Stevens, K. N., Models of phonetic recognition. II. A feature-based model of speech recognition. In P. Mermelstein (Ed.), *Proceedings of the Montreal Satellite Symposium on Speech Recognition,* Twelfth International Congress on Acoustics (1986).

Strange, W., and Jenkins, J. J., The role of linguistic experience in the perception of speech. In R. D. Walk and H. L. Pick (Eds.), *Perception and Experience.* New York: Plenum, pp. 125–169 (1978).

Stroud, D. J., and Hamill, T. A., A multidimensional evaluation of three hearing aid prescription formulae. Presented at the Annual Convention of the American Speech-Language-Hearing Association, St. Louis (November 1989).

Summerfield, A. Q., Some preliminaries to a comprehensive account of audio-visual speech perception. In B. Dodd and R. Campbell (Eds.), *Hearing by Eye: The Psychology of Lip-Reading.* Hillsdale, NJ: Erlbaum, pp. 3–51 (1987).

Summers, W. V., and Leek, M. R., Use of spectral and temporal cues in vowel identification by normal-hearing and hearing-impaired listeners. Presented at the Meeting of Acoustical Society of America, Baltimore, MD (May 1991).

Surr, R. K., Schuchman, G. I., and Montgomery, A. A., Factors influencing use of hearing aids. *Arch. Otolaryngol., 104*, 732–736 (1978).

Thornton, A. R., and Raffin, M. J. M., Speech-discrimination scores modeled as a binomial variable. *J. Speech Hear. Res., 21*, 507–518 (1978).

Turner, C. W., and Robb, M. P., Audibility and recognition of stop consonants in normal and hearing-impaired subjects. *J. Acoust. Soc. Am., 81*, 1566–1573 (1987).

Tye-Murray, N., and Tyler, R. S., Auditory consonant and word recognition skills of cochlear implant users. *Ear Hear., 10*, 292–298 (1989).

Tyler, R. S., Frequency resolution in hearing-impaired listeners. In B. C. J. Moore (Ed.), *Frequency Selectivity in Hearing.* London: Academic Press (1986).

Tyler, R. S., Moore, B. C. J., and Kuk, F. K., Performance of some of the better cochlear implant patients. *J. Speech Hear. Res., 32*, 887–911 (1989).

Tyler, R. S., Summerfield, Q., Wood, E. J., and Fernandes, M. A., Psychoacoustical and phonetic temporal processing in normal and hearing-impaired listeners. *J. Acoust. Soc. Am., 72*, 740–752 (1982).

Walden, B. E., Validating measures for hearing aid success. In G. A. Studebaker and F. H. Bess (Eds.), *The Vanderbilt Hearing-Aid Report: State of the Art—Research Needs* (Monographs in Contemporary Audiology). Upper Darby, PA: E. R. Libby, pp. 188–192 (1982).

Walden, B. E., Demorest, M. E., and Hepler, E. L., Self-report approach to assessing benefit derived from amplification. *J. Speech Hear. Res., 27*, 49–56 (1984).

Walden, B. E., Erdman, S. A., Montgomery, A. A., Schwartz, D. M., and Prosek, R. A., Some effects of training on speech recognition by hearing-impaired adults. *J. Speech Hear. Res., 24*, 207–216 (1981).

Walden, B. E., Montgomery, A. A., Cord, M. T., Demorest, M. E., and Prosek, R. A., Effects of amplification and visual cues on consonant recognition. Presented at the Annual Convention of the American Speech-Language-Hearing Association, New Orleans, LA (November 1987).

Walden, B. E., Montgomery, A. A., and Prosek, R. A., Perception of synthetic visual consonant-vowel articulations. *J. Speech Hear. Res., 30*, 418–424 (1987).

Walden, B. E., Montgomery, A. A., Prosek, R. A., and Hawkins, D. B., Visual biasing of normal and impaired auditory speech perception. *J. Speech Hear. Res., 33*, 163–173 (1990).

Walden, B. E., Montgomery, A. A., Prosek, R. A., and Schwartz, D. M., Consonant similarity judgments by normal and hearing-impaired listeners. *J. Speech Hear. Res., 23*, 162–184 (1980).

Walden, B. E., Prosek, R. A., Montgomery, A. A., Scherr, C. K., and Jones, C. J., Effects of training on the visual recognition of consonants. *J. Speech Hear. Res., 20*, 130–145 (1977).

Walden, B. E., Prosek, R. A. and Worthington, D. W., Predicting audiovisual consonant recognition performance of hearing-impaired adults. *J. Speech Hear. Res., 17*, 270–278 (1974).

Walden, B. E., Schwartz, D. M., Montgomery, A. A., and Prosek, R. A., A comparison of the effects of hearing impairment and acoustic filtering on consonant recognition. *J. Speech Hear. Res., 24*, 32–43 (1981).

Walden, B. E., Schwartz, D. M., Williams, D. L., Holum-Hardegen, L. L., and Crowley, J. M., Test of the assumptions underlying comparative hearing aid evaluations. *J. Speech Hear. Disord., 48*, 264–273 (1983).

Watson, C. S., Time course of auditory perceptual learning. *Ann. Otol., Rhinol., Laryngol., 89* (Suppl. 74), 96–102 (1980).

Weinstein, S., Intensive and extensive aspects of tactile sensitivity as a function of body part, sex, and laterality. In D. R. Kenshalo (Ed.), *The Skin Senses.* Springfield, IL: Thomas, pp. 195–222 (1980).

Weisenberger, J. M., Craig, J. C., and Abbott, G. D., Evaluation of a principal-components tactile aid for the hearing-impaired. *J. Acoust. Soc. Am., 90*, 1944–1957 (1991).

Welch, R. B., and Warren, D. H., Immediate perceptual response to intersensory discrepancy. *Psycholog. Bull., 88*, 638–667 (1980).

Werker, J. F., and Tees, R. C., Phonemic and phonetic factors in adult cross-language speech perception. *J. Acoust. Soc. Am., 75*, 1866–1878 (1984).

Wilson, B. S., Finley, C. C., Lawson, D. T., Wolford, R. D., Eddington, D. K., and Rabinowitz, W. M., Better speech reception with cochlear implants. *Nature, 352*, 236–238 (1991).

Zeng, F.-G., and Turner, C. W., Recognition of voiceless fricatives by normal and hearing-impaired subjects. *J. Speech Hear. Res., 33*, 440–449 (1990).

Author Index

Page numbers in parentheses refer to reference list entries.

Abbas, P., 510, 511, (526)
Abbott, G.D., 515, (528)
Abidin, R., 221, (231)
Able-Boone, H., 227, (231)
Abrahamson, J., 466, (468)
Abrass, 489
Ackerman, B., 59, (69)
Adams, J.W., 218, (231)
Adcock, C., 110, 111, (134)
Adler, A., 377–380, (409)
Aguilar, C., 490, 491, 494, 495, (499)
Ahlstrom, C., 81, (99), 303, (309), 505, (527)
Ahlstrom, J., 303, (309), 505, (527)
Alberti, P.W., 390, 397, 398, 403, (409)
Alcantara, J.I., 506, (525)
Alencewicz, C., 123, 125, (132), 428, (436)
Alexander, G., 76, (98), 243, (257), 302, (308), 494, 495, (498), 505, 507, 508, (526)
Allard, J.B., 12, (15)
Alpiner, J.G., 4, 5, 7, 12, 13, (15), 238, 239, 241, 242, 257, (257), (258), 262, 266, 268, 282, 283, 349, (354), (357), 360, 361, 371, 391, 407, (409), 504, 523, (525)
Amberg, S.M., 507, (527)
Amsel, L., 490, 491, (499)
Anderson, K.L., 182, 186–189, 192, 198, (204)
Anderson, L., 472, (485)
Anderson, R., 138, 158, (164)
Anderson, T.P., 385, 386, (409)
Andrews, J., 22, 32, 164, (167)
Ansbacher, H.L., 378, (409)
Ansbacher, R., 378, (409)
Applebaum, R., 346, (354)
Arana, M., 312, (327)
Ardell, L.H., 511, 516, (526)
Arjona, S., 60, (69)

Armstrong-Bednall, G., 18, (34)
Arndt, P.L., 434, (434)
Arpan, R., 430, (437)
Aryee, D.T.-K., 89, (100)
Aslin, R.N., 121, 122, 128, (132)
Atchley, R., 336, 340, (354)
Aten, J., 141, (164)
Atherley, G.R.C., 238, 240, (258), 390, (412)
Atkins, C., 155, (164)
Atkins, D.V., 222, (231)
Axelrod, 336
Axelsson, A., 254, (257)

Bagi, P., 67, (70)
Bailey, D.B., Jr., 226, (233)
Baker, B., 349, (354), 371
Baker, L.J., 18, (34)
Balkany, T., 60, (71), 422, (434)
Ball, L., 472, (485)
Bally, S., 244, (257), 403, (409)
Balsara, N., 239, 247, 252, (259)
Bandura, A., 378, 381, (409)
Banet, B., 110–112, 115, 119, (133)
Bankson, N.W., 169
Barber, C.G., 248, (259)
Barcham, L.J., 18, (32)
Barker, M.J., 430, 431, (435)
Barley, M., 245, 246, (258), 325, (327), 428, (436)
Barlow, D.H., 375, (409)
Barnes, S., 109, 111, (132)
Barrager, D., 223, (232)
Barrett, C., 377, (409)
Barrett, M., 169
Barta, L., 227, (231)
Barton, L., 152, (165)
Bates, E., 110, (132)
Bavosi, R., 60, 63, (69)
Beattie, R.C., 87, (97)
Beauchaine, K.L., 123, (133)
Beaudry, J., 405, (410)

Beaulac, D., 94, (97), 449, (467)
Bebout, J.M., 19, 24, (32), 89, 94, (97)
Bebout, M., 346, 347, (354)
Beck, A.T., 378–381, (409)
Beck, J., 342, (355)
Beck, L., 88, 94, (97), 441, (467), 503, (526)
Beckman, N., 307, (308), 351, (354)
Beckman, P.J., 217, (232)
Beckmann, N.J., 18, (33)
Beekman, G., (486)
Beiter, A.L., 143, (167), 420, 421, 426–428, 430, 431, (434), 434, (435)
Belal, 333
Belenchia, T.A., 404, (410)
Belgrave, L., 342, (354)
Bell, A.G., 161, (164)
Bell, T.S., 81, (99), 387, (412), 504, (526)
Bellefleur, P.A., 89, (97)
Bender, D., 291, (309)
Benedict, 73
Benguerel, A.P., 248, (258)
Bennett, M., 65, (69)
Bennett, R., 287, 289, (309)
Bennett, S., 348, (354)
Benoit, R., 96, (97)
Bensen, R.W., 251, (258)
Bentler, R., 62, (69), 73, 81, 86, 87, 95–97, (97), (98), (100), 228, (231), 297, 299, 300, (308)
Berg, F.S., 176, 177, 179–181, 191, 193, 196, 198, (204)
Berger, K., 74, (98)
Bergman, B.M., 81, (98)
Bergman, M., 73, (98)
Bergstrom, L., 72, (98)
Berlin, C.I., 73, (98), 181, 182, (205)
Berlin, L., 111–113, 116, (132), 169

Berliner, K.I., 424, (434)
Berliner, K.K., 417, (436)
Bernacerraf, B., 139, (164)
Berne, E., 378–380, (410)
Bernheimer, L.P., 218, (231)
Bernstein, D.K., 153, 163, (164)
Bernstein, M.E., 177, 203, (205), 227, (231)
Berry, G., 89, (98)
Berry, Q., 55, (69)
Berry, S., 126, (134)
Bess, F., 60, 63–65, (69), 70, 73, 74, 88, 89, 98, (100), 178, 181, (204), 334, 345, 348, 350, 351, (354), (355), 490, (498), 507, (525), (527)
Bevacqua, F., 94, (98)
Bevan, M.A., 18, (32)
Bibby, M.A., 222, 225, (232)
Billger, J., 96, (101)
Binney, E., 331, (357)
Binnie, C.A., 20, (32), 247–250, (257), 319, (327), 524, (526)
Binzer, S.M., 423, 430, (437)
Birchley, P., 377, (410)
Birk-Nielsen, H., 238, (258), 390, (411)
Birnholz, J., 139, (164), 166
Biro, P., 149, 153, (167), 168
Bjorklund, A.-K., 403, (411)
Black, J.W., 246, (257), 524, (525)
Black, O., 143, (166)
Black, R.C., 419, (437)
Blackburn, C.C., 318, (327)
Blackwell, B., 340, (354)
Blagden, D.M., 169
Blair, J.C., 176, 177, 181, 185, 186, 192, (204), (206)
Blake, R., 96, (98), 196, (204)
Blamey, P.J., 418–420, 430, 434, (434–437), 506, 516, (525)
Blanchard, K., 35, (45)
Blank, M., 110–113, 116, (132), 152, (166), 169
Blazek, B., 523, (527)
Blechman, E.A., 402, (410)
Blennerhassett, L., 152, (164)
Block, M., 87, (99), 305, (309)
Blood, G.W., 18, (32)
Blood, I., 18, (32), 348, (354)
Bloom, L., 163, (164)
Bluestone, C., 55, 60, 63, 65, 66, (69), 70
Blumberg, 334
Bodner, B., 22, (32)
Bodner-Johnson, B., 223, 230, (231), (232)
Boe, R., 66, (70)
Boehm, A.E., 169
Bohart, A.C., 377, 381–384, (410)
Bolanowski, S.J., Jr., 515, (527)
Bolles, R.C., 339, (354)
Bond, L.C., 186, (205)
Bonfils, P., 67, 68, (69)
Boniface, W.J., 376, 377, (411)
Boothroyd, A., 123–125, (132), 160, (164), 248, 250, (258), 421,

426, (435), 509, 515, (525), (526)
Botwinick, J., 336, 338, (354), (355)
Bouchard, K.R., 393, (412)
Brachman, M.L., 515, (527)
Bracken, A., 169
Brackett, D., 12, (15), 152, (164), (165), 176, 180, 181, 185, (204), (206), 429, (435)
Brackmann, D.E., 417, (436)
Bradley, R., 217, (231)
Bradley-Johnson, S., 157, (164)
Braida, L.D., 95, (98), 500, 506, 507, 511, 514, 516, (525–527), (526)
Brainard, S.H., 387, (410)
Braithwaite, R., 340, (354)
Brammer, L.M., 385, (410)
Brandt, F.D., 244, (257)
Brannon, C., 248, (257)
Bratt, G., 298, (308), 503, 507, (526), (527)
Bray, P., 67, (70)
Brearley, G., 377, (410)
Breeuwer, M., 516, (525)
Breslau, N., 342, (354)
Briery, D., 169
Brimacombe, J.A., 143, (166), (167), 420, 421, 427, 428, 430, 431, (434), 434, (435), (437)
Brinley, J., 338, (354)
Bristol, M.M., 219, (231)
Brockett, J., 239, 244, (259)
Brody, D.S., 22, (32)
Bromwich, R., 217, 226, (231)
Brooks, D., 55, 57, 60, 63, 65, (69), 94, (98), 239, 244, (257), 397, 398, 404, (410), (412), 496, (498)
Brooks, P.L., 516, (526)
Brotman, S.N., 24, (32)
Brown, A.M., 418–420, 422, 423, 431, (434), (435)
Brown, C., 510, 511, (526)
Brown, J., 349, (355), 366
Brown, L., 182, 196, 197, (205)
Brown, W., 293, 294, (309)
Brownell, J., 344, (356)
Bruckner, 336
Bruel, P., 81, (98)
Brummel-Smith, K., 489, (498), 498
Bruner, J.S., 111, (132)
Bryant, M., 293, 294, (309)
Budd, L., 22, (33)
Budinger, A., 293, 294, (309)
Buell, E.M., 161, (164)
Bull, D.H., 128, (134)
Bunch, G.O., 169
Burger, J., 345, (354)
Burke, N., 22, (32)
Burkhard, M., 81, 89, (101), 300, (310)
Burnett, P.A., 422, (436), 511, (527)
Burns, E., 67, (71)

Busby, P.A., 419, (437)
Bustamante, D.K., 500, (525)
Butler, A., 375–377, 382, 387, 394, (413)
Butler, K.G., 179, (206)
Butterfield, E., 477, (485)
Butts, M., 146, (165)
Byrne, D., 74–76, 78, 81, (98), 298, (308)

Caccavo, M.T., 393, 403, (410)
Caldwell, B., 217, (231)
Calkins, A., 293, (309)
Calkins, E., 342, (355)
Calvert, D.R., 178, 182, (206)
Canestri, R., 338, (354)
Cantekin, E., 60, 63, 66, (69), (70)
Carey, L., 482, (485)
Carhart, R., 251, (259), 503, 505, (526)
Carkhuff, R.R., 385, 394, (413)
Carlin, M., 177, (205)
Carlson, E., 94, (98)
Carlson, K., 22, (33)
Carlsson, S.G., 401, 402, (411)
Carmichael, H., 109, (133)
Carney, A.E., 122–125, 127–131, (132), (134), 429, (436)
Carotta, C., 125, 129, 130, (132)
Carpenter, R., 108, (134), 169
Carrow-Woolfolk, E., 169
Carter, E.A., 65, (70), 121, (134)
Cartwright, L., 155, (164)
Cavanaugh, W., 290, (308)
Chandler, D., 72, (101)
Chapman, R., 114, (133)
Chappell, C., 59, (69)
Chellappa, M., 496, (499)
Chen, J., 68, (69)
Chermak, G.D., 13, (15), 523, (526)
Cherry, K., 341, (354)
Chevrette, W., 238, 241, (257), 262, 266, 391, (409)
Chew, R., 87, (98)
Chon, B., 66, (70)
Christopherson, L., 335, (355)
Chung, K., 516, (526)
Cicchitti, D., 342, (354)
Cipollone, E., 94, (98)
Citrenbaum, C., 376, 377, (411)
Clark, 510
Clark, G.M., 418–420, 422, 423, 430, 431, 434, (434–437), 506, 516, (525)
Clark, J., 504, (527)
Clark, J.G., 11, (15), 214, (231)
Clark, L., 343, 346, (356)
Clark, S., 59, (71)
Clark, T., 228, (231)
Clarke, 492, 493, 496, 497
Clarkson, R.L., 230, (231)
Clobridge, C., 325, (327)
Clopton, B.M., 72, (98), (101)
Cluff, L., 345, (354)
Cluver, L., 146, (165)

Clyme, E., 466, (468)
Clymer, E.W., 474, (485)
Coats, A., 67, (70)
Cody, J.P., 177, 203, (205)
Coggins, T., 108, (134), 169
Cohen, 336
Cohen, M.M., 522, (527)
Cohen, N.L., 326, (327), 418, 430, 431, (435)
Cohen, O.P., 230, (231)
Cohen, S., 22, (33)
Cokely, C., 293, (308)
Cole, E.B., 217, (231)
Coleman, J., 342, (354)
Coleman, R., 65, (69)
Collet, L., 67, (69)
Colton, J.C., 508, (526)
Compton, C.L., 92, (98), 443–445, 447, 448, 450, 451, 456, 461, 462, (467), 469
Condon, M., 107, 108, (133)
Cone-Wesson, B., 59, (71)
Constable, C.M., 112, (132)
Conway, D.F., 157, (164)
Conway, L.C., 180, (204)
Conway-Fithian, S., 514, (527)
Cook, D., 378, 382, 386, 393, (410), 483, (485)
Cooper, F.S., 513, (527)
Cooper, J., 333, (354)
Cooper, J.A., 128, (134)
Cooper, J.C., 60, 61, 66, (69), 335, (354)
Cooper, W.A., 79, 81, (99)
Cope, Y., 67, (69)
Coplan, J., 62, 64, (69), 169
Corbin, H., 390, 397, 398, 403, (409)
Cord, M.T., 503, 507, (527), (528)
Cornelisse, L.E., 78, (98)
Corsini, R.J., 374, 375, 377, 382–384, (410)
Corso, 333, 336
Cote, H.A., 502, (526)
Cotton, A.D., (257), 282, 283
Cotton, S., 75, (98)
Coufal, K., 107, 108, (133)
Cowan, R.S.C., 506, (525)
Coward, R., 331, (354)
Cox, R., 76–78, 87, (98), 243, (257), 300, 302, 303, (308), 473, (485), 494, 495, (498), 505, 507–509, (526)
Craig, A., 22, (32)
Craig, J.C., 515, (528)
Craik, F.I.M., 337, (354)
Cram, J.E., 312, (327)
Cranmer, K., 6, (15), 295, 302, 305, (308)
Criswell, E.L., 482, (485)
Crooks, J., 340, (355)
Crowe, T.A., 404, (410), (411)
Crowley, D.J., 224, 225, (231)
Crowley, J., 302, (310), 393, 399, 402–404, (410), 507, (528)
Crump, E.S., 196, (206)
Cullen, J.K., 72, (99)

Culpepper, N.B., 225, 226, (232), 375, (412)
Cunningham, D.R., 14, (15)
Curran, J., 6, (15), 35, (45), 474, (485)
Curtis, B., 42, (45)
Curtis, J., (486)
Curtis, S., 152, (164)
Cutler, S., 331, (354)

Daguio, M., 8, (15)
Dale, P., 108, (132), 139, (167)
Dale, R., 72, (101)
Daly, C., 420, (436)
Daly, J.A., 177, 203, (205), 215, 224, 227, (231)
Dancer, J., 343, 344, (355)
Danhauer, J.L., 18, (32)
Dankowski, K., 430, (435)
Dannemiller, E.A., 402, (410)
Danz, A.D., 524, (526)
Darbyshire, J.D., 89, (98)
Darbyshire, J.O., 224, (233)
Davies, J., 292, (308)
Davis, A.C., 389, (410)
Davis, H., 11, (15), 124, (132), 238, 251, 254, (257), (258), 275
Davis, J., 11, 62, (69), 73, 96, 97, (98), 152, 156, (166), 176–178, 182, (204), 228, (231)
Deal, A.G., 223, 226, (231), (232)
Deans, M., 87, (98)
DeCasper, A., 139, (164)
Decker, T.N., 87, (99)
De Filippo, C.L., 248, (257), 324–326, (327), 429, (435), 524, (526)
De Gennaro, S.V., 500, (525)
Deiner, P.L., 226, (232)
DeJonge, B., 474, (485)
DeLavergne, R., 325, (327)
Delhorne, L.A., 513, 514, 517, (527)
Dell'Oliver, C., 227, (232)
DeMatteo, A., 159, (166)
Demorest, M.E., 23, (32), 243, 244, (257), (259), 355, (356), 382, 387, 391, 392, 399, 401, 405–407, (410), 474, (485), 505, 507–509, (528)
Dempster, J.H., 81, (98)
Dennis, W., 73, (98)
Denton, J., 342, (354)
Dettman, D., 125, 129, 130, (132)
DeVilliers, P.A., 154, (164)
DeVoss, F., 455, (468)
Dey-Sigman, S., 58, 66, (70)
Diabless, D., 22, (33)
Dick, W., 482, (485)
Dickson, H., 60, 61, 66, (69)
Diefendorf, A., 123, (132)
DiFrancesca, S., 152, (164)
Dilka, K., 12, (15), 181, (205)
Dillon, H., 74, 75, 78, 87, (98), 296, 298, (310)
DiMichael, S.G., 380, 399, (410)

Dirks, D.D., 81, 87, (99), (100), 387, (412), 504, (526)
Dixon, R., 338, (355)
Dobie, R.A., 73, (98), 181, 182, (205)
Dodd, B., 246, (257)
Dodds, E., 247, (257)
Donnelly, J., 152, (164), (165)
Dorman, M.F., 430, (435)
Dornan, M.C., 393, (411)
Dowaliby, F., 22, (32)
Dowell, R.C., 143, (167), 419–423, 426–431, 434, (434–437)
Downey, D., 110–112, 115, (135)
Downs, M., 11, (15), 56, 58, 59, 64, 65, 69, (70), 72, 73, 90, (100), 178, 181, 182, 186, (205)
Dreisbach, J.N., 422, (434)
Dublinske, S., 181, (205)
Dubno, J.R., 387, (412), 504, (526)
DuBow, S., 184, (205), 469
Duchan, J.F., 153–155, (165), (166)
Duda, R., 475, (485)
Dukert, L., 490, (499)
Dunckel, D., 66, (70)
Dunn, H.K., 77, (98)
Dunn, J., 66, (70)
Dunn, L.M., 169
Dunst, C.J., 218, 223, 226, (231), (232)
Durieux-Smith, A., 86, (101)
Durlach, N.I., 95, (98), 500, 513, 514, 517, (525), (527)
Dusay, J., 380, (410)
Dychtwald, K., 36, (45)
D'Zurilla, T.J., 402, (410)

Eagles, E., 55, 64, (70)
Eberling, C., 67, (70)
Eccarius, M., 122, 124, (133)
Eddington, D.K., 434, (437), 510, (528)
Edge, R.A., 503, (527)
Edison, T., 41, (45)
Edwards, C., 198, 199, (205)
Edwards, M.L., 163, (165)
Egan, G., 377, 385, (410)
Egan, J.P., 251, (257)
Eichler, J., 60, (69)
Eichwald, J., 64, (70)
Eilers, R., 121, 128, 129, (132), 134, 139, (165)
Eimas, P., 121, (132), 139, (165)
Eisen, N.H., 73, (98)
Eisenberg, R., 65, (69), 139, (165)
Eisenwort, B., 421, (435)
Elbert, E., 251, (258)
Elbert, M., 128, (134)
Elfenbein, J.L., 73, 86, 87, 95–97, (98), (100), 228, (231)
Elfenbeing, J., 62, (69)
Elias, M.F., 339, (354)
Elias, P.K., 339, (354)
Elliott, G., 139, (165)

Elliott, H., 157, (165), 344, (354)
Elliott, K., 139, (165)
Elliott, L., 123, 124, (132), 177, (205), 251, (258), 428, (435)
Elliott, R., 164, (165), (166)
Ellis, A., 378–381, (410)
Elssmann, S.F., 72, (99)
Emery, M., 169
Emmery, G., 378, (409)
Endicott, J., 490, 491, 494, 495, (499)
Engebretson, A.M., 81, (100)
Engelmann, S., 516, (526)
Engen, E., 169
Engen, T., 169
English, B., 6, (15)
English, K., 177, (205)
English, R.W., 378, 386, (410)
Ensher, G.L., 107, (132)
Epstein, N., 394, (412)
Erber, N., 122, 123, 125, 126, (132), 180, 199, (205), 246, 248, (258), 321, 326, (327), 330, 428, 430, (435)
Erdman, S.A., 23, (32), 243, 250, (257), (259), 380, 382, 387, 391–393, 399, 401–407, (410), (411), 474, (485), 518, 524, (528)
Eriksson-Mangold, M., 403, (411), 506, (527)
Erler, S., 23, (33)
Erting, C., 109, (133)
Estabrooks, W., 199, (205)
Estes, C., 331, (357)
Ethol, 333
Evans, J.W., 157, (165)
Evans, L.D., 157, (164)
Evans, W.J., 72, (99)
Ewertsen, H., 238, (258), 390, (411)

Fabry, D., 81, (99), 296, (308), 352, (356), 503, (526)
Fainberg, J., 64, (70)
Fairbanks, G., 238, (258), 390, (411)
Faires, W.L., 94, (99)
Falvo, D.R., 377, 386, 394, (411)
Fant, C.G.M., 503, (526)
Farrar, M.J., 109, 111, (134)
Farrell, W., 290, (308)
Faurqui, S., 18, (33)
Feeley, J., 349, (355), 366
Feigin, J., 79, 82–85, (99), 465, 466, (468)
Fein, D., 332, (354)
Feinmesser, M., 59, (71)
Feitz, L., 340, (356)
Feldman, H., 152, (165)
Fenson, L., 108, (132)
Ferguson, C.A., 128, (134)
Fernandes, M.A., 504, (528)
Festen, J.M., 74, (99), 504, (526)
Fewell, R.R., 222, 223, 226, (231), (232)

Fidell, S., 287, 289, (309)
Field, B., 96, (98), 196, (204)
Fifer, W., 139, (164)
Fifield, D., 74, (98)
Filley, F., 22, (33)
Finger, I., 217, (231)
Finitzo, T., 60, 62, (69)
Finitzo-Hieber, T., 90, (99), 193, (205)
Finley, C.C., 434, (437), 510, (528)
Fino, M.S., 350, 351, (354)
Fischer, R.M., 107, 109, (133)
Fischgrund, J.E., 230, (231)
Fitten, J., 340, (356)
FitZaland, R., 55, (69)
Fitzgerald, E., 161, (165)
Fitzgerald, M.T., 107, 109, (133)
Flahive, M.J., 225, (231)
Fletcher, C., 342, (354)
Flexer, C., 176, 178, 180, 182, 191, 193, 196–198, (205), (206)
Foley, G., 107, 109, (134)
Folkman, S., 389, 390, (412)
Ford, A., 342, (354)
Foster, C., 96, (98), 196, (204)
Foster, R., 169
Fourcin, A.J., 511, (527)
Fox, G.D., 7
Frank, T., 348, (354), 466, (468)
Frankel, B.G., 387, (410)
Frankenburg, W., 56, 68, (69)
Franklin, J.G., 22, (32)
Frankmann, J.P., 251, (258)
Franks, J., 18, (33), 307, (308), 351, (354)
Franz, B.K.-H., 418, 420, 430, 434, (435), (437)
Frazer, G., 62, (71)
Frederick, L.L., 227, (231)
Frederiksen, E., 81, (98)
Fredrickson, J.M., 423, 430, (437)
Freeman, B.A., 91, (98), 465, (468)
French, N., 79, (99), 288, (308)
Freyman, R.L., 502, (526)
Fria, T., 58, 60, 64–66, (69)
Friel-Patti, S., 60, 62, (69)
Fritze, W., 421, (435)
Frost, B.J., 516, (526)
Frueh, F., 325, (327)
Fujikawa, S., 421, (435)
Furness, H.J.S., 89, (99)
Furth, H., 142, (165)

Gabbard, S.A., 94, (100)
Gabrielsson, A., 303, (308)
Gaeth, J.H., 406, (411)
Gagne, J.P., 78, 83, (98), (101), 321, (327)
Gallagher, G., 397, (411)
Gallimore, R., 218, (231)
Gallup, F., 17, (33)
Gambert, 489
Gantz, B.J., 421, 422, 430, (434), (435), 510, 511, (526)

Gardi, J.N., 421, (437)
Gardner, M.F., 169
Garrity, T.F., 386, (411)
Garstecki, D., 12, (15), 20, 21, 23, (33), 257, (257), (327), 330, 344, (354)
Gartner, M., 67, (69)
Garwood, S., 140, (165), 226, (231)
Gary, L.B., 422, (437)
Gasar, A., 22, (33)
Gaschnig, J., 475, (485)
Gatehouse, S., 89, (99), 245, (259), 387–391, 393, 398, (413)
Gates, G., 60, 61, 66, (69), 333, 335, (354)
Gault, R.H., 512, (526)
Gazzanega, M., 140, (165)
Geer, S., 184, (205), 469
Geers, A.E., 123–125, (133), 154, 161, (166), 170, 421, 426, 428, (435), (436), 509, 516, (525), (526)
Geiger, D., 342, (354)
Geis, H.J., 386, (411)
Geist, P., 393, 403, (410)
Gelfand, S.A., 89, (99), (101)
Gellman, W., 391, (411)
Genest, M., 381, (413)
Gentile, J., 238, 240, (259)
George, K.A., 215, 224, 227, (231)
Gerard, L., 338, (354)
Gerkin, K., 57, 58, 59, (69)
Gerrard, B.A., 376, 377, (411)
Geschwind, N., 141, (165)
Getty, L., 404, 405, 407, 408, (411)
Gibbins, S., 148, 158, (165)
Gidden, J.J., 169
Gilhome-Herbst, K.R., 390, (413)
Gillespie, G.G., 393, 399, 402–404, (410)
Gilman, L., 152, 156, (165), 166
Gilmore, C., 243, (257), 302, (308), 494, 495, (498), 509, (526)
Gilmore, R., 448, 466, (468)
Ginsburg, H., 87, (99)
Giolas, T.G., 179, 193, (206), 239, 242, (258), 387, 391, 399, 406, 409, (411)
Gissey, D.M., 431, (435)
Gladstone, V.S., 91, (98)
Glasberg, B.R., 504, (527)
Glascoe, G., 238, 241, (257), 262, 266, 391, (409)
Glass, D.C., 402, (411)
Glass, L., 157, (165), 344, (354)
Glassford, F.E., 182, 196, 197, (206)
Glorig, A., 238, (258), 390, (411)
Goldberg, H., 41, (45)
Golden, D.C., 12, (15)
Golden-Meadow, S., 152, (165)
Goldfried, M.R., 402, (410)
Goldgar, D.E., 158, (167)
Goldojarb, M., 353, (355)

Goldstein, D., 14, (15), 17–20, (33), (34), 255, 257, (258), 470, (485), 505, (526)
Goldstein, M.H., Jr., 516, (526), (527)
Goldstein, R., 65, (71)
Golightly, C.K., 376, 377, (411)
Goodman, A., 11, (15)
Goodman, P., 378, 382, (412)
Goozner, M., 23, 24, (33)
Gordon-Salant, S., 339, (354)
Gorga, M.P., 79, 82–84, 87, (99), 123, (133)
Goss, M., 340, (356)
Goss, R., 216, (231)
Graham, E., 159, (165)
Grammatico, L., 111, (133)
Grant, K.W., 506, 507, 511, 513, 514, 517, (526), (527)
Gravel, J., 90, (98), 465, (468)
Graves, L., 196, (205)
Gray, R.F., 422, 423, (435)
Green, C.L., 216, (231)
Green, K.P., 522, (526)
Greenberg, M., 109, (133), 152, (165)
Greenfield, D.G., 87, (99)
Greenstein, B.B., 73, (99)
Greenstein, J.M., 73, (99)
Gregory, M., 246, (257)
Grieger, R., 378, (410)
Grimes, A., 84, 90, 94, (99), (100), 302, 304, (309), 466, (468)
Grimes, V.K., 228, (231)
Groht, M.A., 161, (165)
Gross, R., 152, (165)
Gruber, H.E., 53, (69)
Grundfast, K., 59, (69)
Gutfreund, M., 109, 111, (132)

Haas, W.H., 224, 225, (231)
Haase, K., 238, 240, (259)
Hackett, T., 298, (309)
Hagberg, N., 74, (98)
Haggard, M.P., 19, (33)
Hall, J.A., 393, (411)
Hallahan, P., 22, (33)
Hallberg, L.R.-M., 401, 402, (411)
Halle, M., 503, (526)
Halliday, M.A.K., 110, (133)
Halpern, C.F., 65, (70)
Halpin, C.F., 121, (134)
Hamby, D., 218, (231)
Hamer, A.W., 223, 226, (232)
Hamilton, J.L., 226, (231)
Hammer, M.A., 177, (205)
Hammill, T.A., 507, (528)
Hammond, L., 91, (99)
Hanin, L., 515, (526)
Hanline, M.F., 221, (231)
Hannley, M.T., 430, (435)
Hanson, M.J., 221, 229, 230, (231), (232)
Harder, J., 94, (99)
Harfield, N., 149, 153, (167), 168

Harford, E., 60, 65, (69), 86, 94, 97, (100), 247, (257)
Harkins, J.E., 451, 454, 456, (468)
Harless, E.L., 345, (354)
Harris, J.D., 44, (45)
Harris, M., 404, (413)
Harris, R., 23, (33), 505, (526)
Hart, F.G., 404, (412)
Hartke, R., 489, (498)
Harvey, M.A., 216, (231)
Hasenstab, S., 139, 140, 142, 143, 146, (165), (166), 169, 223, (232)
Hasher, L., 338, (354)
Haskell, G., 77, (99), 304, (308)
Haskins, H., 123, 124, (133)
Haskins, J., 428, (436)
Haspiel, G., 124, (134)
Haug, M., 342, (354)
Hawes, N.A., 387, (411)
Hawken, P., 36, (45)
Hawkings, J., 123, 125, (133)
Hawkins, D., 73, 74, 79, 81, 83, 86, 87, 89, 91–94, (99), (100), 196, (205), 287, 288, 295, 296, 298–300, 303–307, (308), (309), 319, 325, (327), 465, 466, (468), 503, 507, 522, 523, (526), (528)
Hawkins, J.E., 431, (436)
Haycock, G.S., 162, (165)
Hayes, D., 292, (310)
Hayes, S.C., 375, (409)
Hazlett, J., 178, (206)
Healey, W., 59, (69)
Hedrick, D., 169
Hefferline, R., 378, 382, (412)
Heider, F.K., 524, (526)
Heider, G.M., 524, (526)
Heise, G.A., 321, (327)
Heller, B., 159, (166)
Heller, P.J., 157, (165)
Henggeler, S.W., 221, (231)
Henney, C., 340, (355)
Henoch, M., 392, (410), 493, (498)
Hepler, E., 243, (259), 335, (356), 505, 508, 509, (528)
Heppner, P.P., 402, 403, (411)
Herbst, K., 18, (33), 332, 345, (354)
Hess, J.C., 156, (165)
Hession, C.M., 319, (327)
Hetú, R., 237, (259), 387, 389, 404, 405, 407, 408, (410), (411), (413)
Hicks, B.L., 95, (98)
Higgins, J., 390, (412)
High, W.S., 238, (258), 390, (411)
Himelick, T.E., 422, (436)
Himes, J.H., 13, (15)
Hine, W.D., 89, (99)
Hinrichs, J., 510, 511, (526)
Hipskind, N., 246, (258), 305, (309)
Hirsh, I.J., 251, (258)
Hirtle, P., 290, (308)
Hixon, P., 107, 108, (133)

Hnath-Chisolm, T., 515, (526)
Hochmair, E.S., 512, (526)
Hochmair-Desoyer, I.J., 512, (526)
Hodges, A.V., 423, (436)
Hodgson, W.R., 91, (101)
Hodson, B.W., 151, 163, (165)
Hoene, D., 302, (310)
Hogan, R., 394, (411)
Hohmann, M., 110–112, 115, 119, (133)
Holden, L.K., 420, 430, 434, (437)
Holden, T.A., 420, 430, 434, (437)
Hollenbeck. A., 55, (69)
Holmes, A., 466, (468)
Holmes, D.W., 169
Holmgren, L., 89, (99)
Holstein, C., 216, (232)
Holum-Hardegen, L.L., 507, (528)
Holum-Hardigan, L., 302, (310)
Hood, J.D., 89, (99)
Hoskins, B., 110, (133)
Houghton, R., 302, (309)
Houle, G.R., 226, (231)
House, W.F., 417, (436)
House, W.M., 422, 427, (436)
Howard, D., 477, (485)
Howe, S.W., 87, (99)
Hubbard, R., 343, (355)
Hudgins, C.V., 149, (165), 431, (436)
Hudson, S.P., 83, (101)
Hug, G.A., 242, (258), 272, 350, (355), 390, (412), 494, 495, (498)
Huisingh, R., 169
Hull, C., 55, (70)
Hull, J., 59
Hull, R., 12, (15), 181, (205)
Hultsch, D., 338, (355)
Humes, L., 81, (99), 290, 293, 298, 302, 304, 305, (308), (309), 318, (327), 335, (355), 504, (526)
Humphrey, C., 18, (33), 332, (354)
Hunter, K., 23, (33)
Hurvitz, H., 353, (355)
Hutton, C., 243, 250, (258), 524, (526)

Illich, I., 385, (411)
Inhelder, B., 111, (134)
Ireland, J., 178, (205)
Ireton, H., 62, (70)
Israelite, N.K., 222, (231)
Isrealsson, B., 506, (527)
Itzkowitz, J., 22, (33)

Jackler, R.K., 422, 427, (436)
Jackson, P.D., 404, (410)
Jackson, P.L., 248, 250, (257)
Jacobs, J.F., 151, (166)
Jacobsen, S., 42, (45)
Jacobson, C., 60, 65, 66, (70), 404, (411)

Jacobson, G., 242, (258), 272, 350, (355), 390, (412), 494, 495, (498)
Jacobson, J., 59, 60, 65, 66, (70), 404, (411)
Jakobson, R., 503, (526)
Jamieson, D.G., 78, 80, 83, (101)
Janis, I.L., 22, (33)
Jaquett, Z., 19, (33)
Jarvik, L.F., 341, (355)
Jeffers, J., 245, 246, (258), 325, (327), 428, (436)
Jenison, V.W., 429, (436)
Jenkins, J., 55, (70)
Jensen, H.T., 130, (134)
Jerger, J., 89, (99), 123, 125, (133), 251, (258), 292, 293, 302, (309), (310), 333, 335, (355), (356), 387, 398, 409, (411), (413), 472, (485)
Jerger, S., 123, 125, (133), 333, (355)
Jesteadt, W., 123, (133)
Johansson, B., 139, (165)
Johns, J., 22, (32)
Johnsen, N., 67, (70)
Johnson, C.J., 129, (134)
Johnson, D.I., 398, (410)
Johnson, D.L., 13, (15)
Johnson, H., 152, (165)
Johnson, H.A., 149, (165)
Johnson, R.M., 87, (101)
Jonassen, D., 477, 478, (485)
Jones, B., 170
Jones, C.J., 324, (327), 524, (528)
Jones, K.L., 59, (70)
Jones, L.G., 405, (411)
Jones, R.C., 230, (231)
Jons, C.R., 392, (410)
Jorgenson, C., 169
Jupiter, T., 348, (355)
Jusczyk, P.W., 121, (132)

Kail, R., 111, 115, (133)
Kalikow, D., 251, (258)
Kaminski, J.R., 123, (133)
Kamm, 87
Kampfe, C.M., 214, 215, (231)
Kane, 489
Kane, R., 342, (355)
Kannell, W., 333, (354)
Kaplan, H., 244, (257), 349, (355), 366, 403, (409), (411)
Karasek, A., 125, 129, (132), 465, 466, (468)
Karasu, T., 377, (411)
Karchmer, M., 17, (33)
Karlin, J.E., 431, (436)
Katz, D., 123, 124, (132), 428, (435)
Katz, J., 199, (205)
Kausler, D.H., 338, (355)
Kawell, M.E., 86, 87, (99)
Keith, R., 60, (70)
Kemink, J.L., 427, (436)

Kemp, B., 491–493, 497, (498), 498
Kemp, D., 67, (70)
Kenworthy, O., 59, 60, 62–66, (70), 216, (231)
Kessler, D.K., 421, 424, (436)
Kessler, M., 125, (134)
Khan, L., 151, (165)
Kheriaty, L., (486)
Kielinen, L.L., 387, (411)
Kileny, P.R., 427, (436)
Killion, M., 290, 296, (309)
Kimmell, D.C., 337, (355)
Kimura, D., 141, (165)
Kincaid, G.E., 81, (99), 504, (526)
Kinder, D.L., 94, (100)
King, M., 376, 377, (411)
Kintsch, W., 115, (133)
Kirk, S.A., 169
Kirk, W.D., 169
Kirkwood, D., 7, (15), 284, (309)
Kirn, E., 304, (309)
Kirwin, L., 17, (33)
Klatt, D.H., 503, (526)
Klein, J., 60, 63, 65, 69, (70), (71)
Klockhoff, I., 254, (258)
Klodd, A., 139, (166)
Knutson, J.F., 387, (411), 421, 430, (435), 511, 520, (526)
Kobrin, M., 23, (33)
Koch, D.B., 420, (436)
Koch, E.G., 65, (70), 121, (134)
Kochkin, S., 6, (15), 17, (33), 404, (411)
Koepsell, T., 490, (499)
Konkle, D., 74, (99), 465, (468)
Kopun, J.G., 79, 82–84, 86, 87, (99)
Kotler, 492, 493, 496, 497
Kowal, J., 343, (355)
Kozak, V.J., 170
Kraus, N., 59, (71)
Krauss, M.W., 226, (231)
Kresheck, J., 170
Kretschmer, L., 153, 161, 163, (165), 216, 230, (231), (232)
Kretschmer, R., 153, 161, 163, (165), 216, 217, (232)
Kricos, P., 216, (231), 335, (355), 491, 492, 496, (499), 524, (527)
Kroth, R.L., 214, 227, (231)
Kruger, A., 109, (134)
Kruger, B., 79, 81, 82, (99)
Kryter, K.D., 79, (99)
Kubler-Ross, E., 212, 213, (231)
Kuczwara, L., 139, (166)
Kuhl, P.K., 121, (133), 511, 516, 522, (526)
Kuk, F.K., 352, (356), 430, (437), 510–512, (526), (528)
Kuller, J., 23, (33)
Kuprenas, S.V., 430, (436)
Kuypers, J.A., 22, (33)
Kwiatkowski, J., 22, (33)
Kyle, J.G., 405, (411)

Labov, 155
Lachman, J., 477, (485)
Lachman, R., 477, (485)
Lafayette, R.H., 130, (134)
Lahey, M., 163, 164, (166)
Lalande, N.M., 403, 404–408, (411)
Lamb, A., 478, 480, 481, (485), (486)
Lamb, S., 242, (258), 391, 399, 406, (411)
Lambert, J., 403, 406, (411)
Lambert, P.R., 423, (436)
Lamont, M., 404, (413)
Land, S.L., 22, (33)
Landin, D.P., 91, 93, (101)
Landry, R., 156, (165)
Langer, E., 22, (33)
Langford, S.E., 94, (99)
Lansing, C., 387, 392, (410), (411), 510, 511, (526)
LaRiviere, C., 473, (485)
Larsen, S.Y., 352, (356)
Larson, E., 490, (499)
Lasky, E., 199, (205)
Lass, N., 18, (33), 177, (205)
Laughton, J., 139, 146, 151, 152, 153, 157, 159, 164, (165), (166), 169
Laux, D.M., 19, (33)
Lavin, B., 342, (354)
Lawson, D.T., 434, (437), 510, (528)
Layton, T.L., 169
Lazarus, A.A., 378, 381, 389, 390, (411), (412)
Lazenby, H., 346, (356)
Leavitt, R.J., 180, 193, 196, 197, (205)
Lederman, N., 448, 466, (468)
Lee, F.S., 334, (356)
Lee, J., 348, (355)
Lee, L.L., 169
Leek, M.R., 520, (528)
Lehnhardt, E., 417, (436)
Lenneberg, E., 141, (166), 520, (526)
Leonard, L., 111, 115, (133), 186, (205)
Leopold, I., 336, (355)
Lerman, J., 73, (101), 123–125, (134), 428, (436)
Lerner, E., 342, (354)
Lesner, S., 257, (258), 335, (355), 491, 492, 496, (499), 524, (527)
Letowski, T.R., 351, (355)
Levi, C., 59, (71)
Levine, E., 158, 159, (166)
Levine, H., 55, 64, (70)
Levit, K., 346, (356)
Levitt, H., 326, (327), 501–503, (527)
Levy, L., 19, (33)
Lewis, D., 465, 466, (468)
Lewis, N., 89, (99), 151, (165)
Lewis, R.B., 148, (166)
Lewis, S., 123, 125, (133)

Libby, E.R., 398, (412)
Liberman, A.M., 513, 522, (527)
Lichten, W., 321, (327)
Lichtenstein, J., 345, 350, 351, (354)
Lichtenstein, M., 348, (355), 490, (498)
Liden, G., 86, 94, 97, (100)
Lienberth, A., 470, (485)
Lindblom, U., 254, (258)
Lindgren, B., 60, 62, (69)
Lindkvist, A., 506, (527)
Ling, A.H., 122, 123, (133)
Ling, D., 122, 123, 129–131, (133), 149–151, 162, (166), 178–181, 188, 193, 199, (205)
Linn, M., 23, (33)
Lippman, R.P., 95, (98)
Liske, R., 342, (354)
Lively, S.E., 520, (527)
Loeb, R., 228, 229, (231)
Logan, J.S., 520, (527)
Logan, S., 303, (309), 345, 348, 350, 351, (354), (355), 490, (498), 505, 507, (527)
Logemann, J.M., 95, (100)
Long, V.O., 19, (34)
Longhurst, T., 169, 239, 244, (259), 348, (356)
Loose, F., 96, (100)
Lounsbury, M.B., 67, (70)
Lous, J., 55, 63, (70)
Love, B.H., 376, 377, (411)
Lowder, M., 424, 434, (437)
Lowell, E., 152, (164), 430, (436), 524, (527)
Lucker, J., 55, 65, (70)
Luckner, J., 161, 163, (166), 177, (205)
Lucks, L., 225, 226, (232), 375, (412)
Luetke-Stahlman, B., 161, 163, (166)
Luikart, C., 22, (33)
Lumley, J., 109, (134), 152, (167)
Lund, N., 154, 155, (166)
Lundeen, C., 182, (205)
Lundh, P., 75, (101)
Luterman, D.M., 22, (33), 107, (133), 225, (231)
Lutman, M., 67, (69)
Luttman, M.E., 504, (527)
Luxford, W.M., 417, 422, 426, 427, (436)
Lynch, E.W., 229, 230, (231), (232)
Lynch, J., 152, (167)
Lynch, M.P., 128, (134)
Lyregaard, P., 74, 75, (100), (101), 298, (309)
Lyxell, B., 325, (327)

MacDonald, J., 507, 522, (527)
Mackay, H., 36, (45)
MacKenzie, D., 466, (468)
Mackenzie, K., 81, (98)

Macpherson, B.J., 86, 87, (100)
Macrae, J.H., 89, (100)
Maddox, G.L., 339, (356)
Madell, J., 193, 199, (205), 496, (499)
Madison, L., 22, (33)
Magielski, J., 19, (33)
Maguire, P., 377, (412)
Mahon, W., 72, 95, 96, (100)
Mahoney, G., 217, (231)
Mahoney, T., 64, (70)
Malinoff, R., 350, (355), 494, 495, (499)
Malley, J.D., 94, (99)
Mallinger, C.A., 196, (206)
Malone, C.M., 221, (231)
Mancini, J., 22, (33)
Mandel, E., 60, 63, (69)
Mangham, C.A., 426, 430, (436)
Mangold, S., 506, (527)
Mannie, S., 109, (134)
Manolson, A., 109, (133)
Manuel, S.Y., 522, (527)
Maran, R., (486)
Marascuilo, L.A., 55, (70)
Marchant, C., 60, (70)
Marcus, E., 42, (45)
Margolis, R.H., 87, (100)
Markides, A., 89, (100), 404, (412)
Marquis, M.A., 110, (132)
Marrer, J.L., 20, 21, (33)
Marshall, L., 335, (355)
Martin, D., 470, (485)
Martin, E.L., 422, (436)
Martin, E.S., 502, (527)
Martin, F., 285, 298, 301, 302, (309)
Martin, F.N., 123, (133), 177, 203, (205), 215, 224, 227, (231)
Martin, G., 67, (70)
Martin, L.F.A., 431, (435)
Maslow, A., 492–494, (499)
Mason, D., 290, 305, (310)
Mason, J.L., 516, (526)
Massaro, D.W., 319, (327), 506, 522, (527)
Masur, E.F., 109, 111, (133)
Matkin, N., 62, (70), 72, 73, 89, 91, 94, (99), (100), 182, 188, (205), (206), 225, (232)
Matthess, L.J., 334, (356)
Matthies, M.L., 429, (436)
Mauer, F.J., 333, (355)
Mauer, J.F., 390, (412)
Mauldin, L., 333, (355)
Maurer, J.F., 18, (33)
Maxon, A., 12, (15), 94, (100), 176, 180, 181, 185, 196, 203, (204–206)
May, R., 378, 383, (412)
McAnally, P.L., 163, (166)
McCabe, B.F., 510, 511, (526)
McCaffrey, H., 466, (468)
McCandless, G., 74, (100), 298, (309), 430, (435)
McCarthy, 339
McCarthy, J.J., 169

McCarthy, P., 4, (15), 225, 226, (232), 241, 242, (258), 268, 291, 292, 295, (309), 348, 350, (355), 375, 407, (412), 493, (499), 504, 523, (525)
McClelland, D., 110, 111, (134)
McConkey, A., 112, 122, 124, (133)
McConnell, F., 63, (69), 345, (354)
McConnell, N.L., 169
McConville, K., 73, (99)
McDaniel, D., 303, (308), 473, (485)
McDavis, K.C., 23, (33)
McDermott, H.J., 434, (436)
McGarr, N., 129, (134)
McGee, D., 177, 182, (205)
McGowan, R.S., 128, (133)
McGurk, H., 507, 522, (527)
McKay, C.M., 434, (436)
McKee, B., 22, (32)
McKirdy, L., 152, (166)
Mclauchin, R., 428, (436)
McLinden, S.E., 220, 221, (232)
McLoughlin, J.A., 148, (166)
McSweeney, B., 55, (70)
McWilliam, R.A., 106, (134), 183, 184, 203, (206), 225, (232)
Meadow, K., 109, (133), 152, (167), 216, 229, (232)
Meadow-Orlans, K.P., 392, (412)
Mecklenburg, D.J., 417, 429, (436)
Mehrabian, A., 394, (412)
Meichenbaum, D., 377, 378, 381, (412), (413)
Meier, S.T., 377, (412)
Meline, N.C., 5, 7, (15), 257, 282, 283
Melnick, W., 55, 64, (70)
Meltzoff, A., 121, (133)
Menaghan, E.G., 390, (412)
Mencher, G., 62, (70)
Mendenhall, R., 342, (355)
Menduke, H., 333, (356)
Merzenich, M.M., 421, (437)
Metz, M., 238, 241, (257), 262, 266, 391, (409)
Meyer, D.J., 222, 223, (232)
Mickey, 87
Miettinen, I., 4, (15)
Mikami, K.A., 430, 431, (435)
Millar, J.B., 419, (436)
Miller, G.A., 141, (166), 321, (327), 506, (527)
Miller, J., 114, (133), 156, (166)
Miller, J.D., 515, (527)
Miller, J.F., 169
Miller, L., 110, (133), 163, (167)
Miller, N., 333, (354)
Miller, S., 111, (133)
Miller, S.L., 186, (205)
Millin, J.P., 182, 196, 197, (205)
Mills, J., 58, 66, (70)
Mills, J.H., 89, (100)
Mills, R., 501, (527)
Milne, J.S., 333, (355)
Minifie, F., 139, (165)

Mischook, M., 217, (232)
Mitchell, K.M., 385, (413)
Miyamoto, R.T., 123–125, 130, (134), 422, 428, 434, (436)
Moeller, M.P., 107, 108, 112, 122, 124, (133), 421, (436)
Molfesse, D., 141, (166)
Monson, R., 129, 131, (133)
Montgomery, A.A., 86, 87, (99), 244, 248, 250, (257), 291, 292, 295, 299, (309), 320, 324, 325, (327), 351, (356), 398, (413), 503, 504, 507, 508, 518, 519, 521–524, (527), (528)
Moog, J.S., 123–125, (133), 154, 161, (166), 170, 421, 426, 428, (435), (436), 509, (525)
Moore, B.C., 430, (437), 504, 512, (527), (528)
Moore, J.M., 121, (132)
Moore, J.N., 78, (98)
Moores, D., 147, 160, 164, (166)
Morehouse, C., 59, 60, (70)
Morff, R., 66, (70)
Morford, J., 112, (133)
Morgan, C.M., 18, (33)
Morgan, D.E., 87, (100)
Morgan-Redshaw, M., 222, 225, (232)
Morris, L., 285, 298, 301, 302, (309)
Morse, P., 139, (166)
Morton, M., 341, (354)
Morviducci, A., 94, (98)
Mosak, H.H., 379, (412)
Moses, K.L., 212, 216, (232)
Moulin, A., 67, (69)
Mueller, H.B., 73, 74, 90, (100)
Mueller, H.G., 81, 84, 94, (99), (100), 285, 287, 290–296, 298–300, 302, 304–307, (308), (309), 466, (468), 503, (526)
Mulrow, C., 490, 491, 494, 495, (499)
Myers, D., 478, 480, 481, (485), (486)
Mykleburst, H., 142, (166)
Myres, W.A., 422, (436)

Nabelek, A.K., 334, 351, (355)
Nadol, J.B., 422, (434)
Nance, G., 94, (97), 441, (467)
Naunton, R.F., 89, (100)
Neely, S.T., 123, (133)
Nelson, E., 345, (354)
Nelson, N.W., 154, (166)
Nelson, R.O., 375, (409)
Nelson, T., 477, 478, (485)
Nerbonne, G.P., 502, (526)
Nerbonne, M., 66, (70), 238, 240, 241, 250, (258), (259), 260, 261, 348, 349, (356), 367, 368, 387, 407, (411), (413)
Neuman, A.C., 501, (527)
New, T., 319
Newall, P., 75, 76, (98)

Newman, C., 242, (258), 272, 350, (355), 390, 407, (412), 494, 495, (498)
Nicely, P.E., 506, (527)
Nicholls, J., 111, 112, (135)
Nie, N., 55, (70)
Niebuhr, D., 96, 97, (98)
Nippold, M.A., 153, (166)
Niswander, P.S., 387, (411)
Nittrouer, S., 128, (133)
Noble, W., 238, 240, (258), 387, 390, (412)
Northcott, W.H., 161, (166), 228, (232)
Northern, J.L., 11, (15), 55, 56, 58, 59, 65, (70), 72, 73, 87, 90, 94, (100), (101), 143, (166), 178, 181, 182, 186, (205), 306, 307, 427, (436), (486)
Novick, L., 376, 377, (411)
Nozza, R.J., 186, (205)
Numbers, F., 149, (165)
Nye, C., 89, (101)

Odulana, J., 344, (356)
Oja, G., 239, (258)
Olinger, B., 343, 344, (355)
Oliver, T., 335, (355)
Oller, D.K., 128–130, (133), (134)
Olsen, B., 238, 241, (257), 262, 266, 391, (409)
Olsen, W., 83, 91, (100), 287, 288, (309)
Olsho, L.W., 65, (70), 121, (134)
Olswang, L., 108, (134)
O'Meilia, R.M., 430, 431, (435)
O'Neal, J., 215, 224, 227, (231)
O'Neill, J.J., 245, (258)
Opper, S., 87, (99)
Orchik, D., 66, (70)
O'Reilly, P.P., 246, (257), 524, (525)
Orr, F.C., 159, (166)
Ort, R., 342, (354)
Osberger, M.J., 112, 122–125, 129, 130, (133), (134), 428, 434, (436)
Osborn, J., 196, (205)
Otomo, K., 129, (134)
Ouslander, 489
Ouslander, J., 340, 341, (355), (356)
Over, S.K., 422, (436)
Owen, J., 60, 61, 66, (69)
Owens, E., 242, 244, 251, (257), (258), 326, (327), 391, 399, 406, (411), 421, 424, (435), (436), 523, (527)
Oyer, H., 245, 246, 251, 253, (258), 332, (355)
Oyler, A., 182, (206)
Oyler, R.F., 182, (206), 225, (232)

Paden, E.P., 162, (165)
Palmer, C., 23, (33)

Palmore, E., 22, (33)
Papert, S., 476, (485)
Paradise, J., 55, 60, 65, 66, (69), (70)
Parbo, J., 67, (70)
Parker, R., 375–377, 382, 387, 390, 394, (413)
Parkin, D., 340, (355)
Parkinson, A., 75, 76, (98)
Parving, A., 240, (258)
Pascoe, D., 75, 79, (100), 290, (309)
Patrick, 510
Patrick, J.F., 418–420, (436), (437)
Patterson, C.H., 376, 377, 379, 381, 383–385, (412)
Patterson, K., 343, 344, (355)
Paul, P.V., 138, 151, 163, (166)
Pavlov, I.P., 380, (412)
Pavlovic, C., 79, 81, 86, (100), 290, 300, (308), (309)
Peale, N.V., 35, (45)
Pearson, P., 111, (134)
Pearsons, K., 287, 289, (309)
Peck, L., 246, (257), 524, (525)
Pedersen, J., 334, (356)
Pederson, J., 66, (70)
Peek, B.F., 507, (527)
Pegg, K.S., 250, (259)
Pehringer, J.L., 94, (97)
Pelson, R., 65, (69)
Peltz Strauss, K., 469
Perkins, D., 342, (355), (357)
Perls, F.S., 378, 382, 383, (412)
Perotta, P., 342, (355)
Perrin, K., 59, (69)
Petersen, C.H., 403, (411)
Peters-McCarthy, E.P., 13, (15)
Peterson, J., 337, (356)
Peterson, P.M., 500, (525)
Pettegrew, L.S., 394, (412)
Pfeiffer, E., 491, 496, (499)
Pfingst, B.E., 511, (527)
Phillips, M., 125, (134), 422, (436)
Phillips, P., 346, (354)
Piaget, J., 111, (134)
Pichora-Fuller, M.K., 248, (258), 390, 397, 398, 403, (409)
Pickett, J.M., 502, (527)
Pickles, 318
Pien, D., 152, (166)
Pious, C., 149, 153, (167), 168
Pirozzolo, F., 335, (355)
Pisoni, D.B., 520, (527)
Plant, G., 246, (257)
Plapinger, D., 216, 217, (232)
Platt, F., 96, (98), 196, (204)
Plomp, R., 74, (99), 318, (327), 504, 516, (525), (526)
Pollack, D., 177, 180, 199, (206)
Pollack, M., 225, (232), 242, (258), 296, (310), 380, (412), 423, (436)
Pollock, B., 218, (231)
Pope, M., 123, 125, (134), 422, (436)

Popelka, G., 80, 81, 87, (100), 290, 305, (310)
Powell, A., 217, (231)
Power, D.J., 151, (167), 170
Powers, A., 164, (165)
Prather, E., 169
Pratt, H., 87, (100)
Pratt, T., 23, (33)
Preece, J., 424, (437)
Prescod, S.V., 244, (258)
Press, E., 342, (357)
Preves, D., 95, (100), 296, (309), (310), 474, (485)
Prickett, H.T., 228, (231)
Prizant, B., 108, (135)
Probst, R., 67, (70)
Proctor, A., 516, (526), (527)
Propst, S., 223, 226, (232)
Prosek, R., 86, 87, (99), 248, 250, (259), 299, (309), 324, 325, (327), 503, 504, 506, 507, 518, 519, 521–524, (527), (528)
Prutting, C., 152, (164), (167)
Pujol, R., 67, 68, (69)
Purtilo, R., 377, (412)
Pusakulich, K., 302, (308)
Pyman, B.C., 418, 422, 423, (435–437)

Quigley, S.P., 138, 151, 163, (166), (167), 170
Quirk, J., 340, (355)

Rabinowitz, W.M., 95, (98), 434, (437), 510, 513, 514, 517, (527), (528)
Radecki, S., 342, (355)
Rader, N., 340, (356)
Radvansky, G., 338, (354)
Raffin, M., 152, 156, (165), (166), 507, (528)
Raggio, M.W., 244, (257), 421, (436)
Rahbar, B., 340, (356)
Raiford, C., 332, (355)
Ramji, K., 78, 80, (101)
Ramsdell, D., 140, (166), 180, (206), 493, 494, (499)
Rane, R., 74, (98)
Raskin, N.J., 382, (412)
Rasmussen, G., 81, (98)
Ray, H., 182, 196, 197, (206)
Ray, S., 153, 159, (166), (167)
Reed, C.M., 95, (98), 513, 514, 517, (527)
Reed, M., 159, (167)
Reeder, R.M., 508, (526)
Rees, J.N., 338, (355)
Rees, T., 490, (499)
Reese, L., 240, (259)
Reichert, T., 66, (70)
Reichle, N.C., 219, (231)
Renn, R.J., 516, (526)
Renshaw, J., 123–126, (134)
Rentz, D., 490, 494, (499)

Repp, B.H., 521, 522, (527)
Reynolds, E.G., 251, (258)
Reznick, J.S., 108, (132)
Riding, K., 66, (70)
Ries, P.W., 17, (33), 339, (355), 421, (436)
Riffle, K.L., 336, (355)
Riggs, D.E., 91, (98), 465, (468)
Riko, K., 390, 397, 398, 403, (409)
Ringdahl, A., 254, (257), 403, (411), 506, (527)
Rintelmann, W.F., 89, (100)
Ripich, D.N., 153, 163, (167)
Ritter, R., 87, (101)
Riverin, L., 403–406, 408, (411)
Rizzo, J., 7, (15)
Robb, M.P., 504, (528)
Robbins, A.M., 123–126, 128, (134)
Roberts, M., 522, (527)
Roberts, S.D., 393, (412)
Robins, D.S., 57, 58, (70)
Robinson, C., 217, (232)
Robinson, P.K., 334, (355)
Roche, A.F., 13, (15)
Rodin, J., 22, (33)
Roeser, R., 55, 65, 66, (70)
Rogers, C.R., 378, 382, 383, 385, 394, (412)
Rogers, K., 53, (70)
Rogers, L., 110, 111, (134)
Ronnberg, J., 325, (327)
Rose, S., 111–113, 116, (132), 163, (166), 169
Rosen, S.M., 511, (527)
Rosenberg, B., 384, (410)
Rosenberg, S., 217, (232)
Rosenhall, U., 334, (356)
Rosner, B., 60, (71)
Rosov, R.J., 516, (526)
Ross, L., 89, (99)
Ross, M., 12, (15), 72, 73, 77, 87, 94, (101), 123–125, (134), 159, 161, (167), 176–182, 186, 193, 199, 203, (206), 409, (412), 428, (436), 496, (499)
Rossi, K., 107, 109, (134), 227, 228, (232)
Rossman, R.N.F., 186, (205)
Rothenberg, M., 515, (527)
Rotter, J.B., 22, (33)
Roush, J., 55, (70), 106, (134), 183, 184, 203, (206), 225, (232)
Rovner, J., 24, (33)
Rowland, J.P., 387, (412)
Ruben, R., 60, (70)
Rubinstein, A., 248, 250, (258)
Rupp, R., 60, 63, (69), 333, (355), 390, (412)
Rush, A.J., 378, (409)
Rushford, G., 524, (527)
Rushmer, N., 107, 108, (134), 227, 228, (232), 430, (437)
Russell, W.K., 151, (167)
Ruth, R., 58, 66, (70), 423, (436)
Ryan, S., 67, (70)

Sabo, M.P., 72, (99)
Sachs, M.B., 318, (327)
Sachs, R., 81, 89, (101), 300, (310), 515, (527)
Salisbury, C.L., 219, 220, 221, (232)
Salomon, 345
Salomon, G., 240, (258)
Salvia, J., 148, (167)
Samar, V., 325, (327)
Sammeth, C., 298, (308), 507, (527)
Sandall, S.R., 227, (231)
Sanders, D., 140, (167), 225, (232), 242, 253, (259), 376, (412)
Sandridge, S., 335, (355), 491, 492, 496, (499), 524, (527)
Sarff, L.S., 182, 196, 197, (206)
Sarigiani, P., 228, 229, (231)
Sarvela, J., 344, (356)
Sarvela, P., 344, (356)
Sass-Lehrer, M., 230, (232)
Sataloff, J., 333, (356)
Satterly, D., 109, 111, (132)
Saucedo, K.A., 91, 93, (101)
Scadden, L.A., 387, (412)
Schafer, D., 152, (167)
Schaffer, M., 64, (70)
Scheer, C.K., 248, (259)
Schein, J., 238, 240, (259)
Scherer, P., 170
Scherr, C.K., 246, (259), 324, (327), 524, (528)
Schick, B.S., 106, (134)
Schimpfhauser, F., 342, (355)
Schlesinger, H., 152, (167), 216, (232)
Schmidt, I., 331, (354)
Schmitt, J., 353, (356)
Schneider, B.A., 121, (134)
Schober-Peterson, D., 156, (167)
Schoeny, Z., 140, 146, (165)
Scholl, M.E., 177, (205)
Schontz, F.C., 386, (413)
Schorn, K., 504, (528)
Schow, R., 66, (70), 238–241, 244–247, 250, 252, (258), (259), 260, 261, 347–349, 351, 352, (356), 367, 368, 387–389, 391, 397, 407, (413)
Schubert, E., 242, 251, (258), 391, 399, 406, (411)
Schuchman, G.I., 351, (356), 398, (413), 508, (528)
Schuknecht, H., 333, (356)
Schulman, J., 123, 124, (132)
Schultz, M.C., 514, (527)
Schulz, R., 22, (33)
Schum, D.J., 196, (205), 334, 335, 352, (356), 466, (468)
Schum, R., 62, (69), 73, 86, 87, 91, 92, 96, (98–100), 228, (231)
Schumacher, G., 340, (356)
Schuyler, V., 107, 108, (134), 227, 228, (232), 430, (437)
Schwander, T., 501, (527)

Schwartz, A.N., 337, (356)
Schwartz, D., 65, (70), 74, 75, (99), (101), 250, 252, (259), 302, 303, (309), (310), 324, (327), 340, (356), 504, 505, 507, 518, 519, 524, (527), (528)
Schwartz, R., 65, (70)
Schweitzer, C., 472, (485)
Schweitzer, H.C., 35, 42, (45)
Scott, B.L., 248, (257), 429, (435), 524, (526)
Seaborg, J., 59, (71)
Seal, B.C., 219, (232)
Sedge, R.K., 246, (259), 406, (413)
Seewald, R., 72, 77, 78, 80, 83, 87, 95, 98, (101), 298, (310)
Sefton, K., 156, (165)
Seibert, C.E., 422, (434)
Seligman, P.M., 419, 420, 430, 431, 434, (435–437)
Selker, L., 331, 346, (356)
Serrano-Navaro, M., 312, (327)
Sexton, J.E., 185, (206)
Shadden, B., 332, (355)
Shah, C.P., 72, (101)
Shallop, J.K., 417, 424, 430, 431, (435), (436)
Shanes, E., 339, (356)
Shankweiler, D.P., 513, (527)
Shannon, R.V., 420, (437), 511, (528)
Shapiro, E., 159, (165)
Shapiro, W.H., 326, (327), 430, 431, (435)
Shaw, B., 378, (409)
Shaw, E.A.G., 79, 81, (101)
Sheffler, M.V., 87, (97)
Shenai, J., 59, (71)
Shephard, N., 62, (71)
Shepherd, D., 325, (327)
Shepherd, R.K., 418, (435)
Sherbecoe, R.L., 81, 87, 98, (100)
Sherblom, J., 473, (485)
Sherrick, C.E., 512, (528)
Shipley, K.G., 170
Shontz, F.C., 393, (413)
Shough, L.F., 94, (97)
Shriberg, L., 22, (33), 60, (71), 163, (165)
Shurin, P., 60, (70)
Siegenthaler, B., 124, (134)
Siervogel, R.M., 13, (15)
Sigelman, J.A., 95, (100)
Silman, S., 89, (99), (101)
Silverman, C.A., 89, (101)
Silverman, F., (486)
Silverman, M.S., 72, (98), (101)
Silverman, R.S., 124, (132)
Silverman, S.R., 11, (15), 251, 254, (257), (258), 275
Simeonsson, R.J., 147, 157, (167)
Simkin, J.S., 383, (413)
Simmins, F.B., 511, (528)
Simmons, F., 58, 65, (71), 72, (101), 417, 421, (437)
Simmons-Martin, A., 107, 109, (134), 227, 228, (232)

Simon, C.S., 163, (167), 179, (206)
Sims, D., 248, (259), 325, (327), 421, (437), 474, (485)
Sinclair, J.S., 91, (98), 465, (468)
Singer, B., 455, (468)
Singer, J.E., 402, (411)
Singer, W., 344, (356)
Siqueland, E.R., 121, (132)
Sisco, F., 158, (164)
Sjogren, H., 303, (308)
Skarakis, E., 152, (167)
Skinner, B.F., 380, 391, 393, (413)
Skinner, M., 79, (101), 287, 300, (310), 420, 423, 430, 434, (437)
Smaldino, J., 20, (33), 196, (205), 302, (310), 474, (485)
Smaldino, S.E., 20, (33)
Small, A., 152, (167)
Small, G.W., 341, (355)
Smedley, T., 239, 240, 243, 244, 247, 252, (259), 348, 351, 352, (356), 397, (413)
Smirga, D.J., 19, (33)
Smith, A., 60, (71)
Smith, C.G., 66, (70)
Smith, D.A., 42, (45)
Smith, L., 123, 124, (132), 430, (435)
Smith, L.B., 121, 122, 128, (132)
Smith, M., 22, (33), 68, (71)
Smith, M.C., 315, (327)
Smith, R.D., 3, (15)
Snow, C.E., 110–112, (134)
Snyder, C.L., 337, (356)
Soh, J., 66, (70)
Sohmer, H., 87, (100)
Solomon, D., 342, (355)
Somers, M., 218–220, (232)
Spahr, R., 60, 65, 66, (70)
Sparks, D.W., 511, 516, (526)
Sparks, S.N., 107, (134)
Speaks, C., 251, (258), 387, (413)
Spetner, N.B., 65, (70), 121, (134)
Spinelli, F.M., 153, 163, (167)
Spiro, M.K., 77, (101)
Spitzer, J., 349, 350, (356), 390, (413)
Spivak, L.G., 430, (437)
Sprague, B., 65, (71)
Spretnjak, M., 292, 293, (310), 335, (356)
Spring, D., 139, (167)
Springer, N., 123, 124, (132)
Squier, R.W., 386, 393–395, (413)
St. Clair-Stokes, J., 217, (231), (232)
Staab, W., 296, (309)
Stach, B., 292, 293, (310), 335, (356), 472, (485)
Staller, S.J., 143, (167), 417, 421, 426–428, 430, 431, (434), 434, (434), (435), (437)
Stark, J., 169
St-Cyr, C., 404, 405, 408, (411)
Steckler, J., 8, (15)
Steenerson, R.L., 422, (437)
Stein, L., 59, (71)

Steinberg, J., 79, (99), 288, (308)
Steinkamp, M.W., 170
Stelmachowicz, P., 79, 82–88, 95, (99), (101), 465, (468), 503, (526)
Stenstrom, R., 86, (101)
Stephens, D., 237, (259), 387, 389, (413)
Stephens, K., 251, (258)
Stephens, S., 470, (485)
Stephens, S.D.G., 18, 20, (32), (34), 244, 255, 257, (258), (259), 404, (412)
Sternberg, R.J., 138, (167)
Sterritt, G., 64, 65, (69)
Stevens, J., 68, (71)
Stevens, K.N., 503, (528)
Stevens, S.S., 431, (436)
Stiglbrunner, H.K., 512, (526)
Stoel-Gammon, C., 108, 128, 129, (134)
Stone, A.A., 170
Stone, P., 111, (134)
Stoner, M., 430, (436)
Stormer, J., 59, (69)
Stouffer, J.L., 255, (259)
Stout, G., 430, (437)
Strauss, K.P., 184, (205)
Stream, K.S., 225, (232)
Stream, R.W., 225, (232)
Streng, A., 216, (232)
Strickland, E., 67, (71)
Stroud, D.J., 507, (528)
Stuart, A., (101), 86
Stubblefield, J., 89, (101)
Studdert-Kennedy, M., 128, (133), 513, 522, (527)
Studebaker, G., 81, 88, (100)
Sue, M.B., 170
Sullivan, P., 158, 159, (167)
Summerfield, Q., 504, 507, 522, (527), (528)
Summers, J.A., 227, (232)
Summers, W.V., 520, (528)
Sung, R.J., 91, (101)
Surr, R.K., 252, (259), 351, (356), 398, (413), 508, (528)
Susser, M.W., 387, 388, (413)
Sussman, J.E., 122–124, (134)
Sutton, D., 511, (527)
Svanborg, A., 334, (356)
Swan, I.R.C., 389, 390, 393, 398, (413)
Sweetlow, R., 223, (232), 255, (259), 305, (309)

Taaffe, G., 524, (527)
Tait, C., 55, (70)
Tannahill, C., 240, (259)
Tanner, D.C., 211–213, (232)
Tarter, V., 139, (165)
Tarver, S., 22, (33)
Taylor, S., 343, (356)
Teele, D., 60, 65, (71)
Teele, J., 65, (71)
Tees, R.C., 72, (101), 520, (528)

Tell, L., 59, (71)
Telleen, C., 326, (327), 421, 424, (436)
Teter, D.L., 35, (45)
Thal, D., 108, (132)
Tharpe, A.M., 73, 74, (98)
Thibodeau, L., 91, 93, (101), 353, (356), 465, 466, (468)
Thielemeier, M., 428, (437)
Thomas, A.J., 376, 387, 389, 390, 393, 397, 404, 408, (413)
Thomas, D.D., 219, (231)
Thomas, K., 375–377, 382, 387, 390, 394, (413)
Thompkins, M., 114, (134)
Thompson, B., 475, (485)
Thompson, D.J., 79, 81, (99)
Thompson, J., 338, (354)
Thompson, M., 149, 153, (167), 168
Thompson, W., 475, (485)
Thorn, F., 244, 246, (259)
Thorn, S., 244, 246, (259)
Thornton, A.R., 507, (528)
Thornton, S., 68, (69)
Thorpe, L., 121, (134)
Thwing, E., 62, (70)
Tidwell, R., 218, (231)
Tiegerman, E., 153, 163, (164)
Tillman, T., 90, (99), 193, (205), 251, (259)
Tjossem, T.D., 54, (71)
Tobin, A., 169
Toccafondi, S., 226, (232)
Todd, J., 109, (134), 377, 381–384, (410)
Tomasello, M., 109, 111, (134)
Tonelson, S., 170
Tong, Y.C., 419, (436), (437)
Tonisson, W., 74, (98)
Torpey, C., 96, (98)
Townsend, T., 334, (354)
Trammell, J., 251, (258), 387, (413)
Traynor, R., 403, (413), 474, (485)
Trehub, S.E., 121, (134)
Trezona, R., 490, 496, (499)
Trivette, C.M., 218, 223, 226, (231), (232)
Trout, M., 107, 109, (134)
Truax, C.B., 385, 394, (413)
Tubis, A., 67, (71)
Tucker, F.M., 351, (355)
Turczyk, V., 60, (70)
Turk, D., 381, (413)
Turkat, I.D., 394, (412)
Turnbull, A.P., 227, 228, (232)
Turnbull, H.R., 228, (232)
Turner, C.W., 504, (528)
Turner, R., 59, 62, 67, (71)
Turner, R.J., 390, (413)
Tye-Murray, N., 163, (167), 321, 324, 326, (327), 403, (413), 417, 424, 429, 430, 434, (437), 474, (485), 510, 511, (526)
Tyler, R., 18, (34), 255, (259), 287, (310), 326, (327), 352, (356),

417, 421, 424, 429, 430, 434, (435), (437), 474, (485), 504, 510–512, (526), (528)
Tymchuk, A., 340, (356)

Ulhmann, R., 490, (499)
Upfold, L.J., 59, 64, (71), 81, 177, 182, 203, (206)
Uziel, A., 67, 68, (69)

Vadasy, P.F., 222, 223, (232)
Vaillancourt, M.M., 79, (101)
Valente, M., 298, (310)
Van Dyke, R.C., 89, (97)
Van Hecke-Wulatin, M., 212, 216, (232)
van Kleeck, A., 112, (132)
Van Tasell, D., 81, 83, 91, 93, (99), (100), 196, (206), 287, 288, (309), 325, (327), 352, (356), 465, (468)
Vandali, A.E., 434, (436)
Vane, J.R., 170
Vass, W., 298, (310)
Vassalo, L., 333, (356)
Venditti, L., 94, (98)
Ventry, I., 60, (71), 240, (259), 286, (310), 348–350, (356), 372, 373, 387, 390, (413)
Vernon, M., 158, 159, 164, (167)
Verrillo, R.T., 515, (527)
Vesper, 339
Vestal, R., 340, (356)
Vethivelu, S., 149, 153, (167), 168
Vigorito, J., 121, (132)
Vihman, M., 128, (134)
Vincent, L.J., 219, 220, (232)
Vineberg, S.E., 22, (33)
Violette, J., 94, (101)
Violette, M., 94, (101)
Voeks, 347
Von Almen, P., 176, 177, (204)
VonderEmbse, D., 196, (205)
Voneche, J.J., 53, (69)

Wahlin, B., 403, (411)
Walden, B., 86, 87, (99), 243, 244, 248, 250, (259), 299, 302, (309), (310), 324, 325, (327), 335, (356), 391, 406, (410), (413), 474, (485), 503–509, 518, 519, 521–524, (526), (528)
Waldo, D., 346, (356)
Walker, G., 296, (310)
Wallach, G.P., 163, (167), 179, (206)
Wallber, M., 466, (468)
Walton, W., 55, 63, 64, (71)
Waltzman, S.B., 326, (327), 430, 431, (435), (437)
Wang, M., 340, (356)
Ward, W.D., 387, (413)
Warner, E.O.H., 170
Warren, C., 223, (232)

Warren, D.H., 522, (528)
Watkins, S., 170, 228, (231)
Watson, B.U., 158, (167)
Watson, C.S., 85, (101), 516, (528)
Watson, S.M., 221, (231)
Watson, W., 387, 388, (413)
Watters, B., 290, (308)
Watts, W.J., 250, (259)
Wayman, K.I., 229, 230, (231), (232)
Web, R.L., 418, (437)
Webb, H., 68, (71)
Webb, R.L., 418, (435)
Webster, D.B., 72, (99), (101)
Webster, M., 72, (101)
Weddell-Monig, J., 109, (134), 152, (167)
Wedding, D., 376, (410)
Wedenberg, E., 139, (165)
Weikart, D., 110–112, 115, 119, (133), (134)
Weinstein, B., 238, 240, 242, (258), (259), 272, 286, (310), 332, 343, 346, 348–350, (355), (356), 372, 373, 387, 390, 407, (412), (413), 489–491, 494, 495, (499)
Weinstein, S., 515, (528)
Weisenberger, J.M., 515, (528)
Weisner, T.S., 218, (231)
Weiss, M., 455, (468)
Weissler, L., 129, (134)
Welch, R.B., 522, (528)
Wells, G., 107, 109–112, (132), (134), (135)
Werker, J.F., 520, (528)
Wertz, P., 96, (98), 196, (204)
Westby, C., 110–112, 114, (135)
Westin, B., 139, (165)
Wetherby, A., 108, (135)
Whelan, J.P., 221, (231)
Whitaker, M., 239, 244, (259)
Whitcomb, C., 239, 247, 252, (259)
White, A.H., 170
White, D., 94, (101)
White, M.W., 421, (437)
White, S., 346, (357)
White, S.C., 225, (231)
White, S.D., 77, (98)
Whitehead, L.C., 226, (232)
Whitford, L.A., 420, 430, 434, (435), 506, (525)
Wilbur, R.B., 138, (167)
Wilder, C.S., 17, (34)
Wilderom, C., 342, (357)
Wiley, T., 65, (71), 87, (99)
Wilgosh, L., 222, 225, (232)
Willeford, J., 96, (101)
Williams, D., 224, (233), 302, (310)
Williams, D.L., 507, (528)
Williams, J., 185, (206)
Williams, T.F., 331, 345, (357)
Willot, J.D., 334, (357)
Wilson, B.S., 434, (437), 510, (528)

Wilson, W.R., 55, 63, 64, (71), 121, (132)
Wilson-Vlotman, A.L., 176, 177, (204), (206)
Windle, J., 430, (437)
Windmill, I., 14, (15)
Winslow, R.L., 318, (327)
Winton, P.J., 226, (233)
Wolf, E., 336, (357)
Wolford, R.D., 434, (437), 510, (528)
Wolpe, J., 378, 380, 401, 402, (413)
Wood, C., 4, (15)
Wood, E.J., 504, (528)
Wood, P.L., 405, (411)
Woodford, C., 177, 196, (205), (206)
Woodward, M.F., 248, (259)

Woodworth, G., 510, 511, (526)
Worner, W.A., 196, 197, (206)
Worthington, D.W., 506, (528)
Wray, D., 178, (205), (206)
Wright, B.E., 393, (413)
Wright, J., 377, (409)
Wylde, M.A., 376, 393, (413)
Wynens, M.S., 422, (437)

Yacobacci-Tam, P., 230, (233)
Yahne, C.E., 19, (34)
Yalom, I., 383, (412)
Yanke, R.B., 335, (355)
Yantis, P.A., 10, (15)
Yaseldyke, J., 148, (167)
Ying, E., 149, (167), 199, (206)

Yoder, D.E., 169
Yontef, G.M., 383, (413)
Yoshinaga-Itano, C., 110–112, 115, (135)

Zackman, L., 169
Zacks, R., 338, (354)
Zahorian, S.A., 515, (527)
Zarnoch, J., 60, (71), 349, (357), 360, 361
Zelisko, D.L.C., 78, 80, 83, (101)
Zeng, F.-G., 504, (528)
Zieziula, F., 159, (167)
Zimmerman-Phillips, S., 123, 125, 130, (134), 428, 434, (436)
Zink, G.D., 55, (69)
Zones, J., 331, (357)
Zwicker, E., 504, (528)

Subject Index

Page numbers in *italics* denote figures; those followed by "t" denote tables.

ABX discrimination tasks, 522
Academic performance, *See also* Schools
  impact of hearing and hearing loss on, 177–181, *194–195*
Academy of Rehabilitative Audiology, 5–6
Acceptance, 384–385
  parental, 213
Accessibility
  acoustic, in school, 184
  to private practice offices, 36
  to public accommodations, 27–30
  to public services, 25–27
Accurate Empathy Scale, 394
Acoustic filter effect, 178–179
Acoustic immittance, 65–66
Acoustic phonetics, 188
Acoustic reflex thresholds, 84
Acoustic reflexes, 65
Active learning, 114–115
Activities of daily living, 10–12
Adjustment to hearing loss, 386–390
  age and, 404
  coping and, 389–390
  counseling related to, 376
  course of, 386
  definitions of hearing impairment/handicap and, 387–389, 388t
  factors affecting, 387
  grief cycle and, 211–213
  identifying problems with, 390–392
  mechanisms of, 384–385
  problem-solving exercises for, 399, 400t
Adolescents, hearing-impaired, 3. *See also* Children
Adults, hearing-impaired. *See also* Elderly persons

auditory training for, 325–326
aural rehabilitation group for, 320–322
  benefits of, 320
  determining simple solutions in, 321–322
  goals and purposes of, 329
  outline for, 328
  structure of, 319–320
case study of, 322–323
communication needs of, 404–408
  employment, 404–406
  marriage and family, 406–408
conversation repair for, 320–321
counseling of, 374–409. *See also* Counseling
goals and methods for rehabilitation of, 326, 330
hearing aids for, 284–308
hearing screening for, 238
identification of, 9
individual rehabilitation for, 324
management of, 311–330
nonhearing aid wearers, 323–324
preoperative selection/evaluation for cochlear implants, 421t, 421–424
  audiological evaluation, 423–424, 424t, *425*
  medical/surgical evaluation, 422–423
  patient/family questionnaires, 422, 438–439
rehabilitation services for, 13–14
rehabilitative evaluation of, 237–283
  audiometric assessment battery, 238
  auditory recognition, 249–254

comprehensive screening scale, 255–257
disability/handicap/communication questionnaires, 238–244
overall test battery, 255, 256t
speechreading ability, 24–249
tinnitus, 254–255
speechreading training for, 324–325
Afro-Americans, 230
Age Discrimination in Employment Act of 1973, 30
Ageism, 331–332
Aging, 489. *See also* Elderly persons
  central presbycusis related to, 292, *293*
  chronological vs. physiological, 489
  external ear resonance related to, 81, *82*
  habits in hearing care and, 20
  hearing loss related to, 3, *4*, 333
  models of, 315–316
  psychological changes with, 337–339
    memory, 337–338
    motivation, 339, 491–492, 492t, 498
    slowing and cautiousness, 338–339
  sensory changes with, 332t, 332–337
    audition, 332–335
    body sensations, 336–337
    vision, 335–336
Air conduction audiometry, in candidate for cochlear implants, 423
Alerting devices, 454–456
  determining need for, 464–465
  electronic, 454–456

Alerting devices—*continued*
for emergencies, 28–29, 441
in home, 456–457
mammalian, 456
for recreation/travel, 458–459
in school/college, 457
visual, 455
at work, 457
Alpiner-Meline Aural
Rehabilitation Screening
Scale, 255–257, 256t,
281–283
Altruism, 384–385
American Association of Retired
Persons, 331
American Sign Language, 106, 138
American Speech-Language-
Hearing Association, 6
definitions of hearing handicap/
impairment, 387–389
Guidelines for the Audiologic
Assessment of Children
from Birth Through 36
Months of Age, 54
Guidelines for the Audiologic
Screening for Newborn
Infants Who Are at Risk
for Hearing Impairment,
54, 66
Joint Committee on Infant
Hearing, 54
Americans with Disabilities Act of
1990, 7, 23–31, 184–185,
389
background and legislative
history of, 23–24
effect on audiologic practice,
32
title I: employment, 24–25
title II: public services, 25–27
title III: public
accommodations, 27–30
title IV: telecommunications
relays, 30, 454
title V: miscellaneous, 30–31
Amplification, 320. *See also*
Assistive listening
devices; FM systems;
Hearing aids
for children, 72–105. *See also*
Children
classroom, 196–198
in classrooms, 196–198, 458
nonlinear, 43
personal amplification systems,
445, 446
for telephones, 453
transcranial, 296
Analgesics, 341t
Anger, parental, 212–213
Antihistamines, 341t
Antihypertensive drugs, 341t
Antimicrobial drugs, 341t
Antiparkinsonian drugs, 341t
Architectural and Transportation
Barriers Compliance
Board, 30

Articulation index, 79–80,
288–290, *290*
Artificial intelligence, 503
Assertive patients, 394
Assertiveness training, 380,
399–402
Assessing Linguistic Behaviors,
108
Assessment, 4. *See also* Self-
assessment; specific
instruments
of auditory perceptual
development, 122–126,
123t
computer programs for,
472–474
curriculum-based, 154
of elderly, 347–350, 358–373
of hearing-impaired adults,
237–283
audiometric test battery, 238
auditory recognition, 249–254
comprehensive screening
scale, 255–257
overall test battery, 255
screening, 238
self-report questionnaires,
238–244
speechreading ability,
244–249
tinnitus, 254–255
of hearing-impaired children,
147–149
communicative, 148–149
language, 153–156
preschooler's communication,
108
preschooler's language,
112–114, *113*
rights related to, 148
speech, 150–151
personality, 159–160
psychoeducational, 156–160
of sign language proficiency, 149
of speech development, 54–55,
62, 129–130
Assessment of Children's
Language
Comprehension, 168,
169, 171
Assessment of Phonologic
Processes, 151
Assistive device interview, 323
Assistive devices, 7, 14, 313,
441–467. *See also*
Amplification; Hearing
aids
advantages and disadvantages
of, 29
affordability of, 463
alerting devices, 454–456,
464–465
auditory (assistive listening
devices), 442–451
benefit in school, 181
categories of, 442
compatibility of, 464

cosmetics of, 464
counseling related to, 459
cultural orientation and, 465
determining need for
nonauditory devices, 464
durability of, 464
effectiveness of, 463
to ensure access to public
accommodations, 27–30
to ensure access to public
services, 25–27
evaluation of, 465–466
behavioral assessment, 465
electroacoustic measurement,
465–466
probe tube measurement, 466
speech perception testing, 466
follow-up for users of, 466–467
hearing aid/assistive device
evaluation for, 459–460
hearing aid selection and,
460–463
identification of permanently
installed systems, 29, *29*
mobility of, 463–464
needs assessment for, 456–459
communication needs at
home, 456–457
communication needs at
school/college, 457–458
communication needs at
work, 457
communication needs in
group home, 457
life style, 456
recreation/travel, 458–459
previous experience with, 464
quality/dependability of, 463
role of professional with, 467
selection of, 463–465
telephone devices and systems,
452–454
terminology for, 442
versatility of, 463
visual devices, 451–452
Assistive listening devices,
442–451
hardwired systems, 443–446,
444–445
hearing aid dependent, 443,
446
hearing aid independent, 446
how speech understanding is
improved by, 442–443,
443
microphone placement for, 451
to reduce environmental factors
affecting listening
environment, 442
for telephone, 452–454
use of environmental
microphones with, 451
wireless systems, 446–451
applications of, 446
FM systems, *450*, 450–451
induction loop, 446–449, *447*
infrared, *448*, 449

Atropine, 341t
AT&T Portable Amplifier, 453
Attention, 140
　localization and, 140
　selective, 140
　sustained, 140
Audibility, 178
Audibility index, 290
Audiogram analysis, 150
　count the dot procedure for,
　　290, *290*
　for determining hearing aid
　　candidacy, 286–287
Audiologist
　assistive technology and, 467
　categories of services of, 12
　as children's advocate, 204
　client motivation by, 12, 291
　clinical judgments of, 9–10
　counseling role of, 374–375
　dispensing of hearing aids by, 6,
　　18, 285, 397–398
　education of, 14–15
　effectiveness of counseling
　　provided by, 223–225
　as hearing aid coach, 38–41
　perception of parents' emotional
　　reactions, 215, 224
　relationships with clients, 12,
　　17–32
　　empathic, 393–396, *395*
　　managing difficult patients,
　　　394–396
　　nonverbal cues, 396
　　patient communication styles
　　　and, 394
　　variables affecting, 396
　relationships with hearing aid
　　manufacturers, 37
　role in IEP process, 199
　roles of, 4–5
　school-based, 176
Audiometric testing. *See also*
　　Assessment; specific
　　instruments
　battery for, 238
　for cochlear implant candidate
　　adults, 423–424, 424t, *425*
　　children, 427–428
Audiometric thresholds, 39
Auditory brainstem response, 84
　as screening test, 57, 58t, 64t,
　　66–67
　compared with otoacoustic
　　emission testing, 68, 68t
　cost of, 61, 61t, 67
　recommendations for, 66–67
Auditory deprivation
　effect on speech/language
　　development, 73
　late-onset, 89
Auditory distance, 43
Auditory evoked responses, 84
Auditory learning, 139
　in children with cochlear
　　implants, 143–144,
　　144–145

deficits in, 142–143
evaluation of, 143
hearing impairment and,
　145–146
Auditory nerve evaluation, 423
Auditory Numbers test, 125
Auditory perceptual development,
　119–128
　assessment of, 122–126, 123t
　integrating speech skills with,
　　131–132
　intervention and, 126–128
　normal and interrupted,
　　121–122
Auditory processing, 139–142
　attention, 140
　central deficit in, 291–293, *293*
　　among elderly, 335
　discrimination, 140–141
　organization, 141–142
Auditory recognition, 142,
　249–251
Auditory recognition tests,
　251–254, *253*
Auditory representation, 142
Auditory retention, 141
Auditory sequencing, 141
Auditory Skills Curriculum, 126
Auditory symbolization and
　comprehension, 142
Auditory synthesis, 141–142
Auditory trainers. *See* FM systems
Auditory training, 121, 126,
　249–251
　for adults, 325–326
　after fitting of cochlear
　　implants, 428–430, *429*
　purpose of, 517
　research on, 517–521
　traditional feedback-oriented
　　methods of, 517–521
Auditory-visual integration, 320,
　524–525
Aural rehabilitation. *See*
　　Rehabilitative audiology
Aversion therapy, 380

Balance
　auditory, 44–45
　spatial, 295
Bankson Language Screening Test,
　168, 169, 171
Bare Essentials in Assessing Really
　　Little Kids—Concept
　　Analysis Profile
　　Summary, 168, 169, 171
Bargaining, parental, 213
Barriers to service, 30
BASIC I.D., 381
Baudot code, 454
Behavior
　aggressive, passive, and
　　assertive, 399–400, 401t
　parent-child, 109, 216–218
　slowing with aging, 338–339
Behavior therapy, 378t, 380–381

Behavioral existentialism, 382
Behavioral screening methods,
　64t, 64–65
Behind-the-ear (BTE) hearing aids,
　285, 293–294, 294t, 352
　assistive devices and, 462
　for children, 89
　direct audio input systems for,
　　443
　use with telephone, 460
Better Hearing Institute, 7
Bilateral Contralateral Routing of
　　Signal (BICROS) hearing
　　aids, 296
Binaural squelch, 295
Binaural summation, 73–74, 94,
　295
Biopsychosocial approach, 489
Boehm Test of Basic Concepts,
　168, 169, 171
Bone conduction audiometry, in
　　candidate for cochlear
　　implants, 423
Bone conduction hearing aids,
　90
"Boom boxes," 3
Bracken Basic Concept Scale, 168,
　169, 171
Brain, role in hearing, 42–43
Brainstorming, 116
Bromocriptine, 341t
Brown's stage, 156

California Consonant Test,
　252–254, 256t,
　273–274
Canonical babbling, 128–129
Captioning
　closed, 452
　real-time, 451
Carbidopa, 341t
Cardiovascular drugs, 341t
Carolina Picture Vocabulary Test,
　149, 168, 169, 171
Carrow Elicited Language
　　Inventory, 168, 169, 172
Case management, 13
Central auditory processing
　　deficit, 291–293, *293*
Central Institute for the Deaf
　　(CID)
　Early Speech Perception
　　Battery, 428
　Everyday Speech Sentences,
　　254, 256t, 275–277
　Phase IV procedure, 76, 77t,
　　79–80
　Scales of Early Communication
　　Skills for Hearing-
　　Impaired Children, 168,
　　170
Change/no-change procedure,
　122–123, 125
　for cochlear implant candidates,
　　428
Child Assessment Record, 113

Children, hearing-impaired
Afro-American, 230
amplification for, 72–105
adequate trial period for, 85
benefits/success of, 83–85
binaural vs. monaural, 94
candidacy for, 73–74
effect on residual hearing, 89
FM systems for, 90t, 90–94,
91–93
follow-up of, 96t, 96–97
gain output frequency
response characteristics
for, 74–83
"higher tech" hearing aids for,
94–95
with other physical or mental
impairments, 95–96
output limitation for, 85–89,
87–88
parent counseling about, 96
style issues related to, 89–94
assessment of, 147–149
auditory learning in, 145–146
changing demographics of,
181–183
cochlear implants for, 73, 84,
137
effect on auditory learning,
143–144, *144–145*
counseling with, 229–230
definition of, 11–12
identification of, 9, 53–68. *See
also* Identification
programs
age of, 72
urgency of, 72–73
interventions for, 160–164
components of, 160
educational, 163
goals of, 160
language, 163
learning disabilities, 163–164
purposes of, 161
school placement for,
160–161
speech, 162–163
language assessment in, 153–156
Brown's stage and, 156
language sample procedures
for, 154–155
morphologic mean length of
utterance and, 156
naturalistic settings for, 154
questions for, 153
specific elicitation tasks for,
155–156
tests for, 153–154, 168–175
type-token ratio and, 156
language characteristics in,
151–153, 152t
learning of tactile vocabulary
by, 516
metalinguistics and, 139
new technologies for, 137
number of, 3, 12–13, 181
parental interaction with, 109,
216–218

preoperative selection/
evaluation for cochlear
implants, 424–428
audiological evaluation, 427t,
427–428
medical/surgical evaluation,
426–427
patient/parent questionnaires,
426, 439–440
preschool age, 106–132. *See also*
Preschoolers
psychoeducational assessment
of, 156–160
psychosocial development of,
73, 181, 194–195, 229
school-age, 136–175
self-concept of, 230
speech assessment in, 150–151
speech characteristics of, 129,
149
time demands of caring for,
220–221
with unilateral loss, 73–74
use of hearing aids by, 17
variables affecting rehabilitation
of, 146–147
child-centered, 146–147
school context, 147
Children of hearing-impaired
parents, 406–408
Civil Right Acts of 1964, 25, 30
Classrooms. *See also* Schools
amplified, 458
discourse model for
preschoolers in, 116–119,
117t
listening skills in, 197–198
soundfield FM systems in,
196–198, 457–458
Client-centered therapy, 378t, 382
Client records, 392
Clonidine, 341t
Closed captioning, 452
Coaching, 38–41
Cochlear implants, 7, 13–14,
417–434
as aid to speechreading, 511
auditory training after fitting of,
428–430, *429*
candidate selection for,
421–428, 509, 510
adults, 421t, 421–424
audiological evaluation,
423–424, 424t, *425*
medical/surgical evaluation,
422–423
patient/family
questionnaires, 422,
438–439
children, 424–428
audiologic evaluation, 427t,
427–428
medical/surgical evaluation,
427
patient/parent
questionnaires, 426,
439–440
for children, 73, 84, 137

effect on auditory learning,
143–144, *144–145*
definition of, 417
development of, 417
direct audio input systems for,
443
FDA approval of, 417
future of, 433
3M/House single-channel
system, 417
Nucleus 22 channel system,
417–421
coding strategies for, 419–420
components of, 418
development of, 418
external portion of, 418
MPEAK scheme for, 419–420
programming of, *420,*
420–421
speech processor for, 418
surgical seating of, 418
transmission of digital signals
to, 418
reasons for high level of interest
in, 509–510
results of, 430-
for children, 431–434,
432–433
for postlinguistically deafened
adults, 430–431, *430–432*
single-channel vs. multichannel,
417, 511–512
speech and, 137
vs. tactile devices, 512–513
technical characteristics of,
417–418
training for newly implanted
clients, 510, 516
Codeine, 341t
Cognition, 138
Cognitive behavior modification,
377, 378t, 381
Cognitive status, of hearing-
impaired elderly persons,
490–491
Cognitive therapy, 378t, 379
College, communication needs
related to, 457–458
Color discrimination, in elderly,
336
Common Phrases test, 125, 428
Communication
aggressive, passive, and
assertive, 399–400, 401t
assistive technology to enhance,
441
auditory, factors affecting access
to, 442
counseling as, 376–377
effect of adverse drug reactions
on, 341, 341t
factors contributing to
increasing likelihood of,
314
marital and family, 406–408
model of, 5, *6*
patients' styles of, 394
process of, 316–317

tactile, 513
verbal, 316
Communication and Symbolic
  Behavior Scales, 108
Communication assessment,
  390–392
in children, 148–149
by client, 399
problem-solving exercises for,
  399, 400t
scales for, 108
self-report questionnaires for,
  238–242, 245t
sign language proficiency, 149
Communication Assessment
  Procedure for Seniors,
  349–350, 368–371
Communication assistants, 26, 30
Communication Intention
  Inventory, 168, 169, 173
Communication needs, 441, 493
determination of, 10
in group home, 457
of hearing-impaired adults,
  404–408
at home, 456–457
at school/college, 457–458
at work, 457
Communication Profile for the
  Hearing Impaired, 23,
  239, 239t, 243, 391, 399,
  401–402, 407
Communications Act of 1934, 30
Communications Disorders
  Questionnaire, 344
Compensation, 239–240, 387
Compliance
with medication use, by elderly,
  340
problems with, 386
professional's authoritativeness
  and, 386
Computer-Aided Speechreading
  Training, 249
Computers, 14, 470–485
applications of, 471–474
characteristics of approaches in
  rehabilitation, 484, 484t
devices for monitoring prompts
  of, 455
for evaluation, 472–474
expert systems, 475t, 475–476,
  476
future applications of, 484–485
hypermedia for, 476–482
for notetaking, 452
for patient education, 474
procedural models and,
  470–471, *471–472*
problems with, 474–475
programs and suggested
  readings about, 486
for speechreading training, 249
for treatment, 474
use to close service gap, 470
use with elderly persons, 353
as visual telephone devices, 454
Consonants

characteristics in hearing-
  impaired children, 149
frequency of occurrence of, 251
McGurk effect related to
  perception of, 522–523
recognition of, 251
tests for recognition of,
  251–252, 504
Consumer awareness, 320
Consumer education, 344–345
Consumer rights, 184, 199–200
Contralateral Routing of Signal
  (CROS) hearing aids,
  295–296
for children, 74
Conversation repair, 320–321
Coping, 389–390
Costs
of assistive devices, 463
of auditory brainstem response
  testing, 61, 61t, 67
of binaural vs. monaural
  hearing aids, 295
of early identification programs,
  60–61, 61t-63t
of hearing aids, 18
of hearing services, 8
insurance reimbursement for,
  12, 18
Counseling, 211–231
approaches to, 377–383
behavioral, 380–381
  Bandura, 381
  definition of, 377
  Lazarus, 381
  Meichenbaum, 381
  originators of, 378t
  Wolpe, 380–381
categorization of, 377
cognitive, 378–380
  Adler, 379
  Beck, 379
  Berne, 379–380
  definition of, 377
  Ellis, 379
  originators of, 378t
commonalities among, 384
eclectic, 377
humanistic (affective),
  381–383
  definition of, 377
  May, 383
  originators of, 378t
  Perls, 382–383
  Rogers, 382
for assertiveness training,
  399–402, 401t
attributes of good coach for,
  39–41
as communication behavior,
  376–377
content vs. emotional, 225
converging trends in, 383–386
counselor characteristics and,
  385–386
counselor-client relationship
  and, 385
empathy, 393–396, *395*

managing difficult patients,
  394–396
nonverbal cues, 396
patient communication styles,
  394
variables affecting, 396
definition of, 374–376
effectiveness of, 223–225
for elderly hearing aid clients,
  352–353, 496–497
for environmental awareness
  difficulties, 408
family-centered, 225–227
goals of, 39, 226, 403
group, 408
with hearing-impaired adult,
  374–409
with hearing-impaired child,
  228–229
to identify communication and
  adjustment problems,
  390–392
implications of hearing
  impairment/disability/
  handicap for, 392–393
informational, 376
mechanisms of change in, 384
medical and rehabilitative
  models of, 385–386
multicultural considerations in,
  229–230
of parents of hearing-impaired
  child, 96
personal adjustment, 376
in private practice dispensing
  office, 38–41
for problem solving, 376,
  402–403
vs. psychoanalysis, 378
reimbursement for, 375
related to assistive devices, 459
role of, 374–375, 393
for sharing information with
  parents, 227–228
of spouses/family members of
  hearing-impaired persons,
  407–408
for stress management, 402
vs. traditional hearing aid
  orientation, 396–399
training in, 375
trend toward counseling-
  oriented methodologies,
  501
Count the dot procedure, 290, *290*
"Critical period," 73
Cues
nonverbal, affecting counseling
  effectiveness, 396
secondary, 520
tactile, 512–517
visual, 120, 506–507, 521
  optimized by hearing-
  impaired persons,
  523–524
  tactile devices and, 515–516
  training in use of, 524. *See
  also* Speechreading

Cues—*continued*
  use by normal-hearing
    persons, 523
Cultural influences
  on audiologic practice, 312
  counseling and, 229–230
  on psychoeducational testing,
    158
  on use of assistive devices, 465
CUNY Nonsense Syllable Test,
    250, 302
Curriculum-based assessment, 154

Daycare centers, 219
Deaf perspective, 138
Dementia, senile, 490–491
Denial, 405
  of hearing loss, 286
  parental, 212
Denver Quick Test of Lipreading
    Ability, 246, 247t, 256t
Denver Scale of Communication
    Function, 239, 239t, 241,
    241, 262–267, 391
  Quantified, 490, 495
Denver Scale of Communication
    Function—Modified, 349,
    362–366
Denver Scale of Communication
    Function for Senior
    Citizens Living in
    Retirement Centers, 349,
    358–361
Depression
  among elderly, 490
  parental, 213
Desensitization techniques, 380,
    402
Desired Sensation Level, 76–79,
    77t, *78*, *80*, 89, 102–104,
    298
Developing an Approach to
    Successful Listening
    Skills, 126
Developmental approach, 119–126
Diagnosis of hearing loss. *See*
    Identification programs
Diagnostic Early Intervention
    Program, 107–110
Diagnostic Speech Inventory, 130
Dichotic Sentence Identification
    test, 293
Dictaphone, 457
Digitalis, 341t
Dipheniramine, 341t
Direct audio input, 443, *444*
Directionality. *See* Localization of
    sound
Disability definitions, 387–389,
    388t
Disability measures, 238
Discrimination
  ABX, 522
  acoustic, 141
  auditory, 140–141
  segmental, 141

suprasegmental, 141
Discrimination after Training test,
    428, 431
Discrimination by Identification
    of Pairs test, 124
Discrimination functions, 522
Dispensing of hearing aids, 6,
    18–19, 285–286, 397–398
  consumer confidence and, 398
  in private practice office, 35–49
Divorce, 219
Doctor of Audiology programs,
    14–15
Dyna-Aura Sound Field
    Audiometer, 44

Early Language Milestones, 168,
    169, 173
Early Speech Perception Battery,
    124, 125
Ears
  changes with aging, 333
  sound conveyed by, 42–43
Education and training
  about hearing health care,
    343–345
  after cochlear implantation, 510,
    516
  in assertiveness, 399–402
  of audiologists, 14–15
  auditory. *See* Auditory training
  in counseling, 375
  in geriatric health care, 343
  in-service, 203–204
  in problem solving, 402
  related to hearing care, 20–21
  in speechreading, 19, 246, 249,
    521–525
  in stress management, 402
  to teach child monitoring
    practices for hearing aid,
    96t, 97
Education for All Handicapped
    Children Act of 1975,
    148, 158, 161, 177, 183
Educational audiology, 55,
    176–210. *See also*
    Schools
Educational Audiology
    Association, 176–177
Educational interventions, 163
Elderly persons. *See also* Aging
  alternative hearing health care
    delivery for, 346–347
  audition in, 333–335
  body sensations of, 336–337
  health care costs for, 331
  health care providers'
    relationships with,
    342–343
  medication use by, 340–342,
    341t
  memory of, 337–338
  myths about, 331
  number of, 489
  physical health of, 339–340

slowing and cautiousness of,
    338–339
  vision of, 335–336
Elderly persons, hearing-impaired,
    13, 331–373. *See also*
    Adults
  biopsychosocial approach to,
    489
  central presbycusis in, 292, *293*
  computer-assisted therapy for,
    353
  emotional status of, 489–490
  goals of rehabilitation for, 489
  hearing aids for, 350–353
    benefit of, 292–293, 493–496,
      494t
    counseling about, 352–353,
      496–497
    follow-up for, 352–353
    selection of, 351–352
    use of, 18, 351
  hearing handicap inventories
    for, 348–350
  incidence of, 3
  institutionalized, 23
  locus of control for, 22–23
  motivation of, 339, 491–492,
    492t, 498
  negative stereotyping of, 331
  number of, 331
  outcome indicators in
    rehabilitation of,
    492–493, 493t
  psychological variables affecting
    rehabilitation of, 489–492
  psychosocial consequences of
    hearing loss in, 490–491
  relationship of health and
    rehabilitative audiology
    for, 345–346
  screening of, 347–348
  speechreading training for, 19
ELM scale, 64t
Emergency alerting systems. *See*
    Alerting devices
Emotional reactivity, 394
Emotional status, of elderly, 490
Empathy, 393–396, *395*
Empathy Scale, 394
Employment, 404–406
  accommodations required for,
    24
  under Americans with
    Disabilities Act, 24–25
  communication needs related
    to, 457
  environmental awareness
    difficulties and, 408
  hazards of noise exposure in,
    406
  hearing conservation programs
    and, 405
  reluctance to reveal hearing
    impairment and, 405–406
  underemployment, 404
English as a Second Language,
    138, 153

English Sign Systems, 138
Equal Employment Opportunity
        Commission, 24, 25
Equivalent value exchange, 35
Event analysis, 155
Event-related potentials, 40-Hz, 84
Existential psychotherapy, 377,
        378t, 383
Experiential activities, 119, 120t
Expert systems, 475t, 475–476,
        476
Expressive One-Word Picture
        Vocabulary Test, 168,
        169, 173
    Upper Extension, 168, 169, 173
Eyes, changes with aging, 335–336

Facsimile machines, 454, 464
Familiar Sounds Audiogram, 190,
        190
Family. *See also* Parents
    Afro-American, 230
    counseling centered around,
        225–227
    dynamics of, 218
    effects of environment on
        child's progress, 223
    empowerment of, 226
    guidelines for working with, 220
    impact of hearing-impaired
        adult on, 406–408
    impact of hearing-impaired
        child on, 211–216
        grandparents, 222–223
        parents, 220–221
        siblings, 222
    importance of social interaction
        in, 106, 112
    Individualized Family Service
        Plan for, 109, 199,
        202–203
    language evaluation and
        intervention in, 107–109
    parent-child interaction in,
        216–218
    single-parent, 219–220
    structure of, 218–220
Feasibility Scale for Predicting
        Hearing Aid Use, 390
Fine-tuning, 155
Finger spelling, 513
Fire Protection Equipment
        Directory, 455
FM systems, *450*, 450–451
    advantages and disadvantages
        of, 29
    assessment of hearing aids
        coupled to, 466
    for children, 90–94, 450
        special applications of, 95–96
    electromagnetic interference
        with, 94
    frequencies for, 450–451
    limitations of, 450
    measurement protocols for,
        91–93, *93*

narrow band and wide band,
        450–451
    personal system use in schools,
        196
    receiver coupling methods for,
        91, *92*
    soundfield systems in schools,
        196–198, 457–458
        population for, 197–198
        practical issues related to, 198
        rationale for, 196–197
    technical aspects of, 450
    transmission range of, 450
    transmission system for, 91, *91*
    versatility of, 450
    voice discrimination with, 90t
Frequency response, 297–299,
        299t
    for children, 74–83
    formal selection procedures for,
        298–299
    informal prescriptive procedures
        for, 297–298
    verification of, 301–306
        functional gain, 304
        probe microphone
            measurements, 304–306
        speech-based procedures,
            302–304
Frequency selectivity, loss of,
        318
Freudian psychoanalysis, 378
Functional Auditory Sills Test,
        122
Functional gain analysis, 304
Functionalism, 155
Future directions, 14
    for cochlear implants, 434
    for computer applications,
        484–485
    for research, 500–525
    for school-age children, 164

Gain-targeting formulas, 74–83
Gallaudet University
    National Information Center on
        Deafness, 456
    research on visual alerting
        system, 455
Gentamicin, 341t
Geriatric audiology. *See* Elderly
        persons
Geriatric Depression Scale, 490,
        495
Geriatric Education Centers, 343
Gestalt therapy, 378t, 382–383
Glendonald Auditory Screening
        Procedure, 122, 125, 428,
        432–434, *433*
Grammatical Analysis of Elicited
        Language, 168, 170, 173
Grandparents, 222–223
Grieving cycle, 211–213
    acceptance phase of, 213
    anger phase of, 212–213
    bargaining phase of, 213

denial phase of, 212
    depression phase of, 213
    duration of, 213–214
Group counseling, 408
Group homes, 457

Habilitative audiology. *See*
        Rehabilitative audiology
Hanen Early Language Resource
        Centre, 109
Head shadow effects, 74, 94, 295
Health
    of elderly persons, 339–340
    relationship to rehabilitative
        audiology, 345–346
    self-assessment of, 20
Health insurance, 8, 12
Health Objectives for the Year
        2000, 54
Hearing
    academic performance and,
        177–178
    definition of, 176
    effects of aging on, 332–335
Hearing Aid Compatibility Act of
        1988, 453
"Hearing aid effect," 18
Hearing aid manufacturers
    developing relationships with,
        37
    units returned to, 397
Hearing Aid Performance
        Inventory, 243, 508
Hearing aids, 13, 284–308. *See
        also* Amplification;
        Assistive listening devices
    arrangement of, 294–296
    assistive devices used with,
        461–463, *462*
        evaluation for, 459–460
        hearing aid selection for,
            460–463
    assistive listening devices
        dependent on, 443–446
    balancing sound levels of, 44–45
    "best" fitting of, 505
    binaural vs. monaural, 94,
        294–295
        for elderly persons, 352
    candidacy for, 286–293
        central auditory processing
            deficit, 291–293, *293*
        degree of hearing loss,
            286–290, *288–290*
        patient motivation, 12,
            290–291, 291t, *292*
    for children, 72–105
    circuitry of, 296–297
        automatic signal processing,
            296–297, 352
        compression, 296
        improvements in, 284–285
    client acceptability ratings for,
        508–509
    compatibility with telephones,
        28, 453, 454

Hearing aids—*continued*
  components of selection
      procedures for, 503
  Contralateral Routing of Signal
      (CROS), 74, 295–296
  cost of, 18
  coupled to FM systems, 466
  custom, 285, 293
  delivery systems for, 18–19,
      285–286
  diary for use after purchase of,
      46–49
  dispensing of, 6, 18–19,
      285–286, 397–398
    in private practice office,
      35–49
  ear injury and, 43–44
  for elderly persons, 350–353
    benefit of, 493–496, 494t
    counseling and follow-up for,
      352–353
    motivation to use, 491–492,
      492t
    selection of, 351–352
    underuse of, 351
  electroacoustic features of,
      297–300
    interactions with listening
      environment, 505–506
    SSPL90, 299–300, 300t
    visual cues and, 506–507
  expectations-to-reality gap
      regarding, 41
  fitting for persons with mild
      hearing loss, 284
  frequency of changes in fitting
      of, 508
  gain/frequency response of,
      297–299, 299t
  implantable, 7
  limitations of traditional
      orientation to, 396–399
  loudness mapping for, 43–44,
      44
  malfunction of, 97
  measuring benefit of, 508
    in candidate for cochlear
      implants, 423–424
  observations of client using,
      508
  performance measures for,
      37–38, 38
    in clinic vs. daily
      communication, 507
  prefitting considerations for,
      286–297
  prescriptive fitting of, 285
  probe microphone
      instrumentation and, 285
  programmable, 38, 39, 95,
      284–285, 297
  reasons for lack of use of, 3,
      17–19
  repairs on, 37, 37
  research needs related to,
      503–509
  sales practices for, 19

saturation sound pressure level
      of, 85
  self-report questionnaires about,
      243–244
  shrinking of auditory distances
      by, 43
  stigma associated with, 17–18
  styles of, 293–294, 294t
    for children, 89–94
  usage rates for, 17, 508
  use in schools, 196
  verification of fitting of,
      300–308
    gain/frequency response,
      300–306
    SSPL90, 306–308, 307
Hearing care, 20–22
  knowledge of health care
      providers and consumers
      about, 343–345
Hearing conservation programs,
      186, 187, 405
Hearing ear dogs, 28, 456
Hearing handicap, 10, 237. See
      also Hearing impairment
  definition of, 387–389, 388t
  quantification of, 387
  screening for, 390–392
Hearing Handicap Inventory for
      Adults, 239, 271–272,
      390
Hearing Handicap Inventory for
      the Elderly, 239, 239t,
      240, 242, 286, 350, 351,
      371–372, 390, 407, 490,
      495
    Screening Version, 348, 350,
      373
Hearing Handicap Scale, 238,
      239t–240t, 240, 390
Hearing impairment, 3
  age of onset of, 17–18
  by age range, 3, 4, 333
  auditory learning and,
      145–146
  candidacy for hearing aids
      related to, 286–290,
      288–290
  classification of, 11t, 11–12,
      53–54, 387–389, 388t
  components of, 317–318
    effects of noise, 318
    hearing threshold, 317–318
    loss of frequency selectivity,
      318
  course of adjustment to, 386
  definition of, 10, 11, 237,
      387–389, 388t
  as disabling, 24–25
  in elderly, 331–373
  general effects of, 10–12
  impact on academic
      performance, 178–181
    acoustic filter effect, 178–179
    computer analogy, 179–180
    distance hearing and passive
      learning, 180–181

impact on health status of
      elderly, 345
  incidence of, 3
  incidence of educationally
      significant loss, 182
  mechanisms of adjustment to,
      384–385
  modeled by spectrum shaping,
      504
  perception of psychological
      control and, 21–23
  psychosocial implications of,
      386–390
  self-perception of, 20
  sensorineural, 58–59
  as source of ambiguity,
      314–315
Hearing Industries Association,
      290
Hearing Measurement Scale,
      240–241, 390
Hearing Performance Inventory,
      239t, 242–243, 391, 399
Hearing Performance Inventory
      for Severe to Profound
      hearing loss, 244
Hearing Problem Inventory,
      243
Hearing tests
  demographics of clients having,
      20–21
  in schools, 182
Hearing threshold, 317–318
  aging and, 334
Hierarchy of needs, 492–493
High/Scope curriculum, 116
Hiskey-Nebraska scale, 158
HOLA program, 312
Home health care, 346
HOME Inventory for Infants and
      Toddlers, 217
Hoosier Auditory-Visual
      Enhancement test, 125,
      428
Hotels, 28–29
Hydralazine, 341t
Hydroxyzine, 341t
HyperCard, 477, 481, 486
Hypermedia, 476–482
  conceptual basis of, 477
  development of, 481–482
    guidelines for, 483–484
  elements of, 481
  explanation of, 476–477
  moving about in, 480, 482
  moving into, 477
  organization principles for,
      477–480, 478–481
    structured links, 478–479,
      479
    unstructured links, 479–480,
      480
  programs and suggested
      readings about, 486
  in rehabilitation, 480–481
HyperStudio, 477, 481
Hypoglycemic agents, 341t

Identification programs, 9
  for adults, 238
  costs of, 60–61, 61t–63t
  early, 53–68, 186–188
  educational model for, 54
  for elderly persons, 347–348
  epidemiology of hearing loss
    related to, 58–60
  focus and effectiveness of, 63
  medical/epidemiologic model
    for, 53–54
  in nursing homes, 346–347
  population selection for, 61–63
  psychometric principles of,
    55–58, 56t–58t
  purpose of, 54–55
  in schools, 55, 182, 186–192
  scope of, 63–64
  to screen for hearing handicap,
    390–392
  test selection for, 64, 64t
    acoustic immittance, 65–66
    auditory brainstem response,
      66–67
    behavioral methods, 64–65
    otoacoustic emissions, 67–68,
      68t
  urgency of, 72–73
Illinois Test of Psycholinguistic
    Abilities, 168, 169, 172
Immittance testing, in candidate
    for cochlear implants,
    423
In-service training, 203–204
In-the-canal (ITC) hearing aids,
    284, 293, 352
In-the-ear (ITE) hearing aids, 284,
    293–294, 294t, 352
  assistive devices and, 462–463
  for children, 89–90
  direct audio input systems for,
    443, 461
  use with telephone, 460–461
    acoustic coupling, 460–461
    direct audio input, 461
    inductive coupling, 460
Individual psychology, 378, 378t,
    379
Individualized Educational Plan
    (IEP), 183, 199–200,
    199–202
  components of, 200–201
  hearing management objectives
    for, 201–202
  people-first wording on,
    199–200
  psychoeducational assessment
    for, 157
  purpose of, 199, 200
Individualized Family Service
    Plan, 109, 199,
    202–203
Individualized In-Service Plan,
    203
Indomethacin, 341t
Induction loop, 446–449, *447*
  advantages of, 29, 447–448

disadvantages of, 29, 448–449
  in portion of room, 449
  technical aspects of, 446
  telecoil receivers for, 446–447
  three-dimensional system for,
    448–449
Infrared transmission system, *448*,
    449
  advantages and disadvantages
    of, 29, 449
  frequencies for, 449
  power for, 449
  receivers for, 449
  technical aspects of, 449
Insight, 384–385
Insulin, 341t
Intelligibility, 178
Intelligibility Rating Improvement
    Scale, 243, 494–495
Interaction, 384–385
International Phonetic Alphabet,
    130
Interpersonal Language Skills
    Assessment, 168, 169,
    172
Interpreters, for psychoeducational
    testing, 158
Isoniazid, 341t

Kaufman Assessment Battery for
    Children, 158
Kendall Communicative
    Proficiency Scale, 149
Khan-Lewis Phonological
    Analysis, 151

Labeling functions, 522
Language
  acquisition of, 138
  assessment in hearing-impaired
    children, 153–156
  characteristics in hearing-
    impaired children,
    151–153, 152t
  evaluation and intervention in
    preschoolers, 106–119
    assessment materials/
      strategies for, 112–114
    cognitive approach to,
      110–112, 111t
    collaborative problem-solving
      approach to, 107–110
    intervention strategies for,
      114–119
  interventions for, 163
  signed. *See* Sign language
  tests of, 168–175
Language sampling, 114, 154–155
  spontaneous, 114
Larson Sound Discrimination
    Test, 252, *253*
Laxatives, 341t
Learning
  active, 114–115
  auditory, 139–146

passive, distance hearing and,
    180–181
Learning disabilities
  hearing loss and, 182
  interventions for, 163–164
Leiter, 158
Levodopa, 341t
Lidocaine, 341t
Life style, 456
Ling Five-Sound Test, 122,
    150–151
LinkWay, 477, 481, 486
Lipreading. *See* Speechreading
Listening
  assertive, 317, 320, 323
  in classroom, 198–199
  definition of, 176
  effect of loss of binaural hearing
    on, 317
  environment for, 442
  evaluation of child with
    difficulties in, 209–210
Literacy attainment, 110
Localization of sound, 74, 94, 140,
    295
Locus of control, 22
Long-term care facilities, 346–347
Loudness discomfort level (LDL)
  for binaural vs. monaural
    signal, 295
  clinical measurement of,
    299–300, 300t, *301*
  determining in children, 85–89,
    87–88, 104–105
  measured after hearing aid
    fitting, 306–308, *307*
  SSPL90 selection and, 299–300
Loudness Growth for Octave
    Bands, 43–44, *44*

3M/House single-channel cochlear
    implant system, 417
MacArthur Communicative
    Development Inventory,
    108
Mainstream Amplification
    Resource Room Study,
    National Diffusion
    Network Project study,
    182, 197
Marital issues, 406–408
Maryland Syntax Evaluation
    Instrument, 168, 170, 172
Maslow's hierarchy of needs,
    492–493
Maternal Behavior Rating Scale,
    217
McCarthy-Alpiner Scale of
    Hearing Handicap,
    241–242, 256t, 257,
    268–270, 407
McGurk effect, 522–523
Mean length of utterance, 156
Meaningful Auditory Integration
    Scale, 126
Measures of association, 55

Measures of test operating characteristics, 55–58, 56t-58t, 64t
Medicaid, 8
Medicare, 8, 346, 347
Medications
  adverse effects of, 340–342, 341t
  use by elderly, 340–342
Memory
  automatic vs. effortful encoding for, 337–338
  changes with aging, 337–338
  implicit vs. explicit, 338
  stages in process of, 337
Memphis State University Hearing Instrument Prescription Formula, 76–77, 77t, *78*, 89
Meperidine, 341t
Message decoding, 5, *6*
Message encoding, 5, *6*
Message expression, 5, *6*
Message perception, 5, *6*
Metalinguistics, 139
Methyldopa, 341t
Microphones
  environmental, 451
  placement for assistive listening devices, 451
  types of, 451
Middle ear effusion, 182
  epidemiology of, 59–60
  screening for, 63
Middle latency response, 84
Miller-Yoder Language Comprehension Test, 168, 169, 172
Minimal Auditory Capabilities battery, for cochlear implant candidates
  adults, 424, *425*
  children, 428
Minimal Pairs test, 124–125, 130, 428
Minorities, 230, 312
Modeling, 384–385
Mondini's dysplasia, 427
Monosyllable Trochee Spondee test, 125, 431–432, *432–433*
Morphine, 341t
Motivation, 12, 290–291, 291t, *292*
  determinants of, 491
  of elderly persons, 339, 491–492, 492t, 498
Multidisciplinary team approach, 5, 13, 106, 108
Multimodal therapy, 378t, 381

Narcotic drugs, 341t
National Acoustics Laboratory procedure, 74, 75t, *76*, 77t, 298–299, 299t
National Fire Protection Agency, 455–456

National Information Center on Deafness, 456
National Institute on Deafness and Other Communication Disorders, 7
Noise, 41–42
  assertive control of, 317
  background, 442
  exposure to, 3
  separating speech from, 318, 441
  in work environment, 406
Noncompliance, 386
Nonsense syllable recognition, 504
Nonsense syllable repetition, 130
Nonsense Syllable Test, CUNY, 250, 302
Northwestern Syntax Screening Test, 168, 169, 172
Northwestern University Children's Perception of Speech, 124–126, 428
Northwestern University Word Test Number 6, 251, 252, 256t
Notetaking, 452
  computer-assisted, 452
Notewriting, 452
Nucleus 22 channel cochlear implant system, 417–421. *See also* Cochlear implants
Nursing Home Hearing Handicap Index, 349
  Self Version for Resident, 366–367
  Staff Version, 367–368
Nursing homes, 346–347
  computer-assisted technology in, 353
  hearing aid care in, 353

Observation, during child's play, 114
Omnibus Budget Reconciliation Act of 1987, 346
Otoacoustic emissions, 67–68
  compared with auditory brainstem response testing, 68, 68t
  spontaneous vs. evoked, 67
Otoscopy, 65–66
Outcome indicators, 492–493

Pagers, 455, 458–459
Pain sensitivity, in elderly, 336–337
Paranoia, 392
Parent Behavior Progression, 217
Parent Intervention Method, 107
Parenting Stress Index, 221
Parents. *See also* Family
  counseling with, 96
  directive vs. responsive, 109

  early intervention involvement of, 107–109, 217
  emotional reactions of, 211–216
    acceptance, 213
    anger, 212–213
    audiologists' perceptions of, 215, 224
    bargaining, 213
    denial, 212
    depression, 213
    loss and grief, 211–212
    referral for psychotherapy, 216
    repression of, 214
    variability of, 214–215
  interaction with deaf child, 109, 216–218
  referrals for school services by, 185
  satisfaction with counseling, 223–225
  sharing information with, 225–228
  single, 219–220
  time demands on, 220–221
PBK word lists, 124
Peabody Picture Vocabulary Test—Revised, 168, 169, 172
Pediatric Speech Intelligibility test, 125
Pentazocine, 341t
Percentage of overall agreement, 55, 56t
Person-centered therapy, 378t, 382
Personal amplification systems, *445*, 446
Personality
  assessment of, 159–160
  effect of hearing loss on, 392
  parental, 214–215
Perspective taking, 394
Phonak TC-100, 453
Phonemes, speechreading and, 325
Phonetic Level Evaluation, 129, 150–151
Phonetics, acoustic, 188
Phonologic Level Evaluation, 129, 151
Physicians, 5, 19
  for elderly patients, 342
  knowledge about hearing health care, 343–345
Play observation, 114
Preliteracy development, 110
Presbycusis, 3, 333
  central, 292, *293*
  mechanical, 333
  metabolic, 333
  neural, 333
  phonemic regression and, 504
  sensory, 333
Preschool Language Assessment Instrument, *113*, 113–114, 168, 169, 172
Preschoolers, hearing-impaired, 106–132

auditory perceptual
development in, 121–128
assessment of, 122–126
intervention and, 126–128
daycare centers for, 219
developmental approach to
auditory and speech skills
in, 119–121
integration of auditory and
speech skills in, 131–132
language evaluation and
intervention with,
106–119
cognitive approach to,
110–112, 111t
collaborative problem-solving
approach to, 107–110
goal of, 110
parental interaction with, 216
speech production development
in, 128–131
assessment of, 129–130
intervention and, 130–131
Prescription of Gain and Output,
74, 298
Private practice dispensing office,
35–49
accessibility to, 36
clarity of purpose of, 36–37
contributors to success in,
35–36, *36*
counseling services of, 38–41
essential concepts related to,
41–45
philosophical foundation for, 35
products provided by, 37–38,
38–39
service in, 36–37
Probe microphone measurements,
37–38, 79, 81, 285
to assess FM system
performance, 93, *93*
equipment for, 304
of hearing aid output, 307
pass/fail criteria for, 305
terminology related to, 304,
305t
to verify hearing aid's frequency
response, 304–306
Problem solving, 376, 402–403
exercises for, 399, 400t
Procedural models, 470–471
multidimensional, 471, *472*
problems with, 474–475
unidimensional, 470–471, *471*
Profile of Hearing Aid Benefit,
243, 494–495
Profile of Hearing Aid
Performance, 508–509
Promontory testing, for cochlear
implants, 423, 427
Propoxyphene, 341t
Propranolol, 341t
Pseudohypocusis, 44
Psychoanalysis, 378
Psychoeducational testing,
156–160

administration of, 158
areas of, 157
cultural influences on, 158
difficulties in hearing-impaired
children, 158–159
instruments for, 158
interpreters for, 158
personality assessment, 159–160
purposes of, 157
variables affecting, 157–158
Psychological control, 21–23
Psychometric principles, 55–58,
56t-58t
Psychosocial development, 73,
181, 194–195, 229
Psychosocial implications of
hearing loss, 386–390
in elderly, 490–491, 492t-494t
Psychotherapy, 375–376
Public accommodations,
accessibility to, 27–30
Public Law 94–142, 148, 158, 161,
177, 183, 199–201
Public Law 99–457, 106–107, 177,
183–184, 199, 202, 218,
225, 226, 230
Public Law 101–336. *See*
Americans with
Disabilities Act of 1990
Public Law 101–431. *See*
Television Decoder
Circuitry Act of 1990
Public services, accessibility to,
25–27

Quality of life, of hearing-
impaired elderly, 490
hearing aid effect on, 495–496
Quantified Denver Scale of
Communication
Function, 490, 495
Questionnaire Measure of
Emotional Empathy, 394

Rapid Speech Transmission
Index, 193–196
Rastronics TA-80, 453
Rational-emotive therapy, 378t,
379
Real-ear aided response, 306t
Real-ear insertion gain, 305
Real-ear insertion response, 79,
81, 305, 306t
Real-ear occluded response, 306t
Real-ear saturation response, 79,
306t, 307
Real-ear-to-coupler difference, 79,
81–82, *83–84*, 300, 306t
Real-ear unaided response, 79,
306t
Reality testing, 384–385
Receptive One-Word Picture
Vocabulary Test, 168,
169, 172
Recreation activities, 458–459

Reduced Aspect Feature
Transcription, 128,
130–131
Referrals, 10
by parents, 185
of parents for psychotherapy,
216
by physicians, 343
tests resulting in under- and
overreferrals, 57–58
Reflection of feeling, 396
Reflectometry, 65
Rehabilitation Act of 1973, 25, 27,
177, 184
Rehabilitative audiology
for adults, 13–14, 311–330
components of, 323
goals and methods in, 326,
330
group for, 319–320, 328–329
individual, 324
nonhearing aid wearers,
323–324
approaches to, 13
areas of, 12–13, 19
assessing effectiveness of, 10
audiologist's roles in, 4–5
client attitudes toward, 20
clinical applications of, 312–314
clinical truths about, 311
closing service gap in, 470
competencies for, 16
components of program for, 7–8
current status of, 7–8
definition of, 3–4, 16
determining need for, 9–10
educational directions for,
14–15
for elderly, 331–373
essential components of, 320
factors affecting practice of, 312
goal of, 314, 374
history of, 5–7, 311–312
outcome indicators in, 492–493
participation in services of,
19–20
philosophy of, 12
in private practice dispensing
office, 35–49
relationship to health, 345–346
services of, 4
delivery model for, 8–10, *9*
in schools, 192–193
termination of, 10
Reimbursement, 12, 18
for assistive devices, 467
for binaural vs. monaural
hearing aids, 295
for counseling, 375
by Medicare, 347
Relationship Questionnaire, 394
Research, 10, 14, 500–525
cognitive, 138
conducting within clinical
practice, 375
lack of clinical research,
500–501

Research—*continued*
  on sensory aids, 502t, 502–517
    cochlear implants, 509–512
    hearing aid selection
      procedures, 503–509
    tactile devices, 512–517
  on traditional aural
    rehabilitation techniques,
    517–525
    auditory training, 517–521
    speechreading and auditory-
      visual integration
      training, 521–525
  to validate clinical methods and
    demonstrate clinical
    utility, 501
Reserpine, 341t
Residual hearing
  effect of amplification on, 89
  evaluation in candidate for
    cochlear implants, 423
  maximizing use of, 517
Restatement of content, 396
Revised Speech Perception in
  Noise test, 250
Rhode Island Test of Language
  Structure, 168, 169, 173
Rockford Infant Developmental
  Evaluation Scales, 168,
  170, 174
Room acoustics, 442
Round window stimulation, for
  cochlear implants, 423,
  427

Saturation sound pressure level
  (SSPL), 85–89
  selection of SSPL90, 299–300
  verification of SSPL90, 306–308
Schema-based content units,
  115–116
Schools, 55, 176–210
  communication needs in,
    457–458
  demographics of hearing-
    impaired children in,
    181–183
  fostering of school language by,
    139
  identification programs in, 182,
    186–192
    "failure model," 191–192
    functional audiometric
      information, 188–190,
      208
    history of early hearing loss,
      186–188, 207
    Screening Instrument for
      Targeting Educational
      Risk, 188, *189*
    word identification testing,
      190–191
  IEP in, 199–202
  impact of hearing loss in,
    178–181, *194–195*
    acoustic filter effect, 178–179

computer analogy, 179–180
distance hearing and passive
  learning, 180–181
in-service training in, 203–204
informal language assessment
  in, 154
laws governing audiologic
  services in, 183–185
mainstreaming in, 147, 161,
  176, 177
models of service provision in,
  185–186
  contractual agreement, 185
  modified school- and
    community-based,
    185–186
  parent referral, 185
  school- and community-
    based, 185
  school-based, 185
placements in, 160–161
rehabilitative audiologic services
  in, 147, 192–193
technology to access hearing in,
  193–199
  hearing aids, 196
  listening skills, 198–199,
    209–210
  personal FM systems, 196
  Rapid Speech Transmission
    Index, 193–196
  signal-to-noise ratio, 193
  soundfield FM systems,
    196–198, 450
Screening Instrument for
  Targeting Education Risk,
  188, *189*
Screening Instrument for
  Targeting Educational
  Risk, 188, *189*
Screening Inventory of Perception
  Skills, 123, 125, 127, 428
Self-acceptance, 382, 383
Self-actualization, 382, 493
Self-assessment, 10–11
  by elderly persons, 348–350
  of hearing aid benefit, 508–509
  of hearing aid benefit in elderly,
    494–495
  to identify auditory and
    nonauditory effects of
    hearing loss, 391, 399
  for psychological testing, 391
  purposes of, 239–240
  questionnaires on
    communicative disability,
    238–242, 245t, 286
  research on utility of, 501
Self-Assessment of
  Communication, 239t,
  240, 260, 348, 407
Self-concept, 230
Self-Evaluation of Life Function,
  490, 495
Self-Help for Hard of Hearing
  People (SHHH), 5, 19,
  324, 344

Self-help support groups, 19–20
Semantic development, 151
Sensemaking, 155
Sensitivity, 55–58
Sensorineural hearing loss, 58–59,
  72
Sequenced Inventory of
  Communication
  Development, 168, 169,
  174
Service animals, 28, 456
Service delivery, 8–10, *9*
  alternatives for elderly persons,
    346–347
  for hearing aids, 18–19,
    285–286
  in private practice dispensing
    office, 35–49
  in schools, 185–186
Short Portable Mental Status
  Questionnaire, 490, 491
Siblings, 222
Sickness Impact Profile, 345
Sign language, 138
  assessing proficiency in, 149
  over phone lines, 454
  for psychoeducational testing,
    158
  tactile, 513
Signal-to-noise ratio, 318
  in classroom, 193
  speech spectrum and, 287–288,
    289
Significant Other Assessment of
  Communication, 239t,
  240, 261
SKI-HI Language Development
  Scale, 168, 170, 174
SKI-HI Receptive Language Test,
  168, 169, 174
Social Adequacy Index, 238
Social Hearing Handicap Index,
  390
Social isolation, 391, 402
Social learning methods, 378t, 381
Social workers, 5, 13
Sound
  attributes of, 126–127
  awareness of, 140
  conveyed by ears, 42–43
  distance and, 442
  localization of, 74, 94, 140, 295
Soundfield testing, in candidate
  for cochlear implants,
  423
Spatial balance, 295
Specificity, 55–58
Spectrum shaping, 503–504
Speech
  acoustic and phonological
    redundancy of, 520
  characteristics in hearing-
    impaired children, 129,
    149
  cochlear implants and, 137
  internal representations of
    sounds of, 518–519

interventions for, 162–163
judging intelligibility of,
  303–304
judging quality of, 303, 303t
most comfortable level for, 39
normal decoding of, 521
relationship between pure tones
  and detection of, 188,
  208
Speech development, 128–131
assessment of, 54–55, 62,
  129–130
critical period for, 73
integrating auditory skills with,
  131–132
intervention and, 130–131
normal and interrupted,
  128–129
parent-child interaction and,
  109
stages of, 128
Speech-language pathologist, 467
Speech perception, 517–518, 520
adaptability of, 520
audibility and, 504
by normal-hearing persons, 523
by sensory aids, 503
separating from background
  noise, 318
Speech reception threshold, 284
Speech recognition, 124
assistive listening devices and,
  442–443, *443*
auditory-visual integration for,
  507, 524–525
cochlear implant and, 419, 510
hearing aid selection based on,
  503–504
intersensory discrepancy of, 522
perceptual processes underlying
  auditory vs. visual,
  521–522
stages of, 318–319, 325
  cognitive processing, 319
  interactive processing, 319
  prepositioning, 319
  sensory processing, 319
tactile, 513–517
using secondary cues for, 520
visual only, 521–522. *See also*
  Speechreading
Speech recognition testing
in candidates for cochlear
  implants
  adults, 424, 424t
  children, 427t, 428
in elderly, 334–335
to evaluate assistive devices,
  466
to verify hearing aid's frequency
  response, 302–304
Speech signal processing, sensory
  aids for, 502t, 502–503
Speech spectrum, 287, *288*
articulation index and, 288–290,
  290
intensity range of, 287–288, *289*

long-term average, *78*, 78
Speechreading, 19
analytic and synthetic
  approaches to, 325
assessment of, 244–245
auditory-visual integration
  training and, 524–525
clients' response to training in,
  20
cochlear implant as aid to, 511
computer applications and,
  249
definition of, 244
hearing aid electroacoustic
  features and, 506–507
home self-instruction in, 246
limitations of studies on,
  524–525
maximizing success in
  combination with hearing
  aid, 329
McGurk effect and, 522–523
over phone lines, 454
research on, 521–525
skill in normal-hearing persons,
  523
skills matrix for, 246–247, *248*
steps in process of, 245
tactile (Tadoma), 513–514
training for adults, 324–325
  groups for, 320
visual cues for, 120, 506–507,
  521
Speechreading tests, 245–247, 247t
bisensory evaluation, 247–249,
  249t–250t
for candidate for cochlear
  implants, 424, 424t
limitations of, 246
reasons for use of, 245–246
SPL-ogram, 84, *86*
Stenger test, 44
Stigma of hearing loss, 17–18, 21
Stoic patients, 394, 406
Stress, 402
parental, 221, 227
Stress management techniques,
  402
Structured Photographic
  Expressive Language
  Test—II, 168, 170, 174
Sulfonylureas, 341t
Syntactic system, 151–153
Synthetic Sentence Identification,
  302
Systematic Analysis of Language
  Transcripts, 114
Systematic desensitization, 380

Tactile devices, 512–517
vs. cochlear implants, 512–513
natural vs. electronic methods,
  513–514
Tadoma technique, 513–514
Target to jammer ratio, 42
Task analysis, 114

Teacher Assessment of
  Grammatical Structures,
  168, 170, 174
Teaching Skills Inventory (Version
  2), 217
Telecommunication Device for
  the Deaf (TDD), 25,
  26–28, 454. *See also*
  Telephone devices; Text
  telephones
Baudot and ASCII compatibility
  of, 454
international symbol for, *28*
Telecommunications relay
  services, 30, 454
Telephone, 13, 24–25, 317
questioning job applicants about
  use of, 24
video, 454
Telephone devices, 452–454. *See
  also* Telecommunication
  Device for the Deaf; Text
  telephones
auditory, 452–454
  acoustic telepads/couplers,
    453–454
  in-line amplifiers, 453
  interpersonal assistive
    listening devices with
    telephone interface, 453
  portable amplifiers, 453
  portable induction systems,
    453
  replacement handsets,
    452–453
  telephones designed for
    hearing impaired, 454
  communication assistants for,
    26, 30
  hearing aid compatibility with,
    28, 453, 454, 460–461,
    461
nonauditory, 454
  computers, 454
  TDDs, 26–28, 454
in schools/colleges, 458
for use at work, 457
for use in home, 456
Television
closed captioned, 452
decoding devices for, 452
in hotels and hospitals, 28
use in home, 456
use of hardwired personal
  amplification system
  with, *445*, 446
use of hearing aid dependent
  hardwired systems with,
  444
Television Decoder Circuitry Act
  of 1990, 452
Test for Auditory Comprehension
  of Language—Revised,
  168, 169, 174
Test for Examining Expressive
  Morphology, 168, 170,
  174

Test of Expressive Language Ability, 154, 168, 169, 175
Test of Receptive Language Ability, 154, 168, 169, 175
Test of Syntactic Abilities, 168, 170, 175
Text telephones, 26–27. *See also* Telecommunication Device for the Deaf; Telephone devices
  identification of, 28
  in public accommodations, 28
The Word Test, 168, 169, 175
Three-Interval Forced-Choice Test of Speech Pattern Contrast Perception, 123–126
Threshold of discomfort. *See* Loudness discomfort level
Tinnitus, 254–255
  evaluation for, 255
  grading severity of, 254–255
  management techniques for, 255
  prevalence of, 254
  questionnaire about, 255, 256t, 278–281
ToolBook, 477, 481, 486
Total Communication Receptive Vocabulary Test, 168, 170, 175
Touch sensitivity, in elderly, 336–337
Training. *See* Education and training
Transactional analysis, 378t, 379–380

Transference, 384–385
Travel, 458–459
Trihexyphenidyl, 341t
Tympanometry, 65–66
Type-token ratios, 156

Uncomfortable loudness level. *See* Loudness discomfort level
Underemployment, 404
Universalization, 384–385
University of Iowa Tinnitus Questionnaire, 255, 256t, 278–281
Utley Sentence Test, 246, 247

Vane Evaluation of Language Scale, 168, 170, 175
Ventilation, 384–385
Veterans Administration
  assessment procedures used by audiologists in, 239
  aural rehabilitation program in Los Angeles, 8–10
  Compensation and Pension Examinations of, 11
Vibrotactile stimulation, for children, 73, 84
Visual acuity, of elderly, 335–336
Visual alerting systems, 455. *See also* Alerting devices
Visual devices, 451–452
  closed captioning, 452
  determining need for, 464
  notewriting, 452
  projection techniques for notetaking, 452

real-time captioning, 451
Visual orientation, 523–524
Vocabulary teaching programs, 115
Vocal tract space, 129
Vocational rehabilitation counselors, 13
Vowels
  characteristics in hearing-impaired children, 149
  identification of, 520

Wake-up systems, 455
Wechsler Adult Intelligence Scale—Revised, 158
Wechsler Intelligence Scale for Children—Revised, 158, 159
Word Intelligibility by Picture Identification, 124–126, 428
Word recognition tests, 124–125, 190–191, 249–251, 251–254, *253*
  to assess hearing aids' performance in daily communication, 507
  for child candidate for cochlear implants, 428
  omission errors on, 339
  to verify hearing aid's frequency response, 302
Work. *See* Employment
World Health Organization definitions of hearing handicap/impairment, 387–389